A TEXTBOOK OF

Surgery
for Nurses

Second Edition—Illustrated

EDWARD S. STAFFORD, B.A., M.D., F.A.C.S.

*Associate Professor of Surgery, The Johns Hopkins University; Surgeon,
The Johns Hopkins Hospital; Lecturer in General Surgery, The Johns
Hopkins Hospital School of Nursing*

DORIS DILLER, B.A., R.N.

*Associate Professor of Nursing and Director of the Cancer Control Project,
Skidmore College Department of Nursing, New York City; formerly
Instructor and Supervisor, Surgical Nursing, The Johns Hopkins
Hospital School of Nursing*

W. B. SAUNDERS COMPANY

Philadelphia - London

PREFACE TO
THE SECOND EDITION

SINCE the publication of the first edition, significant advances have been achieved in numerous areas in surgery. Among these are the development of cardiac surgery, the increasing scope of thoracic surgery, improved preoperative and postoperative care of patients, widespread acceptance of the recovery room method, and heightened emphasis on rehabilitation. In order to make room for adequate presentation of these and many other subjects, the authors have omitted the chapters on anesthesia and operating room technic; these last are taught in separate courses in most schools of nursing and good texts are available.

The nursing care of surgical patients is stressed, and the reader will find that the plan for total care in considerable detail is given for each important surgical problem. Some of the original illustrations have been altered, and some new illustrations added in order to increase understanding.

A brief summary has been put at the end of most of the chapters for the purpose of developing an attitude toward the subject matter. The summary is followed by a vocabulary review; in this, the words are selected as much for the purpose of bringing into mind again a particular detail as for the difficulty in spelling. Finally, there is a list of suggested readings, chosen chiefly from the current literature, affording an opportunity to the student who wishes more knowledge in any given subject. For, as the authors stated in the preface to the first edition, the more the nurse knows about surgery, about the aims of the surgeon, and about what has been accomplished in the operating room, the better will she be able to care for the surgical patient.

It will be noted that the subject matter of the various units usually represents a special field of surgery, and often one which is a separate service in the highly organized modern hospital.

Throughout the text the reader will note many references to the excellent textbook on medical nursing by Brown, in which can be found a wealth of nursing detail for patient care in many situations which are entirely applicable to surgical patients, such as oxygen therapy, care in a respirator, and so on. All page references are to Brown, Amy Frances: *Medical Nursing*. 2d Ed. Philadelphia, W. B. Saunders Co., 1952.

Almost all of the new illustrations are the work of Elinor Widmont Bodian.

The chapters on plastic surgery, burns and the breast have been revised by Dr. William Gray Watson of Pittsburgh, Pennsylvania, the chapter on the thyroid and parathyroids by Dr. Robert Lee Payne, Jr., of Norfolk, Virginia, the chapter on ophthalmology by Dr. William Wickham Taylor of Norfolk, Virginia, the chapter on otolaryngology by Dr. Dudley C. Babb of Baltimore, and the chapters on gynecology by Dr. C. Bernard Brack of Baltimore, each of whom was the original author of the chapters mentioned. Dr. Frank J. Otenasek of Baltimore has revised the chapters on neurosurgery.

As before, the authors gratefully acknowledge the helpfulness of the numerous members of the surgical and nursing staffs of The Johns Hopkins Hospital whose advice and aid have been sought.

EDWARD S. STAFFORD
DORIS DILLER

Baltimore, Maryland

CONTENTS

Unit I. THE FUNDAMENTALS OF SURGICAL NURSING

Unit II. NURSING IN THORACIC SURGERY

Unit III. NURSING IN VASCULAR SURGERY

Unit IV. NURSING IN SURGERY OF THE ALIMENTARY TRACT

Unit V. SURGERY OF THE URINARY TRACT

Unit VI. SURGERY OF THE INTEGUMENTARY SYSTEM

Unit VII. DISEASES DUE TO ALLERGY

Unit VIII. SURGERY OF THE ENDOCRINE GLANDS

Unit IX. NURSING IN NEUROLOGIC SURGERY

Unit X. SURGERY OF THE EYE, EAR, NOSE AND THROAT

Unit XI. NURSING IN ORTHOPEDIC SURGERY

Chapter 43. DEFORMITIES OF THE BONES, JOINTS AND MUSCLES 509

Chapter 44. MUSCULOSKELETAL INJURIES 524

Chapter 45. INFLAMMATORY, INFECTIOUS, AND NEOPLASTIC
DISEASES OF THE MUSCULOSKELETAL SYSTEM 544

Unit XII. NURSING IN SURGERY
OF THE REPRODUCTIVE ORGANS

Unit XIII. COMMUNICABLE DISEASE

Unit I. THE FUNDAMENTALS OF SURGICAL NURSING

CHAPTER 1

Introduction

The word surgery is a combination of the Greek words for *hand* and *work*. In ancient times physicians scorned to use their hands for work; hence such manual tasks as were thought necessary in the treatment of a patient were carried out by less exalted individuals. Much of the surgery of antiquity was performed by barbers; indeed the barber's pole is in reality the surgeon's signpost, as it symbolizes a leg encased in a bloodstained bandage. Surgery is one of the special subdivisions of the healing art, and its aims include the relief of pain, the cure of disease, the restoration of function to the crippled limb or damaged organ, and the social and economic rehabilitation of the individual.

The practice of surgery as we know it today owes its existence to fundamental scientific discoveries of the past century. One of these was the introduction of anesthesia. Ether was used by Crawford Long of Georgia, in 1842, but W. T. Morton of Boston, in 1846, really demonstrated the usefulness of this drug. It is difficult today to imagine the agony of the patient during a surgical operation performed without anesthesia, or to realize the obstacles confronting the surgeon in operating upon the screaming, struggling victim.

Another fundamental advance was the application to surgery of the knowledge of bacteria. Following the discovery by Pasteur that putrefaction is due to bacterial contamination, Lister, a British surgeon, realized that suppuration must be a similar process. In 1865 he described a method by which he was able to control bacterial contamination, with the result that wounds did not suppurate. Before that time, infection of wounds was thought essential to healing; in fact, pus was considered laudable and surgeons sought to encourage its formation, even introducing into wounds foreign bodies of various sorts (*setons*) in order to make suppuration certain. In contemplating surgery today it is hard to realize that less than one hundred years ago surgeons dared not enter the abdominal cavity, the chest, or the skull, and that even minor operations were followed by grave infection, with prolongation of convalescence or even death.

More recently, the application to surgery of many new scientific discoveries has opened new fields, and has made modern surgery amazingly safe for the patient.

Antisepsis and Asepsis. During the evolution of modern surgery, certain principles were developed which are essential to its success. One of these is the control of infection. Lord Lister introduced a method which attempted to kill all bacteria that might gain entrance to the wound. This technic was called *antisepsis* (against infection), and consisted in the use of chemical agents which could destroy bacteria. The original method called for the treatment of the patient's skin, the operator's hands, the instruments, and the sponges with a solution of carbolic acid; in addition, an overhead spray diffused droplets of carbolic acid over operative field and operator. Although the success of this treatment in controlling infection was great, it was not complete; also the carbolic spray was uncomfortable and highly irritating, frequently burning the skin of both patient and surgeon. Nevertheless, a beginning had been made, from which it was a logical step to the adoption of aseptic technic. *Asepsis* (without infection) means the prevention of infection by complete exclusion of bacteria. This method resulted from the contributions of numerous

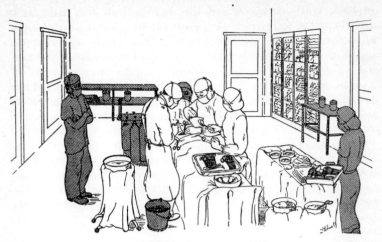

FIGURE 1. Aseptic operating room technic. White surfaces designate what is *clean,* and the shaded surfaces designate the unsterile or *dirty* personnel and equipment. The floor and walls, although unsterile, are not shaded.

surgeons, notably Lawson Tait in Great Britain, Halsted in the United States, and von Bergmann in Germany.

Absolute asepsis, however, is an ideal condition, attained with difficulty. To understand this fact it is necessary to consider the sources of bacterial contamination during a surgical procedure. Disease-producing (*pathogenic*) bacteria are ubiquitous. They may be found on the skin of the patient and on that of the surgeon and his associates. The nose, mouth, and throat of every one are contaminated, as are also the internal surfaces of the respiratory and gastrointestinal organs. Bacteria abound in dust and float in the air; therefore every object that is exposed, be it furniture, clothing, instruments, or dressings, may be contaminated. Since this is so, it is obvious that asepsis is not static, that an object made *sterile* (bacteria free) may not remain so.

Operative Trauma; Hemostasis. Another essential principle is the avoidance of undue trauma. Every surgical operation must be considered an injury to the body; an operative incision is better planned than an accidental one, but both result in wounds which must heal. In order to minimize damage, tissues and organs must be handled carefully and only such manipulation and dissection carried out as are necessary for the success of the operation. Speed in operating, with resultant roughness, is no longer as important as in the preanesthetic days. Adherence to this principle of minimizing trauma aids also in preserving the biologic assets of the patient. Where possible, the functions of muscles, nerves, and organs must be retained. Preservation of the patient's store of blood by the most rigid *hemostasis* (arrest of escape of blood) not only saves life, but also shortens convalescence and reduces complications.

Mental Aspects. Another important consideration is the attitude and mental condition of the patient. A fearful or unnecessarily frightened patient undergoes surgery with an added handicap. Kind, thoughtful treatment and reassurance are essential, for without them permanent damage to the personality may result.

THE NURSE IN SURGERY

The role of the nurse in surgery is not secondary to that of the surgeon; it is equally important. The success of the operation, in fact the very life of the patient, depends upon the reliability of all those engaged in surgical nursing. Without complete honesty, without conscientious attention to details, there will be no asepsis. Following operation patients are often critically ill; complications arise which need immediate treatment, and these must be detected by the constant care and watchfulness of the nurse.

The importance of the personal relation between patient and nurse must be emphasized. Every patient finds himself in a new environment, separated from his home, his relatives, and his routine of life; in addition, he may be—and often is—in actual physical discomfort. It is not surprising, therefore, that such a patient needs reassurance; his comfort and the maintenance or development of his morale depend chiefly upon the nurse. The confidence of the patient is gained by a sincere interest in his family, his occupation, his personal problems, by attempting to mold the hospital routine as far as possible to conform with his mode of life, and by reassuring him concerning his progress. These matters are also the responsibility of the surgeon, but the nurse of necessity spends far more time with the patient. Reassurance is doubly important for a patient who will find it necessary to change his way of living as a result of his injury or illness, as, for example, a patient who has had a limb amputated. There is much that scientists do not understand about life, but it has often been observed that the patient's will to live seems to play a large part in the outcome of an illness. The encouragement of this will to live is as important a contribution to the welfare of the patient as is food, medicine, or any part of the nursing care.

Total Care. The responsibilities of the physician and of the nurse do not cease when the patient is pronounced "out of danger," nor when the incision is healed, nor even when the patient leaves the hospital. Home care, follow-up visits in the home or clinic, programs of instruction, and whatever other nursing measures are needed to ensure the fullest possible rehabilitation of the patient are all essential parts of the idea of total care. In its broadest sense, this concept also includes measures directed toward the prevention of injury and disease.

Since the surgeon and the nurse are working together for the welfare of the patient, they must enjoy mutual confidence and respect. The nurse will carry out the surgeon's instructions, but she will do it better if she understands the surgeon's purpose; he will do well, therefore, to keep the nurse fully informed. Similarly, the patient's welfare is the surgeon's concern, and the patient will profit from intelligent, reliable reports from the nurse to the surgeon. Here, as in all of life, there is no substitute for hard work, honesty and loyalty.

SUMMARY

Careful study of every aspect of each patient is necessary in order to suit the treatment to his needs and to minimize the risk. It is still true that every surgical procedure is hazardous, though today that hazard is in most instances slight. Although there have been many recent advances in surgery, there still remains much that is imperfect or undeveloped, and constant effort must be made to find new facts, new principles, and new methods, as well as to reexamine the old. The aim of surgery is the rehabilitation of the patient; every activity of surgical nursing should be so oriented.

VOCABULARY REVIEW

antisepsis	*pathogenic*	*hemostasis*
asepsis	*sterile*	*rehabilitation*
suppuration	*trauma*	

SUGGESTED READING

1. Gregg, Dorothy: Anxiety—A Factor in Nursing Care. Am. J. Nursing, *52:* 1363–1365 (Nov.) 1952.
2. Keeton, Robert W.: Nutrition and Appetite Training During Illness. J.A.M.A., *151:*253–260 (Jan. 24) 1953.
3. Lais, Barbara Brice: Does Your Voice Defeat You? Am. J. Nursing, *51:*322 (May) 1951.
4. Simmons, Leo W.: The Manipulation of Human Resources in Nursing Care. Am. J. Nursing, *51:*452–455 (July) 1951.
5. Van Schoick, Mildred R.: Emotional Factors in Surgical Nursing. Am. J. Nursing, *46:*451–454 (August) 1946.

CHAPTER 2

Wounds and Healing

WOUNDS

A wound is the forcible solution of the continuity of tissue. It is considered open if the skin has been divided, closed if the continuity of the skin is uninterrupted. Wounds are commonly produced in a variety of ways, so many, in fact, that it is best to classify them according to the injury produced, since that is what determines the manner of healing and the form of treatment, although certain exceptions to this general statement will be noted later.

Open Wounds

Abrasions. In an abrasion the injury is confined to the most superficial layer of the skin (epidermis). It is a common wound of everyday activity, and probably no one has failed to "bark his knuckles" or "scrape his shins." An abrasion is usually caused by a glancing blow, and may be trivial; but often a considerable skin area is exposed to the abrasive agent, as may happen when a person is hurled to the street by collision with a moving automobile. A varying amount of the epidermis may be scraped off; frequently the defects thus produced are filled with small particles of dirt or other foreign material. These particles, if not

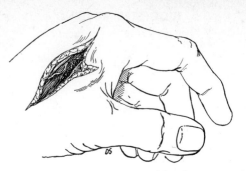

FIGURE 2. Laceration of hand.

removed, retard healing, and may result in unsightly tattoo marks.

Incised Wounds; Lacerated Wounds. These may be considered together, since division of the skin with exposure or possible injury of the underlying structures is common to both. Incised wounds are made by sharp-edged objects, such as knives, glass, or tin cans; lacerations result from the application of a force which tears or splits the skin. Operative incisions are incised wounds, differing from accidental incised wounds chiefly in their purpose and in the conditions under which they are made. The incised wound has regular edges; those of the laceration are usually uneven, with more destruction of tissue.

Avulsed Wounds. An avulsed wound is made by sharp or blunt objects; its characteristic is the loss of tissue. This type of wound is caused by contact with a rapidly moving object, as, for example, a bomb fragment. In an extensive avulsion there may be actual loss of portions of muscles, tendons, nerves and blood vessels, in addition to the overlying skin.

Penetrating (Puncture) Wounds. These follow the introduction into the body of a pointed object, e.g., needle, splinter, nail, ice pick, or of a small object traveling at high speed (e.g., a bullet). These wounds are characterized by a small surface opening which gives no clue to the depth or extent of the underlying damage. In this type of wound the possibility of perforation of underlying organs is great; it is in these wounds also that anaerobic bacteria may grow, since the small surface opening quickly seals over and thus prevents the oxygen of the air from reaching the depths of the wound.

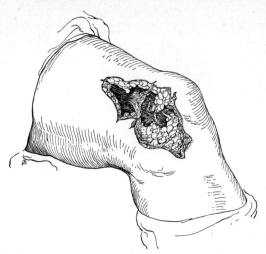

FIGURE 3. Avulsed wound of knee.

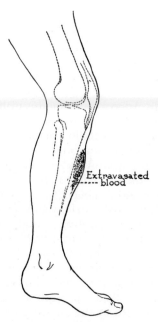

FIGURE 4. Contusion.

Closed Wounds

Blisters. The familiar blister is a simple superficial closed wound. Following chemical, thermal, or frictional irritation of the skin, the damaged epidermis becomes raised and separated from the deeper layer by an outpouring of serum. If the continuity of the superficial epidermis is broken, the wound then becomes an open one.

Contusions. A blow of adequate force on the skin produces a contusion (*bruise*), and swelling and discoloration result from the outpouring of serum and blood which follows this injury to the subcutaneous tissues. A collection of blood (*hematoma*) may form in this way, but more often the extravasated blood is spread diffusely through the tissues in the region of the injury.

Other Varieties of Closed Wounds. Sprains, which result when the supporting ligaments of joints are torn, dislocations of joints, and simple fractures are all closed wounds. Under a variety of circumstances force directed against the chest or the abdomen produces laceration or perforation of the internal organs. That a severe crushing injury may do so is readily understandable; but internal injury following a relatively light blow, without any damage to the overlying skin, is surprisingly common. These closed wounds are known as *subcutaneous injuries* to the chest and abdomen.

HEALING OF WOUNDS

The healing of a wound depends upon the ability of the injured tissues to repair themselves. This in turn depends upon the exact nature of the injured tissues, as well as upon certain more general features, such as the presence of pathogenic bacteria, the physical condition of the patient, his state of nutrition, the location of the wound, and the method of treatment.

The Process of Repair. Immediately following injury to the skin there is bleeding from divided capillaries or larger vessels and outpouring of tissue fluid from opened lymphatics and intercellular spaces. Ordinarily the bleeding ceases in from two to six minutes as a result of clotting of the blood; if not dislodged, this coagulum protects the surface of the wound. Within a few hours white cells (*leukocytes*) from the blood and wandering connective tissue cells begin to move into the blood clot. At the same time the injured capillaries about the wound begin to grow, gradually forming new capillary loops which push their

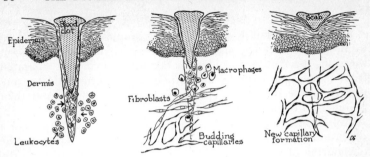

FIGURE 5. Primary healing. The blood clot is replaced first by granulation tissue and finally by scar tissue.

way into the blood clot. This newly formed tissue, composed of capillaries, leukocytes, and wandering cells, has a red velvety or granular appearance, and is known as granulation tissue. It gradually takes the place of the blood clot; much of this is digested and removed, the remainder serves as protection to the external surface of the wound in the form of a scab. At the same time the epithelial cells on the skin surface begin to grow more rapidly and to divide with increased frequency. Spreading into the wound on its surface from all sides, these cells seek to restore the epithelial continuity. When the granulation tissue has filled the defect and the surface is epithelialized, the crust or scab is shed. At this stage the wound appears healed; however, healing is not complete until the granulation tissue organizes into scar tissue. The whole process of repair occupies two weeks or more, depending upon the size of the wound and many other factors.

Primary Healing. Under favorable conditions primary union (*healing by first intention*) occurs. If the edges of an incised wound in a healthy person are promptly and accurately approximated, if bacterial contamination has been slight and is held to a minimum, if there is no foreign material in the wound, and if the wound is protected from movement or other trauma, healing is prompt. Approximation of the wound edges minimizes not only the defect to be filled with blood clot and the gap in the tissues, but also the opportunity for bacteria to enter the depths of the wound. There will be only as much granulation tissue as is necessary to occupy this small space; consequently there will be only a narrow scar. During the healing process there will be less inflammation, less pain, and no discharge of secretion or pus.

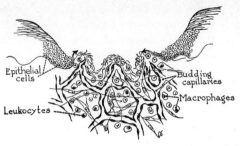

Epithelial cells

Budding capillaries

Macrophages

Leukocytes

FIGURE 6. Secondary healing. Exuberant granulation tissue and slow epithelialization lead to excessive scar formation.

Secondary Healing. The tissues of the human body have a marvelous capacity for repairing wounds under the most adverse circumstances. Secondary union (*healing by second intention*) differs from primary union only in degree; in each, the same fundamental repair process is at work. Wounds in which the tissue edges are widely separated, which may be due either to lack of approximation or to such loss of substance as to prevent approximation, heal slowly. There is a large defect, and consequently a large amount of granulation tissue, resulting in a large scar. Secondary healing is usually accomplished in the face of bacterial contamination, since it is almost impossible to exclude bacteria constantly from an open wound. The reparative process is working at a disadvantage, hence healing is slow, taking several weeks or longer. There is usually inflammation of the injured area, and these granulating wounds are often painful. Serous secretion or purulent discharge commonly occurs. Occasionally wound repair seems to be regressing rather than progressing, or at least to be at a standstill. The explanation of this failure to progress lies in the nature of the factors which influence healing.

Factors Influencing Repair. Certain of these concern the body as a whole; the others are chiefly local. The age and the general health of the patient are important, healing taking place more rapidly in the young and healthy. The presence of a debilitating systemic disease, for example, cancer, tends to delay healing. Since repair is dependent upon the ability of the cells to grow and reproduce themselves, it is obvious that adequate nutrition of the whole body is necessary; especially important are the vitamins. Adequate nutrition of tissues in the vicinity of the wound is equally necessary, and this is accomplished by the circulating blood. Poor local circulation is a common cause of delayed healing. Then, too, the extent of the local damage to the tissues, not only with respect to the amount of tissue damage, but also with respect to the nature of the injured structures, is obviously a determining factor in the repair. Where a wound communicates with the interior of the lung, intestine, or urinary system a permanent opening (*fistula*) often results.

Infection. The healing of wounds is adversely affected by bacterial contamination. There are many varieties of microorganisms distributed widely in nature; some of these are harmful to tissues and produce disease in man. Certain pathogenic bacteria are able to destroy the cells of the body tissues, either by manufacturing a specific poison (*toxin*) or by producing metabolic wastes which are injurious to the living cells. There is great variation in the action of these bacteria and of their poisons upon the different cells of the body. Thus the unbroken surface of the epithelium of the skin or of the mucous membranes affords complete protection against most of these pathogens; it is only when there is a wound, or tiny break in this armor, that a portal of entry is opened. Through this opening, bacteria, if present in sufficient numbers, will penetrate to the subepithelial tissues, which are less resistant. Once present in the tissues of the wound, the bacteria wage war against processes of repair, destroying new cells as well as old. The progress of healing will depend upon the ability of the protective agents of the body to defeat the bacteria.

Foreign Bodies. Healing may also be delayed or prevented by the presence of foreign material in the wound. Certain substances are highly irritating to the tissues; in fact, there are very few materials so inert as to be harmless. Such objects as wood splinters or fragments of cloth not only introduce infection, but are of themselves irritating. Wounds are also subjected to unnecessary injury if the injured part has not been properly splinted or supported, because even slight motion may separate the wound edges, thus interrupting repair again and again before firm union can occur. Too frequent or careless dressing of wounds, or the mistaken use of strong chemicals delays healing by injuring the delicate new cells.

Scar Tissue. Certain elements of the body repair tissue by regeneration; these include epithelium, bone, pleura and peritoneum, peripheral nerves, and some others. Injured or lost epithelium is replaced by new epithelium, indistinguishable from the old, and the same is true of the other tissues in this group, each being able to reproduce itself. Other types of tissue, notably muscle and fascia, do not regenerate, but are replaced by scar tissue. This is also true of various organs of the body in which, despite the regeneration of certain types of cells, the architecture of the organ is not restored, and scarring results. Scar tissue is the end result of the organization of granulation tissue. The wandering connective tissue cells gradually build up dense white tissue which is firm and inelastic. With the passage of time this tissue tends to contract, and thus closes off many of the tiny blood vessels. As a result, scar tissue has poor circulation. Subsequent contraction is likely to cause deformity if the area is extensive. It is important, therefore, to prevent the formation of excess scar tissue.

TREATMENT OF WOUNDS

Certain general aspects of this large subject will be considered here, but the details of the treatment of many wounds will be discussed in connection with the surgery of the various regions of the body. The chief purpose of the surgeon in treating wounds is to promote favorable healing, with as complete repair of all damage as is feasible. The first objective is to save the life of the patient, and this consideration may necessitate the control of hemorrhage and the treatment of shock (Chap. 6). Next comes examination of the patient to determine the local damage and the injury to structures lying beneath the skin. Following this, proper measures are taken to increase the comfort of the patient and to secure optimal repair of the injury.

Open Wounds

Abrasions are treated by cleansing the skin and removing the embedded foreign material. Beneath a nonirritating dressing the skin will heal rapidly.

In treating open wounds that cannot be closed because of loss of tissue (*avulsion*), dressings which are least irritating are used. Sterilized petrolatum gauze is satisfactory when care is taken not to use too much petrolatum, since an excess may prevent escape of secretion and favor maceration of the tissues. The aim in treating these wounds is to secure an epithelial covering as soon as possible in order to hasten healing and to minimize the scar. Plastic grafting procedures are often necessary.

Puncture wounds need little local treatment, as the small surface wound closes and heals quickly, but it is essential to recog-

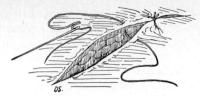

FIGURE 7. Approximation of wound edges by interrupted sutures.

nize and to treat injuries due to penetration of structures or organs beneath the skin. The conditions requisite to the growth of anaerobic bacteria (*anaerobiosis*) exist in such wounds; thus the use of tetanus antitoxin is obligatory unless the patient has been previously immunized. In this latter event, a booster dose of tetanus toxoid must be given.

Cleansing. In dealing with open wounds the first step is to reduce bacterial contamination. The skin about the wound is gently but thoroughly cleansed with soap and water or other detergent, and the wound itself may be irrigated with warm water or physiologic saline solution. The adjacent skin is then treated with a disinfectant, but care must be taken not to use such agents in the wounds, because the resultant destruction of delicate tissue cells would do more harm than good.

Débridement. Foreign material should be gently removed, and all tissue which has been crushed or otherwise devitalized should be excised (*débridement*). This step not only removes material which can serve as a favorable culture medium for bacteria, but also speeds repair, since the wandering cells would have to digest and remove this material before healing could occur. Bleeding is checked (*hemostasis*), as excess blood clot also delays healing.

Closure and Drainage. The tissues are carefully approximated, layer by layer, so that finally epithelium is in contact with epithelium, muscle with muscle, and so on; the defect to be repaired by healing is thus minimized. Undue tension is strictly avoided, for not only will sutures pull out if too tight, but the circulation will be cut off. Where possible, the skin is closed snugly with appropriate sutures; but in the presence of considerable contamination, or where oozing of blood cannot be completely suppressed, a small drain, usually of rubber, is left between the skin edges to facilitate the escape of old blood or wound secretion.

Antitoxin Administration. The tight closure of an open wound affords the proper conditions for the growth of anaerobic bacteria

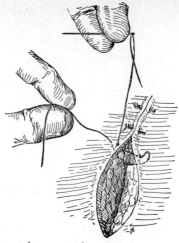

FIGURE 8. Wound closure by means of vertical mattress sutures, affording very accurate apposition of the edges.

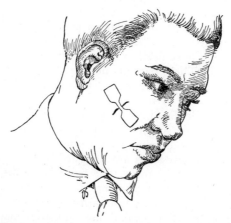

FIGURE 9. Satisfactory approximation of wound edges may be accomplished in an emergency by the use of flamed strips of adhesive.

in its depths. These organisms grow and divide only in the absence of oxygen. One of them is the bacillus of tetanus. Its spores are widely distributed in nature. This pathogen manufactures a poison (*toxin*), a small amount of which is highly fatal to man; fortunately, an antitoxin has been discovered and is available for

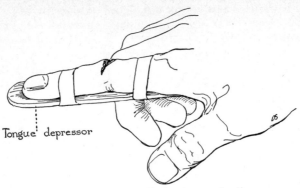

Tongue depressor

FIGURE 10. Proper splinting hastens healing.

use in protecting patients from the effects of this toxin. It is essential, therefore, that patients with wounds in which anaerobic growth is possible shall receive tetanus antitoxin.

In recent years a large part of our population has been actively immunized against tetanus toxin by means of injections of tetanus toxoid, a method similar to that employed in the prevention of diphtheria. All of the members of the armed forces of the United States have been so immunized, and large numbers of children as well. These patients need not be given tetanus antitoxin as a part of the treatment of a wound, but should receive a small booster dose of tetanus toxoid.

Dressings. Sterile dressings are applied and, if the wound is in a region likely to be subjected to motion, a splint is used. The purpose of applying dressings to a wound is to facilitate healing. As far as possible, dressings are designed to protect the wound from mechanical injury, to exclude bacteria, to prevent motion, and to absorb secretion or drainage. Interference with the carrying out of normal functions and with the comfort of the patient should be avoided. For general use, dressings made of several layers of sterilized gauze have been found the most practicable. Although not so soft as cotton, the gauze is more easily separated from the wound and does not leave shreds of material in the wound. Dressings are made large enough to cover a margin of normal skin on all sides of the wound, and thick enough to be protective. They may be held in place by bandages, strips of adhesive tape, or collodion, depending upon the location and the effect desired. Where much drainage is expected, absorbent pads made of sterilized raw cotton are placed outside the gauze dressing, to be changed as often as necessary. Dressings contaminated by purulent drainage must be properly disposed of in order to prevent spread of infection from one patient to the next. A convenient method is to provide paper bags as receptacles for such material; these can later be burned. The same care is taken in the preparation of dressings as in the preparation of the supplies for the operating room.

Redressings. Too frequent dressing of wounds is avoided; in the absence of fever, pain, or other evidence of infection, the wound need not be examined until five to seven days later when the skin sutures are removed. It is important, however, to keep the wound and the dressings dry, as moisture renders dressings permeable to bacteria and macerates the tissues. If there is drainage from the wound, dressings must be changed frequently.

A convenient and practical method of changing dressings in an aseptic manner is by the so-called knife-and-fork technic. For this the surgeon needs the assistance of a nurse and a properly equipped surgical carriage or dressing tray.

The Surgical Carriage. The equipment of the surgical carriage includes sterilized covered receptacles which contain sterilized instruments, gauze sponges, dressings, and towels. In addition, there are unsterile basins, sterile and unsterile bandages, adhesive tape and waxed paper bags, and bottles containing appropriate solutions of Zephiran, ether, acetone and other chemicals of the surgeon's choice. In some hospitals the sterile supplies are individually wrapped or packaged, instead of being placed in large containers. The essential article of the equipment is a long dressing forceps, previously sterilized, which stands in a container filled with a strong disinfectant such as lysol, but with the handle standing above the level of the fluid. By means of this instrument, commonly called a sponge-stick, the nurse may grasp and withdraw sterile supplies or instruments from their containers without contaminating them. Thus by using sterilized instruments in place of unsterile hands, dressings may be performed aseptically. In order to guard against contamination of the sterile supplies remaining in the containers, one must observe the rule that supplies may be taken out but may not be replaced unless the whole container is to be resterilized.

Example: Technic of Redressing an Abdominal Incision. The patient is placed in a position that will give him most comfort and yet be convenient for the surgeon. Undue exposure of the

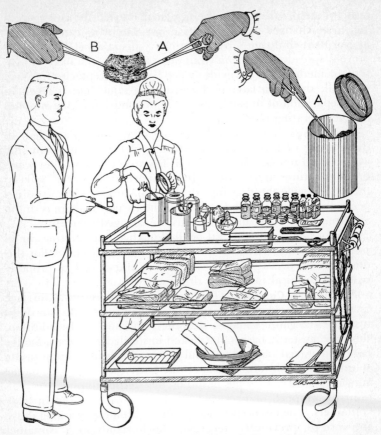

FIGURE 11. The surgical carriage. Inserts show knife-and-fork technic. Note that the ends of the dressing forceps, the dressings, and the interiors of the containers are sterile. Surgical dressings by this method prevent contamination of wound and dressing carriage.

body is avoided. The surgeon removes the dressings, taking care neither to injure the wound nor to inflict unnecessary pain. The old dressing is placed in a paper bag in an unsterile basin at the foot of the bed. The nurse then opens a sterile towel, placing it near the wound. Upon this she deposits with the sterile forceps such instruments and dressings as are needed. The surgeon takes an instrument, usually a forceps, and with it applies the appropriate solutions and the fresh dressings. In this way wound and fresh dressings are in contact only with sterilized instruments, and there will be no contamination of either wound or surgical carriage except through ignorance or carelessness.

Closed Wounds

Closed wounds respond well to conservative treatment. Protection of the bruised surface, together with the application of heat and complete rest, aids repair. Heat is useful in two ways: it increases the circulation and relieves pain. The treatment of sprains, fractures, and subcutaneous wounds of the chest and abdomen, which are closed wounds, will be considered in later chapters.

Bites

The bites of men and of various animals deserve special consideration. In addition to the local injury, the bite may serve to inoculate the patient with the virus of a disease carried by the animal, or with a poison secreted by the animal. When the animals are small and have sharp teeth, small puncture wounds result, with little local damage. Larger animals may inflict wounds in which there is considerable laceration, crushing, and even avulsion of tissue. The mouths of men and of animals are always heavily contaminated with bacteria, so that bites are commonly infected. Human bites produce unusually dirty wounds, a result of the combination of crushed tissue and the bacteria of the human mouth; also to be borne in mind is the possibility of the transmission of syphilis.

In general, the wounds resulting from bites are treated locally as any heavily contaminated wound should be treated, with special attention to cleansing and débridement and with no attempt at closure. Since suppuration, with consequent loss of tissue and delay in healing, is probable, the prophylactic use of antibiotic agents is justified. Daily intramuscular injections of repository penicillin, until serious infection is averted or controlled, is one method of accomplishing this aim.

The bite of a venomous snake may be differentiated from that of a nonvenomous snake either by recognition of the variety of snake or by the appearance of the wound. Venomous snakes have hollow, needle-like fangs through which the venom is injected into the victim, and these puncture wounds are unlike the marks made by the row of teeth of the nonpoisonous snakes. The toxin secreted by venomous snakes is lethal to man if a sufficient amount reaches the central nervous system. The treatment of snake bite consists in the prevention of absorption of the toxin by slashing open the tissues and injecting physiologic saline solution to wash out the toxin. Where the bite is on an extremity, an effort is made to slow the rate of absorption by the intermittent use of the tourniquet, since small sublethal amounts of toxin may be safely metabolized in the body. Neutralization of the toxin by the use of polyvalent antivenin should be tried, and an attempt is made to overcome the paralyzing effect of the toxin by the administration of stimulants to heart and respiration.

War Wounds

The wounds caused by the implements of modern warfare are far more serious than the wounds incurred in civil life, and, furthermore, the exigencies of the battlefield often prevent prompt treatment. The problem which confronts the surgeon is thus vastly different. War wounds are commonly multiple, and there is usually extensive loss of substance. Fractures, if present, are nearly always compound and comminuted. Hemorrhage and shock are conspicuously present. As a rule, such wounds are grossly contaminated by soil, bits of clothing, and other foreign material. The comment may be made that wounds of this nature are not infrequently received in automobile or industrial accidents, and that the results of treatment as carried out in civil life are extremely good; but it must be emphasized that during a battle or an air raid it is not possible to care for all casualties quickly. Thousands of soldiers or noncombatants may be injured in a few minutes; transportation and treatment require time, so that many hours or even days may elapse before a given individual receives any but the most urgent first-aid treatment.

Modern treatment of war wounds begins long before the wound is sustained. Each soldier is actively immunized against tetanus toxin, and cleanliness of body and clothing is emphasized. The first-aid equipment issued to soldiers includes a sterile dressing. The wounded soldier is taken to the nearest casualty clearing station; there, the means for treating shock and for checking hemorrhage are available. The wounded are sorted out (*triage*), so that those in greatest need of surgery will be transported first to the nearest hospital.

At the hospital patients with penetrating wounds of the abdomen and chest and those with head injuries receive treatment first. Next the compound fractures are dealt with, and finally the wounds of soft parts and simple fractures. It is obvious that ordinary closure of soft-part wounds usually is not feasible, as thorough treatment may not be possible until twelve to seventy-two hours after injury. Nevertheless, the use of antibiotic agents, and careful preservation of all viable structures will result in clean granulating wounds which later may be treated by some type of secondary closure, or by plastic reconstruction, so that good functional results will ultimately be obtained.

NURSING CARE

The nurse will often see the injured person first, especially in schools, industry, or in the hospital accident room. Effective first aid requires the performance of numerous acts almost simultaneously. Of nearly equal importance is the cultivation by the nurse of an attitude of calmness, because this last, when combined with obvious efficiency, gives the greatest reassurance to the frightened patient. The nurse must quickly appraise the situation, and, if necessary, commence artificial respiration, take steps to control obvious bleeding, apply sterile dressings to the wounds, summon help, or administer antidotes, as the case may be. Under some circumstances the responsibility for treating minor, superficial wounds, insect bites, and the like may be delegated to the nurse. When the surgeon is needed and has been called, the nurse should gather useful information from or about the patient concerning the circumstances of the injury, and should prepare such sterile instruments and materials as may be needed. She should also attend to the notification of relatives if the patient is a child or a seriously injured adult. She may, in appropriate situations, prepare the tetanus antitoxin or toxoid for administration, and may administer the test dose of horse serum in the conjunctival sac if antitoxin is to be used.

Following the completion of treatment, the nurse may be assigned the job of instructing the patient or his relatives concerning his care, treatments, and return visits. She should not forget, in carrying out these tasks, that the patient and his relatives are likely to be in a highly abnormal state emotionally, and that they are probably quite unfamiliar with the care of injuries and the medical jargon associated therewith. It is best to state the necessary instructions very simply and carefully, and to see that the patient or his relatives can repeat them correctly. Many hospitals have prepared printed instructions to be given to the patient or his relatives. This is a good procedure, but must be accompanied by verbal instructions as well, for there are still some who cannot read or who cannot understand what they read.

SUMMARY

Living tissues naturally tend to repair wounds. The processes of repair are aided by careful approximation of wound edges, by the control of bleeding, by the removal of dirt and devitalized tissue, and by the prevention of bacterial growth. Healing can be retarded by neglect and by overtreatment. Emergency treatment requires calm thinking and prompt, correct action. Although a wound is confined, in a strict sense, to a local area it affects the patient as a whole; therefore, total care is as necessary as the care directed to the wound.

VOCABULARY REVIEW

abrasion	*contusion*	*anaerobiosis*
incision	*hematoma*	*débridement*
avulsion	*extravasated*	*antitoxin*
laceration	*granulation tissue*	*toxoid*
	fistula	

SUGGESTED READING

1. Joergenson, E. J., and Smith, E. T.: Postoperative Abdominal Wound Separation and Evisceration. Am. J. Surg., *79*:282–287 (February) 1950.
2. Kleitsch, William P., and Douglas, Dale W.: Postoperative Wound Disruption. Am. J. Surg., *84*:678–683 (December) 1952.
3. Krause, Marie V.: Nutrition and Diet Therapy in Relation to Nursing, Philadelphia, W. B. Saunders Co., 1952, pp. 223–224.
4. Marshall, Wallace: Some Pathologic Aspects of Cutaneous Wound Healing. Am. J. Surg., *84*:675–677 (December) 1952.
5. Rhoads, J. E., Fliegelman, M. T., and Panzer, L. M.: Mechanisms of Delayed Wound Healing in the Presence of Hypoproteinemia. J.A.M.A., *118*:21–25 (January 3) 1942.
6. Waterman, Donald F., and others: Healing of Wounds in the Presence of Anemia. Surgery, *31*:821–828 (June) 1952.
7. Wolff, William I.: Disruption of Abdominal Wounds. Ann. Surg., *131*:534–553 (April) 1950.

CHAPTER 3

Surgical Infections

The human body is admirably equipped with armor against bacterial invasion; every exposed surface, whether skin or mucous membrane, is covered by a continuous sheet of epithelial cells.

No one can go through life, however, without an occasional break in this armor, and when an opening is made, no matter how small or how temporary, bacteria are always present to take advantage of the opportunity. Once the bacteria are beneath the surface, infection has occurred, and the body must mobilize its defenses against the enemy. Since an important factor in this struggle is the number of pathogenic microorganisms present, the value of cleanliness is apparent. Dirt harbors germs. Those to whom the care of patients with infection is entrusted can hardly escape contact with virulent bacteria, and thus their own safety depends largely upon cleanliness. Regular washing of the hands after such contacts, together with frequent change of clothing, is important. Injury to the hands from unnecessary or rough scrubbing should be avoided, as it is of the utmost importance to prevent breaks in the skin. Visits to patients with uninfected wounds should be made before attending to those with infection.

An occasional postoperative wound infection seems unavoidable, but the occurrence of an infection following the performance of a presumably aseptic procedure indicates a break in technic. For this reason surgeons and nurses must make it their duty to record every postoperative infection, and to investigate fully all the circumstances so that errors in technic can be corrected and carelessness or ignorance exposed. The spread of infection from patient to patient, so common in bygone centuries, is inexcusable now, and must be considered as due solely to the carelessness or inefficiency of those caring for the patients.

Body Defenses Against Infection. The chief antagonists of bacteria are the *phagocytic* (swallowing) white corpuscles of the blood, which can surround and engulf bacteria, and the wonderful chemical substances called immune bodies. These last are found in the blood and in the tissue fluids; some (*antibodies*) have the power to inhibit the growth of bacteria, some (*coagulins*) to cause them to adhere to one another, and others (*lysins*) to dissolve them. The outcome of the struggle depends upon the ability of the body to mobilize and deliver leukocytes and immune bodies. The local concentration of these defenders occurs in the inflammatory reaction, and the old description of inflammation, pain (*dolor*), swelling (*tumor*), redness (*rubor*), and local heat (*calor*), remains adequate. The inflammatory reaction is nonspecific; that is, it may be provoked by irritants other than bacteria. Capillary dilatation results in increased local circulation of blood, producing erythema and local warmth. Leukocytes and serum, spreading among the tissues, cause swelling. The irritation of the local nerves is responsible for the pain and tenderness. The region now contains bacteria, more blood than usual, leukocytes, and tissue fluid. In addition to the swelling, the tissue feels hard when palpated; such abnormal consistency is known as *induration*. The bacteria are surrounded on all sides, and this stage of the infection corresponds to the clinical term *cellulitis*.

Systemic Response. Accompanying the local attack upon the bacterial invaders is a response of the whole body. This, when sufficiently severe to be noticeable, is characterized by a general feeling of illness (*malaise*), fever, loss of appetite, and sometimes headache. The symptoms vary, of course, with the size and condition of the patient, and with the nature and number of the bacterial invaders.

At this stage in the infection at least three different results are possible. The bacteria may be quickly overcome, in which case the inflammation disappears and the infection is over. Or, if the bacteria are more resistant, the infection is localized but proceeds to suppuration. Or again, the bacterial invaders may be stronger than the defense, and the infection spreads.

Abscess Formation. When the infection is not quickly overcome, the leukocytic infiltration about the bacteria increases. If this ring of defenders is successful in confining the bacteria, an abscess forms. During the next period of days or hours, the central mass of bacteria, leukocytes, and cellular debris liquefies as a result of the action of ferments brought by the blood or secreted by bacteria. The presence of this yellowish liquid (*pus*) may be detected by the sudden softening of the central portion of an indurated area, or by the appearance of fluctuation, a sign which is dependent upon the transmission of impulses by an enclosed collection of fluid. Following the evacuation of the pus, the abscess cavity collapses, its walls fall together, and healing occurs exactly as in granulating wounds.

Failure of Local Resistance. The body requires a certain amount of time to mobilize its defenses; often the bacteria are present in such overwhelming numbers that the early local resistance is unable to prevent the spread of infection. On occasion the bacteria gain entrance to the blood, causing septicemia, but the usual mode of spread is either along fascial planes or through the lymphatics. Thus a deep-lying infection—as, for example, an abscess beneath the palmar fascia of the hand—will extend be-

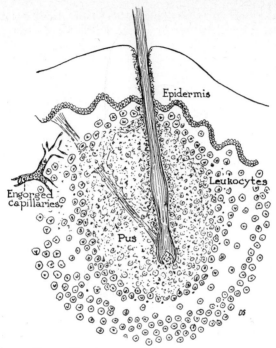

FIGURE 12. The common furuncle (boil).

neath the fascia up into the forearm since there is less mechanical resistance in that direction. Superficial infections are apt to enter the lymphatic system. The nature and function of this system of vessels and glands are considered in some detail later; it is enough to say here that bacteria entering the lymph channels and nodes meet with fierce resistance. The familiar clinical picture of red streaks extending from an infected hand up the arm toward the axilla (*lymphangitis,* Fig. 13), is due to the inflammatory reaction along the lymphatic vessels. It is erroneously known by the laity as "blood poisoning." These vessels drain into the lymph nodes, where further attempts are made to overcome the bacteria. All grades of the inflammatory process may occur in the infection of lymph nodes (*lymphadenitis*), and breakdown with suppuration is common.

Bacterial Invaders. The staphylococcus and the streptococcus are the commonest causes of surgical infection. In general, the

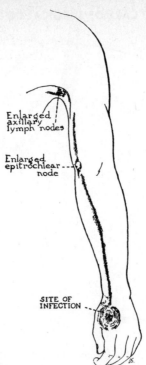

Enlarged
axillary
lymph nodes

Enlarged
epitrochlear
node

SITE OF
INFECTION

FIGURE 13. Lymphangitis and lymphadenitis caused by extension of the infection from the hand.

staphylococcus is more apt to cause localized infection with abscess formation, whereas the streptococcus seems more virulent, producing more profound systemic effects and tending more often to spread through the tissues and the lymphatics. The colon bacillus (*Escherichia coli*), the pneumococcus, and a few others are occasionally encountered in primary infection, but the colon bacillus is often present in wound infections following operations on the gastrointestinal tract. Most of these bacteria live equally well on the surface of the body or in the tissues. Some bacteria, however, thrive only in the absence of free oxygen (*anaerobiosis*); one variety of anaerobic streptococcus produces a particularly destructive and spreading infection. Among the bacteria found in the mouth are certain putrefactive anaerobes, and these play a part in infections due to bites and in pulmonary infections.

NURSING CARE OF SURGICAL INFECTIONS

Infection. The occurrence of unexplained fever or of undue inflammation about a recent wound points to a wound infection. Often the local signs are slight, but usually there are increased tenderness and induration. The early discovery of a wound infection is of the utmost importance, since neglect may lead to a spreading of the process with results that are disastrous to the success of the operation or even fatal to the patient.

It is the purpose of the surgeon to aid the body in its fight against infection, hence certain general measures are undertaken in the treatment of every infection, however trivial it may seem. These measures include enforced rest, not only of the infected part but of the whole body, adequate diet, and relief of pain. Efforts are made to increase the local circulation in the infected area. When pus forms it should be permitted to escape by means of adequate surgical drainage (p. 35), but any surgical procedure which might spread the infection is avoided. The local application of heat and prompt opening of the wound are indicated. Numerous antibiotic and chemotherapeutic agents and prepared immune bodies (*immune serum* and *antitoxin*) are now available, to be used when indicated by the severity and nature of the infection.

Where the infectious process has resulted in considerable destruction of tissue it is advisable to remove the necrotic material; an effective method is by irrigation with Dakin's solution. To be active this solution must be freshly prepared, and it may be used in any wound where there is no danger of hemorrhage, or where no delicate tissue, such as brain, is exposed. Since it is irritating, the adjacent skin must be protected by a layer of grease. In addition to removing necrotic tissue and destroying bacteria, Dakin's solution is a strong deodorant, a quality much appreciated by patient and attendants when a foul, sloughing wound is present. Azochloramid, a more stable and less irritating chemical, may be used in place of Dakin's solution. Further infection of the patient and transmission of the germs to others must be prevented by the proper disposal of pus, dressings and other contaminated articles.

Measures to Improve Circulation. To aid the local circulation of blood, the infected part should be supported at the level of the body. This may best be accomplished by keeping the patient in bed; when the infection is minor, however, such as an infected extremity, placing the infected hand in a sling or elevating the

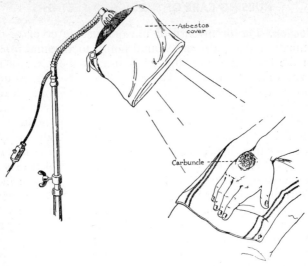

FIGURE 14. Treating an infection by the application of dry heat (carbon filament lamp).

infected foot upon a chair while the patient is seated is helpful. Constricting bandages or clothing should be avoided.

Heat. The local application of heat produces increased blood flow in the area treated, and is also mildly analgesic. Heat may be applied in several ways; dry heat is conveniently obtained from a carbon filament heat lamp, moist heat by the application of hot compresses, or by the immersion of the part in a tub of hot physiologic saline. Heat may also be derived from the use of electrodiathermy. Since heat is a potential source of burns, extreme caution must be observed in the method of its application. The use of electric heating pads is dangerous; serious accidents have occurred from overheating, and electric shock has followed the moistening of the pad. Diathermy requires complicated apparatus and especially trained operators; hence its use is somewhat limited.

DRY HEAT. In using dry heat therapy, numerous considerations must be kept in mind, such as individual differences in resistance to heat, the size of the area to be treated, the energy output (wattage) of the lamp, the size of the reflector, and the distance of the source of heat from the body surface. When equipped with a small reflector, a 300-watt carbon filament lamp (infra-red) (Fig.

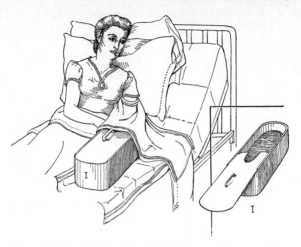

FIGURE 15. Application of moist heat by use of an arm tub.

14) is satisfactory. This lamp has the advantage of producing less light than the thermolite type of lamp, and is thus more comfortable to the patient's eyes. An average distance of 30 inches between lamp and body surface provides sufficient heat, but a safe guide is the sensation of the patient, which should be no more than a feeling of pleasant warmth. When the patient's sensation is not a reliable guide (as with children, mental patients, or in neurological conditions), the nurse's hand at the same distance may be used, or better, a thermometer on the skin surface, with the temperature not over 110° F. Care must be taken so that only a small portion of the total body surface is exposed, since dangerous overheating might otherwise result; periods of exposure should be limited in time (one hour or less) and should be alternated with equal periods of rest.

MOIST HEAT. When moist heat is applied it is well to protect the skin with grease in order to avoid maceration. With a lesion draining infected material, the use of an antiseptic grease, such as 5 per cent ammoniated mercury ointment, is advisable, to prevent wholesale inoculation of the adjacent skin. Hands and feet may be treated by immersion in tubs of physiologic salt solution heated to 105 to 112° F. The temperature may be maintained at that level, or even a little higher if not uncomfortable for the patient.

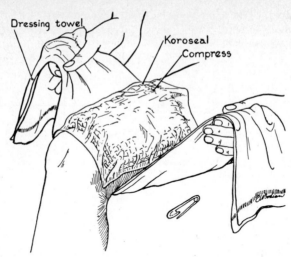

FIGURE 16. Application of moist warm compresses. A sheet of plastic may be used in place of oiled silk.

It is convenient to keep a thermometer at the bedside for testing the temperature of the solution. The maintenance of a fairly even temperature is accomplished by adding solution every half hour. The extremity should be removed from the tub when fluid is added. The solution should be thoroughly mixed before replacing the arm or the leg in the tub in order to prevent a burn. It is difficult to make a patient with a severely infected extremity comfortable; he is often fatigued, irritable, and hypersensitive. Relief at night from the continuous tub may be gained by the application of a hot compress with the part elevated on a pillow. This alternating treatment affords better relaxation since the position in bed is more comfortable; longer intervals of sleep may be obtained because there is less frequent disturbance. Rest lessens ill temper, anxiety, and fretfulness.

Elsewhere about the body, moist heat is derived from the application of compresses. These are made of several thicknesses of any suitable material, usually gauze, are sufficiently large, and are applied directly to the infected area. Sterilization of compresses, basins, and solutions is carried out whenever there is an open lesion or wound. The compresses and solutions are heated to 125° F., following which the nurse, having previously cleansed her hands, wrings out the compress and applies it to the infected area. The compress is then covered with plastic material which extends slightly beyond the edges of the compress, and the whole is held in position by a dressing of bandage or towels. A triangular bandage is often useful for this purpose, as is also a binder. The heat will be maintained at temperatures of 92 to 96° F. throughout the entire compress because plastic materials are excellent insulators. Frequent changing of compresses is necessary to prevent the accumulation of drainage or secretion on the infected surface. At times solutions other than physiologic saline are advisable, and under certain circumstances, usually to prevent damage to delicate tissues, compresses are moistened at intervals without being changed. When compresses are used on healing wounds (granulation tissue) and are changed as infrequently as every four hours, it is advisable to moisten the compress well before removing it, since the underlying tissue may be adherent; unnecessary trauma is thus avoided.

Cold. The use of ice or cold packs has been advocated for the treatment of infections, but there is no physiologic basis for their use. Lowered temperature results in constriction of the blood vessels and a slower cellular metabolism, which are disadvantageous.

Refrigeration. In some situations, however, the use of refrigeration may be a means of saving life. Chilling an extremity by packing it in ice or immersing it in solutions cooled below the freezing point of water has the effect of slowing the circulation locally, lowering the rate of all metabolic processes, and checking bacterial growth and invasion. By this means time may be gained for the regulation of uncontrolled diabetes mellitus in a patient with spreading infection in a gangrenous extremity. Amputation can then be postponed until it can be carried out safely.

Technic of Refrigeration. Before the treatment is begun, the nurse should give the patient a simple explanation concerning it. When the extremity is painful, it is desirable to give the patient an analgesic, such as morphine, at least twenty minutes before the procedure is started in order to prevent excruciating pain at the onset of chilling, before anesthesia is produced by the cold. It is also important that the nurse obtain from the surgeon information as to the exact site where refrigeration is to begin.

To hasten thorough chilling of the deep tissues, surgeons, at times, apply a tourniquet below the level of the intended amputation. To prevent pain due to its application, it is usually not adjusted until twenty minutes after refrigeration is begun.

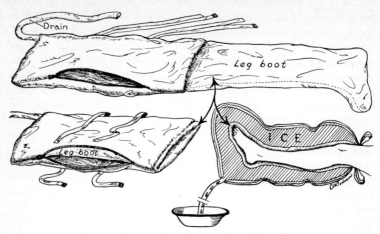

FIGURE 17. Use of plastic boot for refrigeration.

A plastic boot, as illustrated in Figure 17, is most useful. The leg is placed inside the boot, and the tape tied securely around the leg over the outer and inner boot at the level ordered by the surgeon. Finely crushed ice is then inserted through the zipper opening and packed around the leg and foot; the latter is protected by the inner plastic boot. Care should be taken that the leg and foot are uniformly covered with a layer of ice of not less than 3 inches. To help keep the ice in place around the leg as melting takes place, the straps on the outer boot are securely buckled. The drainage tube is extended over the edge of the mattress at the foot of the bed into a basin. A flannel blanket is then placed over the boot to protect the patient's other leg from the cold boot. The bed covers can then be neatly arranged.

This method of refrigeration offers many advantages. Refrigeration may be constantly maintained for as long a period as necessary and there is no seepage of water to make the patient uncomfortable. The flannel lining of the outer boot prevents the condensation of moisture. The patient may be taken to the operating room with the boot in place, and it may be removed without spilling water or ice.

Another method of administering refrigeration is by wrapping a large rubber sheet and a muslin sheet around an extremity, placing the ice between the extremity and the rubber sheet. The ice and rubber sheet are held in place by pinning the muslin sheet. The end of the rubber sheet may be arranged so that the melted ice will drain into a bucket on the floor or on a stool at the foot of the bed. To help prevent seepage around the thigh, the head of the bed should be elevated on shock blocks at a level of 6 to 8 inches. In addition, a strong tape may be securely tied around the sheet and leg at the site ordered by the surgeon. This not only helps prevent the seepage of water but also permits uniform anesthesia where the amputation is to be done. The equipment necessary for this procedure is easily assembled, but it is difficult to add ice. Seepage of water usually takes place in spite of care and it is very difficult to move the patient.

Sulfonamides. Chemotherapy, the treatment of disease by chemical compounds, has long been one of the chief aims of scientific medicine. A development of recent years has been the discovery of the sulfonamide drugs (sulfanilamide, sulfapyridine, sulfathiazole, sulfadiazine, and sulfamerazine). Sulfadiazine is particularly useful in combating infection due to the virulent hemolytic streptococcus. In some way, this drug, while circulating in the blood and through the tissues, seems to inhibit the metabolic activity of the bacteria so that they cease to grow and divide and are thus more easily overcome by the normal defenders of the body, the phagocytic cells. The other members of this sulfonamide group are useful in specific infections and will be discussed in later chapters.

The important considerations in the use of sulfonamide drugs are administration of sufficient amounts early in the disease, careful observation to discover toxic manifestations, and continuous use of the drug until the infection is completely healed.

Toxicity. In certain sensitive persons toxic manifestations, including anemia, fever, skin eruptions, renal damage, and delirium, appear. Nausea and cyanosis are common.

Dosage. These drugs may be administered by mouth or parenterally. The dosage is controlled by frequent estimation of the amount of drug in the circulating blood. Once a satisfactory blood level is established, enough of the drug is given to replace that which is excreted. Sodium bicarbonate in equal amounts is usually administered with the sulfonamides, in order to render the urine more alkaline and thus increase the solubility of the excreted drug. This precaution reduces the frequency of renal damage.

Prophylactic Therapy. Of equal importance is the prophylactic use of sulfonamides. When administered properly before surgical procedures are carried out, these drugs have appeared to prevent infection when it seemed inevitable; this result has no doubt been achieved by increasing the resistance of the tissues, so that larger numbers of contaminating bacteria can be successfully overcome.

Antibiotics. At present, however, the newly available antibiotic agents have largely supplanted sulfonamides in the treatment of infections. That certain substances, manufactured by or derived from growing organisms such as ordinary bread mold, possessed the ability to inhibit bacterial growth has been known for many years. During World War II, stimulated by the urgency of the need, means were devised to mass-produce one of these substances, penicillin. Since then, others have been made available for clinical use, including streptomycin, aureomycin, tyrothricin, bacitracin, chloramphenicol, and Terramycin, and the list is still growing. While each of these agents is effective against a wide variety of pathogenic bacteria, there are some specific indications for their use.

Administration of Antibiotics. One problem that arises from the numerous antibiotics ordered for patients is that so large a portion of the total nursing time available for patient care is thus utilized. Nursing time can often be saved by efficiency in posting the hour of administration. The posting of as many medications as possible to be given at the same time permits the nurse to prepare them for all assigned patients at one time. Preparing injection of two antibiotics in one syringe, such as dihydrostreptomycin and penicillin, results in only one injection, thus lessening discomfort and conserving time. However, combinations of antibiotics should not be prepared in one syringe unless specifically ordered by the doctor. Certain antibiotics are given intramuscularly because there is less pain and better absorption than when given by subcutaneous injection.

Toxicity. The widespread use of antibiotics has disclosed the fact that some individuals are or become specifically sensitized to these agents, whether the antibiotic is administered orally, topically, or parenterally. The sensitivity phenomena produced vary from mild, transitory urticaria (*itching hives*) to such severe symptoms as asthma, dermatitis, edema, spontaneous bleeding, and prostration. The appearance of any of these manifestations is cause for immediate alarm and halting of the administration of the antibiotic in use. Fortunately, an individual who is sensitive to one antibiotic is not necessarily sensitive to others, so that treatment of the infection can be continued by switching to another of these agents. Most of the antibiotics in common use have no toxic effects other than the occasional sensitivity just described, but streptomycin and dihydrostreptomycin, if used over long periods, may cause permanent damage to the inner ear. Loss of hearing and disturbance of gait due to injury to the apparatus responsible for maintenance of equilibrium may follow. Tyrothricin and bacitracin may be used safely only by application to external surfaces, and are not used systemically.

Technic of Surgical Drainage. When suppuration has occurred, evacuation of the pus is in order; general measures and chemotherapy will not accomplish this. If the infection is neglected, the pus may rupture through the skin with spontaneous drainage and cure, or it may burrow through the tissues with consequent spread of the infectious process. Timely incision will provide drainage and prevent this spread. In performing surgical drainage, care must be taken not to damage important structures or to open new channels for the spread of the process. The opening should be made at the most dependent portion of the abscess so as to enlist the aid of gravity in evacuating the pus, and the opening should be maintained until all pus is evacuated. It is for this last purpose that drains, usually of rubber, are employed. During the period of healing, care should be taken to prevent infection of the adjacent skin, which is necessarily exposed to the drainage.

Technic of Isolation. Certain of the bacterial invaders, notably the spore-bearing, gas-forming, anaerobic Welch bacillus and the hemolytic streptococcus, are so easily transferred from the infected patient to any other patient that special precautions must be observed. The transfer of organisms is prevented by means of rigid isolation technic. The infected patient is placed in a separate room, and all the materials needed for his care are kept in that room. As far as possible the nurses and orderlies assigned to the patient treat only him, and they wear gloves, gowns, and masks. All dishes, dressings, and other objects taken out of the room are properly disposed of by immediate sterilization or burning. The dressing cart and utensils used in the care of other patients are never taken into the isolated patient's room. The room and all its contents are disinfected and aired after each occupation.

SUMMARY

The human body defends itself actively against bacterial invasion. Good nursing care supplements and guards against interference with this natural defense. Rest, the application of heat, refrigeration, and antibacterial agents may be used as aids.

VOCABULARY REVIEW

phagocytic	*abscess*	*lymphadenitis*
antibodies	*leukocyte*	*diathermy*
induration	*pus*	*antibiotic*
cellulitis	*septicemia*	*chemotherapy*
malaise	*lymphangitis*	

SUGGESTED READING

1. Preventing Infection in Wounds and Burns. Am. J. Nursing, *42*:1165 (October) 1942.
2. Christopher, Frederick: A Textbook of Surgery. 5th Ed. Philadelphia, W. B. Saunders Co., 1949, pp. 24–63.
3. Kotin, Paul: Techniques and Interpretation of Routine Blood Cultures. J.A.M.A. *149*:1273–1275 (August 2) 1952.
4. Krause, Marie V.: Nutrition and Diet Therapy in Relation to Nursing. Philadelphia, W. B. Saunders Co., 1952, pp. 154–163.
5. McAllister, Sara E., and Pulaski, Edwin J.: A Technic for Dressing Septic Wounds. Am. J. Nursing, *47*:396–398 (June) 1947.
6. Pulaski, Edwin J., and McAllister, Sara E.: Streptomycin Therapy and Infections. Am. J. Nursing, *47*:89–91 (Feb.) 1947.

CHAPTER 4

Neoplastic Disease

A neoplasm is an adventitious growth of new tissue. Once thought to be parasitic upon the human body, neoplasms are now known to be composed of tissue cells originating from those of the person affected. Neoplastic disease seems to be the result of a local disturbance of the natural, orderly growth of cells, as though the usual regulating influences were not functioning properly. Thus the cells of a single region grow more rapidly and divide more frequently than normal, producing a local increase in tissue, or swelling, to which the ancients gave the name *tumor*.

Why tumors form is a subject not yet fully understood. Many theories have been advanced but none of them fits every case, nor is it likely that there is only one cause. One theory, which seems

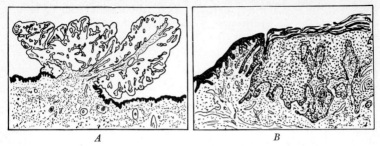

FIGURE 18. *A,* Benign epithelial papilloma; *B,* squamous epithelioma (cancer), showing invasive downgrowth of malignant cells.

to explain the origin of many tumors, holds that the new tissue growth arises as the result of repeated interference with the natural process of repair. The growth of tumors in chronic ulcers and the production of tumors by chronic irritation, particularly by certain coal tar derivatives, are put forward in support of this theory. A second theory is that many tumors arise from small deposits of cells remaining from some developmental stage of the fetus, the embryonic rests. This theory affords a plausible explanation of such tumors as arise from the ovary and testis, and certain cystic tumors which will be discussed later; but no adequate reason is offered to explain why such cells produce a tumor occasionally but not always.

That neoplasms are due to an infectious agent has been suggested, and indeed there is in animals a tumor which is transmissible by a filtrable virus, the Rous chicken sarcoma. No evidence has been discovered, however, to show that any human tumor is transmissible or is due to any known infection.

Whether neoplastic disease is hereditary or not is a subject of controversy. The occurrence of similar tumors in many members of one family is not uncommon: yet such happenings may be coincidental and of no real significance from the standpoint of heredity.

Recently it has been shown that the production and growth of some tumors are influenced by the secretions (*hormones*) of certain of the endocrine glands.

Differentiation of Benign and Malignant Neoplasms. The chief difference apparent between benign and malignant tumors is one of degree. In benign tumors, cellular growth is scarcely less orderly than in normal tissue, and the microscopic appearance

Metastases from
Carcinoma of the Stomach

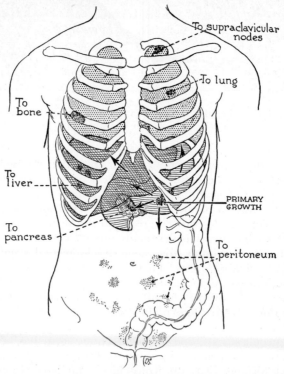

FIGURE 19. Carcinoma of the stomach may spread to the pancreas and peritoneum by direct extension; metastases reach the liver through the
portal vein; lung and bone metastases follow invasion of the blood
stream, but the supraclavicular metastases result from invasion of
the lymphatic system (thoracic duct).

of the benign tumor cell is not different from that of a normal
cell of the same type of tissue. Benign tumors grow slowly and
remain in their original locality. Their effect upon the patient
depends chiefly upon the size attained by the growth. There may
be pain and injury to neighboring structures as a result of the
pressure caused by the expanding growth, but the cells of the
tumor remain distinct, and are separated from the adjoining
tissues by a capsule of fibrous tissue.

Malignant tumors, on the other hand, are characterized by the lack of any restraint of growth. The malignant cells grow rapidly and irregularly, so that in appearance they differ widely from one another and from the original cell type. This characteristic alteration is called *metaplasia*. Even more typical of the malignant tumor cell is its ability to invade the adjoining tissues. No capsule is formed. It was the many-legged appearance of the invasive tumor growth that led the ancients to see a resemblance to the crab; hence the name *cancer*. As a by-product of this invasive ability, malignant tumor cells may be scattered through the body; traveling through tissue spaces, lymphatics, and blood vessels, they produce islands of tumor far removed from the original growth but similar to it in every way. These remote new growths are called *metastases*, and are themselves as malignant as the parent tumor.

By reason of their rapid growth, invasiveness, and tendency to metastasize, malignant neoplasms affect the individual disastrously. A malignant tumor, if allowed to progress, will prove fatal. Death is due to various circumstances, such as erosion of a blood vessel with hemorrhage, or metastatic invasion of the brain or lungs, or interference with the nutrition of the patient as in neoplastic disease of the gastrointestinal tract, or a progressive weakness (*cachexia*) which many malignant tumors, when far advanced, seem able to produce.

Benign tumors, fortunately, are far more common than malignant ones. There is not a person who does not have at least one minor skin tumor, such as a mole, a wart, or a hemangioma. Malignant tumors more often attack older people, although occasionally infants and children have them. Despite recent advances in knowledge, malignant disease continues to be one of the leading causes of death.

NOMENCLATURE

It would be unnecessarily confusing to list even a few of the many names of the different kinds of neoplasms. Tumors are classified according to their appearance under the microscope, and this, in turn, depends upon the type of tissue cell from which the tumor cells arise. The suffix *oma* denotes tumor; thus epithelioma is a tumor of the epithelial cells, and lipoma is a tumor of fat cells. There are certain terms which are of more general usage; thus, carcinoma (cancer) signifies any malignant tumor of epithelial origin; sarcoma signifies any malignant tumor of connective tissue origin; and glioma signifies any malignant tumor of central nervous system origin. The descriptive nature of the various prefixes used, such as *osteo-* (bony), *adeno-* (glandlike), or *chondro-* (cartilage), needs little explanation. The names and cell types of some of the commoner tumors are listed in Table 1.

Tumors often contain a mixture of tissues; examples of this are fibroadenoma of the breast and adenomyoma of the uterus. Another example is the teratoma, a very interesting type of tumor, which probably arises from embryonic cells since it may contain epithelium, connective tissue, hair, teeth, bone, nervous tissue— in a word, all the elements of the body. It is as though the indi-

TABLE 1. *Tumor Nomenclature*

CELL TYPE	BENIGN TUMOR	MALIGNANT TUMOR
Skin epithelium	Wart	Epithelioma
Gland epithelium	Adenoma	Adenocarcinoma
Connective tissue	Fibroma	Fibrosarcoma
Muscle	Myoma	Rhabdomyoma
Cartilage	Chondroma	Chondrosarcoma
Bone	Osteoma	Osteosarcoma
Blood vessel	Hemangioma	Hemangiosarcoma
Nevus cell	Mole	Melanotic sarcoma

vidual had given rise to a maldeveloped twin, or to a bud like that of a plant.

Tumors which arise from the secreting glands of the body are usually functionless, but occasionally an adenoma or adenocarcinoma produces the secretion of the original gland. When the product happens to be a potent hormone, the physiology of the patient is correspondingly affected.

TREATMENT OF NEOPLASTIC DISEASE

Since the cause of neoplastic disease is still unknown, treatment is based upon experience and upon the relief of symptoms as they occur. That the cure of a patient suffering from neoplastic disease can be brought about by the removal of the neoplasm is an old idea, and a correct one. The difficulty lies in the accomplishment of complete removal; moreover, the removal of one tumor does not prevent the development in the same patient of a second, altogether distinct neoplasm.

Benign Tumors. Benign tumors can be completely removed surgically unless the tumor happens to be in an organ or a structure which will not tolerate operation. Fortunately, the occurrence of benign tumors in such locations is uncommon; therefore, benign tumors are curable. The student nurse, however, may rightly inquire into the reasons for the removal of benign tumors, the more so since every person supports a few of them uneventfully. The removal of a benign tumor is justifiably undertaken when it is causing symptoms by virtue of its size and position, or when symptoms are impending as a result of its growth. Endocrine disturbance resulting from the oversecretion of a hormone by an adenoma is likewise good reason for removal. Benign tumors located so as to invite frequent trauma, and those which suddenly start growing rapidly should be removed to forestall the transition of the benign tumor into a malignant one. In addition, the removal of conspicuous, disfiguring tumors is often justified for the cosmetic effect.

Many methods are available for dealing with benign tumors, including surgical excision, desiccation by electrocautery, chemical cauterization, freezing with carbon dioxide snow, and irradiation with x-ray or radium. It is important that a method be used which is adequate, for incomplete removal of a benign tumor will not only fail to cure the patient, but may even add to his trouble by causing the benign growth to undergo malignant degeneration. In evaluating these various methods it is fair to say that the best results follow surgical excision, and that other methods are to be used only when excision is not feasible.

Malignant Tumors. The very nature of malignant tumors constitutes a formidable obstacle to successful treatment. Just as in the case of benign tumors, the cure of a malignant neoplasm depends upon removal or destruction of the entire tumor. The extent of such tumors is not clearly defined, however, since there is malignant infiltration in every direction, and the surgeon may find it difficult to know how much tissue to remove. The occurrence of metastases, moreover, with the resultant growth of remotely situated daughter tumors, obviously precludes all possibility of cure. Added to these difficulties is another dread feature of malignancy, the insidious, symptomless onset of the cancer. Pain or other symptoms do not occur until the tumor has been present for a considerable time, and the unfortunate patient may be beyond all hope of cure before he feels the need of consulting a physician.

It is to be hoped that the time will come when the medical profession will have in its hands a method by which cancer in all stages can be cured. At present, however, the cure of malignant neoplastic disease depends upon early diagnosis, before metastasis has occurred, so that complete surgical removal or destruction by radiation may be accomplished. Many operative procedures for the treatment of neoplastic disease have been developed, and some of these are described in later chapters. A by-product of the accomplishment of nuclear fission and the atom bomb has been the production of radioactive isotopes. Some of these, notably radioactive phosphorus and iodine, are being used experimentally in the diagnosis and treatment of cancer. Many other chemical agents, particularly those capable of affecting the growth of cells, are being studied in the hope of finding some means of aiding the cancer patient who is beyond surgical help.

Cancer Detection. Cancer is dreaded by all, and not without reason. Too often it is this fear which robs the patient of his chance of cure, since many people do not consult a physician when symptoms first appear because they are afraid their suspicions will be confirmed. It is the duty of every nurse to aid the medical profession in educating the public to make the most advantageous use of the facilities now available for the early diagnosis and treatment of neoplastic disease. All uncertainty in the diagnosis of cancer is removed by making use of the simple procedure known as *biopsy* (surgical removal of a small portion of any suspected lesion). Tissue obtained by biopsy, or by needle aspiration, or from secretions is examined under the microscope. There is no hazard, and the information thus gained is of immense value.

NURSING THE PATIENT WITH CANCER

Because cancer is recognized as a major health problem, it is essential for the nurse to have a basic knowledge of the facts about cancer so that she may aid in its control and carry out her responsibilities in the care of the preoperative, postoperative, long-term and terminal patient.

Early diagnosis and early treatment are the principles which are used in the control of cancer. Education directed toward the layman has stressed that the cure of cancer is dependent upon an early diagnosis followed by adequate treatment. The nurse, in her intimate contact with people, is obliged to develop a high index of suspicion concerning cancer. She must discipline her own attitude if she is to be effective and alert to the early signs and symptoms. The seven danger signals which the American

Cancer Society has used effectively in its vigorous effort to teach lay people and professional nurses the signs and symptoms of the commonest forms of cancer should be familiar to every nurse. They are:

1. Any sore that does not heal
2. A lump or thickening, in the breast or elsewhere
3. Unusual bleeding or discharge
4. Any change in a wart or mole
5. Persistent indigestion or difficulty in swallowing
6. Persistent hoarseness or cough
7. Any change in normal bowel habits

Should the patient who has cancer be informed of it? In each instance, the nurse must rely upon the judgment of the surgeon. Some patients do not know they have cancer, prefer not to know it and need not be told. Others know that they have cancer or strongly suspect it, but do not wish to have open confirmation. Most patients, however, are emotionally stable, well-adjusted individuals who frequently have a sound religious faith. They are helped most by being told. They are often no less fearful than the others, but are able to accept the knowledge of cancer better because they are accustomed to keeping their emotions under control and, probably, because they have come to some sort of resignation, at some time or another, about accepting the hazards of living, including cancer.

What should the nurse tell the patient when he asks, "Do I have cancer?" This question should be answered in accordance with the desire of the surgeon, who must carefully instruct the nurse in each situation. An evasive answer serves only to confirm the patient's suspicion. The reason that the nurse frequently does not know what to say is that she is seized with fear. She should be aware that her reactions are transmitted quickly to the patient and, if there is lack of confidence or hesitancy, the patient loses faith. It is, therefore, important that the nurse answer confidently and reassuringly. The more experienced nurse has an unusual opportunity to help the patient when he asks if he has cancer. She may ask calmly and sympathetically, "Why did you ask the question?" or "Do you think you have cancer?" The patient is anxious and is usually very responsive. She frequently learns that the patient knows he has cancer, strongly suspects it, or imagines it and she finds out many things that worry him. When the nurse is a good listener, she can do much to relieve his anxiety by encouraging him to talk; but it is her responsibility to share what she has been told with the doctor so that he may give guidance and support in whatever way may be necessary.

The nursing of patients who have had operations undertaken for the cure of cancer presents the problems incident to the type of operation performed and to the general condition of the patient. In all cases, the teaching of self-care should be carried out in order to encourage self-sufficiency. The first portion of convalescence of the patient who has a laryngectomy, a colostomy or an amputation is often a period of great despair. He feels that he will not be able to adjust to the activities of a normal life. The depression that follows such surgery may be prevented to some extent by proper indoctrination before operation but, when it does occur, it can be overcome by good rehabilitation. Teaching self-care to the greatest possible degree will help the patient master his handicap so that he may again take his place in society. Occupational and diversional therapy help divert the attention and bolster the morale of patients and should be encouraged in all—whether the illness is long-term or relatively short.

Nursing the Patient During Radiation Therapy.[1] Before radiotherapy is begun, the patient should have a good understanding of how the treatments are carried out, what will happen to the tumor and what will happen to him. Winning his confidence with reassurance and good explanation makes him more receptive to treatment.

The reactions from radiotherapy in the treatment of all types of cancer are similar. Radiation sickness is a frequent reaction, usually occurring a few days after treatment is begun. There may be only nausea, but more often there is nausea and vomiting accompanied by lassitude and, at times, prostration. Because a high caloric, high protein diet is important during radiotherapy, frequent small feedings are most easily tolerated. Medications used to control the reaction are vitamin B, sedatives and Dramamine.

When radiation is directed to the abdomen or pelvis, diarrhea may occur. Medications such as bismuth or paregoric may be ordered. The diet for such a patient should be bland.

X-ray, radium and radioactive phosphorus usually bring about fairly severe local reactions depending upon the dosage, the tolerance of the person and the amount of skin and mucosa involved. Mucous membranes become sensitive and tender about the tenth day after treatment is begun and, when such structures

1 Brown, pages 104–112.

as the nasal, intraoral, or pharyngeal lesions are radiated, eating and drinking are painful, the sense of smell is affected and taste may be greatly diminished or changed. Irrigations of the oral cavity and the use of Nupercainal lozenges before mealtime lessen pain and allow the patient to eat with greater comfort. Normal skin undergoes changes similar to that of a degree of a thermal burn. The term "burn" should not be used because it connotes an accident. The erythema which results is an expected reaction. Other reactions are epilation, itching, burning and moist dermatitis.

Before the first treatment is begun, the skin should be bathed with soap and water and any applications of ointment should be removed. In addition, it should be cleansed with ether and/or alcohol. Ointments usually contain metal which will produce secondary radiations and add to the damage caused by the radiation itself. The patient is instructed not to bathe the skin where radiation is applied because heat is applied while bathing. This intensifies the action of x-ray, causing a more severe reaction than should occur. He should be cautioned to avoid any form of light or heat therapy unless it has been specifically ordered by the doctor. Skin reactions usually begin about the tenth day after treatment is started. During the course of treatment, the skin should be kept dry and should not be bathed with soap and/or water. Starch powder allays itching, and blistered areas may be bathed with a weak solution of flavine covered with a dressing of gauze soaked in crude cod liver oil and held in place with a bandage. Clothing should be loose and the bed patient should be encouraged not to lie on the skin which is being irradiated. When the course of radiation is complete, the skin should be kept as dry as possible by dusting with a powder made up of equal parts of zinc oxide, zinc oleostearate and starch. The crusts formed by the repeated applications of powder will peel off spontaneously, usually leaving the skin completely healed after about six weeks.

Discharge of the Patient. During the entire period of hospitalization of the patient, the nurse should keep in mind his eventual discharge. The nurse must be aware of teaching opportunities and must make use of them during her relationship with the patient and his family in order to anticipate future needs by an active program of health teaching. Frequently, she will recognize the need for additional technical and supportive care beyond that which the family can give, such as the need for a social worker or a nurse in the home. The patient may wish a practical nurse or a private duty nurse but, after discharge, additional care can be best provided by referral to the public health nurse. It is wise that the nurse who is going to care for him at home meets him before he leaves the hospital to establish rapport and to learn his needs. Information concerning his care should be explained by the surgeon and nurse at the hospital to provide for continuous care.

Follow-up Care. No patient should leave the hospital without having a clear understanding of follow-up care. The nurse should understand the importance of follow-up, for a cancer patient must continue periodic checkups for his entire lifetime. The care of the terminal patient cannot be sharply differentiated from other care required by cancer patients. The facilities and service for care should be closely coordinated with those available for the treatment of cancer patients. The rate of terminal care patients is approximately one to every four annual cancer deaths. This type of care is most frequently provided for in the home. There are many patients who remain in the home during their entire illness because they prefer to do so. In general, however, about 80 per cent will die in a hospital, having remained at home, on an average, for over half of their terminal care. At present, beds are not sufficiently available and hospital and related institutional facilities cannot be provided to care adequately for all advanced cancer patients. Much work is being done in the study of specific needs of communities to provide necessary services for all long-term illnesses. The majority of patients are in the older age group; therefore, good nursing requires the application of principles used in the care of older people. The open lesions, drainage and odors so commonly thought to be present in terminal cancer occur in less than half the patients. When they do occur, adequate medical attention and good nursing care control them. The fear of pain and the fear of becoming a burden are the emotions which are most common in the patient. Keeping him ambulatory, encouraging occupational therapy, reassuring him by careful attention to his questions all serve to promote a relative peace of mind.

The bed patient frequently becomes depressed, is uncomfortable and expresses the desire not to be disturbed. The nurse should give due weight to his requests but should, nevertheless, carry out nursing care which will ensure the greatest amount of comfort for that day and for the days to come. The most common complications which may develop are decubitus ulcers, hemorrhage, foul odors, starvation and pathologic fractures. Intensive nursing care is necessary to prevent and combat these.

Studies have shown that, on an average, nursing care is required for four hours daily to meet the minimum needs of the patient. In addition, studies have shown that better nursing care reduces the amount of medication necessary for comfort. The complaint of pain should never be ignored, but careful examination with evaluation often indicates a method of therapy whereby the use of narcotics at that particular time may be avoided.

Palliative measures such as x-ray therapy, gastrostomy, colostomy, chordotomy and hormones are used to improve the general condition of the patients. The improvement, although temporary, is almost spectacular at times, especially, when pain has been relieved. When there is no relief of discomfort, these measures may seem unnecessary or even cruel, yet it is possible that tomorrow may bring a means of cure.

SUMMARY

Cancer is one of the most common afflictions of mankind. The nurse takes part in the program to educate the public to recognize the symptoms of cancer and to seek treatment at once. When treated early by surgery and/or radiation, many patients with cancer are cured; unfortunately, the disease is so insidious in onset that it may become incurable before symptoms occur. Even in the late stages, much can be done by skilful nursing to increase comfort and lighten despair.

VOCABULARY REVIEW

neoplasm	*malignant*	*radiotherapy*
carcinoma	*metastasis*	*erythema*
sarcoma	*cachexia*	*palliation*
benign	*biopsy*	

SUGGESTED READING

1. Best, Nelliana: Radio Therapy and the Nurse. Am. J. Nursing, *50:*140–143 (March) 1950.
2. Boeker, Elisabeth H., and Peterson, Rosalie I.: Nursing Care of Patients with Advanced Cancer. Pub. Health Nursing, *44:*463–466 (August) 1952.
3. Cameron, Charles S.: Professional Attitudes and Terminal Care. Public Health Rep., *67:*955–959 (October) 1952.
4. Corrigan, K. E.: Use of Radioactive Isotopes. Am. J. Nursing, *48:*309–310 (May) 1948.

5. Goodman, Joseph I: Nutrition in the Treatment of the Chronically Ill. Am. J. Nursing, *51*:165–166 (May) 1951.

6. Kaiser, Raymond F.: Cancer Control in the United States. Public Health Rep., *67*:877–882 (September) 1952.

7. Ochsner, Alton: Care of the Cancer Patient After He Returns Home. J.A.M.A., *137*:1582–1583 (August 28) 1948.

8. Pendergrass, Eugene: What to Do for the Cancer Patient When He Returns Home. J.A.M.A., *137*:1585–1586 (August) 1948.

9. Peterson, Rosalie I., and Soller, Genevieve R.: Nursing Referral of Patients: A Proposed Two-way Referral Form. Pub. Health Nursing, *43*:628–630 (November) 1951.

10. Steiner, Paul D.: An Evaluation of the Cancer Problem. Cancer Research, *12*:455–464 (July) 1952.

11. Sutherland, Arthur: Psychological Impact of Cancer Surgery. Public Health Rep., *67*:1139–1143 (November) 1952.

12. The American College of Surgeons: Cancer Is Curable: A Symposium. Los Angeles, October, 1948.

13. Thomas, Addie: Typical Patient and Family Attitudes. Public Health Rep., *67*:960–962 (October) 1952.

CHAPTER 5

Nutrition and Water Balance

The surgical patient is not "that appendectomy on Ward A," but is a human being, all of whose biological needs must be considered. Human metabolism, a complex process under normal conditions, is further complicated by illness and the treatment thereof. To provide for the daily output of energy and to make the ever-necessary replacement of worn-out tissue cells, the body requires a constant supply of fuel, which is ordinarily derived from the diet. Although a large proportion of surgical patients, particularly those entering the hospital for elective operation or because of accidental injuries, do not suffer from metabolic imbalance, there remain many in whom the existing disturbance is equal in importance to the surgical problem. The surgeon is most often confronted with acute or chronic starvation due to obstruction of some portion of the gastrointestinal tract. Dehydration, deficient protein in the circulating blood (*hypoproteinemia*), chemical imbalance due to the loss of chloride, sodium, potassium or other electrolytes from the body may occur.

FLUID BALANCE CHART

NAME *John Smith*

WARD *Halsted 5* SERVICE *Surgical* HISTORY NUMBER *218432*

DATE				INTAKE			OUTPUT		
				TIME	FLUID	AMOUNT	TIME	FLUID	AMOUNT
7/17	9 am. Water by bed	1000 cc		6-9 am.	Water.	400 cc	7 am.	Voided	350 cc
				10 am.	Orange-juice	200 cc			
	Per intravenous			11 am.	Glucose	1000 cc	10:15 am.	Vomitus	400 cc
				12 n.	Soup	100 cc			
	1 pm. Water by bed	1000 cc		9-1 pm.	Water	200 cc	1 pm.	Voided	450 cc
				2-pm	ginger-ale	200 cc			
	6 pm. Water by bed	1000 cc		1-6 pm.	Water	200 cc			
				7 pm	Tea	200 cc	6 pm.	Voided	250 cc
	Per intravenous			8 pm.	Glucose	1000 cc	7:30 pm.	Vomitus	300 cc
				10 pm	ginger-ale.	100 cc			
	6 am. Water by bed	1000 cc		6-6 am.	Water	400 cc	11 pm	Voided	400 cc
			total	Mouth	2000 cc	total	Urine	1450 cc
			total	I.V.	2000 cc	total	Vomitus	700 cc
			total	Intake	4000 cc	total	Output	2150 cc

FIGURE 20. Fluid balance chart of patient on fourth day following operation for perforated appendix with peritonitis.

MAINTENANCE OF METABOLIC BALANCE

It is only by careful study and measurement of the actual intake and output that the status of the nutritional and water balance of a given patient may be determined; to do this accurately requires facilities and a period of time not usually available. Fortunately, however, certain readily performed clinical tests furnish data from which a workable evaluation of the patient's status may be obtained. Chemical analysis of a sample of blood will show gross deficiencies of protein or electrolytes; changes from the normal values do not ordinarily appear until the body stores are badly depleted, but either shock or severe hemorrhage may cause temporary alterations. When the kidneys are not damaged by disease, and in the absence of shock or severe hemorrhage which may cause temporary suppression of urine, the amount and concentration of the urine excreted are a sensitive indicator of the state of hydration of the patient.

As a guide to treatment, the surgeon must know the intake and output of patients whom he suspects of imbalance or threatened imbalance. The duty of measuring and recording the amounts is ordinarily a part of the nursing care. A sample chart for recording these data is shown in Figure 20. In the case of a patient who is vomiting, the surgeon can see at a glance the exact amount of fluid intake, and balance this against the urine excreted and the total vomitus, not forgetting to add the insensible loss (respiration and perspiration), which is ordinarily assumed to average 1½ liters in every twenty-four hour period. The amount of fluid necessary to make up a deficit is thus easily calculated.

For those patients who cannot or should not take fluids and food by mouth, several alternative methods of supplying these necessities are available.

Tube-feeding. Tube-feeding (*gavage*) is useful when there is simple inability to swallow, as in the case of unconscious neurosurgical patients. It is possible to administer complete dietary and fluid requirements by this route, although the material must be sufficiently fluid to pass through the tube. The ingredients and composition for a suggested tube feeding containing the daily requirements for an adult are:

eggs	200 gm.	glucose	150 gm.
evaporated milk	600 cc.	orange juice	200 cc.
cream 14 per cent	150 cc.	brewers' yeast	7 gm.
powdered skim milk	50 gm.	strained beef	100 gm.
applesauce	100 gm.		

Two essential precautions must be emphasized: the greatest care must be taken to make certain that the tube is in the stomach and not in the trachea, and an individual feeding must be limited to 500 cc. or less. Larger amounts may cause vomiting, which could be as disastrous for an unconscious patient as pouring the feeding into the trachea; giving the patient 200 cc. of tube feeding every four hours lessens the tendency toward distention and vomiting.

Parenteral Administration of Fluids. This is the introduction of fluids into the body through routes other than the gastrointestinal tract. The fluid used in this type of treatment must be sterile, and must not be harmful to the tissues with which it comes into contact by virtue of either its physical properties or its chemical components. The kind of fluid used varies not only

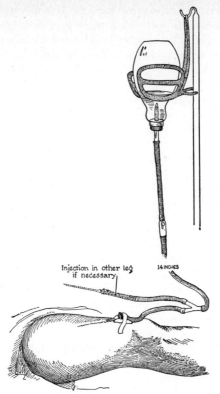

Injection in other leg
if necessary

14 INCHES

FIGURE 21. Apparatus for hypodermoclysis.

with the route by which it is given but also with the therapeutic effect desired.

Subcutaneous Administration. Water, salt, and glucose are absorbed well when introduced by infusion into the subcutaneous tissues (*hypodermoclysis*). The anterolateral aspects of the thighs or the subpectoral regions are the best sites for such infusions, since the subcutaneous tissue there is loosely organized and will take up large quantities of fluid. Upwards of 2 liters in twenty-four hours may be absorbed from a properly given infusion. Physiologic saline solution and a 5 per cent glucose solution are tolerated best. The apparatus consists of a flask, rubber tubing, adapter, and 18 gauge needle, all of which must, of course, be sterile and chemically clean. It is advisable to regulate the flow of solution into the tissues by the height of the flask above the needle. This rate will vary from patient to patient, but a height of 20 to 30 inches will usually suffice to infuse the fluid into the tissues at the optimal rate of absorption, about 100 cc. per hour.

Other essential precautions are the careful disinfection of the skin at the site of injection, the avoidance of injury to important structures in inserting the needle, the application of sterile dressings, and adequate fixation of the needle. A needle improperly placed in the subpectoral region may penetrate the chest wall with puncture of the lung, or with introduction of fluid into the pleural cavity followed by collapse of the lung. The continuance of an infusion after twenty-four hours increases the possibility of infection entering along the needle tract, and it is therefore advisable to start a new infusion in a new location should further fluid be necessary. There is always some discomfort at the site of the infusion, and in some patients the pain is intolerable, constituting one of the chief disadvantages of this form of therapy. This discomfort may be minimized by avoiding overdistention of the tissues with fluid. The addition of an enzyme, hyaluronidase, to the solutions has been found to promote more rapid absorption of the fluid by the tissues.

Peritoneal Administration. Physiologic saline solution, with or without 5 per cent glucose, is sometimes injected into the peritoneal cavity. Under normal conditions fluid is well absorbed by the peritoneum, but this method is almost entirely limited to infants with thin abdominal walls. Since the hazard of puncturing intestine or bladder is considerable, the use of intraperitoneal injection should be limited to certain infants in whom other routes are not feasible.

Intravenous Administration. The parenteral route of fluid administration used most widely at present is intravenous infusion (*venoclysis*). This method for introducing needed substances into the body has been one of the most valuable means of improving surgical results since the development of asepsis. A prime requisite is the ability to insert a hollow needle into a vein without unduly damaging the vein. Although it was once looked upon as a difficult procedure, with a little practice the technic is simple. In many hospitals intravenous therapy has already been delegated to the nursing staff. Although the actual administration of an intravenous infusion is simple, great care must be

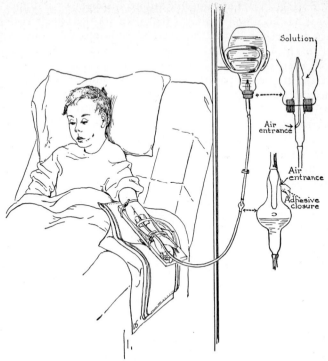

Solution

Air entrance

Air entrance

Adhesive closure

FIGURE 22. Apparatus for venoclysis. The splint straps must be tight enough to hold the arm, but not to occlude the veins or rubber tubing.

taken in the preparation of the apparatus and the fluids to be used, as well as in the choice and amount of fluid and the rate of injection.

Attention to certain details will facilitate the technic of intravenous therapy. An 18 or 20 gauge needle with a sharp point but short bevel is the most satisfactory, but smaller needles must be used for small veins even though the rate of flow will be slower. The use of a splint to immobilize the arm or leg is important, since in that way the needle will not be dislodged by a sudden movement on the part of the patient. The injection of bubbles of air must be avoided, as serious or even fatal air embolism might result (see Chap. 15). The apparatus need consist only of a flask, pure rubber or cellophane tubing into which a visible-drip tube has been interpolated, and an adapter to fit the needle (Fig. 22). This simplification of apparatus is important since it has been amply shown that many of the febrile reactions which formerly followed intravenous infusions were due to failures to clean the apparatus. Small particles of dirt or lint or blood, even though sterilized, may act as *pyrogens* (fever producers). In the preparation of the set, simple washing is not sufficient; the component parts must be *chemically* clean. Solutions and containers must be chemically pure and sterile. In order to take the special precautions necessary to prevent febrile reactions it has been found advisable in most hospitals to establish a central unit for the preparation of the intravenous outfits and fluids. Other hospitals make a practice of purchasing fluids and intravenous sets already prepared. Some of these use plastic or cellophane tubing, which is to be used only once.

Following each use the apparatus must be completely dismantled. The rubber tubing is boiled three to five minutes in 1 per cent sodium bicarbonate solution, rinsed thoroughly in hot water, then rinsed in freshly distilled water. Glassware is placed in a rack where it is dipped in boiling 4 per cent sodium triphosphate solution, then dipped in boiling water. Hot water followed by freshly distilled water is then circulated through each piece by means of suction. The set is reassembled and checked for any particle of any kind in the tubing by examination under fluorescent light. Tubing which has lost its elasticity should be replaced.

It is essential to prepare all new rubber tubing before using, because of the sulfur content. A good method is to run hot sodium hydroxide solution through the tubing for one-half hour, followed by 1 per cent acetic acid for neutralization. The tubing is then washed in hot tap water, and hot tap water is run through the tubing for one hour. Finally, freshly distilled water is run through the tubing. Disregard of the proper cleaning and preparation of the sets will be followed by reactions.

The fluids commonly used in intravenous therapy include whole blood, plasma, saline and glucose solutions in various concentrations, solutions of protein hydrolysates, and certain therapeutic agents which may be dissolved in water or added to the above solutions. It is possible to use hypertonic (concentrated) solutions in intravenous therapy without damaging tissues, because the chemicals, if injected slowly, are rapidly diluted in the flowing blood stream, but care must be taken lest the wall of the vein be damaged or the solution be spilled outside the vein; occlusion of the vein or tissue necrosis may follow these accidents.

It is unnecessary to warm these solutions before using them; in fact they may be used as taken directly from the refrigerator. There is indeed some danger in applying heat to such solutions since one or more of the chemical constituents may be altered.

The choice of the fluid, the amount to be given, and the rate of administration depend upon the need of the individual patient, and are naturally the surgeon's responsibility. Just as in any type of treatment, the nurse should ask for exact directions. It should be borne in mind that intravenous fluids given too rapidly or in too large amounts may seriously embarrass the circulation, causing heart failure; these precautions are particularly important for the aged and for those who may already have heart disease. The rate of flow is measured in drops per minute, and is controlled by a thumb-screw clamp on the tubing. Authorities differ somewhat as to the rate of flow that is advisable, but ordinarily there is no advantage in speed. If the circulating blood is loaded with additional fluid too rapidly, the excess will be quickly secreted by the kidneys and much of the value of the treatment may be lost. In the treatment of hemorrhage, where the immediate restoration of the total blood volume is important, rapid injection may be advisable.

Among the advantages of the intravenous method of fluid administration are the inherent efficiency, the relative freedom from pain, the means of adding to the blood volume quickly, and the wide variety of substances which can be used. The disadvantages include the necessity for careful preparation of equipment and fluids, occasional difficulty in performing venipuncture, and the danger of circulatory embarrassment. It is now possible to maintain a patient in metabolic balance by intravenous therapy alone for short periods of time.

Continuous Intravenous Drip; Use of Cannula. When the condition of the patient necessitates continuous and exacting regulation of intravenous fluids, the surgeon may place a cannula or a polyethylene tube into the vein because of the difficulty in keeping a needle in position. It is convenient to have the necessary equipment assembled and autoclaved in readiness. A satisfactory set includes a cannula, knife blade and handle, hemostats, mouse-tooth forceps, iris scissors, iris forceps, towel clips, fine intestinal needles threaded with black silk, No. 25 x ⅝ hypodermic needle, 2 cc. Luer syringe, 20 cc. Luer syringe, medicine glass, gauze sponges, 2 inch bandage and sterile adhesive tape. Polyethylene tubing is available in sizes which accommodate various gauges of intravenous cannulae. Soaking new tubing in aqueous solution of benzalkonium chloride solution 1:1000 for eighteen hours is a satisfactory method of sterilization. A suitable vein is exposed through a small incision. An opening is made into the vein, about 10 cm. of tubing is introduced into the vein and a ligature is applied about the vein and tubing. The tubing is then fastened to the extremity with sterile adhesive tape. This is done because there is some tendency for the streaming current of fluid and blood to draw the tubing entirely into the vein. The intravenous cannula is then fitted into the tubing. Splinting the extremity is useful and, with careful attention, the venoclysis may be continued for several days.

SUMMARY

One of the factors contributing to the safety of modern surgery is the recognition of the entire needs of the individual patient. Deficiencies of water, salt, and other chemical constituents of the body may occur as the result of disease or incident to surgery; these deficiencies must be prevented or overcome. When a patient cannot take fluids or food by mouth, water and other essential chemicals must be administered by other routes.

VOCABULARY REVIEW

metabolism	*parenteral*	*cannula*
dehydration	*hypodermoclysis*	*venipuncture*
electrolyte	*venoclysis*	*glucose*
gavage	*pyrogen*	

SUGGESTED READING

1. Bayles, Spencer, and Ebaugh, Franklin G.: Emotional Factors in Eating and Obesity. J. Am. Dietet. A., *26*:430–434 (June) 1950.
2. Cooper, Lenna F., Barber, Edith M., and Mitchell, Helen S.: Nutrition in Health and Disease. 11th Ed. Philadelphia, J. B. Lippincott Co., 1950, pp. 68–116.
3. Dericks, Virginia C.: Measuring and Recording Oral Fluid Intake. Am. J. Nursing, *47*:319–320 (May) 1947.
4. Elman, Robert: Fluid Balance from the Nurse's Point of View. Am. J. Nursing, *49*:222–224 (April) 1949.
5. Elman, Robert, and Weichselbaum, T. E.: Pre- and Postoperative Parenteral Maintenance of Electrolyte Balance with Salt Mixture Containing Sodium, Potassium, Chloride and Phosphate. Ann. Surg., *135*:145–288 (February) 1952.
6. Gentry, Martha E., and Swanson, Florence L.: A Psychological Aspect to Weight Control. Am. J. Nursing, *52*:849–850 (July) 1952.
7. Lloyd, Ruth E.: Integrating Nutrition and Diet Therapy. Am. J. Nursing, *51*:473–476 (July) 1951.

CHAPTER 6

Hemorrhage and Shock

HEMORRHAGE

Blood is normally contained within the walls of the arteries, the veins, and the capillaries, escaping only when an opening is made in one of these. This abnormal escape of blood, or bleeding, constitutes a *hemorrhage,* and the size of the hemorrhage—that is, the amount of blood lost—depends upon the circumstances of the bleeding. Arterial bleeding is characterized by the forceful spurting of bright red blood; blood escaping from a vein is darker, and flows out with less force but often with equal rapidity; capillary bleeding is less rapid than either of these, with a relatively slow oozing of bright red blood. The kind and size of hole in the vessel wall, the number of vessels opened, and the patient's blood pressure influence the rate of blood loss.

Bleeding in association with an open wound is usually external, but internal bleeding is fairly common as a result of penetrating wounds or subcutaneous injuries, and is incidental to certain abnormal conditions produced by disease. An internal hemorrhage may occur in any of the body cavities or organs, and recognition of such a concealed hemorrhage is difficult. The coagulating mechanism is altered in vitamin K deficiency and in hemophilia. In addition, there are other diseases in which there is a tendency to spontaneous hemorrhage or to prolonged bleeding: these include the leukemias, purpura, and sickle cell anemia. Thus, before performing an operation, it is important to discover whether the patient has a tendency to bleed abnormally, for not only must proper precautions be taken, but this additional hazard must be duly weighed in considering the advisability of attempting operation.

Mechanism. There is scarcely an aspect of surgery which has received more attention and study than hemorrhage, and still there remains much to be learned. Nevertheless, the following points seem established: As blood is lost the body makes a great effort to compensate for this loss. Storage depots of blood in the spleen and the bone marrow are called upon, and fluid is drawn from the tissues; the vessels contract, and the heart pumps faster in an effort to make a smaller volume of blood perform the necessary tasks of supplying oxygen and other nutrition to the cells and removing carbon dioxide and other wastes. As the hemorrhage continues, a critical point is reached at which the total volume of the circulating blood is so reduced that the mechanics of the pumping system fail, and the oxygen-carrying capacity of the blood is insufficient. Investigators are not yet agreed as to what factor plays the chief part in the ultimate collapse, and it is probable that it is the result of the combined action of all of them. Whether a patient can withstand a hemorrhage depends upon the portion of his total blood volume which has been lost, upon the rate of loss, and upon his ability to compensate for loss. Thus, a large healthy person might successfully stand the slow loss of a considerable amount of blood, whereas a small debilitated person might not survive a rapid loss of only a small amount.

Symptoms and Signs. Patients who are bleeding severely complain of faintness, giddiness, and thirst. They are restless and pale, and breathe with increasing rapidity and depth, as though hungering for more air. The body temperature may fall a degree or two below normal while the pulse increases in rate though diminishing in force. A sudden increase in pulse rate is often the first sign of concealed bleeding. If the bleeding remains unchecked the blood pressure falls rapidly and the pulse at the wrist becomes imperceptible. At this point the bleeding may cease because the low blood pressure permits clotting of the blood, thus closing the opening in the vessel, and the patient may rally; or the hemorrhage may have exhausted the reserve of the patient so that, despite cessation of bleeding, he becomes comatose and dies.

Treatment of Hemorrhage

The first step in treating hemorrhage is to stop the bleeding (*hemostasis*). Before discussing surgical methods employed in hemostasis it is well to consider the wonderful protective mechanism for this purpose with which the human body is endowed. Blood has the property of coagulating, forming a firm adherent mass or clot which if undisturbed will occlude an opening in a vessel. Except under unusual circumstances blood does not clot while circulating in the vessels; but when it has escaped into a wound the necessary reaction takes place. Coagulation normally requires only three or four minutes. If the bleeding is so free and rapid that the escaping blood is quickly washed out of the wound there is at first no chance for coagulation; later, as the blood pressure falls and the rate of flow lessens, clotting may occur with resultant cessation of bleeding. When arteries or veins are divided completely, coagulation is favored because the open end of the vessel both retracts and contracts from the action of the elastic tissue in its wall; the more dangerous bleeding is usually associated with a partly divided vessel, when retraction is impossible. It is beyond the scope of this work to consider the theories of coagulation and the details of its complex mechanism, but interference with the normal functioning of this mechanism is of great importance in surgery.

Administration of Vitamin K. Deficiency of vitamin K results in altered coagulation, a condition commonly encountered in the newborn and in patients with biliary duct obstruction. In these instances the clotting may be brought to normal by administration of the vitamin either parenterally or by mouth, in which latter case bile salts must be taken as well in order to promote absorption of the vitamin from the intestine.

Electrocoagulation. Hemophilia is another condition in which severe or often fatal hemorrhage occurs as a result of failure of the blood to coagulate. Fortunately not very common, this disease is confined to the male sex, and is hereditary, the bleeding tendency being transmitted only by the female. There appears to be a congenital absence of some essential factor in the coagulation process, and thus far modern science has not supplied the missing substance. Electrocoagulation with high frequency cautery has proved the most valuable means of controlling hemophilic bleeding.

Methods of Arresting Hemorrhages. *Hemostasis*—that is, the prevention of loss of blood by the control of bleeding—is essential in surgery; nevertheless, the most skilful surgeon may suddenly be confronted with dangerous bleeding in the course of an operation. Then, too, hemorrhage may result from a postoperative mishap or infection, or from disease, or may be caused by an accidental injury. The prompt control of bleeding saves lives; but although speed is essential, haste is dangerous, for ill-considered measures may not only fail of their purpose but may actually damage important structures or introduce infection. The means

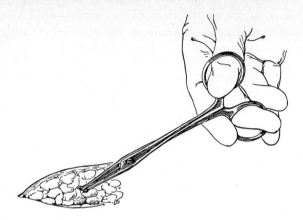

FIGURE 23. Clamping a vessel by a hemostat.

to be employed depend upon the exigencies of the situation, and range from the deliberate and direct application of a fine artery forceps (*hemostat*) to the use of the bare fingers. The prime consideration is to bring about the occlusion of the bleeding vessel. During the course of an operation the surgeon may temporarily control bleeding by the application of hemostats, by the use of a tourniquet on an extremity, by manual pressure, or by packing with gauze; but at the end of the procedure the divided vessels must be occluded by ligature or suture, although capillary oozing from a large surface may be treated by packing.

Tourniquet. When hemorrhage occurs outside of the operating room, elsewhere in the hospital, on the street, or in the home, the life of the patient may depend upon the ability of the bystanders to render first aid. Bleeding from an injured arm or leg may be controlled by the application of a tourniquet; but in every instance the tourniquet must be applied above the elbow or the knee, closer to the trunk than the wound, and tightly enough to stop bleeding. A tourniquet placed below the elbow or the knee will not occlude the vessels which lie between the two bones of the forearm or the leg. If not sufficiently tight, a tourniquet will constrict only the veins, thus serving to encourage bleeding. Soft rubber tubing makes an ideal tourniquet, but in an emergency anything that can be used to constrict the extremity will do—a handkerchief, a stocking, or a belt. Studies have shown that

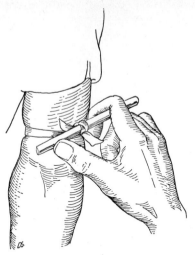

FIGURE 24. An emergency tourniquet.

narrow tourniquets are less damaging to tissue than wide ones, and that tight tourniquets, properly applied, may be left in place for several hours without fear of injuring the tissues which are temporarily deprived of circulation.

Manual Compression. Manual compression of large arteries which run superficially may serve to check bleeding, especially in wounds of the head and neck (Fig. 25). When the emergency is extreme it is far better to plunge one's fingers into a wound than to watch the patient bleed to death.

Internal Hemorrhage. *Conservative Treatment.* The treatment of internal hemorrhage, such as that from an ulcer of the stomach, is of particular importance. In general, two courses of action are open, conservative treatment or operation. Conservative treatment is selected for those patients in whom operation is inadvisable, or when it seems likely that the hemorrhage may not be prolonged. The patient is kept in a quiet room, with the foot of the bed elevated. Sedatives are given, and often an ice-cap is placed on the affected region. Food and fluid by mouth are withheld, as are parenteral fluids, since it is not desirable to stimulate the intestinal tract, and since a low blood pressure favors coagulation at the site of the hemorrhage. In many instances the bleed-

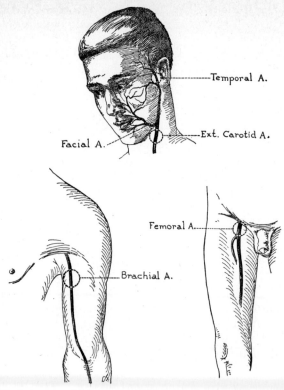

FIGURE 25. Points at which the application of digital pressure will suppress bleeding from large arteries.

ing ceases spontaneously, and the patient may then receive fluid and transfusions; but when the bleeding continues to a dangerous degree, immediate blood transfusions may be necessary.

Operative Treatment. If it seems obvious that the patient is bleeding rapidly from a source which is accessible to surgical intervention, operative treatment is advisable. For such contingencies a large amount of blood is held available for transfusion (*blood bank*), a rapid operative procedure is carried out with a view to checking the bleeding immediately; when that has been done large transfusions are given to replace the blood which the patient has lost.

Blood Transfusions. The best agent for counteracting the systemic effects of hemorrhage is whole blood. The idea of infusing new vigor into a sick person by introducing the blood of a healthy person is an old one, but transfusion has been practically possible only since the beginning of this century. The problems involved are three: the compatibility of the donor's blood with that of the recipient; the prevention of coagulation during transfer; and the exclusion of bacterial and other contamination.

Blood Groups. Human beings are divided into four groups on the basis of blood compatibility, Groups O, A, B, and AB. (No known animal blood is compatible with that of human beings.) These groups are differentiated by the specific reaction of the blood serum of the members of each group upon the red cells of the members of other groups.

BLOOD TYPING AND CROSS-MATCHING. The test to distinguish blood types is simple. A centrifuge is used to separate the red cells from the serum, and a few red cells suspended in normal saline solution are added to a drop of known Group A serum, and a few to a drop of known Group B serum. These preparations are examined under the microscope for agglutination (forming clusters of cells). The red cells of Group O are not agglutinated by either serum, those of Group AB are agglutinated by both, whereas those of Group A are agglutinated only by the B serum, those of Group B only by the A serum. This test is known as grouping. In preparing for a transfusion the blood of the prospective recipient is typed; then his serum and red cells are cross-matched with those of a prospective donor of the same group. If there is no agglutination or hemolysis (dissolution of red cells) the matching is satisfactory, and the donor's blood is suitable for that recipient.

Rh Factor. Despite careful cross-matching a number of serious reactions were observed after transfusion, particularly after multiple transfusions, although the donor's blood was thought to be compatible and had previously been given successfully to the patient. This mishap may now be prevented. Studies made in the past few years have shown that the blood of most people (about 85 per cent) possesses a substance known as the Rh factor. These persons are considered Rh positive, and those who do not have it are Rh negative. Rh positive blood may be safely administered only once to an Rh negative recipient, because the Rh negative individual is thereby sensitized to the Rh factor. A second Rh

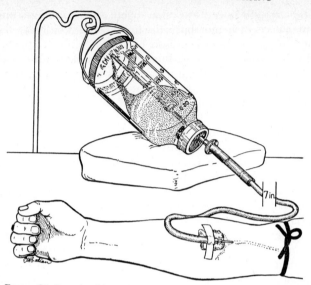

FIGURE 26. Drawing blood from the donor in indirect transfusion.

positive transfusion to an Rh negative recipient is likely to cause serious or even fatal reaction.

The Rh factor, in common with the other factors of blood grouping, is an inherited characteristic. An interesting and most important effect of this is the sensitization of an Rh negative mother by the blood of an Rh positive fetus, so that the first transfusion from the necessarily Rh positive husband and father might result in serious consequences. The agglutination produced in this reaction is delayed, and is observed only after the cross-matching has been incubated for several hours. The safest procedure at present is to use only Rh negative donors for Rh negative recipients, unless it is known that the contemplated transfusion is the recipient's first, and that the latter, if a woman, has never been pregnant.

Methods of Transfusion. The problem of transferring the blood from donor to recipient is managed in two different ways: the so-called indirect method in which an anticoagulant is added to the blood as it is drawn from the donor; and the direct method in which the transfer of blood is carried out so rapidly that coagulation does not occur. There are advantages and disadvantages in both methods, but the advantages of the indirect method make it the general choice.

INDIRECT TRANSFUSION. The apparatus needed is the same as that for an intravenous infusion with the addition of a needle and tubing for drawing the blood into the flask. Similar precautions as to sterility and cleanliness are necessary. An amount of an anticoagulant (usually 5 per cent sodium citrate) sufficient to prevent clotting is first drawn into the flask; then the desired amount of blood is taken from the donor's vein and the flask is gently agitated to ensure mixing of the blood with the citrate solution. The flask may then be sealed and stored, or the blood may be given at once, just as any intravenous treatment is given. It is unnecessary to warm blood before injecting it even though it has been taken directly from the ice box; in fact, there is danger of altering the blood if heat is applied. The chief advantages of the indirect method are: (1) the blood may be stored, thus making a large supply of blood available for immediate use; (2) the blood may be administered rapidly or slowly as dictated by the need of the patient; (3) it is unnecessary to keep donors on hand, waiting for an emergency; and (4) the whole transfusion can be managed by a single worker.

DIRECT TRANSFUSION. There are several technics for performing direct transfusion, but one of the simplest is the multiple syringe method. This requires at least three workers, patient and donor must be on adjacent stretchers, and the apparatus needed consists of needles, three-way stopcocks, and about a dozen 20 or 30 cc. Luer syringes.

A venipuncture is performed on both donor and recipient; one worker then draws a syringeful of blood, detaches the syringe from the stopcock, and hands it to a second worker who injects the blood directly into the recipient. The third worker receives the used syringes, washes them in sterile physiologic saline solution, and thus prepares them for the first worker. In this way the transfer is accomplished before the blood can coagulate.

The advantages of the method are that no special apparatus or solutions are required, and that the blood is unchanged in any way. Disadvantages include the need for a team of trained workers, the undesirability of having the donor or donors on hand or in the operating room, and the necessity for speed, which means that the blood cannot be given slowly.

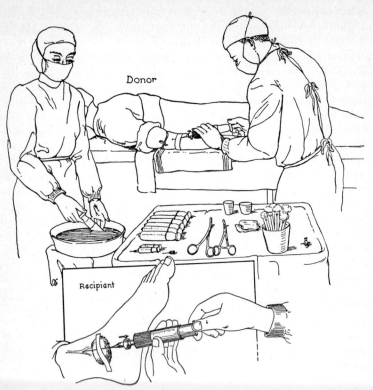

Donor

Recipient

FIGURE 27. Direct transfusion by the multiple syringe method. The whole procedure is carried on with aseptic technic.

Blood Banks. The value of a large store of blood which is ready for immediate use is obvious. Thousands of lives were saved in World War II because an improved technic of handling and storing blood had been developed. Blood for a bank may be obtained from the relatives or friends of patients, or from volunteer donors. Care is taken that the blood drawn for the bank, as for all transfusions, comes from healthy nonsyphilitic, nonmalarious donors. In addition, the donor must be carefully questioned concerning recent attacks of jaundice or other symptoms suggestive of hepatitis. The blood is collected in flasks containing citrate solution, and these, after being sealed and properly labeled as to group, are stored in a special refrigerator at 35° F. By adding fresh blood as the bank is drawn upon, a constant supply is maintained, and in an emergency blood can be had for a patient as soon as the matching can be performed, which is a matter of minutes. There is deterioration of the red blood cells after a few days, however, and if the blood has not been used in two weeks the red cells are discarded. The plasma (blood from which the red cells have been removed) can then be kept for a long time, provided, of course, that there is no bacterial contamination. Plasma can be dried, after which it can be stored indefinitely; it is ready for use when dissolved in the proper amount of sterile distilled water. In some banks plasma to be stored is frozen; it is thawed immediately before use.

SHOCK

This term serves to designate a state of collapse from which the patient may not recover unless prompt measures are taken. The clinical appearance of the profoundly shocked patient is not difficult to recognize, but incipient shock is often not detected. This is unfortunate, for here as in many other conditions, early treatment is far more successful than late. At times the onset of shock is abrupt; but often it may be recognized by a slight acceleration of pulse rate, by a small drop in the systolic blood pressure, or by the patient's sudden restlessness or complaint of uneasiness. In a late stage the severely shocked patient is apathetic, his respirations are shallow or sighing, and the pulse is rapid, feeble, and disappearing in quality. The skin is moist, pallid, even cyanotic, and the body temperature falls. The blood pressure is low, often so low that it cannot be recorded.

Ordinary fainting (*syncope*) resembles shock in some ways, particularly in the sudden collapse with loss of consciousness and fall in blood pressure. This condition is apparently due to a sudden circulatory collapse resulting from nervous stimulation and differs from shock in being quickly reversible. Most patients recover completely following the simple procedure of lowering the head.

Although the clinical condition of shock has been recognized for a long time, it was the experience in caring for wounded soldiers in the war of 1914–1918 which led to the serious investigation of this condition, an investigation which is still being vigorously prosecuted. As a result of these studies it has become apparent that shock is caused in many ways—by severe trauma, hemorrhage, burning, prolonged anesthesia, and others. Interestingly enough, shock develops as a result of many conditions which are not surgical, some of which are pneumonia, coronary thrombosis, and hyperinsulinism. A practical way to consider shock is to realize that any circumstances or diseases which cause a person's death may in the same way cause shock, which is, after all, the ultimate stage of living. There are many observable alterations in the physiology of the shock patient, and it is not yet certain which of them are causes and which are effects; all are closely related, and each helps the others to form a vicious circle from which it is difficult to extricate the dying patient.

Treatment of Shock

Improvement in the treatment of shock has not kept abreast of the volume of experimental study of the condition, and the best treatment is still prevention. Through adequate study of each patient before operation, the proper measures can be taken to see that he is in the best possible condition. The loss of blood and of other body fluids should be kept to a minimum, and any loss of significance must be promptly replaced before the loss plays a part in producing shock. Obviously, it is not possible in every instance to prevent shock, particularly when the condition develops as the result of an accident or other injury.

When shock is present it must be treated vigorously by every means available. Care must be taken to remove the causes or to lessen their effects, as by splinting fractures to prevent further trauma, checking bleeding, or relieving pain. Circulatory stimulants are indicated, such as caffeine, epinephrine, ephedrine, Coramine, Levophed, and the like, but may not help materially. Transfusions of large amounts of blood constitute the best treatment when reduction of the circulating blood volume is the predominating cause. When blood is not immediately available, the intravenous injection of plasma or of dextran solution may be of temporary benefit. The patient should be placed in a tilted bed, with feet elevated, so as to favor circulation to the brain, and careful attention paid to his airway, in order to aid respiratory exchange as much as possible. Treatment with oxygen may be helpful. It must be constantly borne in mind that a shocked patient may reach a certain critical point in his downward course after which no therapeutic measures will successfully break the

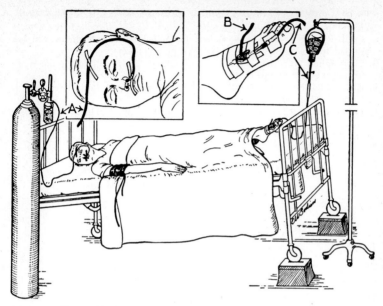

FIGURE 28. Arrangement of equipment in shock therapy.

vicious circle of changes and death will be inevitable; hence the need for prompt recognition and immediate treatment.

SUMMARY

Bleeding is always serious; the rapid loss of considerable blood may be lethal. The nurse must recognize external hemorrhage and the signs of internal bleeding and know what to do immediately. Blood is the best replacement for blood lost. Shock is a dangerous condition produced by serious hemorrhage and by injury or disease. Measures undertaken to combat shock are successful only when begun early.

VOCABULARY REVIEW

hemorrhage	*tourniquet*	*hemolysis*
coagulation	*transfusion*	*Rh factor*
hemophilia	*agglutination*	*plasma*

SUGGESTED READING

1. Blalock, Alfred: Principles of Surgical Care: Shock and Other Problems. St. Louis, C. V. Mosby Co., 1940.

2. Brown, Ivan W., Jr.: Present Status of the Rh Factor. Am. J. Nursing, *48:*14–17 (January) 1948.
3. Cecil, Russell L., and Loeb, Robert F.: A Textbook of Medicine. 8th Ed. Philadelphia, W. B. Saunders Co., 1951, pp. 1211–1214.
4. Christopher, Frederick: A Textbook of Surgery. 5th Ed, Philadelphia, W. B. Saunders Co., 1949, pp. 13–17.
5. Kirby, Charles: The Clinical Use of Blood and Blood Derivatives. Am. J. Nursing, *50:*88–90 (February) 1950.
6. Lam, Conrad R.: What Is Shock? Am. J. Nursing, *51:*116–117 (February) 1951.

CHAPTER 7

Preparing the Patient for Operation

On entering the hospital the patient finds himself in a new world. He is confronted with strange sights, sounds, and smells which, if they do not actually frighten him, at least do not add to his peace of mind. The necessary preoperative examinations, the drawing of blood, or the questions of the house surgeon may shake his confidence by suggesting that his condition is not yet well understood. Furthermore, few patients anticipate an operation with pleasure, though many are resigned or conceal their true feeling. Children do not hide their honest terror, and it is well to realize that many adults experience the same emotion beneath an apparently calm exterior. To explain away the strangeness, to maintain the confidence of the patient in his surgeon, to encourage and support, are duties of both the nurse and the surgeon; but these duties will fall largely to the nurse since she will be constantly with the patient.

Routine Preoperative Examination. A complete survey of the patient's physical condition must be made before operation, not only for the purpose of establishing the proper diagnosis, but also to avoid unnecessary complications. An acute respiratory infection or a recent exposure to such an infection warrants postponement of all but emergency procedures. Such systemic disorders as diabetes mellitus, heart disease, and nephritis must be discovered so that the proper measures may be taken. As has been stated, dehydration and dietary deficiencies must be corrected. Study of the patient's blood is made with particular reference to possible anemia or alteration of coagulation. It is obvious that the discovery of any abnormality other than that for which the operation has been proposed calls for reconsideration of the whole situation, and may necessitate a change in the plan for the patient.

Hygiene. Since the presence of bacteria on the patient's skin is a source of wound contamination, the personal cleanliness of the patient is important. The number of bacteria on the skin may be reduced by a thorough bath the evening before operation and by freshly laundered clothing. Long hair of women should be plaited into two braids. The hair of all patients is covered with a muslin cap either in the ward or on arrival in the operating room. This is done for protection and cleanliness.

The value of adequate rest is obvious, and except in an emergency the patient should have a night of sound sleep before operation. To secure this rest often necessitates the use of sedatives, the most useful of which are the barbiturates.

Shaving. The skin of the operative field must be shaved before operation. The exact area to be shaved will depend on the nature of the operation and the custom of the surgeon. In general, it is better to shave too large an area than too small. Hair prevents adequate skin disinfection, may act as a foreign body if caught in a wound, and adds to the discomfort caused by removing dressings.

The area should be shaved carefully with a sharp razor; the general direction for drawing the razor should be the one in which the hair naturally inclines. It is often necessary to go over the area two or three times in order to remove all hair. In order to avoid misunderstanding, the nurse in charge of preparing a patient will do well to ask for specific shaving instructions, even to the marking of the area to be shaved.

Preparation for Anesthesia. In the matter of preparation a distinction may be made between those patients who are to have general or spinal anesthesia and those who are to have local infiltration anesthesia. For the last-mentioned, unless an extensive procedure is planned, the preparations already described are sufficient. All other patients should be sent to the operating room with the stomach as nearly empty as possible. The importance of this point cannot be exaggerated. It is nearly impos-

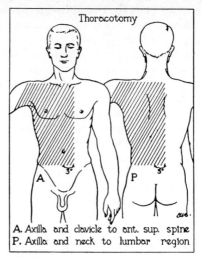

FIGURE 29. Preoperative shaving in thoracic surgery.

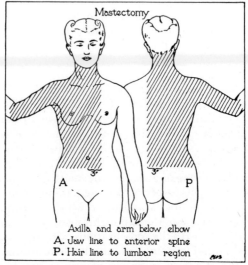

FIGURE 30. Preoperative shaving in radical mastectomy.

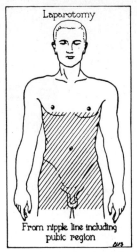

FIGURE 31. Preoperative shaving in abdominal surgery.

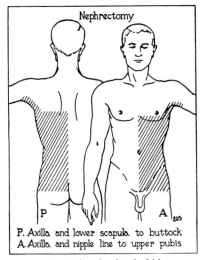

FIGURE 32. Preoperative shaving in kidney surgery.

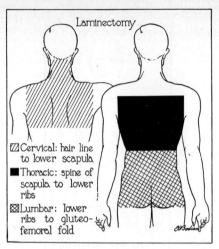

FIGURE 33. Preoperative shaving in spinal surgery.

sible to induce anesthesia smoothly when the stomach is full, and vomiting will almost always occur with the consequent dangers of aspiration and physical overexertion. Moreover, nausea and vomiting often occur during the period of recovery from anesthesia, and here again the value of an empty stomach is demonstrated. The hazard and inconvenience of a full stomach when that organ itself is to be operated upon, scarcely need mention. These patients, therefore, are not permitted to have solid food for at least eight to twelve hours before operation, and should not be allowed to have any liquid, including water, for at least four hours before the induction of anesthesia. It is quite helpful to place signs on the bed showing, in bold-face letters, "Nothing by Mouth"; this serves as a reminder to personnel who may not realize that the patient is being prepared for operation. Patients who, as a result of their condition, may not be deprived of fluids during this period should receive the necessary fluids by parenteral routes. At times, especially with obstructions of the stomach or intestinal tract, it is necessary to pass a tube into the stomach in order to make sure that it is empty. In most hospitals routine preoperative orders specify that food and fluids be withheld; but the vigilant cooperation of the nurse is needed, as patients not

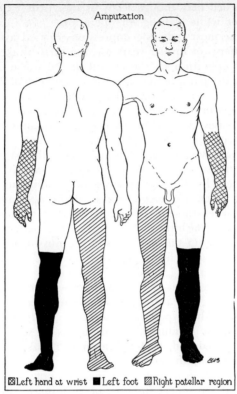

Amputation

☒Left hand at wrist ■Left foot ▨Right patellar region

FIGURE 34. Preoperative shaving in surgery of the extremities.

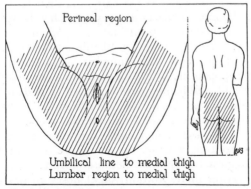

Perineal region

Umbilical line to medial thigh
Lumbar region to medial thigh

FIGURE 35. Preoperative shaving in perineal surgery.

confined to bed may thoughtlessly or designedly search for and obtain water while waiting for operation.

One of the most indelible impressions carried away by many surgical patients of former years was the early awakening on the morning of operation by the arrival of the nurse or attendant armed with the paraphernalia of the ritual enema. The value of emptying the colon and rectum immediately before attempting surgical procedures on these structures cannot be denied; but in most other cases the preoperative enema is unnecessary, or at least should be given the night before operation.

Preanesthetic Medication. The comfort of the patient, the task of the anesthetist, and the hazard of operation may all be favorably influenced by the intelligent use of certain drugs. The value of sedatives to ensure adequate rest before operation has been mentioned; when these are given, particularly the more powerful and long-acting barbiturate derivatives, the patient should not be permitted to get out of bed, and the nursing staff should so arrange matters that he is disturbed as little as possible until called to the operating room.

Atropine. Atropine is given to patients who are to undergo general anesthesia. The average adult should receive 0.6 mg. of atropine sulfate by hypodermic injection about twenty minutes before anesthesia is induced. By this means the secretion of saliva and mucus is reduced, leaving the mouth and the air passages dry. Absorption of the anesthetic agent is thus favored and the hazard of aspiration lessened. During long operations it is sometimes necessary to repeat the dose of atropine in order to maintain a dry airway.

Scopolamine. In recent years many anesthetists have come to prefer scopolamine in place of atropine. They believe that this drug does not render the bronchial secretions quite so viscid as does atropine, thus lessening the likelihood of the formation of the mucous plugs which cause pulmonary atelectasis (collapse of the lung). Scopolamine, in addition, produces in many patients a definite sense of well-being (euphoria), which adds to the ease of anesthetization. The usual dose of this drug, in the form of hyoscine hydrobromide, is 0.3 mg. for the average adult.

Morphine. The use of morphine in preparing the patient for operation is routine, whether the procedure is to be done under general or regional anesthesia. Because morphine has a powerful depressing action in respiration, small doses (8 or 10 mg.) are given if general anesthesia is to be used; the effect accomplished will be to quiet the patient, allay fear, and render induction of anesthesia easier. When local anesthesia is contemplated, however, larger doses (12 or 16 mg.) are indicated because of the effectiveness of morphine in relieving or dulling pain.

Care of Valuables. All loose articles such as jewelry, hairpins, eye-glasses, and false teeth must be removed and placed in safe-keeping. This is done not only to prevent damage or loss of these articles, but also to safeguard the patient from the hazard of aspirating loose dental appliances. Rings which cannot be removed easily, or when there is objection to their removal, may be left on the fingers; in either event a narrow tape is tied to the ring and fastened securely around the wrist, care being taken not to obstruct the circulation. The nurse should always try to persuade the patient to remove all rings except the wedding band. Valuables, such as a pocket watch or a wallet containing several dollars, are often kept at the bedside of the patient. Unless the nurse specifically asks the patient concerning his valuables before he goes to the operating room, he will most likely forget about them because of anxiety and apprehension of the forthcoming operation. The nurse should assume the responsibility for these valuables. A safe way to care for them is by placing them in an envelope made of heavy paper, with spaces for the patient's name, the name of the nurse who takes the valuables, and the patient's signature when the valuables are returned. The envelope should be placed in the hospital vault or a place especially prepared for this purpose by the hospital.

Legal Consent. The surgeon must obtain the consent of the patient before anesthesia is induced or operation is performed. In some states verbal consent is sufficient; but much better protection is afforded the surgeon and the hospital if an operative permit is signed by the patient or his guardian. It is the nurse's responsibility to see that this important legal formality has not been overlooked.

Final Preparation. When the patient awakens on the morning of operation, he is usually anxious and apprehensive. Making him understand that those who care for him are genuinely interested in him will build up confidence. This may, in part, be accomplished by carefully explaining in a calm and reassuring manner the details of the care given him. It is usual for the family to visit the patient before he goes to the operating room. The

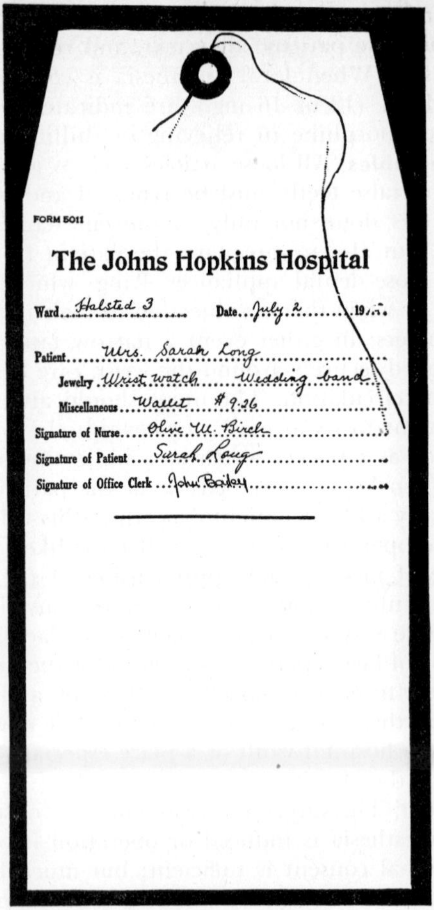

FORM 5011

The Johns Hopkins Hospital

Ward....*Halsted 3*....   Date...*July 2*.......19....

Patient.....*Mrs. Sarah Long*............

Jewelry *Wrist watch....Wedding band*

Miscellaneous...*Wallet $ 9.26*...........

Signature of Nurse.....*Olive M. Birch*........

Signature of Patient....*Sarah Long*..........

Signature of Office Clerk...*John Bailey*...........

FIGURE 36. Envelope for patient's valuables.

feeling of dependency, mingled with fear of the unknown, make both patient and relatives especially alert and sensitive at this time to the way in which the nurse and other personnel take care of him. Every consideration shown fosters confidence, pleasant associations and cooperation. In ordinary circumstances, the nurse knows the time that the patient is scheduled for operation. She is, therefore, able to make a plan so that his care can be carried out calmly and efficiently and so that, at the same time, the needs of other patients can be met. The nurse must not lose sight of the importance that this event has for the individual patient even though she has taken care of innumerable other preoperative patients. She should guard against giving the impression that this is just another patient. The latter should be made to feel that, because his nurse has taken care of many patients, he is fortunate to have an experienced nurse with a deep interest in him.

Just before going to the operating room there are certain details of care which are essential. For the comfort and convenience of both patient and surgeon, it is always important to make certain that the patient has voided just before leaving the ward. The patient is clothed in long cotton flannel boots and short cotton flannel gown, open in the back. A sufficient number of blankets should be used to avoid undue exposure of the patient while he is wheeled through draughty corridors, but care must be taken not to use so many covers that he is made to perspire.

In some hospitals the clinical record is taken to the operating room by the nurse who accompanies the patient; in others an attendant from the operating room collects all charts the first thing in the morning. The nurse should review the clinical chart to see that it is complete before it is sent to the operating room. The patient is finally taken to the operating room in his bed or on a previously prepared stretcher. In most instances, the family is not permitted to go to the operating room but exceptions, at times, must be made when those who take care of the patient think it advisable.

While accompanying a patient to the operating room, the nurse should try to do all she can to prevent tension. Preventing the orderly from wheeling the stretcher too rapidly, carefully guiding the stretcher so that the elevator is entered with ease and talking only to the patient, except when directions are necessary, will demonstrate to the patient that he has the full attention and interest of the nurse; these are essential for good supportive care. The nurse must not leave the patient until the anesthetist has obtained from her the patient's name, the preoperative medication, and the exact time it was given; when the anesthetist assumes charge of the patient, the nurse may return to the ward. It is desirable to close the door of the anesthesia room in order to protect the patient from the noises in the corridor, the con-

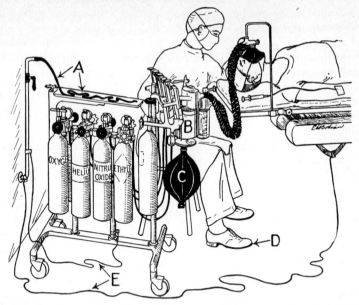

FIGURE 37. The administration of general anesthesia. Note suction equipment (*A*); soda lime absorber (*B*) ; breathing bag (*C*) ; conductive soles (*D*); and grounding wire to reduce explosion hazard (*E*).

versations and, also, from seeing the transportation of operating room equipment. All of these things seem routine to the nurse but, to the patient, these may actually cause terror. It is during the last few moments before anesthesia is induced that many patients are most in need of reassurance, an essential service which must be rendered intelligently and faithfully.

SUMMARY

In preparing a patient for operation, the concept of caring for the entire individual is again emphasized. The operative area is shaved, but the psychologic preparation of the patient is far more important. Careful stock is taken of the physical condition of the patient and proper medication is given. Legal obligations such as consent to operation and care of valuables must not be overlooked. A good nurse brings to the operating room a confident, calm patient.

VOCABULARY REVIEW

atropine *scopolamine* *morphine*
 hyoscine hydrobromide

SUGGESTED READING

1. Coller, Frederick A., and DeWeese, Marion S.: Preoperative and Postoperative Care. J.A.M.A., *137:*455–461 (November 5) 1949.
2. Mason, Robert L., and Zintel, Harold A.: Preoperative and Postoperative Treatment. Philadelphia, W. B. Saunders Co., 1947.
3. Meehan, Rose: Understanding the Preoperative. Am. J. Nursing, *42:*1289–1290 (November) 1942.
4. Krause, Marie V.: Nutrition and Diet Therapy in Relation to Nursing. Philadelphia, W. B. Saunders Co., 1952, pp. 222–223.

CHAPTER 8

Postoperative Nursing Care

Patients who have had minor procedures under local anesthesia ordinarily do not require special care, but all others, particularly those who have had general anesthesia, must have constant nursing attention until they are fully conscious. In some hospitals, it is still the custom to return the patient to the ward or to his room immediately after operation, where he receives care from a nurse employed by him or assigned to him for this special duty. Other hospitals, however, have established a recovery room or ward equipped and staffed for the particular purpose of rendering special care to patients during the immediate postoperative period. The advantages of this latter method are many.

RECOVERY ROOM

Under ideal conditions, the recovery room is located on the same floor as the operating room suite and should, if possible, actually be one of the units of that suite. The size of the recovery room depends upon the daily load of the operating room. The most satisfactory arrangement is the unit designed for the accommodation of four patients; this is the number of patients which can be most efficiently cared for by one nurse. Multiples of this

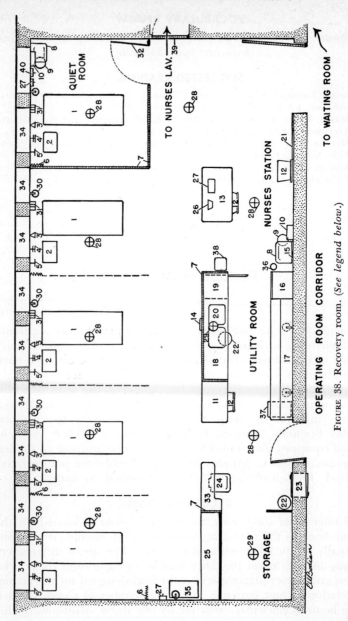

FIGURE 38. Recovery room. (*See legend below.*)

1. Hausted stretcher
2. Bedside cabinet
3. Oxygen outlet
4. Sphygmomanometer
5. Suction outlet
6. Cubicle curtain
7. Partition to ceiling, part glass
8. Lavatory
9. Waste paper receptacle
10. Paper towel dispenser
11. Table
12. Straight chair
13. Executive type desk
14. Clock
15. Mirror
16. Locked wall cabinets
17. Shelf with cabinets
18. Work counter
19. Refrigerator under counter
20. Double compartment sink
21. Bulletin board
22. Sanitary waste receptacle
23. Two-way laundry chute
24. Clinical sink with bedpan flushing attachment
25. Storage cabinet
26. Telephone outlet
27. Nurses' calls with emergency call button with duplex receptacle
28. 500-Watt indirect lighting units
29. 200-Watt semi-direct lighting
30. Single receptacle 30 amps.
31. Heavy duty electrical outlet
32. Glazed door
33. Shelf
34. Windows
35. Dressing cart
36. Fire extinguisher
37. Treatment table
38. Water cooler
39. Door with one-way vision glass
40. Hook strip

unit can be used when larger numbers of patients are to be cared for.

At the conclusion of an operative procedure carried out under general anesthesia, the still unconscious patient is carefully transferred to a stretcher and wheeled by the anesthesiologist directly to the recovery room. The stretcher used is specially equipped for the proper positioning of the patient, and has adjustable sides to prevent the patient from falling. Poles can be attached to hold the flasks of blood or intravenous fluids, and the wheels of the stretcher can be locked solidly. The patient remains on the stretcher during his stay in the recovery room. The stretcher is wheeled into one of the specially prepared spaces; immediately at hand are oxygen equipment,[1] suction apparatus, mouth gag, tongue forceps, and airway (breathing tube). Also available is the equipment for measuring the patient's blood pressure. In convenient cupboards are stored drugs, solutions, dressings, pillows, basins, linen, such emergency items as sterile

[1] See Brown, pages 119–150.

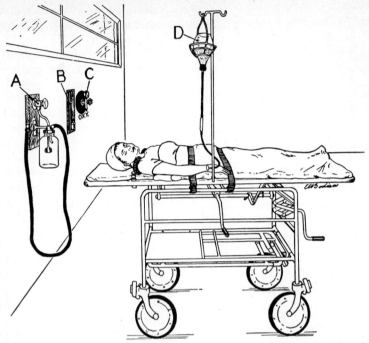

FIGURE 39. Recovering from anesthesia. *A*, suction; *B*, sphygmomanometer; *C*, oxygen; *D*, intravenous fluids.

sets for performing tracheotomy and intravenous cut-downs, and other sterile supplies such as syringes, needles, intravenous equipment and the like.

The anesthesiologist delivers the postoperative orders, as well as the patient, to the recovery room nurse and the latter then assumes responsibility for the care of the patient.

ROUTINE CARE DURING RECOVERY FROM ANESTHESIA

The stuporous or partly conscious patient is unable to help himself effectively; indeed, he may even add to his difficulties by involuntary or ill-controlled movement during the period of restlessness and confusion which occurs as he awakes. As the patient eliminates the anesthetic agent from his body he passes through the same stages as during induction, but in reverse order. Muscle

NAME _John. Smith_
WARD _Halsted 3_   DATE _May 14_   19____

HOURS	TEMP.	PULSE	RES'N	URINE	STOOL	DRAIN	MEDICINE AND TREATMENT	NOURISHMENT	REMARKS
10:30		140	32						From a.r. unconscious
									Pulse thready, noisy
10:40		138	30						respiration, with much
									mucus in throat. Face flushed.
10:50		136	30						Skin hot and moist
									Dressing clean
11: am		132	28			0			Nasal tube connected to suction
									Patient restless, trying
									to pull out tube.
11:15		130	28						
									Venoclysis started, running
									at 120 drops per minute
11:30		128	26				Turned Coughed		
							Morphine Sulfate 12 mg (h)		Patient fully conscious,
									complaining of pain in
11:45		124	26						abdomen. Dressing clean
									Water by bed 1000 cc.
									Placed in Fowler's position
12 noon	103.6	120	24						Comfortable – Suction
							Turned Coughed		running well–pulse stronger
1 pm.		124	22						Sleeping
							Turned Coughed		
2 pm		118	24						Moderate amount of foul
							Turned Coughed		drainage on dressing
							Glucose 5%	1000 cc ⎫	I.V. treatment ended
							Normal Saline	500 cc ⎬	Taking water well
3 pm		116	24				intravenously		Suction running well
				1/350cc			Turned Coughed		Voided
4 pm.	102	110	22			400cc			Restless, complaining of
									pain — pulse rapid but
							Morphine Sulfate		good quality. Skin dry
							12 mg (h)		

FIGURE 40. Postoperative chart (bedside notes) following operation for perforated appendix with peritonitis.

tone and reflexes are regained; and at this time painful sensation from the operative wound may stimulate the patient, causing restlessness or other poorly coordinated movement. Unless carefully guarded, he may roll out of bed or may pull off his dressings. Nausea and vomiting are of frequent occurrence, and it will require the utmost vigilance and skill on the part of the nurse to prevent aspiration of vomitus and soiling of the dressings or bedclothing.

The nurse must be able to determine accurately the state of consciousness of the patient. The appearance of involuntary motion and swallowing or blinking presage a return to consciousness. So, too, does response to painful stimulus; as, for example, groaning or moving when strong pressure is made by the finger between the ribs. In many instances the patient's sense of awareness can be aroused quickly by informing him that he has had his operation. When he registers surprise it is evident that he is becoming more alert. A patient is not fully conscious, however, until he responds promptly to his name, answers questions coherently and correctly, and performs coordinated movements in response to definite requests. It is only when the patient is fully conscious that the nurse may safely leave the bedside.

Bedside Notes. During the recovery period the nurse must carry out simultaneously three assignments: the observation of the patient, the performance of necessary treatments, and the recording of both. To be observed are the character and rate of the respiration and pulse, the behavior of the patient, and the condition of the operative field. Treatment includes maintenance of adequate respiratory exchange, maintenance of the patient in the desired position, protection of the operative field, medication as ordered, assistance with transfusions or other procedures undertaken by a house surgeon, and reassurance of the patient. An accurate and up-to-the-minute record is kept on a suitable chart so that the surgeon may determine at a glance the condition of his patient.

Maintenance of Respiration. The student nurse who would learn how to facilitate the breathing of an unconscious patient should first observe someone who is sleeping naturally. She will note that such a person breathes regularly, slowly, and deeply. The color is good, and the respiration is quiet and seemingly effortless. Assuming that the person under observation is lying on his back, it will be seen that his mouth opens and his jaw drops as muscular relaxation accompanies deepening sleep. At

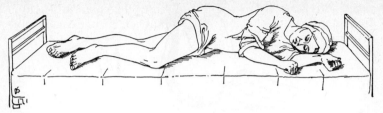

FIGURE 41. Position recommended for the patient recovering from general anesthesia. Note that head and mouth are dependent.

the same time the muscles of the soft palate relax, and the quiet breathing becomes a noisy snoring. There is now partial obstruction to free breathing, and it is apparent that the person is making more effort, chiefly on inspiration. In addition, the tongue may fall back and overlie the upper opening of the larynx (glottis), thus effectively blocking the ingress of air. When this occurs a loud snoring inspiration is suddenly cut short, and the sleeper makes a forceful inspiratory effort, accompanied by congestion or even cyanosis of the head and neck. It is as though he was suddenly being choked; that, of course, is exactly what has happened, although the obstruction to the passage of air is internal and due to displacement of the relaxed tongue. The stimulation caused by this choking awakens the sleeper, who then shifts his position. A patient, however, under the influence of an anesthetic which has relaxed his muscles and paralyzed his reflexes, does not awake, nor can he change his position but will die of asphyxia unless quickly aided.

The student nurse will also note that unanesthetized patients who sleep on the side or the abdomen, so that the face is inclined downward, are able to sleep deeply without snoring or other evidence of respiratory obstruction. The ideal position, therefore, for the patient during recovery from anesthesia is the lateral or, better still, the prone position, one arm and shoulder elevated, face to the side and down as illustrated in Figure 41. Obviously, this position also facilitates the drainage of vomitus, mucus, or blood from the mouth and nose, whereas the unconscious patient lying face up on his back will certainly aspirate any fluid that collects in his mouth. The nature and the location of the surgical procedure often prevent the use of the prone position, but only rarely is it impossible to place the patient on his side, or at least to turn the head to the side.

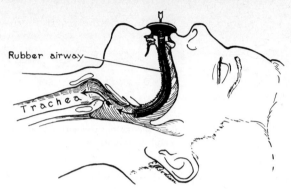

FIGURE 42. Sagittal section showing breathing tube in position, holding tongue forward, permitting free passage of air into the trachea.

The appearance of noisy or labored respiration, cyanosis, or gurgling in the mouth or throat is the signal for the nurse to act, and act quickly. A brief period of asphyxia is fatal to a very ill patient, especially to one who is already suffering from anoxia due to hemorrhage and/or shock. The aspiration of a large quantity of blood or stomach contents results in drowning, but aspiration of even small amounts produces serious and often fatal pneumonitis. The mouth and throat must be kept reasonably dry, therefore, and this may be done by placing the patient's head in the proper position for drainage, by suction, and by wiping out the mouth with dry gauze. The nurse should next investigate the position of the tongue; if necessary, she should grasp the tip firmly with gauze or with the proper tongue forceps and pull it well forward. Before this maneuver it is advisable to insert a gag gently between the jaws to prevent the patient from biting his tongue or the nurse's fingers. In addition to pulling the tongue forward, the nurse may be obliged to support the patient's jaw firmly until muscle tone returns, in order to prevent recurrence of the obstruction.

An indispensable device for holding the tongue in the proper position is the metal or hard-rubber airway, illustrated in Figure 42. It is curved to fit over the tongue and, being hollow, permits free exchange of air. As consciousness and the gag reflex return, the patient will no longer tolerate the airway in the mouth, and it must be removed.

During anesthesia or during the recovery from anesthesia, a

patient may suddenly stop breathing as the result of an overdose of the anesthetizing agent or from asphyxia. Artificial respiration given promptly and adequately may restore breathing and save the patient's life. A preliminary of vital importance is to grasp the tongue quickly, holding it well forward to maintain a clear airway through mouth and glottis at least; this maneuver in itself may serve to start the patient's breathing. If the asphyxia is due to aspiration, the throat and trachea must quickly be cleaned out by suction. Rhythmic, slow, manual compression of the patient's chest is then carried out, alternating with periods of relaxation. It is important to be certain of the passage of air into and out of the lungs, for unless there is exchange, no results are to be expected. Artificial respiration should be performed slowly, since a rapid rate might cause excessive loss of carbon dioxide, thus depriving the respiratory center of its usual stimulant.

Pulse Rate and Blood Pressure. The observation of the patient's pulse needs little comment. Any increase in rate or decrease in quality is important as a sign of possible hemorrhage or shock, and the surgeon should be informed at once of such changes. In many hospitals, nurses have been taught to take blood pressure readings and are instructed to take them at regular intervals during the recovery period, a policy which should receive all possible encouragement.

The blood pressure is measured by the use of a sphygmomanometer. The rubber arm cuff is wrapped snugly about the upper arm, and is inflated until the pressure reading is about 200 mm., unless the patient is suspected of having a higher pressure than that. Using a stethoscope, the nurse listens for the sound of the pulse over the brachial artery. This is readily located by placing the bell of the stethoscope in the *antecubital fossa* (*elbow*). The pressure is gradually released, 5 or 10 mm. at a time, by means of the release valve on the rubber bulb. The pressure reading noted upon the first appearance of the sound of the pulse is considered to be the systolic pressure; the reading obtained when the pulse sound is at maximum intensity (loudness) is the diastolic pressure. The nurse should repeat the reading to check its accuracy. Another check is the palpation of the radial pulse, which should appear just at the time the sound becomes audible.

Protection of Operative Field. Care is taken that the patient does not disarrange his dressings or damage his wound by movement. The dressing should be inspected at regular, frequent intervals so that bleeding or discharge of secretion may be promptly noted and reported. Vomitus, sputum, or other excretions are also carefully inspected, and the presence of blood is reported. The vomiting of a large quantity of blood following removal of the tonsils, for example, may be the first evidence of a serious hemorrhage from the operative site. If there should be sudden gross bleeding from a fresh wound the nurse should immediately apply pressure, or a tourniquet when the wound is on an extremity. The surgeon is, of course, notified at once.

Administration of Narcotics. As the patient emerges from anesthesia, whether local, spinal, or general, sensation gradually returns, and with it there is increasing pain. The pain varies, naturally, with the location and extent of the operation and with the sensibility of the individual. The partly conscious patient is rendered vaguely uncomfortable by pain, and thus becomes restless. It is at this time that the administration of narcotics for the relief of pain should be begun. For this purpose the most effective are the various derivatives of opium, including morphine, Pantopon, Dilaudid, Schlesinger's solution, and codeine. The choice of drug and the dose depend upon the patient's size and need; since there are individual idiosyncrasies to some of these drugs, there is no single drug which is suitable for every patient. Full consciousness brings with it full appreciation of the pain which inevitably follows most surgical procedures, and narcotics must usually be given at regular intervals (four to six hours) during the first twenty-four hours. After that time most patients become increasingly comfortable, so that milder drugs may be used and the interval between doses lengthened. It is important that patients get adequate sleep; in securing this the long-acting barbiturates are useful, although it must be remembered that they do not relieve severe pain.

RETURN TO WARD

Certain preparations must be made before the patient is returned to the ward from the recovery room. The bed is freshly made and is arranged for the efficient handling and protection of the patient.

The need for a plentiful supply of fresh air is obvious, but the patient should be protected from drafts and from rapid changes in the temperature of his surroundings. It must be remembered that overheating may produce dangerous loss of fluid and electrolytes.

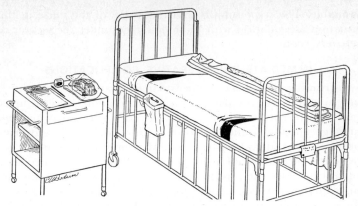

FIGURE 43. Postoperative bed.

The patient is returned to his own room or ward from the recovery room when he has fully regained consciousness and if the recovery room staff considers that his general condition is satisfactory. He is transferred from the stretcher to his own bed and the postoperative orders are turned over to the nurse in charge who then assumes responsibility for the care of the patient.

Procedures which increase the patient's comfort are frequent changes in position, massage of the back, and bathing of the face and hands. A quiet room and occasional reassurance are appreciated. Visitors should be discouraged for, at this time, the social amenities are very tiring to the patient. Relatives, of course, have the right to visit a critically ill patient, and must be apprised of his condition; but they should receive tactful instructions not to disturb him or to interfere with necessary treatments. On occasion, religious observances must be permitted at the request of the patient or his relatives. Such requests must be honored promptly and willingly, even though the nurse does not share the patient's faith, and though the routine may suffer temporary dislocation.

There are many hospitals which have not as yet organized recovery rooms; in these, the patient will be returned to his own bed from the operating room. It is imperative that such patients receive continuous nursing attention until fully conscious. All of the supplies and equipment mentioned above must be readily available. The responsibility and the duties of the nurse in this situation are identical with those described under the section on recovery room.

IMMEDIATE POSTOPERATIVE COMPLICATIONS

In reading these pages there is danger that the student nurse may wonder how any patient survives operation, since so much can happen. Fortunately, however, the great majority of patients undergo anesthesia and operation without difficulty, recovering promptly and almost without aid. It is only the occasional pa-tient who needs special assistance; yet all must be treated with equal care since there is no certain way of knowing in advance in which patient a complication will develop. The observant nurse, however, knowing what to expect, is able to recognize and to deal with whatever problem may arise.

Hemorrhage; Shock. These have already been considered, as also has been their treatment (Chap. 6). It is important to remember that either or both may develop hours or days after the operation. There are certain well-defined symptoms and signs characteristic of bleeding after surgical procedures limited to particular regions of the body, such as the brain and the neck, which will be discussed in later chapters.

Pulmonary Complications. The prevention of aspiration pneumonitis has been discussed.

Atelectasis. Of equal important is the prevention, early diagnosis, and treatment of collapse of the lung (*atelectasis*). This condition is generally due to the obstruction of a bronchus by a plug of thick mucus, with consequent absorption into the blood of the air from the obstructed portion of lung. The development of atelectasis is favored by insufficient movement of the chest and diaphragm; following injury to or operation upon the chest or upper abdomen, movement is painful, and the patient consciously or unconsciously restricts the respiratory excursion.

The trachea and upper air passages are usually aspirated carefully by the anesthesiologist at the conclusion of the operation. If necessary, this can be repeated later in the recovery room. When the patient regains consciousness, he is required to cough and breathe deeply several times at hourly intervals for at least twelve hours. Turning the patient regularly facilitates better drainage of all parts of both lungs and encourages their movement in respiration. Proper relief of pain in the operative site is also most helpful in securing adequate respiratory motion.

SIGNS. The onset of atelectasis is characterized by rapid, labored respiration, increased pulse rate, cyanosis, and fever. The characteristic physical signs and the appearance of the x-ray film will differentiate atelectasis from concealed hemorrhage or other complications.

TREATMENT. Treatment includes immediate examination of the trachea and the bronchi by means of the bronchoscope, with removal of the offending plug of mucus. The patient should be encouraged to cough, and when no bronchoscope is available a hard slap on the back may dislodge the plug. Frequent change of position is also helpful. By change of position is meant a radical alteration at frequent intervals. The patient is turned on the left side for an hour, then on the right side for an hour, then on the back, so that no one part of the lungs is dependent for a long period of time. Change of position for definite and specified periods prevents inadequate expansion and pooling of secretions. Collapse of the lung—always a serious complication, since oxygenation of the blood is interfered with and since pneumonia nearly always follows—may be fatal if a sufficient amount of the lung is affected.

Pneumonia. Pneumonia is still a frequent postoperative complication, but the mortality resulting from it has been reduced enormously since the introduction of the sulfonamide drugs and antibiotics. Often developing in patients who have an infection of the upper part of the respiratory tract, or who have recently had one, pneumonia is likely to follow operations about the upper abdomen or procedures which necessitate a long period of anesthesia. It is especially apt to occur in the elderly or the debilitated patient, and is of more frequent occurrence in cold weather.

PREVENTION AND TREATMENT. Prevention includes the postponement of operations upon patients having respiratory infections, frequent change of position after operation, and, in the case of elderly patients, getting them out of bed as soon after operation as is feasible. The treatment of postoperative pneumonia is not different from that employed in other cases of pneumonia.

Complications Other Than Pulmonary. *Abdominal Distention.* Distention due to accumulation of gas in the stomach and intestines follows nearly every intra-abdominal operation (*laparotomy*). It is curious that distention occurs also after operations other than abdominal, as, for example, after thoracic or orthopedic surgery. It is this condition which is responsible for the "gas pains" described by the lay person. Distention is the result of a partial and temporary derangement of intestinal activity; normal intestinal contraction (*peristalsis*) and muscle tone fail, permitting the intestines to distend. Ordinarily the distention persists only for a twenty-four to forty-eight hour period, at the end of which normal peristalsis returns. When not contraindicated by the nature of the operation, enemas, the passage of a rectal tube, and the use of such drugs as Prostigmin are helpful.

Psychosis. Delirium following operation is not uncommon. The fear which delirious patients have is heightened by their postanesthetic confusion, the strange surroundings, and their physical weakness and discomfort. When chronic alcoholism is a factor, the use of thiamine hydrochloride is usually effective, but in all cases adequate rest and reassurance are the chief aids in promoting recovery. Constant surveillance is necessary to prevent accidents, as delirious patients may get out of bed or even attempt to leave the hospital, but actual physical restraint usually adds to their terror. The least deviation from normal behavior should arouse the nurse's suspicion. Early evidence of delirium usually consists in mental confusion, visual hallucinations such as "seeing bugs crawling in the bed," or a suspicious attitude on the part of the patient toward the medicine or diet offered by the nurse.

SUMMARY

The period of recovery from general anesthesia is fraught with dangers to the patient. During this time he needs and must have constant and expert nursing. The organization of a recovery ward, staffed by specialists in this area of surgical nursing, is of great value in making surgery safe for the patient.

VOCABULARY REVIEW

consciousness	*anoxia*	*atelectasis*
asphyxia	*airway*	*delirium*
cyanosis	*hallucination*	*sphygmomanometer*
aspiration		

SUGGESTED READING

1. Booth, Shirley C.: Recovery Room Service. Am. J. Nursing, *51*:359 (June) 1951.
2. Krause, Marie V.: Nutrition and Diet Therapy. Philadelphia, W. B. Saunders Co., 1952, pp. 86–93.
3. Leithauser, Daniel J.: Early Ambulation. Am. J. Nursing, *50*:203–206 (April) 1950.

4. Matthews, Thelles B.: Surgical Recovery Room. Am. J. Nursing, *51*:669 (November) 1951.

5. Michelsen, Olaf: Nutritional Aspects of Antibiotics. J. Am. Dietet. A., *29:* 221–229 (March) 1953.

6. Schafer, Margaret K., and Galbraith, T. P.: Recovery Room Services. Hospitals, *26*:65–74 (Nov.) 1952.

CHAPTER 9

Convalescent Nursing Care
and Rehabilitation

To say that a patient is convalescent is not to imply that he no longer needs nursing care. Indeed, many patients need more care at this time than at any other, particularly those who have a readjustment to make, as after an amputation. Other patients, once the discomfort of the first few days is over, become bored and rebellious. The morale must be bolstered, and in this task intelligent nursing is essential. The patient's interest in himself and his problems is acute, and he is quick to detect and to resent any lessening of his nurse's attention.

Diet. A patient recovering from operation must not be deprived of sustenance. At first, particularly when some portion of the gastrointestinal tract has been operated upon, certain restrictions are necessary, but deficiencies must be made up by parenteral administration of fluids. Experience has shown that it is futile to offer patients anything more than water until the postanesthetic nausea has abated; in many clinics cracked ice is permitted, but some surgeons feel that tap water is less nauseating and more refreshing. The majority of patients, however, may be fed as rapidly as food is tolerated. There need be no dietary limitations following minor procedures under local or spinal anesthesia, however, and full diet is also permissible on the day following minor operations under general anesthesia.

Distention commonly follows major surgical procedures, particularly those on the chest and abdomen. In the case of patients in whom distention is likely to develop it is advisable to restrict them to fluids during the first forty-eight hours and to increase the diet gradually. In general, ginger ale and other carbonated beverages are tolerated better and seem to cause less distention than fruit juices or milk. When distention occurs, the diet should be restricted to fluids without milk until active peristalsis returns.

In feeding postoperative patients, the best results may be obtained by suiting the diet as far as possible to the individual's need and taste.

Early Ambulation. Early ambulation is not a new procedure but its use is much more widespread than was formerly the case. Primitive peoples have never enjoyed the luxury of remaining in bed; it was usual, for example, for a woman to return to work in the fields a few hours after the delivery of her child. The movement toward the early ambulation of patients was given much impetus by the experiences of World War II. The scarcity of hospital beds and the exigencies of the transport of the wounded convinced many surgeons that postoperative patients suffered no injurious effects and actually seemed to derive benefit from this treatment.

Although it was hoped that early ambulation would decrease vascular complications, such as thrombophlebitis and pulmonary embolism, this has not proven to be true. Among the benefits noted, however, have been an improvement in appetite, better maintenance of muscular tone and a more rapid return to a state of well-being. It must be emphasized that the term ambulation should mean actual walking; the patient who is merely transferred from a sitting position in bed to a sitting position in a chair cannot be said to have been ambulated.

The patient who has undergone a minor surgical procedure, even though it has been under general anesthesia, usually experiences no difficulty in getting out of bed and walking about without restriction. This is not the case, however, following major surgery. In the latter event a wise preliminary to ambulation is to have the patient sit upright on the side of the bed. After a few minutes of this he should be encouraged to swing his legs. In the event that his head remains clear and he feels strong, the patient should be assisted in standing on the floor and should be encouraged to take a few steps about the room on the arm of his nurse, after which he may return to bed. If, on the other hand, the patient becomes light-headed or pale after a few minutes of sitting on the side of the bed, he should be permitted to lie down. Ambulation should be postponed and a second attempt made later in the day. Most patients will gain confidence rapidly and will soon be able to perceive the benefit derived; patients particularly appreciate the early acquisition of lavatory privileges. Some patients need much encouragement and reassurance, and special efforts should be made with these in order to discourage any tendency toward chronic invalidism. It is difficult at times to differentiate between the patient who is reluctant and the patient who is too ill to walk; if in doubt, the nurse should seek definite instructions from the surgeon.

Early ambulation does not exert any deleterious effect on wound healing. The patient should be told that movement may be painful but will not be injurious.

Late Postoperative Complications. *Dehiscence.* Occasionally complete breakdown of the wound (*disruption* or *dehiscence*) may happen, due variously to improper wound closure, to lack of immobilization, or to malnutrition of the patient. A sudden discharge of straw-colored or blood-stained fluid which soaks the dressing over an abdominal wound should lead the nurse to suspect wound disruption. The surgeon should be called at once, and the patient should be kept as quiet as possible, since movement might result in forcing a portion of the intestine through the open wound (*evisceration*). The correct surgical treatment is immediate resuturing of the wound.

Vascular Complications. Postoperative inflammation and occlusion of the veins (thrombophlebitis) of the pelvic organs and legs, together with the dread sequel, pulmonary embolism, are discussed in Chapter 15.

Bedsores. A serious complication, and one which is usually preventable by good nursing, is the development of bedsores (*decubitus ulcers*). The debilitated or paralyzed patient moves so little that there are long periods of pressure on the skin over the bony prominences upon which he lies. This pressure prevents adequate circulation of the blood, causing local starvation of the tissues and, in time, necrosis. Sponge rubber or air-filled cushions help to prevent and relieve pressure over the sacrum and hips. Rings of cotton wrapped with gauze bandage placed under the heels, the elbows, the ear or the back of the head relieve pressure in these regions. Whenever the patient has many bony prominences, or when he is emaciated or debilitated, he can be more easily cared for by placing him on a sponge or air-filled mattress. The presence of moisture, especially when due to incontinence, aids in the maceration of the superficial epithelium, so that bacteria readily gain entrance. The addition of such infection hastens the necrotizing process, and before long the skin sloughs away, leaving a painful, infected, open wound. Whenever there is incontinence of urine, hourly delivery of the urinal to the male patient or the bedpan to the female patient may at times keep the bed dry. It is well to use a large pad to absorb the urine. Cleansing the back, buttocks and genitalia each time there is soiling helps to prevent bedsores. After the back, the buttocks and the genitalia have been washed with soap and water, a massage of the back, especially over the sacrum, with soap lather stimulates the circulation and cleanses the area thoroughly. It also serves as an alkalinizing agent to the skin. This may be alternated with massaging with a rubbing lotion or 50 per cent alcohol followed by the use of dusting powder of zinc stearate, powdered boric acid, or talcum. Continual urinary incontinence makes the problem of preventing decubitus ulcers even more difficult. In such cases, a retention catheter is usually inserted. Incontinence of feces can be controlled in many cases by the administration of an enema each morning. Telltale reddening always appears as the first sign of an impending bedsore, and should cause the nurse to redouble her efforts to keep the patient in such positions as to prevent pressure and maceration of the skin. To heal such an ulcer is a difficult task.

Baths. During the first days after operation bed baths are usually given. Following the removal of sutures and the complete healing of the incision showers or tub baths are permitted.

The first tub bath should be approached cautiously, as immersion in too warm water may cause the weakened person to faint. It is advisable to use cool water and to limit the time the patient is in the tub to only three or four minutes at first; a nurse or attendant must, of course, be constantly present.

Orientation of Patient Toward Recovery. It is not surprising that many patients, after an operation, are apprehensive about the future; they wonder about the success of their operation, whether they will recover fully, whether unpleasant symptoms may return to plague them, whether they will be disabled in some way, whether they have cancer, whether their doctor is telling them the complete truth, and so on. Such fears and doubts are common and may loom large enough to cause frank depression, or lesser effects such as anorexia, decreased tolerance to pain, and insomnia; lack of cooperation in treatments or in following a program of ambulation or exercises may be other manifestations of inner apprehension. The surgical nurse must cultivate a carefully controlled attitude toward the patient, and must school herself to make every conversation, treatment, or other contact with the patient an opportunity to direct the patient's thoughts toward recovery. She must somehow convince the patient that the surgeon and the nurse know that the patient will recover fully; that unpleasant symptoms and pain are usual, temporary, and can be relieved; that proper cooperation and adequate effort on the part of the patient are as essential as any part of the treatment of the disease or injury; and that the patient can overcome any handicap, with proper help; and, finally, that such help is available and will be forthcoming. It is essential that the nurse guard against becoming irritated or angered by the patient; she must remain calm and objective, cheerful, friendly, sympathetic, and firm.

Total Care. Care is not complete until the patient has received maximum benefits. In the case of a person who is perfectly well one day, has acute appendicitis the next, is operated upon, up walking about the day after, and back on the job in ten days, the problem of total care is quite simple. Such a patient only needs a few words of advice concerning removal of the dressing, diet, and the resumption of full activity. Other patients present more complicated problems, and it is only possible to present here a general method of handling them. The plan, of course, must be laid out by the surgeon, and he will designate which portions are to be carried out by the nursing staff, and which by other personnel such as social service workers, physical therapists. occupational therapists and dietitians. The plan of care must be fully understood by the patient and his family; this involves a job of instruction in which the nurse usually takes part. When the patient is ready and able to leave the hospital, arrangements must be made to continue all phases of the plan as laid out. The plan of total care ceases to operate only when the patient has reassumed his place in society, or has taken the place most compatible with his disability, or, if incurable, has finally succumbed to his disease.

Rehabilitation. This important phase of total care applies chiefly to two categories of patients: those who have been disabled by illness for so long that they must be retrained physically and mentally to regain full useful activity; and those who have acquired a permanent disability to which they must adjust mentally and for which they must accommodate physically. An example of the first category might be a patient finally subjected to definitive surgery after a long period of chronic invalidism due to peptic ulcer. A patient who has lost a leg might exemplify the second category. More will be found in later chapters on the subject of rehabilitation in specific situations.[1]

SUMMARY

Early ambulation has proved to be valuable in accelerating convalescence. Among the late complications of surgery are wound dehiscence, thrombophlebitis, pulmonary embolism, and decubitus ulcer. A plan of total care should be made for all patients except those with minor illnesses of brief duration. Rehabilitation is an important feature of total care in patients who are expected to recover from their illness.

VOCABULARY REVIEW

dehiscence	*decubitus ulcer*	*disability*
evisceration	*ambulation*	*orientation*
	rehabilitation	

SUGGESTED READING

1. Carn, Irene, and Eleanor W. Mole: Continuity of Nursing Care. Am. J. Nursing, *49*:388–390 (June) 1949.
2. Covalt, Nila K.: Early Exercise for the Convalescent Patient. Am. J. Nursing, *47*:544–546 (August) 1947.
3. English, O. Spurgeon: Psychosomatic Medicine and Dietetics. J. Am. Dietet. A., *27*:721–725 (September) 1951.
4. Krause, Marie V.: Nutrition and Diet Therapy. Philadelphia, W. B. Saunders Co., 1952, pp. 223–225.
5. Sebrell, W. H.: Nutrition—Past and Future. Nutrit. Reviews, *11*:65–68 (March) 1953.
6. Zahler, Anastasia M.: Decubitus Ulcers. Am J. Nursing *49*:385 (June) 1949.

[1] See Brown, pages 36–57.

CHAPTER 10

Introduction

Physiology. The organs of the respiratory system provide for the introduction of oxygen from the air into the circulating blood and for the escape of carbon dioxide from the blood to the air. This gaseous exchange is called *external respiration,* in contradistinction to *internal respiration* which is the exchange of gases that takes place between the blood and the tissue cells.

The upper respiratory tract includes the nasopharynx, larynx, and associated structures (ears, paranasal sinuses, tonsils, and vocal cords). For many years the diagnosis and treatment of surgical disease of the upper respiratory tract has been the province of specialists in that field (*otolaryngologists*). Diseases of this tract are treated in the section on Otolaryngology.

During inhalation, air enters the respiratory tract through the nose (or, at times, the mouth) and is drawn successively through the pharynx, larynx, trachea, bronchi, and bronchioles, finally reaching the tiny saclike and elastic alveoli of the lungs. The exchange of gases takes place in the alveoli; oxygen, carbon dioxide, and other gases pass freely through the contiguous alveolar and blood vessel walls. During exhalation, gases from the alveoli pass through the tract in the reverse direction and are expelled from the body.

The movement of air into and out of the lungs is accomplished by contraction and relaxation of the diaphragm and the intercostal muscles. The effect of muscular contraction is to increase the capacity of the thorax, for the diaphragm moves downward and the intercostal muscles pull the ribs upward and outward. The lungs, being elastic, expand as the thorax enlarges, and air flows in. Upon relaxation of the diaphragm and intercostal muscles the thorax collapses, the lungs are compressed, and air is expelled. At the end of exhalation there is still a large quantity of air in the lungs (*alveolar air*), since the extent of thoracic collapse is limited by the bony ribs, the sternum, and the spine.

The respiratory movements of the chest exert important effects upon the other intrathoracic organs (the heart and the great vessels) as well; these are discussed elsewhere (Chap. 15).

Vital Capacity. The volume of air which can be exhaled following the deepest possible inspiration is known as the vital capacity of the individual (2 to 3 liters in the average adult). It may be measured in a spirometer or breathing bag. Disease or injury may greatly diminish the vital capacity, an occurrence of grave significance, since a large reduction will diminish the amount of oxygen available for the blood. During ordinary respiration the volume of air inhaled at each breath is much less than the vital capacity; this volume is known as the tidal air, and amounts to 300 or 400 cc. It is obvious, therefore, that the ventilation of the lungs is a fractional process: a small amount of fresh air is added to and mixed with the alveolar air at each inspiration, and an equally small amount of used air is expelled with each exhalation.

Intrapleural Pressure. The thorax is lined with a smooth, glistening, serous membrane (the parietal pleura), which is continuous with the covering of the lungs (the visceral pleura). The parietal and visceral pleural surfaces are normally in continuous and direct contact, permitting frictionless slipping during the movements of the thorax and lung. There is, however, a potential pleural cavity, but separation of the pleural surfaces occurs only as a result of disease or injury. By inserting a sterile needle through the chest wall the intrapleural pressure may be measured by means of a water manometer. The normal pressure is negative, and fluctuates slightly with breathing, diminishing during inspiration.

Pneumothorax. Following injury, or as a result of disease, air may enter the pleural space, separating the lung from the chest wall (pneumothorax). The most important consequence of this is the reduction in size of the lung, with resultant diminution in the vital capacity of the patient. In the same way the lung capacity is reduced by the presence in the pleural sac of serous fluid (*hydrothorax*), of blood (*hemothorax*), or of pus (*empyema thoracis*).

When no opening in the thoracic wall is present, a constant quantity of air in the pleural space may compress the lung wholly or in part; the vital capacity is thereby reduced but the intra-thoracic mechanics are not greatly altered. This is a closed pneumothorax and, if the quantity of air is not too large, respiration will be adequate. If, on the other hand, an opening in the chest wall exists, air may enter or leave the chest through that opening during respiratory movements; the amount of air will depend chiefly upon the size of the opening and the duration of the condition, unless as a result of previous disease the visceral and the parietal pleura are adherent. If the opening is of such size as to admit more air to the pleural sac during inspiration than can gain entrance to the lung through the bronchus, the lung will quickly and completely collapse (*atelectasis*). The vital capacity of the patient is thus rapidly and drastically reduced; to make matters worse, the mediastinal structures are normally elastic enough to permit some displacement, so that even the lung on the opposite side may be severely compressed. Such diminution of vital capacity is intolerable, and the patient will die rapidly from progressive asphyxia.

Prevention. Until a method was evolved for preventing collapse of the lungs in the presence of an opening in the chest wall, surgical approach to the intrathoracic organs was attended by a forbidding mortality. This problem has now been solved by employing an intratracheal tube or a tightly fitted face mask connected to an apparatus capable of introducing oxygen and anesthetic gases under positive pressure. In this way the lungs may be mechanically inflated and deflated, just as one inflates and deflates a rubber balloon. Ventilation of the lungs is carried on for the patient during that part of the operation in which the chest is open; at the conclusion of the procedure the lungs

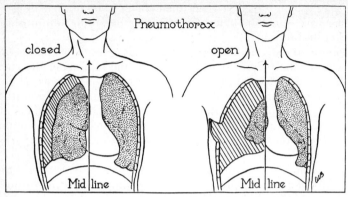

FIGURE 44. *Left:* Closed pneumothorax; *right:* open pneumothorax. Note the complete collapse of lung and shift of mediastinum, partially compressing lung on opposite side in case of open pneumothorax.

are inflated at the moment the wound is finally closed, and the patient is then able to carry on for himself.

Tension Pneumothorax. Occasionally air enters the pleural space through a small opening in the thorax, or through a leak in the lung, in such a way that a quantity of air enters the pleural sac during each inspiration, but, because of the nature of the opening, the air is unable to leave during exhalation. This results in a progressive accumulation of air (tension pneumothorax) which, if unchecked, will eventually produce as severe collapse of the lungs as would an open pneumothorax. Tension pneumothorax may develop insidiously, moreover, giving no indication of its presence until the condition of the patient becomes suddenly alarming. Death by asphyxiation quickly results unless the pressure of air inside the pleural cavity (but outside of the lung) is relieved. Any sudden increase in difficulty in breathing, or any change in color occurring under circumstances that might permit the development of tension pneumothorax, should be noted at once. The surgeon is summoned, and oxygen must be given to the patient pending his arrival.

Obstruction of the Bronchus; Bronchial Fistula. Following complete obstruction of the trachea or both of the main bronchi, the patient is asphyxiated; unless this state is quickly relieved, death results. Obstruction of one bronchus or of a branch bronchus may be survived, however, and collapse (*atelectasis*) of

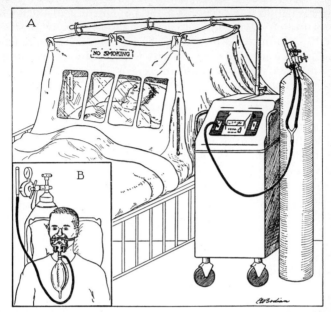

FIGURE 45. *A,* Oxygen tent; *B,* patient receiving oxygen through BLB mask.

that portion of the lung supplied by the obstructed bronchus is the result, because the air remaining in the alveoli of the obstructed segment is rapidly carried away by the circulating blood.

As a result of disease, injury, or operation, an opening (fistula) may form between a bronchus and the pleural cavity, or between a bronchus and the external chest wall. In the first instance a closed pneumothorax, of the tension variety, is a result. In the second case, air is inspired and exhaled through the external opening at every breath.

It is to be remembered that some pathogenic bacteria are constantly present in the respiratory tract; they are sucked into the lungs with each inspiration. An almost inevitable consequence of atelectasis or fistula, therefore, is infection.

Roentgenography; Oxygen Therapy. No introductory discussion of the respiratory system would be complete without the mention of roentgenography and oxygen therapy. The diagnosis of pulmonary lesions has become marvelously accurate as a result of the use of x-rays; by making successive films the surgeon is able to study the progress of the patient in a manner far superior to that afforded by physical diagnosis. The use of oxygen, whether administered by mask or by tent, has saved innumerable patients in whom the vital capacity was so reduced that ordinary air could not supply amounts of oxygen adequate for saturation of the circulating blood.[1]

SUMMARY

The movement of air into and out of the lungs is essential to life. Impairment of this function because of disease or injury results in respiratory embarrassment leading, if severe, to asphyxia. Openings in the chest walls, leaks in the lung or bronchi, and obstruction to the latter are dangerous. Oxygen therapy is life-saving.

VOCABULARY REVIEW

vital capacity	*atelectasis*	*mediastinum*
tidal air	*asphyxia*	*oxygen*
pneumothorax	*bronchus*	

SUGGESTED READING

1. Cooper, Lenna, Barber, Edith M., and Mitchell, Helen S.: Nutrition in Health and Disease. 11th Ed. Philadelphia, J. B. Lippincott Co., 1950, pp. 288–289; 490–494.
2. Christie, Arthur C.: Mass Screening Techniques for Chest Diseases. J.A.M.A., *151*:114–117 (January 10) 1953.
3. Lacy, Marvin, and Hitchcock, Marie Owen: Retained Secretions Following Thoracic Surgery. Am. J. Nursing, *51*:607–609 (October) 1951.
4. Poppe, J. Karl, and James, Ruby B.: Intratracheal Suctioning. Am. J. Nursing, *45*:538–540 (July) 1945.

CHAPTER 11

Thoracic Injuries

The majority of thoracic injuries respond readily to simple, conservative treatment. Injuries to the chest are of grave significance only when disturbance of the respiration is caused, when serious hemorrhage occurs, or when the element of infection is introduced. Severe chest wounds are likely to be com-

[1] See Brown, pages 119–150.

plicated by all of these factors. Simple contusions, abrasions, and lacerations of the chest wall which do not involve the deeper structures are treated just as are those occurring elsewhere about the body, and do not merit special consideration.

BLUNT FORCE INJURIES

Fracture of one or more ribs is the usual consequence of a heavy blow or fall upon the chest. Broken ribs constitute a very painful injury, but are not in themselves serious. Such fractures heal readily, and the only treatment necessary consists in measures to relieve the pain which accompanies each respiratory movement. Splinting of the injured area by means of adhesive strapping, or preferably by the use of a snug bandage of an elastic material such as stockinet, will minimize the movements of the bone ends and thus relieve the pain. Morphine or other narcotics may also be given, provided the patient's respirations are not depressed, and it is certain that the signs of other injury will not be masked by the effect of the narcotic agent.

Puncture of the lung or tearing of the intercostal blood vessels often accompanies the fracture of a rib, the injury being caused by the momentary displacement inward of the jagged bone end. It is highly important, therefore, to realize that severe intra-thoracic damage may complicate a blow upon the chest, even though there is little external evidence of violence. When such damage occurs, the treatment is the same as for penetrating wounds of the chest.

A far more serious and often fatal type of injury follows severe compression of the chest. This injury may be produced by crushing, as in a mine cave-in, or by the blast of a nearby explosion. Great numbers of the lung alveoli and capillaries are ruptured by the sudden terrific squeezing of the chest. For this accident, rest and the administration of oxygen are the best treatment. The internal damage is often so extensive, however, that death quickly follows from a combination of hemorrhage and asphyxiation.

PENETRATING WOUNDS

In civil life the chest wall is penetrated in various ways, usually by a revolver bullet, a knife, or an ice pick. Such wounds are occasionally self-inflicted, but are seldom accidental in the ordinary sense of that word. The relatively low mortality rate occurring in these injuries in civil life is not necessarily a tribute to the skill of the surgeon; it is an index to the widespread lack of accurate anatomical knowledge and the lack of accurate aiming in the heat of attack. In war, penetrating wounds of the chest are followed by a far higher mortality rate, due, no doubt, to the frequent occurrence of multiple wounds (e.g., those caused by machine guns and high explosives), to the occurrence of large wounds (such as those from high explosives and bayonets), to the accuracy of aim which practice brings, and to the unfortunately unavoidable delay in securing surgical aid.

Any wound which has penetrated the skin of the chest wall, or, for that matter, the skin of the adjacent neck or abdomen, should be suspected of being a penetrating wound and must be treated as such until the wound is absolutely proved to be nonpenetrating. It is astonishing how much internal damage can be accomplished through a tiny, innocent appearing, external wound. The examiner may readily peer into the depths of a large wound and see that the chest wall has been penetrated, or he may hear air passing in and out (*sucking wound*), or he may feel the characteristic crepitation of air bubbles which have been forced into the deeper tissues by the respiratory movements (*subcutaneous emphysema*); but simple examination of the wound which has none of these characteristics will not serve to prove nonpenetration. The color of the patient, the character and rate of respiration, the pulse rate, the blood pressure level, and the percussion and auscultation of the chest are as important considerations as inspection of the wound, for careful observation of these will afford a means of gauging the nature and extent of an intrathoracic injury when one is present. When circumstances and the condition of the patient permit, accurate information may be secured by fluoroscopy.

Treatment. The proper treatment for a penetrating wound of the chest consists in adequate disinfection and closure of the wound, administration of tetanus antitoxin, or tetanus toxoid if the patient has been previously immunized, and careful observation of the patient's progress. If his general condition remains good, with adequate maintenance of blood pressure level and no respiratory distress, no additional immediate treatment is necessary other than rest in bed.

Sucking wounds must be closed without delay, or, if too large for closure, the opening must be quickly packed with an airtight dressing so that the open pneumothorax is converted at once into a closed pneumothorax.

In nearly every patient who has received a penetrating chest wound, there is *hemopneumothorax* (air and blood in the pleural sac). When the signs of rapid and progressive hemorrhage are apparent, simple treatment will not suffice, and it is necessary to open the chest at once (*thoracotomy*). The source of the bleeding must be found, the bleeding checked, and the blood which has been lost must be replaced by adequate transfusion. In most patients, fortunately, the bleeding will not be so severe; recovery is aided by prompt and repeated aspiration of the blood from the pleural cavity. This procedure (*thoracentesis*), carried out by inserting a needle through the chest wall between two ribs, is necessary so that the blood will be removed before it clots and thus permanently compresses the lung.

If the hemothorax has already clotted, the clot can be liquefied by the use of the enzymes streptokinase and streptodornase, which have the power to liquefy fibrin. In cases of neglected or unsuccessfully treated hemothorax, it still may be possible to achieve expansion of the compressed and constricted lung by an operation (*decortication*) in which the lung is exposed and the old, organized clot peeled off.

Complications. Since bacteria are present in the lungs, and since they may also be introduced through the wound, infection is a frequent complication. The resulting infectious process does not differ greatly from other types of empyema thoracis, and its treatment is, in general, the same as for the other types (Chap. 12). Infection is suspected when a rise in temperature and an increased leukocyte count are noted, usually forty-eight to seventy-two hours after injury. The diagnosis is made by examining and culturing fluid obtained from the chest by aspiration with a needle (*thoracentesis*).

Wounds of the heart are not infrequent in penetrating wounds of the chest. The diagnosis and treatment of these are discussed in Chapter 17.

DIAPHRAGMATIC HERNIA

The diaphragm serves as the dividing wall between the thoracic and abdominal cavities. Ordinarily, there are openings only for the passage of the esophagus, the aorta, the vena cava, lymphatics and nerves. Abnormal openings may result from developmental failure during fetal life, or can be produced by injury or infection. Such an abnormal opening or defect in the diaphragm will permit abdominal contents (stomach, omentum, colon, small intestine) to enter the thoracic cavity. If the opening is large there may be serious compression of the lung, interfering with respiratory function just as does a pneumothorax. Other symptoms, particularly those of intestinal obstruction, may result from the displacement and twisting of the abdominal organs involved.

Operative treatment is required to relieve the symptoms and save life. Repair of a diaphragmatic hernia includes replacement of the abdominal organs and closure of the defect in the diaphragm. The procedure is tolerated well even by the newborn infants. Nursing care is given as after any thoracotomy; usually the patient will also be treated with continuous gastric suction to prevent abdominal distention (see p. 243).

NURSING CARE

The patient who has a thoracic injury usually is admitted through the emergency room. It is desirable to place him near the nurses' station to facilitate close observation and care.

If it is the patient's first admission to a hospital he may not only be frightened by his pain and condition but also by his new surroundings. His family must be notified and asked to come to the hospital. The nurse should give explanations and answer questions in a calm and reassuring manner to try to reduce the anxiety and apprehension which usually exist in both patient and family.

The temperature, pulse, respirations and blood pressure should be taken as soon as he has been made comfortable in bed. Rest, quiet and the control of pain are essential; usually morphine or some other narcotic is ordered. There may be great variation in the appearance of patients with thoracic injuries but the principles of care are the same for all; modifications are made according to the needs of the patient. Because his condition may change rapidly, the nurse must observe him frequently for change in color or cyanosis, more rapid or weak pulse, difficulty in breathing, subcutaneous emphysema or a drop in blood pressure. Any change in the vital signs of the patient should be called to the attention of the surgeon immediately.

Routine care given to a patient on admission includes bathing the patient but this should be postponed until his condition is fully evaluated and permission is given by the surgeon. Antibiotics are usually ordered and, when administered to a patient who has been in an accident which invariably makes him dirty, special care should be taken in cleansing the skin before the intramuscular injection is given. Usually a liquid diet is permitted and increased to a normal diet according to the patient's tolerance, but when the patient is very ill, or if there is a question of abdominal injury, fluids and solid food are usually withheld.

The patient who has difficulty in breathing is given oxygen. Explaining the value of the oxygen as a means of making him more comfortable before attempting to administer the treatment, and also explaining very simply when the apparatus is applied, lessens apprehension and increases cooperation. A sterile thoracentesis set is kept near the patient in case of sudden need for the aspiration of fluid or air from the chest.

During the convalescence, routine care including good physical care, instruction of good health habits and direction of diversional and occupational therapy should be given. Learning to know the patient, to develop awareness of his needs and to help him meet them in order to prepare him for a more healthful life, are criteria of good care. Before discharge, instructions concerning his return visit to the doctor and his home care should be clearly explained and written out for him.

SUMMARY

Thoracic injuries are always dangerous. Careful observation of the patient will permit early detection of loss of blood or interference with respiration. Oxygen therapy and thoracentesis are regularly employed.

VOCABULARY REVIEW

sucking wound *hemopneumothorax* *decortication*
subcutaneous *diaphragm* *thoracentesis*
emphysema *thoracotomy*

SUGGESTED READING

1. Carter, B. Noland, and Giuseffi, Jerome: The Use of Tracheotomy in the Treatment of Crushing Injuries of the Chest. Surg., Gynec. & Obst., *95*:55–64 (January) 1953.
2. Christopher, Frederick: A Textbook of Surgery. 5th Ed. Philadelphia, W. B. Saunders Co., 1949, pp. 847–851.
3. Coleman, Frank P.: Traumatic Hemothorax: Decortication in the Treatment of the Chronic Infected Type. Arch. Surg., *50*:14–18 (January) 1945.
4. Lindsey, Monette: Traumatic Thoracic Surgery. Am. J. Nursing, *44*:1029–1032 (November) 1944.

CHAPTER 12

Suppurative Disease of the Lung and Pleura

LUNG ABSCESS

An abscess in the functioning substance (*parenchyma*) of the lung presents much the same pathologic appearance as an abscess elsewhere. Preceded by a stage of bacterial invasion, tissue *necrosis* (death) and local resistance combine to produce a central core of pus surrounded by a wall of inflammatory granulation tissue. Sooner or later the contents of the enlarging abscess cavity rupture into a small bronchus, and as a result of this the patient coughs persistently, producing large amounts of foul purulent sputum. Despite the constant drainage of pus into the bronchus, an abscess cavity in the lung may show little tendency to collapse and heal, due in large part to the noncollapsible nature of the thoracic wall. As is to be expected, the infectious process causes a systemic response: the patient has fever and leukocytosis, feels badly, and loses weight.

Solitary abscess of the lung occurs, but multiple abscesses are somewhat more common. The causative agent cannot be incriminated in every instance, but abscesses are known to follow the aspiration of irritating substances (often foreign bodies, such as a peanut, chewing gum, pins) or purulent material from tonsillar or dental infections, and from retained foreign bodies such as bullets, shell fragments, or bits of clothing received in a wound. Lung abscesses are also produced by bacteria carried into the lung by the circulating blood (blood stream infection, *septicemia*), and by direct extension into the lung of a suppurative process originating outside the lung. Because of the nature of the bacteria, lung abscesses are usually productive of the foulest pus. The putrefactive nature of the infection is due to the presence of organisms, both aerobic and anaerobic, ordinarily found in the mouth; although the mouth bacteria may not be the initial cause of the abscess, as secondary invaders they soon dominate the picture.

112

Nursing Care of Lung Abscess

Prevention. As always, the best treatment is prevention. The known incidence of pulmonary abscess following tonsillectomy and dental extraction makes it imperative to prevent aspiration of material from the mouth or pharynx during those procedures. This is best accomplished by placing the patient with head down and feet elevated, and by careful use of the suction apparatus. In fact, aspiration must be guarded against in all patients undergoing general anesthesia, and in those unconscious from other causes.

General Measures. Clinical experience has shown that about one third of acute pulmonary abscesses heal spontaneously during the first three months. It is wise, therefore, to treat all early, acute cases conservatively, using such measures as rest in bed, amplified diet, transfusion, antibiotics, and postural drainage. The remainder of the patients do not improve, but show progression of the lesion. Fever and cough persist, larger amounts of pus are produced, and the patient becomes thin and weak. Early in the disease, examination of the chest reveals the signs of pulmonary consolidation; later there is cavity formation. This is best demonstrated by roentgenography. The chronic stage may last months or years, death finally resulting from hemorrhage (caused by erosion of a pulmonary vessel), extension of the abscess into the pleural space (*empyema*), or spread of the infection through the blood stream, commonly to the brain. About half of the patients suffering from chronic pulmonary abscess can be cured by surgical means.

Coughing. The patient should be encouraged to cough, and to continue coughing, for the bringing up of as much as possible of the pus will empty the abscess cavity, thereby aiding in the collapse and healing of that cavity.

Technic of Postural Drainage. Postural drainage is a most useful treatment, but is often poorly understood by nurses and ineffectually carried out by patients. To properly perform it, the patient is positioned so that his head and trachea are dependent and the abscess cavity is uppermost. The exact location of the abscess determines whether the patient must be on his back, chest or side. When the patient is correctly positioned, the pus will have a downhill path from the abscess cavity to the mouth. The purulent material, however, is viscous, and may not flow rapidly; therefore the patient must be made to remain in the proper posi-

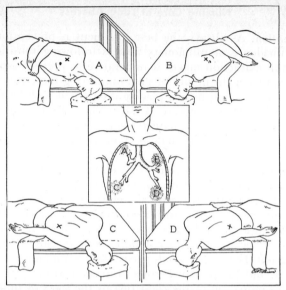

FIGURE 46. Proper positions for postural drainage of pulmonary abscess in
right upper lobe (*A*), left upper lobe (*B*), right lower lobe (*C*),
and left lower lobe (*D*).

tion for twenty to thirty minutes despite his discomfort, and must
be encouraged to cough vigorously and frequently the while.
Morning and evening sessions usually suffice, but more may be
required if the output of pus is large.

Measuring and Disposal of Pus. The purulent expectoration is
naturally highly infective, and patients must be provided with
suitable containers so that its proper disposal can be accomplished. It is important, also, that the twenty-four hour volume
be measured, as the progress of the disease may thus be gauged.
A graduated waxed cardboard box fitted with a cover is a good
container for collection and measurement of the sputum. The expectoration has a very foul, nauseating odor and should be removed immediately. The best method of disposal is burning.
For this purpose sawdust is added to the material and the container wrapped in several thicknesses of newspaper.

Bronchoscopic Examination. The bronchoscope has been
widely used in treating pulmonary abscess. This instrument, a

metal tube equipped with an electric light, can be passed through the mouth and larynx into the trachea, and by means of it the mucous membrane lining the respiratory tract can be inspected as far down as the main bronchi. Suction can be used, and many different medicaments have been instilled, but with little success. Postural drainage properly carried out is far more satisfactory. Following bronchoscopic examination the patient may complain of sore throat and may cough a great deal, but these complaints are temporary.

Nursing Care of Patients Having Bronchoscopy. In preparing the patient for bronchoscopic examination nothing is given by mouth for at least six hours prior to the time of the procedure. This helps prevent vomiting, which would not only interfere with the examination but might lead to aspiration. The patient should be told what to expect at examination to prevent apprehension and encourage cooperation.

Before the patient leaves for the examining room, a barbiturate is usually ordered and, in many instances, morphine and/or atropine are also given. False teeth are removed and the patient is transported on a litter or in bed.

Either cocaine or tetracaine hydrochloride is used to anesthetize the pharynx. These drugs are cerebral stimulants, but in large doses will cause depression of the central nervous system. The sedatives given before examination counteract the stimulating effects of these anesthetic agents and help prevent laryngeal spasm.

Following bronchoscopy, the nurse must observe the patient closely for slowed respirations and cyanosis. Giving the patient oxygen through an oronasal mask is helpful in combating the reaction.

The patient should be told that he must not take anything by mouth for at least two hours, so that aspiration because of the anesthetized pharynx may be prevented.

Surgical Treatment of Lung Abscess. The removal of the diseased portion of the lung (*segmental resection*) is now the safest and most satisfactory method of dealing with lung abscess. In some instances, this may mean the removal of one lobe (*lobectomy*), and occasionally the removal of the entire lung (*pneumonectomy*). The operation, its complications and dangers, and the postoperative care are the same as in the treatment of bronchiectasis, and are described in the discussion of that condition.

In most patients, the result of the removal of the diseased lung is dramatic, with recession of fever, immediate disappearance of cough and sputum, gain in strength and weight, followed by a return to normal life.

BRONCHIECTASIS

Bronchiectasis is a pathologic condition of the lung characterized by progressive enlargement of the tiny bronchioles. There is, in addition, a considerable degree of chronic inflammation of the involved portion of the lung, attributable in part, certainly, to secondary infection. A common complication of other pulmonary diseases, bronchiectasis is often the result of the obstruction to the bronchi that follows the growth of a lung tumor, the enlargement of a lung abscess, or the swelling of tuberculous lymph nodes. Bronchiectasis also occurs as a primary disease, without demonstrable cause. In this primary form of the disease the initial lesions are usually found in the lower lobe of one or both lungs.

It is important to realize that primary bronchiectasis is a disease of young people; the onset is usually in the second or third decade of life. The patient notices a chronic hacking cough that is often thought at first to be due to "chronic bronchitis"; weeks or months later the cough becomes productive of increasing amounts of foul smelling sputum. In the early stages most of the sputum is coughed up in the morning on rising; later, expectoration is more frequent and large in amount. At first there is little systemic disorder, but after months or years, loss of weight, fever, anemia, and clubbing of the fingers appear.

Enlargement of the distal phalanx of the fingers (*clubbed fingers*) is a curious phenomenon which has been observed since the days of Hippocrates. It is known to occur in association with any form of chronic pulmonary disease, but no adequate explanation has been offered.

The clinical diagnosis of bronchiectasis is a difficult one, since the symptoms are so similar to those of pulmonary tuberculosis. Bronchoscopic examination often discloses the bronchus from which the pus is coming, and the introduction of a radiopaque substance (Lipiodol) into the bronchus affords a means of outlining the enlarged bronchioles on the x-ray film. When untreated, the disease is slowly progressive, and the patient dies after a few years as the result of hemorrhage or spread of the infection.

Treatment of Bronchiectasis

Until recent times the treatment of bronchiectasis was far from satisfactory. General hygienic measures, change of climate, the eradication of possible foci of infection such as infected teeth, tonsils, or sinuses, and bronchoscopic treatments all had extensive trial with but indifferent results. Fortunately, however, the development of thoracic surgery has brightened the outlook for those afflicted with this disease. In those patients in whom the process has not spread beyond the lower lobes of either or both lungs, the surgical removal of the affected portions brings about a cure.

Segmental Resection. The term segmental resection means the removal of a portion of pulmonary tissue which comprises an anatomic unit, such as an entire lobe, or that portion of a lobe served by a branch of the lobar bronchus.

General anesthesia is induced in the usual manner, and then a tracheal tube is inserted, making it possible for the anesthetist to control accurately the oxygenation and inflation of the lungs and to aspirate secretions or blood from the trachea and bronchi. Some surgeons prefer to enter the chest anteriorly, others prefer the posterior approach. Difficulty is encountered if the lung is adherent to the chest wall, as the dissection necessary to free the affected lobe often causes brisk bleeding. The branches of the bronchus, pulmonary artery, and pulmonary vein to the diseased segment are carefully identified, isolated, and divided. This makes possible the removal of the diseased portion of the lung.

Great care must be exercised in closing the bronchial stump, for a leak will result in disaster. It is, of course, necessary to ligate the branches of the pulmonary vessels securely. Before the chest wall is sutured the remaining portion of the lung is inflated by the anesthetist, and, remarkably enough in most instances, the cavity will be nearly filled. A soft rubber catheter is introduced into the chest through a separate, tiny stab wound, and is placed so that its tip lies in the space formerly occupied by the removed segment. To prevent the entry of air into the chest, the outer end of the catheter is securely closed by means of a clamp.

The operation is ordinarily performed quickly and without shock, but it is naturally a wise precaution to have blood available. At the conclusion of the procedure the anesthetist aspirates the bronchial tree and removes the tracheal tube.

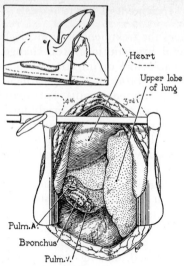

FIGURE 47. Lobectomy. The left lower lobe has been removed, the vessels ligated, and the bronchus sutured. Insert shows location of incision.

If the disease is bilateral the operation may be attempted on the opposite side about three months later.

Nursing Care Following Segmental Resection. In preparation, the following equipment should be assembled: the routine postoperative unit, oxygen therapy equipment and sterile "water seal" suction apparatus. Oxygen therapy is begun immediately and is usually continued for twenty-four to forty-eight hours or until the patient breathes easily without increased rate of respirations.

Before attaching the chest catheter to the suction apparatus, as illustrated in Figure 51, the whole system should be tested. Clamping the tubing that leads to the catheter and turning on the suction should produce bubbling of water in bottle 2. Such a suction drainage system withdraws the effusion of serosanguineous fluid, which varies from 200 to 500 cc. after intrathoracic operations, and provides for detection of bleeding. A clamp is attached to a piece of cotton tape at the head of the bed so that if any of the bottles breaks or if the suction fails in any way the chest catheter may be clamped off immediately. The bottles should be placed no less than 18 inches below the level

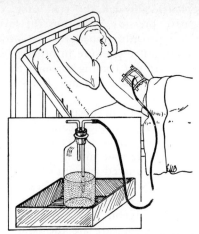

FIGURE 48. Straight drainage under a fluid level. End of tube from chest is beneath fluid level; second tube through bottle stopper is open. Bottle is placed in box on floor.

of the catheter in the chest. Placing the bottles in a sturdy container, such as a wooden box, helps prevent breakage. The oscillation of fluid in the tube leading to the catheter is assurance that the system is functioning properly. The position of the chest catheter should be checked at regular intervals to be certain that it has not worked loose. When the system does not seem to be working properly, it should be carefully examined for loose stoppers and kinks in the tubing, especially the tubing leading to the patient. The nurse should observe the type of drainage and call the doctor if there is excess bleeding. The bottles are arranged so that bottle No. 1 contains a measured amount of sterile water or normal saline, with glass tube under fluid to which the catheter in the patient's chest is attached; it provides a reservoir for the collection of fluid. Air-tight continuity by means of connecting links of rubber tubing between the bottles and the source of suction provides an entirely closed system of drainage with suction. The air vent provided by the long glass tube in bottle No. 2 makes it possible to control the amount of negative pressure exerted upon the chest. This is done by altering the length of tubing beneath the water level. If the negative pressure above the level of water in bottle No. 2 exceeds the height of the column of water in the immersed portion of the vent tube, air will be sucked into the bottle through the vent tube, therefore maintaining the negative pressure at a constant level. Needless to say, the mechanism providing suction must produce a slightly greater amount of negative pressure in order to keep the system working. If bubbles are not coming through the vent tube, one may suspect that the negative pressure is less than the desired amount.

When the drainage is to be measured, which is usually ordered every twelve hours, the chest catheter is clamped off, the suction is turned off, the "water seal" bottle is emptied, the contents measured, the bottle and tubing are resterilized, and the bottle is filled with the ordered amount of sterile solution. After reattaching it to bottle No. 2 and to the chest catheter, suction is applied and the clamp is released.

In some cases, the surgeon may order simple "water seal" drainage. The principles of care are the same as when suction drainage is used.

Frequent turning and coughing are usually ordered; these may make the patient uncomfortable but are essential in preventing atelectasis and pneumonia. Analgesics should be given to keep him comfortable and to lessen pain while coughing. Holding a towel firmly around the chest to add support is useful while the patient is coughing. When the patient does not cough deeply, it may be necessary to stimulate the cough reflex by suctioning through the nostril into the pharynx by means of an electric aspirator. Steam inhalations are helpful in loosening and thinning viscid mucus.

Fluids are administered intravenously until the patient is able to take the necessary amount by mouth. Antibiotics are given intramuscularly.

The patient is gotten out of bed according to his condition. It may be as soon as the third day but often he may remain in bed much longer.

A high caloric, high vitamin diet is increased as tolerated and routine convalescent care is given as described previously under thoracic injuries.

In the absence of complications, the chest catheter is removed in two to four days and the operative wound heals per primam. The chest is usually examined by x-ray several times during the first week.

The activities of such a patient are gradually increased while he is in the hospital and when he goes home he is advised to exercise according to his tolerance. The convalescent period varies with the individual. The rapidity of recovery seems to decrease with increasing age of people; the young person frequently is very active before leaving the hospital. Excessive exercise such as swimming is usually forbidden temporarily. These patients are not handicapped in leading a normal life. A mother is able to take care of her children and carry out the household duties, and the office worker can resume his work. Only when the person has done work involving strenuous physical labor does it seem necessary that he be advised to change to another type of work.

Complications. The mortality rate among carefully selected and prepared patients is low, far lower than the rate for the disease if untreated. Fatalities occur nevertheless, and are nearly always due to one or more of the three serious complications of pulmonary resection. These are hemorrhage, tension pneumothorax, and infection; of the three, infection is the most common, the most difficult to prevent and the hardest to cure.

HEMORRHAGE. The symptoms and signs of hemorrhage following lobectomy are the same as those of concealed hemorrhage elsewhere, but the diagnosis is made somewhat more easily when bright blood appears in the drainage tube. If the bleeding is rapid or persistent the surgeon must reopen the chest to control it. Large blood transfusions are often necessary. The appearance of small amounts of old blood in the drainage tube, however, may be expected as a matter of course, as there is nearly always a small amount of blood in the chest cavity at the conclusion of the operation.

INFECTION. A problem always confronting the thoracic surgeon is the rate and completeness of healing of the bronchial stump. The healing of this structure depends somewhat upon its size, for small bronchial branches heal more rapidly and more readily than do the main branches or the stem bronchus. Infection invariably follows even the most minute leak in the bronchial closure, and, of course, air will also pass through the opening. If the leak occurs in the first seventy-two hours after operation, before the remaining lung becomes adherent to and seals over the stump, not only will infection be spread throughout the pleural cavity but the grave condition of tension pneumothorax will be produced. This state must be discovered at once as the application of negative pressure to the drainage tube may prevent mediastinal shift and asphyxiation. Prompt treatment is imperative because death may occur within a few minutes after the onset of the symptoms.

A leak in the bronchial stump occurring after the stump has become sealed off by surrounding lung tissue is less serious. Pneumothorax is thus prevented, and the infection is localized. Sometimes the infection will drain spontaneously through the bronchus, with expectoration of the pus; at other times it must be drained surgically. The whole problem of treatment of these postoperative infections of the chest is more properly discussed with the treatment of empyema thoracis.

EMPYEMA THORACIS

Empyema thoracis is the term used to designate the occurrence of pus in the chest, and does not, in itself, indicate the amount of pus or the source of the infection. Acute empyema thoracis is the result, variously, of the introduction into the pleural space of infective material from the outside, as in a puncture wound; or of the spread to the pleural surface of an infection within the lung, as in pneumonia, tuberculosis, or pulmonary abscess; or of an infection occurring as a complication of an intrathoracic operation. Since this is so, it is obvious that the nature of the empyema and its treatment will depend upon the nature of the underlying cause, Chronic empyema thoracis is the usual consequence of an acute case improperly treated or neglected.

Postpneumonic Type. One who has seen under the microscope a slide prepared from a pneumonic lung will recall the abundant bacteria that are present in the lymphatics beneath the pleural surface of the lung. It is not surprising, therefore, that some of these bacteria gain entrance to the pleural space, and, indeed, in nearly every case of pneumococcal pneumonia, fluid containing pneumococci is present in the pleural space during the height of the disease. In the majority of instances, particularly when chemotherapy is used, the infection is quickly overcome, the bacteria are killed, and the fluid is absorbed. In some, however, the bacteria gain the upper hand, and the infected portion of the pleural sac then resembles an abscess. The pleural surfaces about the collection of pus become greatly inflamed, thickened, and adherent, forming a typical abscess wall. The size and location of the empyema cavities vary greatly: a massive empyema may involve nearly the entire pleural space, whereas a small empyema cavity may be located anywhere about the surfaces of the lung and may contain only a few cubic centimeters of pus.

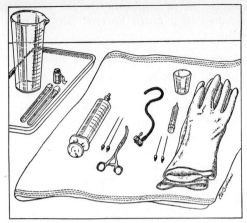

FIGURE 49. Set-up for thoracentesis. Flask of procaine, medicine glass, small syringe and fine needles are for procaine infiltration anesthesia of chest wall. Large syringe, three-way stopcock, and large gauge long needles are for thoracentesis. Graduate is for measurement of volume of fluid aspirated, and sterile tubes are for collection of samples for culture and other studies.

The character of the wall of the empyema cavity is of great importance. Early in the disease the wall is delicate and easily torn, so that improper treatment may permit spread of the disease, with further collapse of the lung. Later, however, the empyema wall becomes so firm and rigid that expansion of the lung is prevented even after evacuation of the pus, and a chronic empyema is formed. It is apparent, therefore, that the optimal time for the treatment of empyema falls between these extremes.

The occurrence of empyema is suspected clinically when a patient recovering from pneumonia has an unexpected rise in temperature or complains of pain in the chest. Often the characteristic physical signs of fluid can be elicited; but when the collection of pus is small or deeply situated there may be no signs. Roentgen ray examination of the chest nearly always discloses the empyema, especially if a series of films has been made showing the progress of the pneumonia. An absolute diagnosis of empyema thoracis rests upon thoracentesis with the discovery of pus on aspiration. Decisions as to the time and form of treatment are based on the character of the pus obtained. All such specimens should be saved, therefore, so that comparisons may be made.

The widespread use of antibiotics in the treatment of pneumonia has resulted in a much lowered incidence of postpneumonic empyema.

Treatment of Acute Empyema Thoracis

There are several methods of treating acute empyema thoracis, and it is only fair to say that most of these methods produce excellent results when used by surgeons who properly understand the principles of treating empyema and the limitations of the various methods. The underlying principle for treatment, as in any abscess, is the evacuation of the pus in such a way and at such a time that the cavity will be collapsed.

Technic of Open Drainage. In this method a large opening is made directly through the chest wall into the empyema cavity. After the abscess is located, an incision is made and a short segment of rib removed. This procedure is readily carried out under local anesthesia, and, in the case of a very ill patient, can be done in the ward. A large soft rubber tube is inserted, and copious dressings are applied. At first there is a rapid fall in temperature and profuse drainage. After two or three days the drainage subsides, the patient's appetite improves, and he may soon get out of bed. The tube is gradually removed, and in three to four weeks the wound is healed.

The most important considerations are to operate at the optimal time, and to make the opening in the proper location to provide dependent drainage. The time for operation is determined by the character of the pus. When the pus is the thickness of pea soup, it can be safely assumed that the walls of the cavity are strong enough to prevent collapse of the lung when the chest is opened. (Collapse would cause both spread of the infection and further reduction of an already impaired vital capacity.) If the pus is too thick to drain readily, the cavity may be gently irrigated once or twice daily with normal saline or Dakin's solution.

The student may well ask how it is that the lung reexpands in the presence of an open pneumothorax. This mechanism has thus far defied exact solution, but it is a fact that in properly treated patients the lung does expand and the cavity is obliterated. The best explanation offered is that the granulation tissue of the cavity walls becomes organized into scar tissue, after which the usual contraction of scar tissue takes place, and the lung is pulled back into position against the chest wall.

The advantages of open drainage are the simplicity and direct-ness of the method, the absence of complicated apparatus, and the simplicity of the after-care. The patient need not be long confined to bed or hospital. The only disadvantage, the fact that drainage cannot be safely instituted as soon as the empyema appears, is more apparent than real; for, should it prove neces-sary, large amounts of pus can be easily removed by aspiration (*thoracentesis*) until the time is ripe for operation.

Open drainage may be employed even in bilateral empyema, provided care is taken to postpone operation until the walls of the cavities are sufficiently fixed.

Nursing Care. For irrigation of the cavity the patient is turned slightly toward the unaffected side. After removal of the dressings a sterile curved basin is placed against the chest, under the in-cision, for the collection of the return flow of pus and fluid. The solution which was ordered is introduced into the cavity through the rubber tube by means of a sterile Asepto syringe. To ensure more complete drainage, the patient should be turned toward the affected side before the application of dressings. Following the irrigation, the area around the tube and the incision should be cleaned by sponging. Benzalkonium chloride 1:1000 is a satis-factory solution for this purpose. The dressing is made by placing four or five sterile fluffs around the tube and over the incision, then covering them with a large sterile cotton pad. When fre-quent change of dressings is necessary, the use of Montgomery straps[1] prevents the irritation of the skin and the discomfort to the patient incident to the frequent removal of adhesive. Two of these adhesive straps are fastened on either side of the dress-ing and tied over the dressing.

The drainage is sometimes irritating to the skin. In such cases the area directly surrounding the wound should be protected by boric or some other mild sterile ointment. The soiled dressing should be wrapped in several thicknesses of newspaper before being burned; the basin used for the collection of pus should be emptied immediately, then washed and boiled.

Technic of Closed Drainage. Closed drainage is carried out by introducing a small rubber tube, usually a 16 F. catheter, through

---

[1] Montgomery straps are made by cutting 2-inch adhesive tape in strips about 10 inches long. Three or four inches of the adhesive at each end is folded on it-self. Cotton tape about 6 inches long is tied through a hole made in the double thickness of adhesive. Toothpicks, inserted in the end of the double adhesive, joined by rubber bands, may be used instead of cotton tapes.

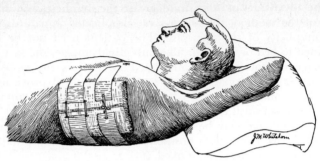

FIGURE 50. Drainage dressing held by Montgomery straps. The upper strap is
fastened by cotton tapes, the lower by elastic bands over toothpicks.

a trocar which has been inserted between the appropriate ribs
into the most dependent portion of the empyema cavity. The
operation is easily and quickly performed in the operating room
or in the patient's bed. It must be pointed out that the procedure
is a "blind" one: the operator cannot see the tissues through
which he is forcing the trocar. The drainage of deeply situated
or small collections of pus, therefore, is attended by both difficulty and danger. The catheter is, of course, closed by means
of a clamp until it can be connected to the apparatus ordered by
the surgeon, for the chief difference between the open and closed
methods of drainage lies in the careful prevention of an open
pneumothorax in the closed method.

A number of common mishaps are encountered in using the
various closed drainage systems. Sooner or later there will be
leakage of pus and/or fluid about the drainage tube; this can be
sometimes corrected by changing the tube to one of larger size.
The drainage tube is often plugged by thick pus or lumps of
fibrin, a complication requiring constant watchfulness and re-
sourcefulness. The fibrin-dissolving enzymes, streptokinase and
streptodornase, may be used to make the pus thin. Sometimes a
clot of fibrin acts as a flapper valve over the inner opening of
the catheter, so that fluid may enter but may not leave the cavity.
This complication has occasionally resulted in rupture of the
cavity with consequent collapse of the whole lung. Air may
enter the apparatus through faulty joints, but in some instances
air escapes into the cavity through the development of a bronchial fistula. Such a fistula may result from the destructive effect

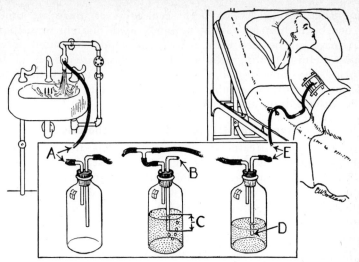

FIGURE 51. Suction drainage. Note that this is a closed system. *A*, Source of suction; *B*, pressure regulator (amount of negative pressure is determined by distance *C*); *D*, drainage bottle; *E*, tubing to patient.

of the infection, or from the mechanical pressure against the lung of an improperly placed drainage tube.

Nursing Care. The use of all apparatus for drainage should be clearly understood by the nurse before she attempts to care for the patient. Care of the apparatus may be summarized in three rules: Keep the tubing clear, allow no air to enter, measure and record the drainage. In emptying the drainage bottle the nurse must be certain that the tube leading to it is clamped off tightly to prevent the entrance of air into the tube. The drainage tube is kept under fluid in the collection bottle when straight drainage is used. The exact amount of pus collected is calculated by subtracting from the total drainage (1) the amount of fluid placed in the bottle plus (2) the amount of irrigating fluid introduced into the cavity.

The formation of a bronchial fistula presents a serious problem when closed drainage is used. Not only are the dynamics of the apparatus upset, but also there is opportunity for the irrigating fluid to run into the bronchial tree, causing continual coughing at best, or drowning at worst. When possible, open drainage is the simplest method of treating an empyema complicated by a bronchial fistula. As has been seen, however, there are times when open drainage cannot be safely used. Straight or suction drainage can be used without irrigating fluids, and often prove most useful in dealing with bronchial fistulas. Care must be taken to use very mild suction, since it is not hard to suck the lung around the drainage tube in such a way as to close the tube off without draining the empyema.

Treatment of Chronic Empyema Thoracis

The modern treatment of acute empyema thoracis should seldom allow a case of chronic empyema to develop, but there are always a few hardy patients who do not seek medical aid during the acute stage. The patient with chronic empyema usually presents a small draining sinus in the chest wall overlying a cavity which is easily demonstrable in the x-ray film. Such a patient has, as a rule, no constitutional symptoms, and may have led a normal active life for months or years except for the annoyance of the purulent drainage from the sinus. The inflammatory tissue walls of the chronic empyema cavity may be a centimeter or more thick, and are as tough as cartilage.

Until recently the only method of dealing satisfactorily with this condition was to choose or devise a plastic procedure (*thoracoplasty*) which had for its object the obliteration of the cavity. This involves the resection of ribs, the excision of the thick scar tissue, or the implantation of pedicled flaps of muscle and skin. Experience has shown, however, that operative removal of the thickened wall of the cavity by peeling it off the underlying lung is a highly successful method of promoting healing in chronic empyema, as the freed lung quickly reexpands to fill the cavity. Bronchial fistulas often complicate chronic empyema, but will usually heal if the cavity is obliterated.

Treatment of Other Forms of Empyema Thoracis

Infection of the Pleural Space Following a Penetrating Wound. This is not uncommon, and the resultant empyema may be treated satisfactorily in the same manner as postpneumonic empyema.

Intrapleural Rupture of Abscess. A particularly grave form of empyema is that which results from the spontaneous rupture into the pleural cavity of a pulmonary abscess. In this instance there is a sudden overwhelming infection, usually of the entire pleural sac, complicated by the presence of a bronchial fistula. Not only is the lung likely to be collapsed, but also a tension pneumothorax exists. To make matters worse, the type of infection is usually highly virulent and *mixed* (composed of numerous varieties of bacteria). Adequate treatment, then, must include immediate drainage, relief of the tension pneumothorax, prevention of an open pneumothorax, and the administration of antibiotics.

The proper diagnosis is not difficult. The sudden appearance of high fever, prostration, pain in the chest, cyanosis, and dyspnea in a patient suspected of having or known to have a lung abscess points to intrapleural rupture of the abscess. The physical signs of fluid and air in the pleural space (*hydropneumothorax*) are usually present, and x-ray is needed only for later confirmation. The mortality rate is high, but prompt treatment saves many lives. Closed drainage should be instituted at once.

Postoperative Empyema. In postoperative empyema the treatment depends upon the nature of the previous operation. If all or nearly all of the lung is still present, the treatment does not differ from that which is used in postpneumonic empyema, except that a bronchial fistula will nearly always be present. Infection following the removal of the whole lung is extremely troublesome to treat, since the entire pleural cavity is infected and there is no simple method of collapsing or filling that space. In the event that open drainage, irrigation, and antibiotic therapy are unavailing, a plastic procedure to collapse the cavity is necessary.

SUMMARY

Lung abscess, bronchiectasis, and empyema thoracis are the common suppurative infections of the lung and pleurae. Successful treatment requires a combination of general medical care, antibiotics, and surgery. In the nursing care of these patients skills in the technics of postural drainage, "water seal" suction drainage, and in the care of oxygen therapy equipment are necessary.

VOCABULARY REVIEW

bronchoscopy	*Montgomery*	*thoracoplasty*
bronchiectasis	*straps*	*pneumonectomy*
lobectomy	*bronchopleural*	
empyema	*fistula*	

SUGGESTED READING

1. Bickford, Ellinor, and Budd, Esther: Pulmonary Resection. Am. J. Nursing, 52:40–41 (January) 1952.
2. Bugden, Walter F.: Pulmonary Resection. Am. J. Nursing, 52:38–39 (January) 1952.
3. Carr, Duane, and Robbins, S. Gwin: Streptokinase and Antibiotics in the Treatment of Clotted Hemothorax. Ann. Surgery, 133:853–866 (June) 1951.
4. Pulaski, Edwin J., and White, Thomas T.: Streptomycin in Surgical Infections; Lung Abscess and Empyema. Ann. Surg., 128:312–318 (August) 1948.
5. Touroff, A. S. W., Nabatoff, R. A., and Neuhof, H.: Acute Putrid Abscess of Lung. J. Thoracic Surgery, 20:266–271 (August) 1950.

CHAPTER 13

Surgery of
Pulmonary Tuberculosis

Of the various forms of human infection with the tubercle bacillus, pulmonary tuberculosis is the most common, and is one of the major causes of death. The student nurse, during the course of her study of medical diseases, has already become familiar with the clinical picture, the diagnosis, and the general medical care of the patient who has pulmonary tuberculosis.[1] She is also well aware of the importance of early case-finding on a community-wide basis, and of the need for isolation of the infectious patient. The treatment of pulmonary tuberculosis is primarily medical; new and promising chemotherapeutic and antibiotic agents are under extensive trial. There are, however, indications for surgical therapy in this disease.

COLLAPSE THERAPY

In pulmonary tuberculosis the lung is the site of the infection; it is therefore to the lung that specific measures to produce physiologic rest are directed. The first of these is to teach the patient to control and minimize coughing. With practice and perseverance this ordinarily violent movement of the diaphragm and other muscles of respiration can be reduced to one that is barely perceptible.

[1] See Brown, pages 985–1026.

The regular activity of the lung is breathing; since one must breathe to live, it would seem impossible at first glance to put the lung at rest. Experience has shown, however, that if the patient restricts his physical activity and thus reduces to a minimum the oxygen need of his body, a small amount of healthy lung is sufficient to oxygenate the blood. The student can get a rough idea of the minimum amount of lung needed by contrasting the volume of air ordinarily inspired by a person at rest (300 to 400 cc. per breath) and the vital capacity (2 to 3 liters normal average). Furthermore, the lung, in common with most of the organs and tissues of the body, possesses the ability to increase its capacity for work: one lobe may, in time, be able to accomplish nearly as much oxygenation of the blood as was originally accomplished by the whole lung.

In order to rest an affected hand, a patient may wear his arm in a sling; he may refrain from speaking to rest the vocal cords; but no one can voluntarily restrict the activity of one lung. This must be done by means of artificial collapse of a part or all of the lung, and it is the accomplishment of this collapse that is the principal aim of nearly all the surgical procedures undertaken for the cure of pulmonary tuberculosis.

The ideal type for collapse therapy is the patient who has an early infection limited to one lung, and in such a case the prognosis is good. Even in patients with advanced tuberculosis of one lung much can be accomplished. The collapse of a tuberculous cavity in the lung may convert an "open" lesion into a "closed" one; the patient thus ceases to expectorate large quantities of virulent tubercle bacilli and is no longer highly infective both to himself and to others. In mild cases of bilateral disease a partial bilateral collapse is often successful, but in advanced tuberculosis of the lungs the outlook is grave and collapse therapy is usually not feasible.

The general condition of the patient is a matter for careful study; tuberculous patients, as a rule, are sicker than they appear, and withstand poorly any surgical procedure or postoperative complication.

The use of the roentgen ray in diagnosing and following the clinical course of the tuberculous patient is probably the most important modern contribution to the subject. By means of repeated fluoroscopic examinations and regular x-ray film studies, it is possible to make early diagnoses and to follow in exact detail the results of collapse therapy.

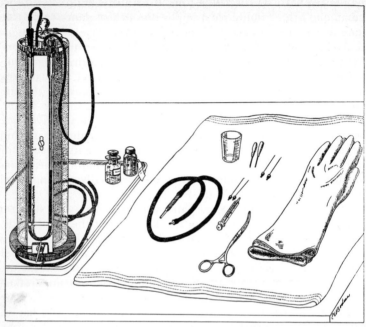

FIGURE 52. Set-up for administering artificial pneumothorax.

Technics of Pulmonary Collapse

The methods for obtaining pulmonary collapse are: (1) pneumothorax; (2) oleothorax; (3) phrenic nerve block; (4) pneumonolysis; and (5) thoracoplasty.

Pneumothorax. The simplest and most effective means of collapsing part or all of a lung is the induction of artificial pneumothorax. After infiltration of the chest wall with procaine, a needle is carefully introduced into the pleural space and a measured amount of air is slowly injected. The lung is thus pushed away from the inner chest wall. Certain precautions are necessary. Strict asepsis must be observed, although the air that is used is ordinarily not sterilized, there being too few pathogenic organisms in a small amount of clean air to cause an infection. A pressure of only a few millimeters of water should be used to inject the air, for a high pressure may tear adhesions or the lung itself, causing hemorrhage or infection, or both. The amount of air used on the first occasion should be limited to 300 to 500 cc., since the patient must be permitted to adjust himself gradually to the reduction in his vital capacity. The amount of pulmonary collapse is visualized under the fluoroscope or on x-ray films, and at further sittings additional amounts of air are introduced until the desired amount of collapse is obtained. The air thus injected is slowly absorbed by the pleura, and it is necessary, therefore, to add more air from time to time, usually at intervals of six weeks to three months.

The advantages of this method for obtaining collapse are its simplicity and ease; the collapse need not be permanent (when the lesion is healed the affected lung may be allowed to expand and resume its normal function); and in favorable cases a more complete collapse of the lung can be secured than by any other method.

On the other hand, the impermanence of the method is at times a disadvantage: there is necessity for refills, and the collapse is not constantly maintained. Furthermore, the presence of pleural adhesions may make the collapse incomplete or impossible. There is also the not too remote possibility that a massive empyema will result from the introduction of pathogenic bacteria or from the tearing of a delicate adhesion between the pleura and the lung. By and large, however, artificial pneumothorax is safe and successful; it is used widely and, in fact, so commonly that it is scarcely regarded as a surgical procedure.

Pneumoperitoneum. Another method used to obtain collapse of the pulmonary tissue is pneumoperitoneum. Large amounts of air are introduced by needle into the peritoneal cavity. This air naturally rises into the subphrenic spaces if the patient is upright, and will push the diaphragm upward into the thorax. As in pneumothorax, the air is gradually absorbed and refills are necessary.

Oleothorax. The necessity for refills inherent in a program of treatment by means of artificial pneumothorax led to the trial of substances other than air for compression of the lung. The ideal material would be nonabsorbable, fluid, and light in weight. In some clinics a light paraffin base oil is used. Following the successful induction of collapse by means of artificial pneumothorax, an equal amount of oil is substituted for the intrapleural air. Refills are unnecessary. Even the most inert substances are somewhat irritating to the pleura, however, and adhesions form which render reexpansion of the lung impossible, should it be later desired; there is also the difficulty of completely removing the oil.

An additional real danger lies in the presence of so much foreign material if empyema should occur. This method is not widely used at present.

Phrenic Nerve Block. The paired phrenic nerves serve as pathways for the impulses which control the activity of the powerful diaphragmatic muscles. Arising from the fourth and fifth cervical nerves, the phrenics are deeply situated in the neck, pass into the mediastinum along with the great blood vessels, and then course down to the diaphragm on either side. Division of one of the phrenic nerves results in flaccid paralysis of the diaphragm on the same side. The paralyzed diaphragm balloons upward, and the volume of the pleural cavity on that side is thus much reduced. This makes available an additional means of furthering the collapse of a lung.

Paralysis of the diaphragm is second only to pneumothorax in value, and is used to secure collapse in patients who have had unsuccessful or only partly successful pneumothoraces. Some authorities, indeed, are of the opinion that phrenic nerve block should be used in conjunction with nearly all pneumothoraces as well as in the unsuccessful ones.

Fortunately for the surgeon there is one portion of the phrenic nerve which is readily accessible. After procaine infiltration of the skin at the base of the neck, a small incision is made just above and parallel to the inner portion of the clavicle. The phrenic nerve is here easily exposed and identified. In the case of patients who have a good prognosis, with expectation of using the lung after the lesions are healed, the procedure of choice is to crush the nerve thoroughly without dividing it. Immediate paralysis of the diaphragm results, but it is not permanent since the nerve will regenerate in six to nine months. In the case of those needing permanent collapse, however, the nerve is divided (*phrenicectomy*) and a segment of it removed so that regeneration is effectively prevented. In competent hands the operation is without risk, and can be performed almost without regard to the general condition of the patient. After phrenic nerve block, the patient is kept flat in bed with no exercise for twenty-four hours; he is not even permitted to feed himself. By thus reducing the patient's activity, respiratory activity is held to a minimum, affording optimal conditions for elevation and fixation of the paralyzed diaphragm.

Pneumonolysis. In some patients the accomplishment of a satisfactory collapse is prevented by adhesions between the lung

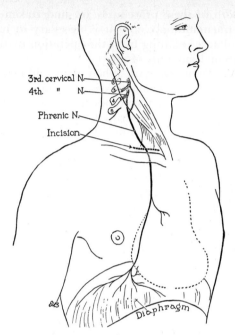

3rd. cervical N.
4th.   "   N.
Phrenic N.
Incision

Diaphragm

FIGURE 53. Phrenic nerve block.

and the inner chest wall. When such adhesions are few in number, the surgeon may undertake their division (*pneumonolysis*) so that a better collapse can be obtained. In performing an open intrapleural pneumonolysis the chest is opened and the adhesions are divided under direct vision; this method has the advantages afforded by good exposure so that bleeding and injury to the lung may be avoided, but has the disadvantage of being a rather severe procedure to carry out on ill patients. Closed intrapleural pneumonolysis is performed by inserting into the pleural space a cystoscope-like instrument equipped with cautery and light; adhesions are divided by means of the cautery. This operation is readily accomplished under local anesthesia, even in very ill patients, but has certain inherent disadvantages: not all adhesions are accessible, and there may be great difficulty in controlling bleeding. A risk attendant upon both methods is that of infection, for often the lung is drawn up into the adhesive band so that bacteria may be spilled into the pleural sac upon division of the band. Both of these procedures are undertaken as adjuncts to artificial pneumothorax, and it is necessary to maintain the additional collapse resulting from the operation by the introduction of additional amounts of air.

Extrapleural Pneumonolysis. When many and dense adhesions prevent intrapleural pneumonolysis, the procedure of extrapleural pneumonolysis is sometimes undertaken. In this operation an attempt is made to strip the parietal pleura from the inner surface of the intercostal muscles and ribs, thus forming an extrapleural space into which air may be introduced to maintain collapse. As a rule, this radical procedure is poorly tolerated by ill patients, and is therefore seldom used.

Extrapleural Thoracoplasty. As a final method of obtaining collapse of the lung the surgeon can carry out plastic procedures upon the chest wall (*thoracoplasty*) which actually reduce the capacity of the chest. A number of different methods have been evolved, but the essential feature of all of these is the removal of some part of the bony thoracic cage, permitting the soft parts of the chest wall to fall in upon the lung.

Thoracoplasty is a major surgical procedure, and an irrevocable one; therefore the greatest care must be used in selecting the proper patients and in choosing the proper time for operation. Patients with progressive unilateral tuberculosis, in whom all other forms of collapse therapy have been unsuccessful or are impossible, are suitable for thoracoplasty. An advantage of the procedure is that it may be divided into multiple stages, so that no more need be attempted at one time than the patient can tolerate.

By careful preparation the patient is gotten into as good general condition as possible. Phrenic nerve block should, of course, be carried out before thoracoplasty, in order to secure the maximum degree of collapse. Selection of the time for operation is based upon such considerations as the patient's temperature, pulse rate, weight, hemoglobin, and mental attitude. Preparations should be made for blood transfusion. General or local anesthesia may be used. The incision is usually made between the inner border of the scapula and the spine, and is carried down around the lower angle of the scapula. The heavy muscles are divided, and the scapula is then easily retracted laterally, giving good exposure of the posterior portions of all the ribs. Beginning at the upper end, segments of the ribs are removed, the utmost care being taken not to enter the pleural space, or to traumatize the lung in any way. The attempt is made to remove as much of

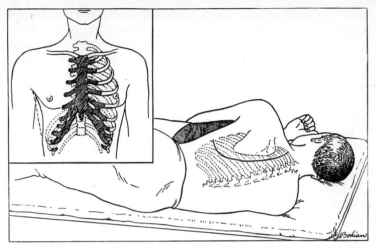

FIGURE 54. Position of patient on operating table and location of incision for left thoracoplasty. Insert shows final result of right thoracoplasty; despite extensive removal of ribs there is little outward evidence of deformity.

each rib as possible, from the vertebral attachments posteriorly to the costal cartilages anteriorly. In very ill patients the operation is terminated after the removal of two ribs, but stronger patients may tolerate the removal of three or four. The scapula is replaced, the muscles and skin are sutured, and a snug dressing is applied to compress the chest wall as much as possible. The patient's condition is estimated by his pulse rate, blood pressure, and color; significant change in any of these is a warning to stop the operation at once. The comfort of the patient and the degree of collapse after operation are increased by the use of sandbags or a bag containing buckshot. Some surgeons prefer to have the patient lie with the operative side down, upon correctly placed sandbags, while other surgeons prefer to have the operative side uppermost, weighted down by a saddle-shaped bag of shot.

Intervals of two to three weeks between stages are the most satisfactory, since a shorter time does not permit full recovery of the patient, and a longer interval tends to lessen the degree of ultimate collapse because there is some regeneration of the ribs from the periosteum which is not removed. Strong patients in good condition will tolerate a two-stage thoracoplasty, but very ill patients will require three or more stages. The same incision is used for the later stages.

The final result is a permanent one, and the degree of collapse is considerable, although not quite so complete as with the most successful pneumothoraces.

There is great deformity of the chest, but this is not too obvious when the patient is clothed. When the patient has regained sufficient strength, the outward appearance of this deformity can be largely overcome by the use of exercises designed to strengthen the muscles of the back, thus preventing undue curvature of the spine and lowering of the shoulder on the operative side.

Complications. Despite every precaution, serious complications often follow thoracoplasty. Surgical shock may occur, and is best treated by prevention, that is, by stopping the operation before the patient becomes shocked. Postoperative hemorrhage is uncommon. Cyanosis due to the sudden reduction in vital capacity is of frequent occurrence, and is treated by the use of the oxygen tent or mask. Fat embolism occurs occasionally as the result of the multiple rib resections. Spread of the tuberculosis may take place if the lung has been traumatized. Infection of the wound and empyema are also serious though infrequent sequelae of the operation.

Combined Thoracoplasty and Segmental Resection. In recent years more radical operative procedures have been carried out in selected patients. Since the upper portion of the upper lobe of the lung is most often involved, it has seemed beneficial to remove the diseased portion of the lung in combination with extrapleural thoracoplasty. This has the great advantage of eradicating the focus of infection and thus eliminating the possibility of spread of the disease.

Nursing Care of Patient with Thoracoplasty. The patient admitted to the surgical unit usually comes from a tuberculosis sanatorium where he has had excellent teaching in proper self-care. He is well aware that the uncovered cough, the contact of his hand with his mouth and the contamination of other areas by his hands are the greatest hazards in the spread of the bacilli. He has learned the importance of procedures necessary to protect others from infection. His spirits are usually low. He knows that thoracoplasty is his last chance for collapse therapy and cure. He heard much in the sanatorium about deformity following thoracoplasty and must be reassured early about methods for overcoming this.

Isolating him in a room from surgical patients with other conditions is essential. In caring for him all personnel must conscientiously carry out respiratory isolation technic to protect themselves and the other patients against infection.

After being accustomed to the association with many other patients at the sanatorium, this complete isolation brings on loneliness unless there is adequate diversional therapy. Providing the patient with a radio, reading material and an appropriate form of occupational therapy for use before operation and during the periods of convalescence will help him to pass the time.

Preoperatively the care depends on the various examinations, supportive therapy and instruction which the surgeon orders according to the individual patient. Usually it includes x-rays, the collection of sputum specimens, vital capacity tests and bronchoscopy. Antibiotics and a high vitamin, high caloric diet with adequate fluid intake are essential. Frequently the patient is taught abdominal breathing by the physical therapist. The force of the abdominal muscles against the viscera pushes up the diaphragm to allow for exchange of air from the lower lobes of the lungs. At least three days before operation, teaching the patient the essentials of good posture while sitting up and lying in bed is begun by the physical therapist and/or nurse. There is need for the patient to understand the criteria of good posture so that the direction of activity between stages and after operation is met with cooperation in order to keep the disfigurement at a minimum.

The immediate preoperative care for all stages is similar to other types of chest surgery. In addition to the usual postoperative unit, oxygen equipment is necessary and it is advisable that an aspirator be close at hand.

Following operation, the patient is placed in the lateral position. If the patient's blood pressure is low, the foot of the bed should be raised. He should be turned every hour for the first twelve hours and every two hours thereafter. Some surgeons order the patient to be turned only on the side of operation and the back, while others permit him to turn on either side. The rate and quality of the pulse, the blood pressure, the color of the patient and the dressings should be observed as for any patient with chest surgery; unfavorable signs and symptoms should be immediately reported to the surgeon. The chest should be exposed frequently the first day to observe the respirations of the patient to insure that exchange of air is normal. Paradoxical respirations, in which the weakened chest wall is sucked in during inspiration, may occur and must be reported immediately.

The patient must be made to cough each hour. The nurse

should give analgesics and splint the wound with the palm of her hand to help prevent pain while coughing. When coughing is not forceful enough, pharyngeal suctioning with an aspirator will stimulate coughing and also remove excess mucus.

Intravenous fluids are administered at intervals until there is adequate intake by mouth; antibiotics are given as ordered. The diet is increased according to the tolerance of the patient. Oxygen therapy is usually discontinued after twenty-four hours or when breathing is easy without an increase in rate of respiration or dyspnea.

It has been found that giving the patient special attention such as turning him, rubbing his back and reassuring him at regular intervals will lessen the demand for medications to relieve pain. To withhold medications when necessary should be guarded against, but good nursing care directed toward making the patient feel that those caring for him are interested, without any demands from him, tends to lessen tension, gives him peace of mind and seems to lessen pain.

Usually, on the third day following each stage of the thoracoplasty the nurse or physical therapist assists the patient in exercising the arm on the operative side. The exercises are limited to the tolerance of the patient and must not be carried out when there are signs of dyspnea. He should be encouraged to move freely in bed and to move his arm in all directions, increasing his activities according to his tolerance. At first weariness takes place with only a small amount of motion; encouragement and reassurance are necessary. As his condition improves, appealing to his sense of pride and emphasizing that people with good posture command respect and admiration from others are worth while in raising his morale. Placing a large mirror on the wall, where he may observe himself while sitting up in bed, not only makes him more conscious of his position but also enables him to practice posture toward better alignment.

He is usually permitted out of bed for short periods of time between operations. This not only helps raise his morale but also tends to improve muscle strength.

He is usually transferred to the sanatorium about ten days after the last operation. Each patient's activity is increased according to his condition, but, by and large, he is quite inactive and recuperates as a bed patient for the first three months after his return to the sanatorium. After this, he is permitted out of bed. Gradually his activities are increased and bed rest is decreased so that after another two to six months he is permitted to return home. During his whole convalescence he is encouraged to maintain good posture.

None of these patients are permitted to return to work until one year after the operation. The work that they may do is often restricted to that which is sedentary or that which requires a minimum amount of exertion. However, many patients have been able to increase their activities remarkably.

Frequent check-ups by the doctor are emphasized so that close follow-up care may be given. These people can lead useful and reasonably normal lives.

TUBERCULOUS EMPYEMA

Tubercle bacilli may gain access to the pleural space either by direct spread from the lung, or as the result of tearing the tuberculous lung during the performance of any of the surgical procedures that are undertaken to produce collapse. The empyema caused by the tubercle bacilli is apt to be low grade rather than fulminating, but it is progressive and very resistant to treatment. The walls of the empyema cavity are made up of typical tuberculous granulation tissue, and become enormously thickened and scarred, contributing to the difficulty of the cure. The various forms of surgical drainage do not constitute adequate treatment for tuberculous empyema and, indeed, are likely to be harmful, for secondary bacterial invaders may enter the drained cavity and cause a mixed infection.

Tuberculous empyema should be suspected when the symptoms and signs of fluid in the pleural space appear in patients who are known to have active pulmonary tuberculosis. Examination of the fluid serves to differentiate empyema from a simple pleural effusion, a condition that often accompanies early tuberculous activity but tends to disappear with the onset of healing. The most successful treatment consists in collapsing the empyema cavity by thoracoplasty, care being taken not to enter the empyema cavity during the procedure. If the cavity is broken into, tuberculous infection of the wound results and may be extremely troublesome to clear up. In favorable cases the empyema will heal, but the percentage of cures is far lower than in the other forms of empyema.

The rupture into the pleural space of a tuberculous cavity causes a fulminating, highly fatal form of empyema, similar in most respects to that which follows the spontaneous intrapleural rupture of a pulmonary abscess. In this instance the tuberculous infection is complicated by a secondary mixed infection of great virulence, and at times by a bronchial fistula. In these cases immediate surgical drainage is necessary to save the patient's life even though the course of the tuberculous infection is little influenced. This can be dealt with later if the patient survives the initial mixed infection.

TUBERCULOSIS OF THE RIBS AND STERNUM

These lesions are nearly always secondary to pulmonary tuberculosis, and often are caused by direct extension of the disease from the lung to the bones and cartilages of the thoracic cage. There is first a little swelling of the affected part, but no pain or redness. Gradually the typical "cold abscess" of tuberculosis develops; fluctuation appears but still there is no pain. Aspiration of the lesion yields thick creamy pus from which the tubercle bacilli can be recovered. Finally, if the lesion progresses, the overlying skin becomes red, shiny, and thin; ultimately rupture occurs, and pus is discharged. Unlike other abscesses, this lesion does not heal following drainage or rupture: a draining sinus remains.

As in all forms of tuberculosis, healing depends upon the patient's resistance. In favorable cases the lesion may regress, finally healing with only a scar left to mark the site. In addition to general measures directed toward the improvement of the patient's condition, healing may be expedited by the surgical excision of the infected portion of bone or cartilage where this is feasible.

SUMMARY

Nursing the patient who is having surgery for pulmonary tuberculosis constitutes a great challenge, for these patients are long-term problems, are critically ill, and require much reassurance, and instruction as well as regular nursing care. The need for careful isolation technic is emphasized. Collapse of the diseased lung tissue is the goal; removal of the diseased segment combined with collapse of the space previously occupied by this segment is receiving extensive trial. Antibiotic agents have improved the outlook greatly.

VOCABULARY REVIEW

sanatorium	*extrapleural*	*dyspnea*
pneumonolysis	*paradoxical*	*thoracoplasty*
artificial	*respiration*	
pneumothorax		

SUGGESTED READING

1. About the New Anti-tuberculosis Drugs. Am. J. Nursing, *52*:574 (May) 1952.
2. Ellison, Bess M.: Nursing Care in Collapse Therapy. Am. J. Nursing, *50:* 473–475 (August) 1950.
3. Getz, H.: Nutrition and Tuberculosis. Nutrition Review, *5*:97 (April) 1947.
4. Kezar, Vera: Tuberculosis with Pneumonectomy. Am. J. Nursing, *49:*188– 199 (March) 1949.
5. Riley, Arnold O., and Longhurst, Grace M.: Pulmonary Decortication. Am. J. Nursing, *52*:878–880 (July) 1952.
6. South, Jean, and Jones, Frank T.: Tuberculosis Control in the General Hospital. Am. J. Nursing, *52*:1094–1095 (Sept.) 1952.
7. Tetbrock, Harry E., Fisher, Martin M., and Mamlok, Eric R.: The New Drug —Isoniazid. Am. J. Nursing, *52*:1342–1344 (Nov.) 1952.

CHAPTER 14

Neoplastic Disease
of the Respiratory Organs

The entire respiratory tract is lined by epithelial cells which are subjected to nearly as much wear and tear as are the epithelial cells of the skin. It is not surprising to find, then, that epithelial tumors of the respiratory tract are common. There are several different types of epithelial cells among the myriads which form the lining of the respiratory tract and, therefore, there are several kinds of epithelial tumors, some of them benign and others malignant.

The lungs, pleura, and mediastinum are also extremely common sites for metastases from tumors located elsewhere, because of the constant return of blood and lymph from the other organs and the extremities.

PRIMARY NEOPLASMS OF THE BRONCHI AND LUNGS

Tumors of the lung occur in patients of all ages, but are more common after the fourth decade of life. The usual first complaint is a persistent nonproductive cough. Expectoration of blood (*hemoptysis*) is another frequent symptom. The quantity is ordinarily small, and great care must be taken to discover the origin of the blood, since slight bleeding from the nasopharynx or gums is common. A sensation of constriction or oppression in the chest may occur; at times there is actual pain. Later, if the tumor is malignant, loss of weight and weakness (*cachexia*) are noted. An early, small neoplasm is not readily detected by physical diagnosis or roentgenography. As the tumor becomes larger, or when the changes incident to obstruction of a bronchus occur, physical signs and x-ray evidence appear. Another common occurrence is the formation of fluid in the pleural sac (*hydrothorax* or *pleural effusion*); such fluid often contains blood and, at times, recognizable tumor cells.

Since the onset of pulmonary tumors is usually insidious, many patients have no complaints until the tumor has been present for a considerable time. In many cases it is also most difficult to find out whether the patient has a tumor or tuberculosis, a matter of great importance since the treatment of the two conditions is so different. Careful examination of the sputum is necessary. Bronchoscopy is a routine procedure, and will reveal tumors situated in, or adjacent to, the trachea and the main bronchi. When the growth can be seen, a small portion is removed for study (biopsy). When no tumor is visible, further information can be obtained from roentgen films made after the introduction of Lipiodol into the bronchial tree. Irregularities in the bronchial outlines and obstructions of the bronchi or bronchioles are thus visualized.

Benign Tumors. A common tumor arising from the lining of the trachea or the bronchi is the benign epithelial *papilloma*. A tiny tumor of this sort growing in the trachea or stem bronchus may cause a most distressing cough; fortunately most of these small papillomata can be destroyed successfully by *fulguration* (electric cauterization) through a bronchoscope. Biopsy and an exact diagnosis must be made before treatment, because malignant tumors do not respond favorably to such therapy.

When situated in a smaller bronchus, the papilloma cannot be seen, and is likely to be untreated until it is large enough to obstruct the small bronchus, so that the first symptoms and signs are those incident to the resultant bronchiectasis. The proper treatment under these circumstances is the removal of the involved segment of the lung.

Cancer of the Lung. Prior to 1933 cancer of the lung was a uniformly fatal disease; in that year Graham successfully removed a cancerous lung and thereby cured the patient. Since then much knowledge has been gained in regard to the technic of complete removal of a lung (*total pneumonectomy*). Primary carcinoma of the lung is nearly as common a disease as carcinoma of the stomach, and is similarly difficult to cure because the tumor grows insidiously and without symptoms: diagnosis is seldom made before the growth has extended beyond the confines of the organ from which it has arisen. These tumors do not respond well to radiation therapy, and until some better means is discovered, the patient's best chance lies in the early diagnosis of the disease followed by prompt removal of the affected lung. It is, of course, true that if the tumor involves the trachea or the mediastinum, or has invaded the pleura or the chest wall, or if there are metastases elsewhere, removal of the lung will not be curative.

Total Pneumonectomy

The removal of an entire lung is indeed a formidable procedure, but when carried out properly the mortality rate is low and the discomfort and disability surprisingly little. As a result of this operation, all of the exchange of gases between the air and the circulating blood must be carried out in the remaining lung.

Anesthesia. During the operation, the anesthesiologist must be able to control respiration at all times; this necessitates the use of an intratracheal tube and the use of positive pressure while the chest is open. Since there is ventilation of but one lung, the anesthetic agents used must necessarily permit the use of a high concentration of oxygen.

Operation. Most surgeons prefer the posterior approach. The pulmonary artery and the pulmonary veins are carefully isolated, ligated and divided. The main bronchus is also divided, and the stump tightly closed by suturing. The whole lung is then removed from the pleural cavity, together with adjacent mediastinal lymph nodes. The chest wall is closed tightly without drainage.

The student may well ask what occupies the space in the chest formerly filled by the lung. A large part of that space is obliterated by a gradual shifting of the mediastinal structures toward the operative side, and by the elevated position of the paralyzed diaphragm. The cavity remaining, however, is still large, and eventually comes to be filled by a curious tissue, like Swiss cheese, probably the end result of the coagulation and organization of tissue fluid that gradually accumulates there. If, on the other hand, the cavity becomes infected, as may happen when the bronchial stump leaks, healing does not follow simple drainage of the infection: it is necessary to collapse the cavity by means of some type of thoracoplasty.

Complications. This undeniably hazardous operation is likely to cause some degree of surgical shock, and intravenous fluid, preferably whole blood, should be administered during the procedure. Just as after lobectomy, the most serious complications are hemorrhage and leaking of the stump of the bronchus; following pneumonectomy, however, either hemorrhage or infection, or a combination of these is much more dangerous, since the vessels involved are very large ones, and since an infectious process will spread through the entire pleural space. The possible development of a tension pneumothorax must be constantly borne in mind.

Nursing Care. The patient who has cancer of the lung is usually an older person than one who has a resection for bronchiectasis. The general principles of care are the same but, because of the difference in age and a greater physiologic disturbance caused by pneumonectomy, certain aspects of care should be emphasized.

For the first few days, the patient is encouraged to lie only on the operated side and the back to prevent the accumulating fluid in the pleural cavity of the operated side from forcing the mediastinum towards the unoperated side.

The use of oxygen therapy is required for a longer period of time but rarely more than four days. It is judicious to leave the equipment at the bedside for a twenty-four hour period after it is discontinued while the patient is given a trial without oxygen.

The nurse must be especially careful in the administration of parenteral fluids, because of the danger of overloading the circulation, with resultant pulmonary edema. The rate of flow of the fluid should not exceed 50 drops per minute unless specifically ordered. The older the patient, the more necessary is this precaution. Symptoms of this complication are dyspnea, frothy sputum and rales in the chest. The patient should be encouraged to take an adequate amount of fluid by mouth as soon as he has recovered from anesthesia; this will obviate the need for parenteral fluid and thus will minimize the danger of embarrassing the circulation.

Occasionally the surgeon drains the cavity through a catheter into a water seal bottle, but usually the fluid is not removed. Changes in respirations should be noted and dyspnea or cyanosis should be reported immediately.

The advantages of early ambulation are obvious but an older person who has had his entire lung removed should not be forced out of bed too soon. The surgeon will allow the patient to be up according to the individual case.

Prevention of atelectasis in the remaining lung is aided by encouraging the patient to cough and breathe deeply to force out the accumulated secretions. Intratracheal aspiration may be necessary.

A high caloric, high vitamin, high protein diet should be given. Encouraging the patient to eat is essential so that weight loss and strength may be regained.

During the convalescent period in the hospital, which is usually not less than two weeks, the patient should be taught the essentials of good posture. Abdominal breathing exercises have been helpful by lowering the diaphragm and thus increasing the vital capacity.

Before the patient leaves the hospital, a return appointment to the surgeon should be made. Follow-up care is essential and the patient should have an explanation concerning this.

Guidance for activities during the period of convalescence should be outlined for the patient. Gradually, exercise may be increased but only according to tolerance. The patient finds that dyspnea comes on very quickly at first, but that this decreases greatly after several months of convalescence. Many patients are able to resume work, when not physically strenuous, and enjoy an active life.

NEOPLASMS OF THE MEDIASTINUM AND CHEST WALL

The mediastinum contains such important structures as the heart, the great vessels, the trachea, the esophagus, the thymus, and many lymph nodes. If one excepts tumors of the trachea and esophagus, it is a fact that the great majority of the remainder of mediastinal tumors are the result of secondary (*metastatic*) invasion of lymph nodes by malignant tumors arising elsewhere in the body. For such a condition, obviously, surgery affords no hope of cure. Benign tumors of the mediastinum do occur, however, and are usually dermoid cysts, arising probably as the result of some mischance during fetal development.

Tumors of the mediastinum do not, as a rule, produce any symptoms until they reach sufficient size to encroach upon the adjacent structures, and these symptoms vary depending upon which structures are involved. The first complaint may be a cough, from pressure on the trachea, or there may be difficulty in swallowing due to pressure upon the esophagus. A feeling of substernal weight or oppression is not uncommon. Examination usually shows enlargement of some portion of the mediastinum, which is confirmed by the x-ray film.

The surgical removal of benign tumors of the mediastinum is accomplished with but little risk, and cure is permanent. The same operative approach is used as for pneumonectomy.

Since the chest wall is composed of skin, muscles, bone, cartilage, nerves, and blood vessels, it is not surprising that there is a considerable variety of neoplasms. In general, these tumors are the same as those arising from similar tissues elsewhere in the body, and must be diagnosed and treated in the same way. In the past, the surgeon was somewhat limited in the removal of malignant neoplasms of the chest wall by the fact that extensive defects in the chest wall were not compatible with life since the mechanics of intrathoracic pressure were altered. It is now possible to remove a large portion of the chest wall, replacing the ribs and muscle with tantalum mesh. This nonreactive metal prosthesis serves to stabilize the thoracic wall, permitting normal respiration.

SUMMARY

Pain in the chest, persistent cough, and bloody sputum may be symptoms of cancer of the lung. If discovered early, cure is attainable by removal of the lung, an operation which is attended by surprisingly little disability afterward.

VOCABULARY REVIEW

hemoptysis	*pneumonectomy*	*tantalum mesh*
papilloma	*dermoid cyst*	*pulmonary edema*

SUGGESTED READING

1. A Cancer Source Book for Nurses. American Cancer Society, Inc., New York, 1950, pp. 82–84.
2. Cancer Nursing. National Cancer Institute and N. Y. State Dept. of Health, 1950, pp. 56, 74.
3. Graham, Evarts A.: Considerations of Bronchiogenic Carcinoma. Ann. Surg., *132*:176–187 (August) 1950.
4. Overholt, R. H.; and Schmidt, I. C.: Silent Phase of Cancer of the Lung. J.A.M.A., *141*:817–820 (November 19) 1949.
5. Sweet, Richard H.: Thoracic Surgery. Philadelphia, W. B. Saunders Co., 1951, pp. 171–179.

CHAPTER 15

Circulatory Disturbances:
Thrombosis; Embolism; Gangrene

Physiology of Circulation. The circulating blood brings the necessities of life to the cells of the body, and takes from them the products of metabolism. To maintain the circulation is the task of the vascular system. The powerful rhythmic contractions of the heart pump the blood into the aorta and the large arteries which arise from it; the elasticity of the thick muscular walls of these vessels helps to force the pulsating stream of blood into the smaller arteries and arterioles. The blood finally reaches the numerous tiny capillaries. These have thin walls, and are so arranged that the blood which courses through them moves at a relatively slow rate, which allows time for the exchange of chemicals between the blood and the tissues.

The blood in the capillaries drains into venules, which are tributaries of the larger veins that accompany the main arteries;

149

finally the blood reaches the great veins which empty into the heart. Veins have thin walls in contrast to arteries, and the blood is impelled through the veins not so much by the pumping action of the heart as by a combination of other means. The force imparted to the stream of arterial blood by the heart gradually diminishes until there is only a slight impulse left when the blood passes out of the capillaries into the venules; consequently, venous pressure is much lower than arterial pressure. But blood must be returned to the heart as rapidly as it is pumped out, since, obviously, the heart could not keep up its output without an equal inflow. There are at least three factors contributing to the solution of this problem: the large size of the veins as compared with the arteries, the squeezing action of the muscles of the body, and the sucking action of the chest during inspiration.

Since venous pressure is low, one might wonder why the blood in the veins does not reverse the direction of its flow during expiration, especially when the intrathoracic pressure is suddenly increased as in coughing or sneezing; the force of gravity, too, in the dependent arms or legs tends to pull the blood away from the heart. In order to prevent the occurrence of retrograde blood flow, some veins are supplied with valves. These are small cuplike projections which are held against the wall of the vein as long as the blood moves toward the heart. If the flow begins to reverse, the lumen is closed by these delicate valves which are filled by the flow of blood, much as an umbrella is filled out by a sudden gust of wind. Retrograde flow does not occur when the valves are competent.

Despite the wide distribution of the blood in the capillary vessels throughout the body, a supplemental network is necessary. The chief arteries and veins might be likened to the highways which connect great cities; the capillaries would then represent the main street of a city. Not every resident lives on a main street, however; and not every cell of the body is situated along the wall of a capillary. Each cell, nevertheless, must receive its share of the chemicals carried by the blood, and must have an outlet for its products. This service is rendered by a system composed of the myriads of minute spaces between cells (*tissue spaces*) and the lymphatic channels with which they communicate. *Lymph* (or tissue juice) is a colorless fluid which in composition closely approximates blood serum. It may, in fact, be blood serum which has left the vascular system through the thin walls of the capillaries. In any case, adequate exchange of chemicals, including oxygen, takes place between the circulating blood and many of the cells of the body through the mediation of this tissue fluid.

Much of the tissue fluid returns to the circulating blood through the capillary walls, but some of it collects in the tiny thin-walled lymph vessels. These are widely distributed, and the lymph vessels of each part of the body drain into the lymph nodes of that region. Eventually lymph is returned to the vascular system, either into the blood vessels of the lymph nodes or directly into the veins.

The arteries and the veins, especially the smaller terminal vessels, are richly supplied with nerves. These nerves emanate from the sympathetic division of the autonomic nervous system; thus stimuli which activate the sympathetic system affect the tone of the muscle fibers in the walls of blood vessels. Stimulation of the nerves by such a drug as ephedrine causes, in most instances, contraction of the vessels, with a consequent diminution of the blood flow to the affected areas, whereas paralysis of the nerves, as by procaine, permits dilatation of the vessels with attendant increase of blood flow.

An additional fact of importance, and one which is peculiar to the vascular system, is the arrangement of collateral vessels. By means of the frequent communications between the smaller branches of the main arteries and veins respectively, the vascular system is able in most regions to overcome the effect of an obstruction to the circulation. Thus, following the occlusion of a large artery or vein at one point, the blood may be "detoured" around the obstruction through the communicating branches above and below the obstruction. There are, however, certain regions where adequate collateral circulation does not exist, and some arteries which are terminal arteries, the occlusion of which leaves the affected area without blood supply.

The relationship between the flow of blood through the lungs (*pulmonary circulation*) and the flow through the rest of the body (*systemic circulation*) may be compared to the numeral 8, the upper loop representing the pulmonary circuit, the lower loop representing the systemic circuit, the heart being located at the intersection. It is at once apparent that all blood returning from the body is pumped into the lungs, and all from the lungs into the rest of the body.

The course of blood returning from the stomach, intestines, pancreas, and spleen is unique in that the blood passes through the liver before returning to the systemic circulation. The large

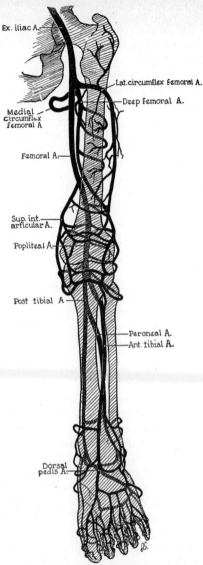

Ex. iliac A.

Lat. circumflex femoral A.

Deep femoral A.

Medial circumflex femoral A

Femoral A.

Sup. int. articular A.

Popliteal A.

Post tibial A

Peroneal A.

Ant. tibial A.

Dorsal pedis A.

FIGURE 55. Diagram of arteries of leg to show the extensive collateral circulation by means of anastomoses between major vessels.

vein, with its tributaries, which collects this blood and delivers it to the liver is the *portal vein,* and this intermediary circuit is called the *portal circulation.* The blood in the portal vein is low in oxygen content, but the liver has a supply of freshly oxygenated blood from the hepatic artery. The blood from the portal vein and the blood from the hepatic artery are ultimately combined inside the liver, leave that organ by way of the hepatic vein, and rejoin the general circulation.

The lymph vessels which drain the tissues of the intestines are known as *lacteals.* These lymphatics are tributaries of a large lymph channel, the thoracic duct, which runs parallel to the spine and finally reaches the left subclavian vein, into which it empties its accumulated lymph. This lymph is known as *chyle,* and contains much fat.

THROMBOSIS

If the delicate endothelial lining of the vessels is intact, the flowing blood does not coagulate; following damage to the vessel wall by accident or from disease, however, a blood clot forms over the injured portion. This coagulation of the blood within the lumen of a vessel (*thrombosis*) is the first step in the process of healing the injury. The blood clot (*thrombus*) acts to protect the damaged wall and to prevent escape of blood if there is an opening in the vessel wall. Successive layers of blood coagulate over the surface of the original clot, producing the characteristic laminated appearance of a fresh thrombus. The lumen of the vessel is filled by the coagulum and the flow of blood is obstructed. Just as in a wound, organization of the thrombus into granulation tissue occurs as the second stage of healing; finally the organized thrombus is transformed into scar tissue. In the scar tissue small channels which permit the passage of blood may be formed (*recanalization*), but rarely is the original capacity of the vessel restored.

The walls of arteries and veins may suffer injury as the result of a blow, a sudden violent twist or pull, or a wound. Bacterial invaders are capable of damaging vessel walls and when the injury is the result of infection the thrombus is often contaminated, with subsequent abscess formation. There are systemic diseases, too, such as arteriosclerosis, thromboangiitis obliterans and others, which affect the walls of the blood vessels. Extremes of heat or cold and certain chemical poisons must also be included in the list of causes of vascular damage.

EMBOLISM

Occasionally a portion or all of a thrombus becomes dislodged and is swept along in the current of the flowing blood until the vessel is too narrow to permit further passage of this plug (*embolus*). There is especial danger when the thrombus originates in one of the peripheral veins, as the embolus passes through the heart into the pulmonary circuit, thus blocking the flow of blood through a portion of the lung (*pulmonary embolism*). Massive pulmonary embolism usually causes sudden death.

Dislodgment of a thrombus is not the only source of embolism, for anything that can plug a vessel will produce the same result upon gaining entrance into the blood. In endocarditis small portions of the diseased heart valves are a frequent cause of embolism. *Fat embolism* sometimes occurs following a severe fracture, as a result of the entrance into the blood of drops of fat from the bone marrow.

Air embolism is well known, too, and is encountered when there is sudden and great reduction in the atmospheric pressure. It occurs in workmen leaving the high atmospheric pressure of underground excavations (*caisson disease*) and in aviators who ascend too rapidly. The symptoms and signs of this condition, known as "the bends," are due to numerous small embolisms from bubbles of air in the blood, just as bubbles appear in a bottle of ginger ale when the cap is removed. The treatment of air embolism from this cause is, of course, to place the patient at once in a high pressure chamber, with resultant return of the air into solution in the blood. The pressure is then slowly lowered, permitting the patient to release the excess air through the lungs. Air embolism also follows the accidental introduction of air into the venous circulation during the course of pneumothorax or pneumoperitoneum therapy.

Embolectomy. Solid emboli must be removed surgically when there is sufficient disturbance of the circulation to justify the risk entailed. The operative removal of an embolus (*embolectomy*) calls for great refinement of technic, since thrombosis is as likely to occur after an operative procedure upon a blood vessel as after any trauma.

Surgeons have long been attracted by the possibility of saving the life of a patient who has a massive pulmonary embolism. On theoretical grounds the removal of the embolus from the pulmonary artery before death occurs is possible, and it has been carried out in a few instances. Unfortunately, there has been no great success in these attempts, largely because the patient dies in two or three minutes, before the surgeons can be assembled and the preparations made. Unless further embolism occurs, patients who survive pulmonary embolism for fifteen minutes or longer usually recover without operative treatment.

Anticoagulants. During the past few years new drugs have been made available which have the ability to alter the natural coagulability of the blood. Chief among these are heparin and Dicumarol. Depending upon the amount of these agents administered to the patient, the clotting of the blood may be delayed, or even temporarily abolished. As might be expected, however, such potent drugs as these are not without their dangers. It was hoped that anticoagulant therapy would find its greatest use in the prevention and treatment of thrombosis and embolism, but so far as surgery is concerned, these agents have not met expectations and continue to be in the nature of experimental drugs.[1]

GANGRENE

When obstruction to the flow of blood through an artery occurs, the tissues supplied by that artery are subjected to a resultant decrease in blood flow (*ischemia*). The degree of ischemia and, therefore, the degree of reduction of the oxygen and other vital supplies depend upon the ability of the collateral vessels to furnish the affected area with blood. When there is no collateral circulation, as in a terminal artery, or when the collateral vessels are affected by the same disease as the main artery, as in arteriosclerosis and other generalized vascular diseases, the tissues are likely to suffer great damage. Prolonged deficiency of arterial blood supply results in starvation of the tissues. The affected part becomes cooler, and is usually pallid or cyanotic. The skin becomes dry, glossy, and inelastic, and muscular atrophy occurs, with consequent scarring. Ulceration is common, and wounds are slow to heal. As might be expected, there is decreased resistance to the entrance and spread of infection.

When the arterial circulation is inadequate, the cells of the affected part die, and this frank mortification of a portion of the body is called gangrene. A line of demarcation appears between the viable and the dead tissue; the gangrenous portion becomes black, shriveled, dry, and finally sloughs away. This description

[1] See Brown, pages 450–451.

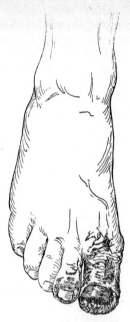

FIGURE 56. Dry gangrene.

applies to the type known as *dry gangrene*. When infection is present the necrotic tissues are boggy, purulent, and foul (*moist gangrene*).

It is important to note that since gangrene, or death of tissues, follows the loss of an adequate supply of arterial blood, it is a potential complication of any disturbance which results in decreased arterial flow.

PHLEGMASIA ALBA DOLENS; LYMPHEDEMA

Blocking of veins, resulting in obstruction to the drainage of blood from the affected region, produces "white swelling" or "milk leg" in the terms of the layman. Since the lymph vessels empty into the venous system, a lymphatic obstruction usually accompanies venous block, with consequent lymphedema. At first there are swelling and pallor; later the tissues become boggy with the accumulation of fluid in the distended lymphatic and tissue spaces, and such areas pit on pressure, as does a soft pillow. There is no rapid death of tissues, but gradually the incomplete removal of waste products and the prolonged pressure of the insufficiently drained blood and lymph injure the less hardy cells. Widespread scarring results, producing a brawny hardness; finally the skin may break down, and painful, chronic ulcers are formed. Chronic lymphedema is called *elephantiasis*.

The collateral vessels of the venous and lymphatic systems are far more abundant than those of the arterial system, consequently a complete venous or lymphatic obstruction is uncommon. The changes seen in phlegmasia alba dolens and in lymphedema are therefore the result of inadequate drainage of the tissues, rather than absence of drainage.

Gangrene or edema may thus occur as the local result of circulatory disturbance although a variety of pathologic conditions may be responsible for the disturbance.

VASOSPASM

Recent investigations of peripheral circulatory disturbances have shown the importance of nervous control over the muscular tone of blood vessels. Muscular contraction (*spasm*), with consequent reduction of the caliber of the vessel, is associated with nearly all pathologic alterations of the vessels; indeed, there is one disease, Raynaud's, in which the symptoms are due entirely to vasospasm without apparent abnormality of the vessels.

The control exerted over the blood vessels by the sympathetic nervous system is an integral part of the everyday physiology of the individual, since digestion, the regulation of body temperature, and physical activity, to mention a few functions, are dependent in part upon the proper adjustment of blood flow. Vasospasm due to or in association with disease is serious, however. For example, spastic contraction of the already partly blocked vessel serves only to increase the obstruction, and spasm of the adjacent portions of that vessel acts to diminish the efficacy of the collateral branches.

DIAGNOSTIC PROCEDURES

The story of the patient's complaints and the record of his previous health and habits constitute the first information to be gathered. Such complaints as numbness, discoloration, or coldness of the extremities and cramps or swelling of the legs suggest circulatory disturbance. The age is significant; degenerative vascular disease is common in the aged, but in the young, vascular abnormalities are usually congenital, traumatic, or spastic in origin. Often the initial symptoms occur during pregnancy or as a complication of some serious but unrelated illness. Inquiry must be made as to the use of tobacco, because it seems probable that vasospastic diseases are aggravated by nicotine.

In the examination of the patient much accurate information can be obtained about the peripheral vessels, for some of them can be visualized, many others can be easily palpated, and a good estimate of the functional ability of the vessels of the extremities can often be formed from the appearance of those parts. Thus the condition of the blood vessels of the retina can be observed directly by means of the ophthalmoscope, and many of the large arteries and veins of the neck, arms, and legs may be felt by the examining fingers. Enlargement, thickening of the vessel wall, tenderness, and increased or decreased amplitude of the pulsations are discovered in this way. Inspection of the hands and feet may show swelling and abnormal color; palpation may reveal altered temperature and tissue consistency.

Certain vascular lesions are accompanied by a noise (*bruit*), which is termed a *murmur* when audible and a *thrill* when sufficiently forceful to be felt. The bruit is due to vibrations set up by the action of the pulsating blood stream. Often the patient is aware of the murmur or thrill, and it may be the chief complaint.

Simple, easily performed tests of vascular function yield data of great value when correctly interpreted. Pressure applied to the fingernail or toenail causes blanching, and the speed of return of the normal color following release of pressure is a good indication of the adequacy of the arterial supply. Oscillometry affords a method of more accurately determining the blood flow through an extremity. This is carried out by carefully observing the changes in volume of the extremity or part accompanying each beat of the arterial pulse.

The competence of the valves of the saphenous vein in the leg can be determined by elevating the leg to empty the veins, applying a tourniquet to the thigh just tightly enough to constrict the superficial veins, and then lowering the leg. If the saphenous vein remains empty the conclusion may be drawn that there are no incompetent communicating branches below the tourniquet; release of the constriction will permit rapid retrograde filling of the vein if the valves are inadequate. The patency of the deep veins of the leg is determined by observation of the leg during exercise following the application of a tourniquet to the thigh while the veins are distended. The superficial veins will become less distended if the deep veins are open, but must perforce remain engorged if the blood cannot leave by way of the deep veins.

The part played by vasospasm in disturbances of the peripheral vascular flow may be measured by studies of the skin temperature of the extremities under carefully regulated conditions. This type of examination should be carried out in a room equipped for the maintenance of a constant cool temperature. It has been found that vasodilatation with consequent rise in surface temperature will normally occur in all the extremities upon immersing one arm or one leg in a basin of warm water. This response is lessened or is absent in an extremity suffering from arterial occlusion. Following this preliminary study a procaine nerve block is performed upon the sympathetic nerve supply to the affected extremity; in this way the vasomotor fibers are paralyzed and the vasospasm is relaxed. The temperature studies are then repeated and the results compared with the first study; any difference between them is the effect of vasospasm.

The presence or absence of sympathetic nervous system hyperactivity may be determined by the presence or absence of sweating. A more refined test is accomplished by the measurement of the skin resistance to the conduction of measured electric currents.

Roentgenograms of the extremities will disclose the calcification of arterial walls which, when present, is characteristic of advanced arteriosclerosis. Decreased density of the bones accompanies prolonged circulatory deficiency, and x-ray films may also show bony defects due to the presence of abnormal blood vessels. A method has been devised, moreover, to visualize the blood vessels directly by injecting into them a radiopaque solution. Arteriograms and venograms are readily made and afford direct, accurate information on the size, potency, and course of vessels. Catheterization of the great vessels and even of the chambers of the heart is now a routine procedure in patients suspected of certain lesions; this will be discussed at greater length in Chapter 17.

SUMMARY

A knowledge of the physiology and mechanics of the circulation is essential in surgical as well as in medical nursing. Thrombosis is the natural response to the injury of a blood vessel. Arterial obstruction leads to gangrene; venous obstruction may cause elephantiasis or death from pulmonary embolism. Hyperactivity of the sympathetic nervous system produces vasospasm.

VOCABULARY REVIEW

collateral	*ischemia*	*anticoagulant*
chyle	*lymphedema*	*arteriogram*
thrombosis	*vasospasm*	
embolism	*bruit*	

SUGGESTED READING

1. Allen, Arthur W.: Management of Thromboembolic Disease in Surgical Patients. Surg., Gynec. & Obst., *96*:107–113 (Jan.) 1953.
2. Bauer, Gunnar: Combatting Thrombosis and Pulmonary Embolism. Am. J. Nursing, *47*:589 (September) 1947.
3. Cassell, Melvin: Treatment of Post-thrombotic Syndrome by Interruption of Superficial Femoral Vein. Arch. Surg., *61*:540–553 (September) 1950.
4. Homans, J.: Deep Quiet Thrombosis in the Lower Limb. Surg., Gynec. & Obst., *79*:70 (July) 1944.
5. Krause, G. Lynn: Varicose Veins, Diagnostic Treatment. Am. J. Nursing, *53*: 71–72 (January) 1953.
6. Vetter, Frances C.: Varicose Veins, Nursing Care. Am. J. Nursing, *53*:71–72 (January) 1953.
7. Proudfit, Fairfax T., and Robinson, Corinne Hogden: Nutrition and Diet Therapy. 10th Ed. New York, The Macmillan Co., 1951, pp. 500–503.

CHAPTER 16

Peripheral Vascular Disease

ANEURYSM

When the muscular and elastic tissues of the wall of an artery are weak, the continual hammering of the pulsating blood produces a dilatation or widening of the artery at the weak spot. The weakening of the arterial wall may be the result of trauma, either from a direct penetrating wound or from a sudden violent pull on the vessel. Destruction of tissue as the result of infection may also weaken the wall; syphilis is a frequent cause since the spirochetes of syphilis have a special tendency to attack arterial walls. Another common type, the congenital aneurysm, is the result of abnormal development of vessels during the fetal stage.

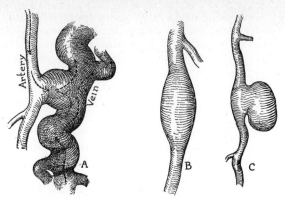

FIGURE 57. *A*, Arteriovenous fistula; *B*, fusiform aneurysm; *C*, saccular aneurysm.

The diagnosis of aneurysm is usually not difficult, as the symptoms and signs are produced by the mechanics of the condition. There is local pain, and there may be erosion of adjacent structures due to the pressure of the aneurysm. When superficially located, the pulsating enlargement of the artery is easily felt, and there is usually an audible and palpable bruit synchronous with the pulse. In the case of a large aneurysm of some duration, enlargement of the heart and elevation of the blood pressure occur because the thin-walled aneurysmal sac is easily expanded and does not aid the heart in propelling the blood. As a matter of fact, the aneurysm acts as a pressure vent, so that a considerable portion of the arterial pressure is lost and it is therefore necessary for the heart to work harder in order to supply the rest of the body. The blood supply of the tissues beyond the aneurysm is affected severely because the cushioning effect of the easily dilated aneurysm acts to diminish the flow of blood through the artery beyond that point. Ischemia and gangrene, therefore, are potential complications.

The best treatment for an aneurysm is surgical removal, for in this way the "pressure vent" is removed and the work of the artery now occluded by operation may be taken up by the collateral circulation. Removal is not always possible, however, as aneurysm may occur in very large arteries, or even in the aorta. The use of grafts to reestablish the continuity of a large vessel or of the aorta is a new method which offers much promise.

An abnormal communication or fistula sometimes occurs between a large artery and a large vein (*arteriovenous aneurysm*), either as the result of a small puncture wound, or because of abnormality of development. Arterial blood flows directly into the vein, with consequent enlargement of the thinner walled vein which is not designed to withstand the force of arterial blood pressure. Here, too, the mechanics of the circulation are upset; this short circuiting increases the work of the heart and diminishes the blood supply beyond the aneurysm. The thrill or bruit is usually continuous, rather than intermittent, and is called a "to and fro murmur," often resembling the purring of a cat. The ideal treatment is the closure of the fistulous communication; when this is not possible, division of artery and vein above and below the point of communication is necessary. On the other hand, the prompt recognition and proper treatment of vascular damage in penetrating wounds serve to prevent the occurrence of aneurysms.

VARICOSE VEINS

As has been stated, the thin-walled veins are not able to withstand much pressure; when subjected to the abnormal pressure of retrograde flow they quickly enlarge and become longer, dilated, and tortuous, and are then varicose. As a rule the deep veins are not affected since the overlying muscles and fascia support their thin walls, but the superficial veins lying immediately beneath the skin do not have that support. Varicosities occur in the esophagus and in the rectum (*hemorrhoids*), and will be discussed later, but except for them varicosities are practically limited to the greater and lesser saphenous veins of the legs and their tributaries. When a person is in the upright position the weight of the column of blood in the veins, extending from the heart down the legs, is considerable, and it is not surprising, therefore, that the delicate valves of the veins occasionally give way, permitting the formation of varicosities.

Varicose veins are often painful, causing a burning, aching sensation. Unless the deep veins have been occluded, or unless there is ulceration and infection, there is usually little or no swelling of the leg and foot. In longstanding, severe varicosities the tissues suffer damage as a result of the prolonged venous backpressure and poor drainage. Ulceration of the skin is common, and usually occurs at the lower end of the area drained by the greater saphenous vein, the region just above the inner aspect of the

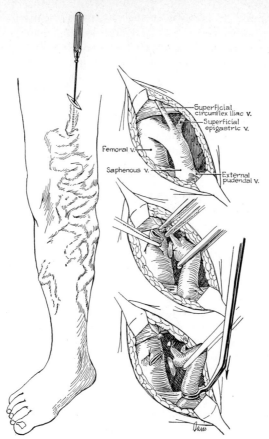

FIGURE 58. Treatment of varicose veins, showing exposure and division of the saphenous vein at its junction with the femoral vein. The saphenous vein is then removed by stripping.

ankle (*medial malleolus*). These ulcers will not remain healed while the varicosity persists, and in longstanding ulcers there is so much scar tissue formation that plastic surgical procedures are usually necessary in addition to treatment of the veins.

The modern treatment of varicose veins combines ligation of the veins at or below the incompetent valves and communications with the deep veins, and removal of the varicosities distal to the points of ligation, a step accomplished by stripping (see Fig. 58). These procedures can be performed under local or general anesthesia. In either case the patient is required to get out of bed and walk shortly after operation, and frequently thereafter. Elastic pressure dressings are applied to the operated limbs, from toe to above the knee; these dressings are removed and reapplied when they become disarranged or loose. The patient may leave the hospital as soon as recovery from anesthesia is complete.

Instructions for home care include the application of the elastic bandages, avoidance of wetting the operated legs in bath or shower until the wounds are healed, and the making of an appointment for the return visit.

PHLEBITIS

Since inflammation of a vein is almost always accompanied by thrombosis, the double name *thrombophlebitis* is often used. As elsewhere in the body, inflammation may be the result of infection, or of the action of other noxious agents such as irritating chemicals, or of trauma. Often thrombosis and thrombophlebitis occur without any apparent cause, especially after abdominal operations; and it has been variously assumed that operative trauma, the position or the inactivity of the anesthetized patient with resultant stasis of venous blood, dehydration, or a low grade infection might be the cause. This type of phlebitis is usually found in the iliac veins and their tributaries, the pelvic and femoral veins, and is the most common source of pulmonary embolism.

When caused by infection or trauma, phlebitis also occurs in the upper extremities, the head, and the neck, and the abdominal cavity. Thrombophlebitis of the lateral sinus or of the jugular vein is a dreaded sequel of mastoid infection, and *pylephlebitis* (infection of the portal vein) sometimes follows appendicitis. An abscess may form in a thrombosed vein. Thrombosis is sometimes found in the mesenteric vessels which supply and drain the intestines. This condition obviously is very serious since gangrene of the intestines results.

Thrombosis constitutes the first step in the process of healing the inflamed vein; nevertheless, the obstruction of the vein augmented by the occlusive effect of regional venospasm will seriously affect the venous drainage of the region. Phlegmasia alba dolens appears, as does lymphedema, since lymphatic obstruction follows venous blocking. The inflamed vein is usually very tender, and, if it is superficial, there will be local heat and redness. At times mild fever and other systemic symptoms appear.

In most instances of venous obstruction the collateral vessels are able to take up the burden. When very large deep veins are affected, or when the thrombosis extends for a considerable distance, the effect of the obstruction is more pronounced, and the regional swelling is greater and more lasting. The healing of phlebitis is often characterized by recanalization of the vessel with partial return of function.

The occurrence of phlebitis following an operation may be suspected when there is tenderness in the calf muscles or pain there upon dorsiflexing the foot (Homans's sign), and confirmed by examination of the legs. Often the swelling is so slight as to be missed altogether unless careful measurements are made; it is helpful if the circumference of the legs has been measured before operation. Iliac or femoral thrombophlebitis is also a frequent complication of pregnancy.

Conservative treatment is usually advocated for patients with acute phlebitis. Rest in bed, with position favoring the maximal drainage of the affected part, is advisable. This can be best achieved by elevating the foot of the bed 6 inches. Massage is strictly forbidden as there is real danger of dislodging thrombi, thus causing embolism. An additional precaution is the avoidance as far as possible of sudden straining, including coughing, sneezing, or straining when using the bedpan. Care must be taken to avoid pressure of the bedclothes upon the affected part. The use of hot or cold applications is common, but there is little reason to believe they are efficacious. Some surgeons advocate immediate ligation of the vein in order to prevent embolism. When the venous drainage is affected, it is advisable to block the sympathetic nerve supply of the regional veins, which relaxes venospasm and not only improves the circulation but also relieves pain. Anticoagulant therapy is thought by some surgeons to be useful in limiting the extent of the disease.

Healing may take place with disappearance of all symptoms, but often the venous obstruction persists and permanent damage follows. Probably the most useful measure in treating postphlebitic swelling of an extremity is tight bandaging accompanied by exercise. Proper care of this sort in the early stages may prevent such sequelae as varicosities and ulceration.

ARTERIOSCLEROSIS

"Hardening of the arteries," as this condition is known to the layman, is found in many people over 40. The cause is as yet unknown. The walls of arteries become thick, inelastic, scarred, and even calcified, resulting in serious impairment of the peripheral circulation. Since the disease generally affects the whole arterial tree, the collateral vessels are damaged too. Arteriosclerosis, moreover, is a progressive disease. Although vascular damage occurs anywhere in the body, the surgeon is chiefly concerned with sclerosis of the arteries supplying the legs, because this is a common cause of gangrene.

The usual symptoms are coolness and discoloration of the toes and feet and cramps in the legs. The cramps come on characteristically after walking a short distance, and disappear upon resting (*intermittent claudication*). This symptom is due to the narrowing of the arteries so that the blood supply to the muscles of the legs, which is sufficient during rest, becomes inadequate during exercise when the muscles need an increased blood flow. Examination of the legs may show all of the manifestations of deficient arterial supply, and usually the superficial arteries feel hard and do not pulsate. Calcification of the vessel walls is often apparent in x-ray films. The foot is usually no warmer than room temperature, and does not warm up when attempts to produce vasodilation are made. Vasospasm is present in arteriosclerosis, but in advanced cases there is so much organic damage that little or no relaxation is gained by interruption of the nervous control. In patients having severe sclerosis, frank gangrene of toes or foot appears.

For many years the frequent observation of gangrene of the lower extremities in patients having diabetes mellitus fostered the belief that the diabetes caused the gangrene. It is known now that the so-called diabetic gangrene is due to arteriosclerosis, which in patients with diabetes occurs at a younger age and progresses more rapidly than in those without diabetes. Circulatory disturbances in patients having diabetes are the more serious because of the lower resistance to infection which is always associated with diabetes.

The treatment of legs with impaired circulation as a result of arteriosclerosis consists in attempting to improve the collateral circulation and in preventing damage from external causes such as trauma or infection. The activity of the patient must be restricted to that amount which can be accomplished without causing symptoms. In the early stages some of the circulatory impairment is due to vasospasm, and in patients in whom this can be demonstrated a sympathetic block (*lumbar sympathectomy*) is helpful.

The appearance of gangrene signifies failure of the circulation, and removal of the dead portion is indicated. Occasionally this process is limited to the loss of a toe or two, but when most of the foot is gangrenous, experience has shown that amputation at a higher level may be necessary in order to make sure that the tissues at the site of operation have enough circulation to heal.

THROMBOANGIITIS OBLITERANS (BUERGER'S DISEASE)

This disease is characterized by an inflammation of arteries and veins. All the usual features of inflammation may occur, including severe pain, tenderness, and circulatory disturbance as a result of both thrombosis and severe vasospasm. The cause of this disease is unknown. In contrast to arteriosclerosis, Buerger's disease affects relatively young persons, usually men of 20 to 35. It is uncommon in women. Healing occurs following the period of acute arteritis and phlebitis, and the ultimate condition of the circulation depends upon the amount of vascular damage and the number of collateral vessels which have escaped the inflammation. In most cases there is residual pain and circulatory impairment varying from minimal cramps and coolness to gangrene. The vessels of the legs are more commonly affected than those of the arms.

Treatment is designed to relieve the symptoms, to bring about favorable conditions for healing of the vessels, and to improve the circulation. Since much of the pain and circulatory disturbance is due to vasospasm, the operations which interrupt the nervous control of the diseased vessels (*sympathectomy*) are often effective.

Thromboangiitis obliterans was once known as the "tobacco smokers' disease" because many patients suffering from it were heavy smokers. It is not likely that tobacco smoking causes the disease, but it is certain that nicotine produces vasospasm and aggravates spasm already present. Patients who have vascular disease, therefore, should never smoke.

RAYNAUD'S DISEASE

Curiously enough, this disease usually affects the vessels of the arms and hands, and is more common in young women. The cause is not known, nor are any pathologic alterations of the vessels found. Vasospasm is the sole feature of the disease and to it may be ascribed all of the symptoms and signs. Coldness and cyanosis of the hands, particularly in cold weather or when the patient is under some nervous strain, appear early. Pain and severe circulatory deficiency of the fingers occur later; loss of nails and gangrene of the fingertips are not uncommon. In some patients there is thickening of the skin of the body (*scleroderma*), a condition thought to be related to the vasospasm. As might be expected, operative interruption of the sympathetic nervous control of the vessels relieves the symptoms and prevents further progress of the disease. The vasospasm of Raynaud's disease can be relieved in some patients by the use of drugs which inhibit or paralyze sympathetic nervous system activity.

SCALENUS ANTICUS SYNDROME

Symptoms similar to those of Raynaud's disease are sometimes caused by the presence of a cervical rib. This congenital abnormality pinches the subclavian vessels and the brachial plexus, causing circulatory deficiency and neurologic disturbances in the arm and hand. A similar picture may result from spasticity of the anterior and middle scalene muscles in the neck. Cure in either case results from the surgical division of these muscles, and it is not necessary to remove the rib.

NURSING CARE IN CIRCULATORY DISTURBANCES

In dealing with an extremity suffering from impaired circulation it is important to realize that trauma is poorly tolerated and that healing is difficult. Resistance to bacterial invasion is low. Cleanliness aids in compensating for the lowered resistance to bacterial invasion, but the methods employed must be so gentle as not to injure tissue. Scrubbing must be avoided. Maceration of the skin leads to infection, and must be prevented by keeping the extremity dry. Alcohol is useful for this purpose, and should be applied after the limb has been gently bathed with mild soap and water. Particular care should be taken of the nails, and of the spaces between the toes, in order to avoid the creation of portals of entry for infection.

A defective circulation cannot compensate for sudden changes in temperature; thus the extremity is more susceptible to burning and freezing. No precaution must be neglected in protecting the limb rendered fragile by disease; chilling even a limited part of the body will produce vasoconstriction. In cold weather warm gloves and proper protection for the head, ears and neck are imperative. Woolen socks and comfortably fitting shoes loosely laced are best for the ambulatory patient.

The patient should be taught methods to produce generalized vasodilation such as immersion of the arms in water heated to 109° F. twice daily, or the application of a heating pad to the abdomen for thirty minutes twice a day. Simple exercises which increase the circulation are: elevation of the feet for one minute, a horizontal position, with toes and ankles flexed, for three minutes, and the legs dangling over the side of the bed for two minutes. A patient with thromboangiitis obliterans should be encouraged to drink three or four liters of water daily to increase the blood volume and reduce the viscosity of the blood.

Explicit directions should be given concerning the diet. A vitamin-high diet including large amounts of fresh uncooked fruits and vegetables, milk, and butter is essential.

Elevation of the extremity to the level of the heart favors the circulation. There should be no constricting bands or clothing. Support of the limb must be adequate without local pressure points which might result in ulcers. An even, warm temperature should be maintained. An electrically heated cradle may be used to accomplish this, provided care is taken not to burn the patient. In summer, an ordinary cradle may be used to keep the bedclothes off the legs and feet.

Massage is forbidden, because not only is there danger of loosening thrombi, but the skin, which is now less resistant, may be damaged.

The morale of these patients is often very low because they have much pain and have usually been ill and incapacitated for a long time. Improvement, furthermore, takes place slowly, and the nurse must support the patient's will to recover. Smoking is not to be tolerated, but other possible forms of diversion short of the use of narcotics should be encouraged. Drug addiction is a complication to be avoided if possible. Careful observation as to which drugs or combinations of drugs are most effective is helpful in reducing the total amount necessary.

SURGICAL PROCEDURES

Perhaps the simplest and earliest operation performed on a blood vessel was phlebotomy (*venesection*), a procedure only occasionally used now. It was easy for the surgeon to incise a vein, but the patient did not always profit by the subsequent loss of blood. The ancients also knew how to stop the flow of blood by tying a thread (*ligature*) about a vessel, but this relatively simple operation, called ligation, was first put on a sound basis by Larrey, the surgeon of Napoleon's armies. It is now one of the essential procedures of operative surgery.

Although it was truly a great advance when surgeons learned to save life by ligating a bleeding artery, further steps have been taken. A successful technic has been devised for suturing a wound in a vessel, and also for bringing together the divided ends of a severed vessel (*anastomosis*). More recently it has been found possible to transplant portions of arteries and veins to replace segments of injured or diseased vessels; indeed portions of arteries may be frozen by special technics and preserved in readiness for use when needed.

AMPUTATIONS

The surgical removal of a part or all of a limb is not primarily an operation upon the vascular system, but it is discussed at this time because it is frequently necessitated by the presence of gangrene. A proper amputation removes no more of a limb than is necessary, and yet is designed to leave nothing which may require further surgical treatment. The level of amputation for gangrene is determined by the condition of the circulation, for it is essential to place the operative wound in viable, healthy tissues. The surgeon must also take into account such technical considerations as the formation of a stump which can bear weight painlessly and which will be so placed as to enable the patient to make the most effective use of an artificial limb (*prosthesis*).

The simple guillotine or circular amputation is performed when infection is present, as in moist gangrene, or when contamination is inevitable, as in modern war. In this operation a circular incision is made, and skin, muscles, and bone are divided at the same level. Blood vessels and nerves are ligated but no attempt is made to close the wound. As might be expected, healing is prolonged in this type of amputation and secondary operations are usually necessary; but the tissues have a better opportunity of overcoming infection, drainage is free, and there is no chance for the growth of anaerobic bacteria.

It is in this last kind of situation that refrigeration of the extremity proves its value. If this technic (described on p. 31) has been used, the amputation is performed while the extremity is being permitted to thaw out, and no other anesthesia is necessary.

Circumstances permitting, a plastic type of amputation is far

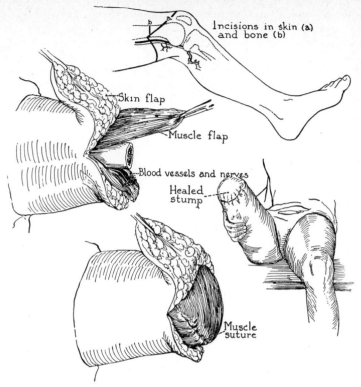

Incisions in skin (a) and bone (b)

Skin flap

Muscle flap

Blood vessels and nerves

Healed stump

Muscle suture

FIGURE 59. Thigh amputation.

more satisfactory. The incision is designed to provide appropriate skin flaps. The bone is resected at a level slightly higher than that at which the muscles are divided, and the anterior and posterior groups of muscles and tendons are brought together over the bone end. The skin flaps are sutured in such a way that the scar is remote from the region intended for weight bearing. Blood vessels and nerves are dealt with as in the guillotine type of amputation.

Nursing Care. To lessen edema and for comfort, the stump is elevated on a pillow after operation. Because oozing, and perhaps bleeding, will occur, it is advisable to protect the pillow with a rubber case. Many surgeons require that the stump be kept in full sight from twenty-four to forty-eight hours after operation to eliminate a failure to discover a sudden hemorrhage. A tourniquet should always be instantly available. It is convenient to have it tied to the foot of the patient's bed. If the patient is incontinent of urine or feces the dressing should be covered with a waterproof substance, such as waxed paper, rubber tissue, or oiled silk, secured around the leg above the stump with adhesive to prevent contamination. Skin traction is applied to the limb after a guillotine amputation to pull the skin down over the stump. The traction may be rigged up with a pulley and a weight, or it can be more simply arranged by the use of a Thomas splint with elastic traction or a turnbuckle fastened to the distal end of the splint. This latter arrangement permits greater freedom of motion; in fact, it is then possible for the patient to be allowed out of bed without discontinuing traction. Occupational therapy is useful in diverting the patient's attention during convalescence and in restoring his morale.

Operations upon the blood vessels, including amputation, are occasionally complicated by severe hemorrhage. This may occur in the first few hours after operation, sometimes as a result of the breaking of a ligature or a suture. Immediate application of a tourniquet or pressure bandage is indicated; and if the bleeding is severe, exploration of the wound should be carried out so that the bleeding vessel may be ligated securely. Hemorrhage may also take place several days after operation; this is usually due to infection, with erosion of the vessel wall or of the thrombus. The treatment is the same as for immediate postoperative hemorrhage.

A dreaded complication of amputation for gangrene is infection with the anaerobic gas-forming Welch bacillus. Sudden fever and acceleration of pulse rate should warn the surgeon of the onset of such an infection. Because of the relative frequency of infections, antibiotic therapy is used routinely as a prophylactic measure.

Rehabilitation of the Amputee. In civilian life the patient who has undergone an amputation usually is discharged from the hospital as soon as the wound is healed, so that most of the job of rehabilitation must be carried on during his convalescence at home. This is in contrast to the practice in the hospitals of the Veterans Administration and of the Armed Forces; in those facilities the patient receives care as an inpatient until maximum benefit is achieved. Good results can be obtained by either method, although the latter is more costly.

The goals to be achieved are: (1) convincing the amputee that he can and must make the effort to accept his misfortune and overcome his handicap; (2) teaching him to use his prosthesis; and (3) training him, if necessary, in a new vocation by which he can earn a living. It is the first of these goals with which the nursing personnel is mainly concerned, as specialists usually take over the actual training program which begins when the wound is healed.

Most patients are badly depressed immediately after an amputation. Doctor and nurse alike must encourage the patient, always emphasizing the achievements which it is possible for the patient to realize and stressing the necessity for effort on the part of the patient. As rapidly as possible the patient is encouraged to become self-reliant, so that he can see for himself that he will not be permanently dependent, or an object of pity. Learning to move himself about in bed, giving his own bath, getting from bed to chair, and the like are devices to be utilized. In discussing the future, the subject of goals that can be attained should be handled in a realistic manner, and individualized to suit the patient. It is amazing to observe how well young patients can adjust to the situation and how they can overcome severe handicaps; older patients, as might be expected, do these things less well and it is better not to plan too ambitious a program for them.

SYMPATHECTOMY

The treatment of vasospasm in association with vascular disease requires surgical attack upon the sympathetic nervous system, in order to divide the nerves which carry the impulses causing spasm. To relieve vasospasm in the arm, for instance, it is necessary to divide the sympathetic fibers which lie along the upper thoracic vertebrae (*dorsal sympathectomy*). For vasospasm of the leg, *lumbar sympathectomy* is performed.

Dorsal Sympathectomy. Incision is made between the spine and the scapula on the affected side, and a small portion of the second rib is removed. The sympathetic ganglia and nerves can then be exposed and divided. A frequent complication of dorsal sympathectomy is perforation of the pleura with consequent collapse of the lung. Cyanosis, dyspnea and fever should be reported to the surgeon. Upon regaining consciousness the patient may complain of severe pain because of trauma to the pleura. Opiates are given to relieve this distress. Frequent turning and coughing help to prevent pneumonia.

Lumbar Sympathectomy. This is the operation performed for the relief of vasospasm of the leg. Through a small lateral abdominal incision, dissection behind the peritoneum proceeds until the sympathetic ganglia lying along the lumbar vertebrae are exposed. The lumbar ganglia are removed and the fibers divided. When the operation is correctly performed the peritoneal cavity is not opened, and thus some of the complications attendant upon laparotomy may be avoided. There is often discomfort beginning the day after operation because of abdominal distention. This may be relieved by an enema followed by hourly intramuscular injection of 0.3 mg. of Prostigmin for three doses, and by the passage of a rectal tube. Hourly turning should be encouraged to prevent further distention.

Sympathectomy for Relief of Essential Hypertension. This is carried out in the same manner, although the surgeon attempts to interrupt the sympathetic fibers of the vessels of the abdomen as well as those of the extremities. Essential hypertension is a highly fatal syndrome, the cause of which is not known. It attacks those in the third and fourth decades of life, and is characterized by a progressive elevation of the blood pressure. Since stimulation of the vasomotor nerves causes constriction of the peripheral vessels, resulting in a rise in systolic blood pressure, it seemed likely that the interruption of the vasomotor fibers might permit lowering of the blood pressure. When this can be accomplished, progressive and irreparable damage to the kidneys, peripheral arterioles, heart and brain may be prevented or postponed. The right and left sides are usually denervated in two stages; the second operation is performed eight or ten days after the first.

Nursing Care. The patient with malignant hypertension has been carefully selected by physician and surgeon as being a suitable candidate for operation. Such a patient should be kept on bed rest and every attempt should be made to provide a pleasant and relaxing atmosphere; a private room away from the noise and distractions of a busy ward is helpful. Good preoperative care also necessitates that the nurse take the time to discover the fears and worries of the patient. Encouraging him to talk, and listening attentively, will win confidence and release tension. A tactful question injected into the conversation, every now and then, may help the patient to unburden himself. The nurse will find that she really needs to say very little and that reassurance comes to the patient when he can "talk things out."

The immediate preoperative preparation is the same as that for any patients being prepared for general anesthesia.

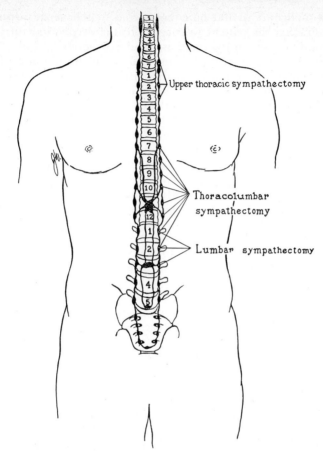

FIGURE 60. Diagram of sympathetic ganglia to show location of sympathectomies performed to relieve vasospasm of extremities and to relieve hypertension.

Following operation, the patient is usually placed in the lateral position and, when the blood pressure is low, shock blocks are placed under the foot of the bed. Frequent reading and recording of the blood pressure, pulse, temperature and respirations are essential. The large incision in the back and the trauma to the pleura are the cause of the severe pain which the patient invariably has upon reacting from the anesthesia. Morphine or other analgesics should be administered to relieve this distress. Encouraging the patient to cough, breathe deeply and turn are essential in preventing atelectasis and pneumonia.

Since there is often a profound drop in blood pressure which is accompanied by faintness, dyspnea and dizziness when the patient is placed in an upright position, it is wise to test his reaction and accustom him gradually to the sitting position. High Fowler's position should be attempted several times each day, beginning several days after operation. The day before the patient gets up he should sit on the edge of the bed with his legs dangling. He should be taught that a quick change from the prone to the upright position will usually result in dizziness and faintness for some time after operation; by moving slowly and dangling he may avoid this discomfort. Symptoms of faintness always disappear when the patient lies down. Dizziness and shortness of breath are relieved by walking but may return when the patient stands still for only a few minutes.

Various methods may be used to lessen these symptoms. The application of elastic bandages from instep to knee may prove effective but in severe cases a girdle or abdominal binder should also be worn. Additional support may be gained by wearing a piece of sponge rubber, 3 by 5 inches, over the lower abdomen inside the girdle. The leg bandages are usually discarded after a few weeks, but the girdle is often left on for several months. Girdle neuritis occurs at times and may last several weeks. Analgesics are usually given according to the severity of symptoms.

Throughout the postoperative period the nurse should instruct the patient in self-care suitable to his particular needs. On leaving the hospital, he should feel confident that he is able to control the uncomfortable symptoms by understanding what to do.

Both the physician and surgeon will take part in the follow-up care of the hypertensive patient, which is a long-term problem that requires regular evaluation and attention to old and new symptoms.

SUMMARY

In general, the effect of peripheral vascular disease is to deprive the part of the body served by the diseased vessels of adequate circulation of blood. Surgical procedures are directed first at improving the flow of blood; failing in this objective, surgery is then employed to remove the dying or dead tissue. Good nursing care includes the instruction of patients in self-care, the prevention of narcotic addiction, aid to patients in giving up the use of tobacco, and much attention to morale building and rehabilitation as many of these patients will have a permanent disability to which they must adjust.

VOCABULARY REVIEW

aneurysm	*ligation*	*guillotine*
varicosity	*sympathectomy*	*thromboangiitis*
thrombophlebitis	*amputation*	*obliterans*
claudication	*prosthesis*	

SUGGESTED READING

1. Fedder, Helma: Nursing the Patient with Sympathectomy for Hypertension. Am. J. Nursing, *48*:643–644, 1948.
2. Glover, John R. The Major Amputations. Am. J. Nursing, *50*:544–549 (September) 1950.
3. Here's an Idea: Am. J. Nursing, *50*:555 (September) 1950.
4. Moskopp, Mary-Elizabeth, and Sloan, Joan: Nursing Care for the Amputee. Am. J. Nursing, *50*:550–555 (September) 1950.
5. Spinney, Jean McDonald: Buerger's Disease. Am. J. Nursing, *49*:119–122 (February) 1949.
6. Swan, Marguerite: Leg Amputation with Refrigeration Anesthesia. Am. J. Nursing, *47*:415–416 (June) 1947.
7. Smithwick, Reginald H., and Kinsey, Dera: Surgical Treatment of Hypertension. Am. J. Nursing, *47*:153–155 (March) 1947.

CHAPTER 17

Surgery of the Heart and Great Vessels

Enveloped completely in the pericardial sac, the heart is situated in the lower midportion of the thorax (*inferior mediastinum*). It is not difficult to expose the heart surgically, but in order to do so it is necessary to open the chest. All of the considerations discussed in connection with thoracotomy (Chap. 11) are therefore applicable.

CONDITIONS REQUIRING CARDIAC SURGERY

Heart Wounds. The treatment of heart wounds has proved to be a successful field of cardiac surgery. A large wound of the heart causes death very rapidly, either from loss of blood externally or into the pleural cavities, or from disorganization of the heart action. If, on the other hand, the opening in the pericardial sac is small, blood pumped out of the heart wound is confined within the sac; the amount of blood lost is thus limited, and death does not occur at once. As the blood accumulates in the pericardial sac, however, the heart is compressed (*cardiac tamponade*), producing the classic triad of low arterial pressure, high venous pressure, and a quiet heart. Unless the compression of the heart is relieved, the cardiac action becomes progressively feeble and finally ceases. Rapid diagnosis and immediate treatment are needed. Tamponade is relieved by evacuating the blood from the pericardial sac. Unless vital portions have been damaged, wounds of the heart heal readily when sutured in the proper manner. Pneumothorax, hemothorax, and laceration of the lung and intrathoracic vessels often accompany heart wounds, having been produced by the same agent (e.g., stab or gunshot) and must be dealt with as outlined in Chapter 11. The need for large transfusions is obvious.

Cardiac Standstill. Occasionally during the induction of general anesthesia, or during the course of an operative procedure the normal rhythmic contractions of the heart cease, presumably due to a sudden failure of the intrinsic nerve impulse conduction system of the heart. When this occurs, the flow of blood abruptly stops and anoxia rapidly develops; without oxygen, the cells of the brain are irreparably damaged within five to ten minutes and death ensues. In many instances, the heart beat can be restored and the life of the patient saved by prompt action. The heart is quickly exposed by an incision through the chest wall, or through the diaphragm if the abdomen is already open, and the surgeon massages the heart carefully and rhythmically. This, if done properly, restores the flow of blood and relieves the anoxia. Oxygen and artificial respiration are usually administered by the anesthetist. Procaine may be injected into the heart, and electrical stimulation may be necessary. Often the rhythmic contraction returns spontaneously after a few minutes of massage.

Cardiac massage is not invariably successful, and there is a high mortality rate in cardiac standstill. Sometimes the heart beat is restored after an interval which is longer than the survival time of the cells of the brain which have been deprived of oxygen; then consciousness is not regained although the patient may live for some time.

Many hospitals keep on hand special equipment for dealing with this emergency, including oxygen equipment, sterile instruments for opening the chest, electrical stimulating equipment, the necessary drugs and syringes, and electrocardiographic equipment.

Acute and Chronic Pericarditis. Many cardiac conditions once considered exclusively medical in nature are now being attacked surgically with success. Surgical drainage should be performed in cases of acute suppurative pericarditis, just as in any pyogenic inflammation. There have not been many cures, chiefly because patients with suppurative pericarditis also have other and less favorable lesions. Chronic constrictive pericarditis, on the other hand, offers a better chance of surgical cure. In this condition the action of the heart is badly hampered by thick scarring and calcification of the pericardium, the result of the healing of a pericardial inflammation, usually secondary to rheumatic fever or tuberculosis. The surgical removal of large portions of the scarred pericardium liberates the heart, permitting it to expand and contract effectively. The operative mortality is high, but the risk is justified since the untreated patient faces certain death after months of invalidism, while the successfully treated patient may return to a normal life.

Congenital Heart Lesions. *Pulmonic Stenosis.* A brilliant recent advance has been made in extending the benefits of surgery to "blue babies," who, as a result of a congenital malformation of the heart which does not permit adequate circulation of the blood through the lungs, suffer from insufficient oxygenation of the blood. The most common variety of malformation is the tetralogy of Fallot; there are four defects in the heart but the most important is the narrowing of the orifice of the pulmonary artery (*pulmonic stenosis*). The children who have this congenital abnormality do not grow properly and are doomed to an early death unless successfully treated surgically. They are cyanotic, cannot tolerate exertion; blood studies show a high red cell count (*polycythemia*) and a low degree of oxygen content.

In 1945, Blalock and Taussig reported the first successful results obtained by performing an operation they devised to shunt the blood around the narrow pulmonary orifice. One of the large branches of the aorta, usually the right subclavian artery, is

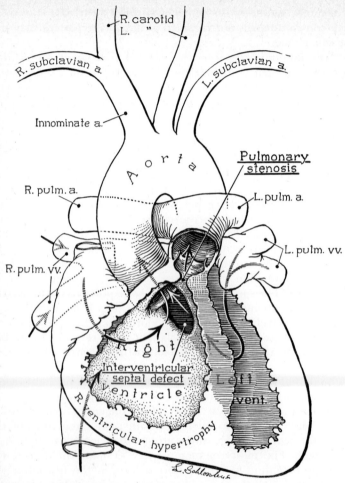

FIGURE 61. Diagrammatic sketch of heart and great vessels of "blue baby."
(By permission of *Surgery, Gynecology and Obstetrics*.)

connected (*anastomosed*) to the pulmonary artery. The immediate result is dramatic, with rapid disappearance of cyanosis and
intolerance to exercise. The late results are equally impressive.
Thousands of children all over the world who would have been
dead without operation are now leading relatively normal lives,
growing and developing properly.

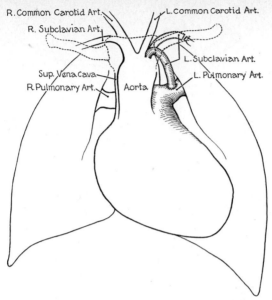

FIGURE 62. Blalock operation: left subclavian artery anastomosed to left pulmonary artery. (By permission *Journal of the American Medical Association*.)

Patent Ductus Arteriosus. A second common congenital cardiovascular malformation is a persistent patent (open) ductus arteriosus. This structure, which is a large, open communication between the aorta and the pulmonary artery, is present normally in the fetus to permit the circulation of blood which is oxygenated in the maternal placenta rather than in the nonfunctioning lungs of the fetus. The ductus normally closes during or shortly after birth, but in some individuals it remains open permanently. In the past, most of these unfortunates died young, but the outlook has been changed completely by the success of modern surgery. The patent ductus is ligated; the results have been excellent.

Coarctation of the Aorta. In this congenital lesion, the thoracic aorta is narrowed or closed. Usually, the narrowing involves only a very short segment. The patient who has this condition suffers from elevated blood pressure (*hypertension*) in the upper part of the body, and low blood pressure (*hypotension*) in the lower portion of the body. The treatment consists in removing (*resect-

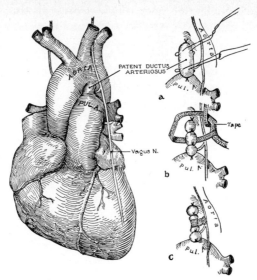

FIGURE 63. Steps in ligation of patent ductus arteriosus.

ing) the narrowed segment and performing an end-to-end anastomosis of the aorta. The mortality of the operations is now reasonably low and the result highly satisfactory. Although coarctation is a congenital lesion, the symptoms do not make themselves known, as a rule, until the patient is in the second or third decade of life; without operation, few of these patients live beyond 30 years of age.

Surgery of Acquired Valvular Heart Disease. Rheumatic fever, syphilis, and bacterial infection often leave damaged heart valves in their wake. The valves become thick and narrowed, and usually leak. Direct surgical attack is now being made on these diseased valves in patients who otherwise would die of cardiac failure. The best results thus far have followed surgical treatment of mitral stenosis. In one technic, the surgeon introduces his finger into the heart and dilates the valve; in another technic, a punch instrument (*valvulotome*) is inserted into the heart and a portion of the diseased valve cut away.

Portal Hypertension. Obstruction to the flow of blood through the portal vein from the stomach, spleen, and intestines to the liver (and ultimately into the vena cava) results in elevation of the pressure in the portal vein and its tributaries. Cirrhosis of the liver is probably the most common cause of this condition; other causes are Banti's disease, and thrombosis of the portal vein. As the pressure in the portal venous system rises, the collateral communications into the systemic veins of the body enlarge. Among the major collateral channels are the esophageal veins and the hemorrhoidal veins. Serious hemorrhage from either source can occur, and is often a cause of death in these patients. Another complication of portal hypertension is the accumulation of large amounts of fluid in the peritoneal cavity (*ascites*).

Following the pioneer work of Blakemore, surgeons may now perform a by-pass or shunting operation; by joining the portal vein or one of its major tributaries to a systemic vein, a way is opened for the blood to by-pass the obstruction in the liver. Portacaval anastomosis (joining the portal vein and the inferior vena cava) relieves the portal hypertension and its complications, but, when the hypertension is due to cirrhosis, the underlying disease of the liver usually continues unchecked, the patient ultimately succumbing to hepatic insufficiency.

NURSING CARE IN CARDIAC SURGERY

The patient who is a candidate for cardiac surgery has usually spent many days at the hospital as an outpatient while physical examination, blood studies, fluoroscopy, x-rays and electrocardiogram were done. In addition, in some patients, heart catheterization[1] and angiocardiogram are carried out. For either of these procedures, the patient is usually admitted to the hospital.

Heart Catheterization. Preparation for heart catheterization or angiocardiogram consists of withholding fluids and food for two hours prior to the treatment to prevent nausea and subsequent vomiting. Morphine and scopolamine are administered about twenty minutes before the patient is taken from the ward. If there is restlessness during the procedure Nembutal is usually given. Patients are occasionally given general anesthesia but usually the previously mentioned sedation suffices.

The nurse has had only a brief time to make friends with her patient, frequently a child, and it is often rather difficult to win full cooperation. She usually gives very few explanations concerning his treatment when he is under 5 years of age unless the questions which he asks indicate that he is able to understand. To the older child, the nurse explains simply and in a matter-

[1] See Brown, pages 264–265.

of-fact manner that he will have pictures taken of his chest, that blood tests will be done, and that he will ride on the stretcher to see the doctor. If an adult, she questions him to find out if he understands what will be done.

After the patient returns to the ward the temperature, pulse and respirations are observed for any irregularities and, if so, the doctor should be notified. Nausea may occur following the procedure. To minimize vomiting, fluids and food are withheld for about two hours.

Such a patient is usually discharged from the hospital but may return later after a complete evaluation has been made of all the findings and the cardiologist has recommended him for surgery.

Preparation for Operation. When the patient is admitted for surgery, the nurse should familiarize herself with his history as shown on the chart, giving special attention to the description of the patient's attributes, habits, interests and limitations. Repetition of details already given may be disheartening and discouraging to the patient or family, suggesting a lack of coordination within the institution. Therefore the plan of care of the patient should be based on information received from the history with such additional details as are volunteered by the family and the patient.

The anxiety and problems of the patient and his family must be recognized by the nurse. Friendliness and patient listening will do much to foster confidence and peace of mind. The surgeon responsible for the care of the patient has talked to the family and explained the operative treatment in full detail, but if the nurse is questioned concerning technics she should again refer the family to the surgeon to promote a better understanding.

Preoperative treatment consists of protecting the patient from infection, forcing fluids to an adequate intake and in establishing a friendly relationship between the patient and the ward personnel. It is desirable that the nurse who is to give the postoperative care learns to know him best.

The immediate preoperative care consists of the usual treatment with special emphasis on the provision of a good night's sleep. Nembutal administered the evening before operation not only induces sleep, but also lessens tension and anxiety the morning of operation. Water is given until only a few hours before operation; the adequacy of the intake must be watched, especially when the patient has polycythemia. In the morning, it is usually inadvisable to have parents see the child because of the transmission of fear and apprehension that would inevitably take place; however, each patient must be considered individually and no general routine applies to all. Sometimes provision can be made for the parents to see the child without him seeing them. In other cases, the child has adjusted well enough to his new situation so that a visit from parents would not increase his anxiety.

The wishes of an adult patient should be respected as should those of his family. They find comfort in each other's company and the time of waiting to go to the operating room passes quickly while they visit with each other. It is desirable for the patient to remain in bed because the sedative administered the night before may cause dizziness if the patient gets up. Also the effects of the drug in allaying anxiety will be prolonged if activity is kept at a minimum.

Postoperative Care. In general, the preparation to receive all patients following cardiac surgery and their immediate care is similar. In addition to the usual postoperative unit, the following equipment should be available:

1. Oxygen tent
2. Suction machine, tray with No. 10 and No. 12 French catheters, and container with sterile water
3. Sterile water-seal drainage bottle, rubber tubing and glass connecting tubes
4. Stethoscope and sphygmomanometer
5. Standard equipment for intravenous therapy, intravenous saline and 5 per cent glucose
6. Emergency medicine tray containing caffein sodium benzoate, adrenalin, aminophylline, Digalen, sterile needles and syringes, solution for clean up, tourniquet and adhesive tape
7. Arm board and padded restraint to restrain leg into which intravenous is running
8. Steam inhalator
9. Shock blocks

When the patient returns to the ward, the nurse should read the report of the operative procedure and the record of fluids and medications given, and should observe his general condition. The doctor's orders should be read carefully and carried out. The use of oxygen, usually ordered by tent, will aid in slowing the heart and respiratory rates. The temperature in the tent should be maintained between 68 and 70° F. and the concentration of oxygen should be at least 50 per cent.

The patient is usually under light anesthesia, and therefore semiconscious on arrival from the operating room; the nurse should, at her earliest convenience, restrain the foot to insure against the dislodgement of the continuous intravenous infusion which was started in the operating room. Further restraint is not advised and is seldom necessary.

Thereafter the nurse counts the patient's pulse and respirations, noting the volume, regularity and rate of the pulse, the depth, ease, rate and rhythm of respirations. These are usually taken and recorded every fifteen minutes for two to four hours, then every hour. It is suggested that the femoral pulse be taken whenever possible because it is more accessible when the patient is in a tent, it prevents oxygen leakage, is frequently more easily obtainable and is less disturbing to the patient.

Dyspnea, increased respiratory rate, grunting respirations, pain on inspiration, cyanosis or increase of cyanosis and flaring at the nostrils are symptoms which should be watched for; when these occur the doctor should be notified.

The blood pressure is usually taken every half hour for six hours, then every hour for six hours and thereafter according to order; this will depend upon the condition of the patient and the nature of the operation. If the patient is in an oxygen tent, the nurse takes the pressure on the arm the first time and checks it on the leg in the popliteal space at the same time. If the readings are almost the same, the pressure may be taken on the leg thereafter unless it becomes unstable, in which case it should be checked on the arm. The instability of the blood pressure should be reported to the doctor.

The temperature is taken every hour for at least two hours and thereafter every four hours if there is no fever. However, when whole blood has been administered it should be taken every hour for four hours after the treatment is started. Any rise or fall of over a degree, either sudden or gradual, should be reported.

The next observation is the patient's state of consciousness. A quick response is desirable; when the patient does not respond within an hour after operation the doctor should be notified. The movement of extremities should be checked carefully. If there has been cerebral damage as the result of cerebral thrombosis during the operation hemiplegia may be present. Paralysis may occur in varying degree. The nurse should ask the patient to squeeze his hands, show his teeth, and wiggle his toes, in order to elicit abnormal signs. Any deviation of the eyes should also be noted.

The dressing should be observed frequently for bleeding. The drainage from the catheter in the chest should be observed and the apparatus cared for exactly as described on page 118.

Turning and coughing are encouraged for all patients every hour for the first twelve to twenty-four hours. Mucus is removed by suction and, if coughing is not sufficiently forceful, endotracheal suction is indicated. The nurse can help the patient greatly in lessening the pain of coughing if she exerts some pressure with the palm of her hand over the operative area. When the mucus is very tenacious, steam inhalations are ordered; this makes the mucus less viscid and allows easier expectoration. The patient is usually kept flat in bed for the first day, or until the blood pressure is stable. After this, he is frequently more comfortable with the head of the bed raised to a 20 to 30 degree angle.

Infrequently laryngeal edema occurs. This is characterized by labored respirations having a wheezing, crowing sound and signs of inspiratory retraction of the chest. Tracheotomy may be necessary.

An adequate fluid intake is important. The surgeon orders the amount of intake that he desires the patient to have within twenty-four hours. Since the patient receives intravenous fluids until he is able to take by mouth the full amount ordered, the nurse must keep careful check on the amount of fluid the patient receives by all routes. Furthermore, the nurse must know the amount that the patient should receive by mouth and vein each hour. When the patient increases his amount by mouth, the drops per minute of the intravenous infusion should be reduced accordingly or vice versa. Allowing the patient more fluid than is ordered may result in pulmonary edema and cardiac decompensation. Water in small amounts, 30 to 50 cc., should be offered each half hour soon after the patient reacts from anesthesia. Other liquids and solid foods are added when the patient seems able to tolerate them.

The output of urine is carefully measured and recorded. A decreased amount is an early sign of cardiac decompensation. Pulmonary edema is characterized by dyspnea, orthopnea, wheezing respirations, cyanosis and frothy sputum.

The site of the intravenous cannula should be observed closely for swelling, redness, heat and pain; these signs may indicate the onset of infection or phlebitis, and should be reported to the doctor.

Antibiotics and ascorbic acid are usually administered to all patients to prevent infection and aid healing.

Pain in the chest generally lasts for twenty-four hours in children and sometimes longer in adults, varying with their threshold of pain. Restlessness and pain are relieved by barbiturates, such as Nembutal and Luminal, and narcotics. When narcotics are used the nurse must be on guard against depressed respirations, especially when these are administered to a child.

The requirement for constant nursing care is usually twenty-four to seventy-two hours, but varies with each patient.

Careful consideration should be given the family during this immediate postoperative period. Allowing them to see the patient as soon as the operation is over, and at least three times a day briefly, helps allay anxiety and apprehension. To permit them to see the patient, even if only for a five-minute period or less, gives them assurance that everything is being done for their loved one that is possible.

Special Considerations

Cardiac Injuries. The care described under thoracic injuries on page 108 is applicable. In addition, preparation should be made for measurement of the venous pressure and for pericardial aspiration. The sterile articles essential for tapping the pericardium are: heart needles, 10 cc. Luer syringe, 50 cc. Luer syringe, rubber gloves, sponges and procaine, $\frac{1}{2}$ per cent solution.

The patient's pulse should be felt frequently, with particular attention to the volume and regularity. An increase in the pressure within the pericardial sac causes the pulse to become more feeble. When there is a decrease in volume, the surgeon should be notified immediately.

Chronic Constrictive Pericarditis. The patient is usually an adult who is admitted to surgery through the medical service where he has undergone treatment for the temporary relief of his ascites, dyspnea and edema. His pulse is feeble before operation and he complains of a feeling of general weakness.

Following operation he is cared for like other patients with cardiac surgery but with special attention to the volume of the pulse. It is convenient to have a venous pressure apparatus in readiness since the surgeon will measure it at intervals.[1] The soft and undistended abdomen, the increase in pulse volume, and general increase in strength are the evidences of improvement which the nurse observes during convalescence.

Ambulation depends entirely on the condition of the patient; sometimes it is begun on the third day, and sometimes not until the fourteenth day.

Congenital Heart Disease Including Tetralogy of Fallot and Pure Pulmonic Stenosis. The cyanotic child or adult who comes for surgery has frequently been an invalid, leading an abnormal life physically and emotionally. The physical limitations have restricted his social contacts with others of his own age. The physical problems manifested usually result in overprotection by parents or guardians. This produces dependency, immaturity and insecurity in the patient, regardless of age.

While in some the mental development may be retarded, others may appear precocious. The child who has normal mental faculties often seems beyond his years in his mannerisms and speech because of continual association with well-educated adults. Because of the constant companionship and vigilance, the parents may seem oversolicitous, overanxious, and apprehensive.

In reviewing the records of many of these children, one finds that it is not uncommon for the child and mother to have slept in the same room since the birth of the baby; a 4 or 5 year old child is still drinking from the bottle; and the diet is usually inadequate. Behavior problems such as severe temper tantrums, kicking, spitting, biting, and other attention-getting devices, and immature response to situations are also common. The mother is usually aware of the diet and behavior problems but states that when she tried to correct them, the child became so agitated that she feared the child would die if she pursued them. Tantrums would bring on increased cyanosis, dyspnea and unwillingness to eat or drink. These she attempted to avoid and in so doing she "spoiled" the child.

In view of the problems presented in each case, the nurse learns to understand the parents and child and in this way has a basis for beginning reeducation. The problems that such a patient has must be dealt with gradually, and teaching includes both parent and child. A good time to begin is on admission. Taking the child and parents to the playroom where they may see

[1] See Brown, pages 262–263.

how well the other children can work and play together and explaining the play program may serve as a start to establish rapport and confidence. If admission is at mealtime, it affords the parent the opportunity to see how well children eat together. When possible, the child should be allowed to eat with them, thus placing him in a normal routine.

During the course of admission the nurse should avail herself of the opportunity to question the mother concerning habits of diet, sleep, elimination and play. If he is partial to certain foods, arrangements should be made with the dietary department to try to obtain them. The mother should be questioned about his elimination and toilet training. Frequently the child has his own expressions for the desire to void and defecate and if the nurse is cognizant of these, there is a greater tendency to preserve and maintain good habits taught at home. The child learns the vocabulary of the hospital after a few days' companionship with other children so that this problem soon vanishes. Since most of these children have very poor teeth, good mouth care is especially essential. If the dietary habits are extremely poor, and the behavior problems are intense then it is usually not advisable to try to change them before operation. To encourage the child to take adequate fluids, in the manner to which he is accustomed, is more important, preoperatively, than the fact that the child has not attained the proper behavior level for his age. The mother, in such cases, will also be less anxious and fearful if she is assured that the child will be cared for in the manner that she has described. Winning the confidence of the parents and the friendship of the child should be the goal of the nurse to insure an adequate basis for the care of such a child.

The fluid intake and output is carefully measured and an adequate intake is maintained in order to prevent cerebral thrombosis which may occur from dehydration and high polycythemia.

Following operation, the pulse is taken in the arm opposite to the side of operation whenever the subclavian artery is used, as in the Blalock-Taussig technic, since no pulse can be felt on the affected side. The arm may feel slightly cooler, but no attempt should be made to warm it.

The child usually resists movement of the arm on the side of operation. He should be encouraged to use the arm, exercising it by raising it, and by walking the wall with the fingers to help prevent deformity.

Behavior reeducation and emotional readjustment cannot be fully accomplished during the patient's brief hospitalization but a start should be made. The usual hospital convalescence is from two to three weeks, depending on the condition of the patient. During this time there is often a great change in the personality of the child. He becomes more alert, takes an interest in other children, learns to take his turn, and learns that he is no longer the center of attention as he was at home and when first operated upon.

As the appetite of the child improves an attempt should be made to teach him to eat a balanced diet. Eating with other children, having the nurse explain that a combination of all food helps to make him well, withholding dessert until he has eaten some of the food on his plate, serving food sieved, chopped or prepared to suit the child are methods which have proved effective. The child who is still drinking from the bottle when over a year old, and who is physically capable of drinking from a cup or glass, should be taught to do so as soon as his condition permits. Suggestions to meet this problem are: an attractive cup, the use of drinking straws, encouraging him to eat and drink with the other children and as they do.

The nurse should make use of her contacts with the parents throughout the child's stay. They should be informed of any training that is being done and of the progress made.

Behavior problems mentioned earlier must also be met when present. Temper tantrums seldom appear following operation but when they do there are several ways to deal with the situation. Ignoring the incident as much as possible, or if the behavior becomes intolerable to the group, isolating him where he can do no harm to himself or others usually curbs this tendency.

Toilet training should be started as soon as possible by establishing a definite time for toilet care. Commendation for good habits is also very helpful.

Before the patient leaves the hospital, the parents are given definite instructions concerning his activities. Activities of adult patients are restricted for one month; parents are advised to let their child find his own limit in exercise, which is usually the point when he becomes short of breath. He cannot enter into competitive games. Whenever necessary, the doctor will refer the patient to a child guidance clinic convenient to his home. Not all children and parents need this service but, by and large, the child has a better chance to develop into an emotionally stable person when both parent and child understand what should and should not be done.

Patent Ductus Arteriosus. The physical and emotional development of adult or child with this condition usually has not deviated far from normal. In general, he may appear a little more frail and may have been somewhat overprotected because of his susceptibility to infections.

Progress following surgery is rapid in uncomplicated cases. The patient may be out of bed the second or third day. In some clinics he is permitted to go home after a week; in others, he convalesces in the hospital from twelve to fourteen days.

The patient is instructed to increase his activity gradually and, after three months, all restrictions are removed. The doctor carefully emphasizes the importance of prophylactic penicillin therapy if he has any minor surgery such as a tooth extraction, or if he contracts a respiratory infection. An infection during the first six months may cause subacute bacterial endocarditis which, in turn, could result in reopening of the ductus arteriosus.

Coarctation of the Aorta. This healthy-appearing person usually exhibits normal emotional stability. When an adult, the shoulders and trunk are large in comparison to the somewhat underdeveloped lower half of the body. The child does not manifest any appreciable abnormality in physique.

Following operation the blood pressure is taken in the arm and the leg and recorded accordingly. If there is a drop, it should be called to the attention of the surgeon immediately, as this may mean a leak in the anastomosis of the aorta. After the second day, it is taken once daily for seven days.

The adult male frequently has difficulty voiding for the first twenty-four to thirty-six hours. Urinary retention and discomfort should be reported. The patient is relieved either by a retention catheter or repeated catheterization until he is able to void.

Complete bed rest for this patient is usually continued for twelve to fourteen days and he leaves the hospital about a week later.

Physical activity instructions vary according to surgeons; some are more conservative than others in permitting exercise. Very minimal activity for three months, gradually increased to normal within another three months, is satisfactory for many patients.

Mitral Stenosis. The patient who has severe mitral stenosis is obviously ill. He develops fatigue and dyspnea with only slight exercise; he often has edema, especially of legs, ankles, and feet. He has been under the care of a physician for some time and has been referred to the surgeon to alleviate the increasing heart failure. The severity of the illness varies but fairly often such a patient has been incapacitated to such a degree that he is an invalid on bed rest when he comes to operation. It is therefore important to learn to know him by evaluating his way of life as manifested by his activities, his interests, his work and his restrictions.

Following operation, bed rest is continued for at least two weeks. Lethargy and fatigue are apparent. A quiet atmosphere, careful observations of the vital signs, and meticulous personal care should be provided not only while under constant observation but also during the whole convalescent period.

As the patient's strength increases, diversional therapy such as reading material supported on a book rack, or some hand work requiring very little activity, should be provided. A radio is also a helpful adjunct.

Such a patient is carefully followed after discharge by both surgeon and physician in order to determine the cardiac status and guide the patient's activities accordingly.

SUMMARY

Modern surgery has achieved its most brilliant success in accomplishing by operative means the repair of cardiac injuries, of congenital defects of the heart and great vessels, and of abnormalities resulting from disease. The technics are difficult and the nursing care of these patients demands special skill, patience, and constant alertness.

VOCABULARY REVIEW

tamponade	portacaval	cardiac standstill
stenosis	anastomosis	polycythemia
tetralogy of Fallot	pericarditis	valvulotome
coarctation	patent ductus arteriosus	angiocardiogram

SUGGESTED READING

1. Blalock, Alfred, and Ravitch, Mark: A Consideration of the Non-operative Treatment of Cardiac Tamponade Resulting from Wounds of the Heart. Surgery, *14:*157–162 (August) 1942.
2. Blalock, Alfred, and Taussig, Helen B.: The Surgical Treatment of Malformationes of the Heart. J.A.M.A., *128:*189–202 (May) 1945.

3. Gross, Robert: Surgical Management of the Patent Ductus Arteriosus. Ann. Surg., *110*:321–356 (September) 1939.
4. Gross, Robert: Surgical Correction for Coarctation of the Aorta. Surgery, *18*:673 (November) 1945.
5. Holman, Emile: Surgical Treatment of Tuberculosis Pericarditis. Arch. Surg., *61*:266–272 (August) 1950.
6. McClure, Catherine T.: Guest in the House. Am. J. Nursing, *49*:775–777 (December) 1949.
7. Potts, Willis J.: Tetralogy of Fallot. Am. J. Nursing. *47*:298–300 (May) 1947.
8. Price, Constance Garside: Mitral Stenosis. Am. J. Nursing, *51*:72–74 (February) 1951.
9. Stallman, Dorothy P.: Nursing Care in Cardiac Catheterization. Am. J. Nursing, *49*:215 (April) 1949.
10. Stevens, Marion: Visitors Are Welcome on the Pediatric Ward. Am. J. Nursing, *49*:233 (April) 1949.
11. Wallace, Mildred: Care of the Child with Tetralogy of Fallot. Am. J. Nursing, *52*:195–198 (February) 1952.
12. Wallace, Mildred, and Feinauer, Violet: Understanding a Sick Child's Behavior. Am. J. Nursing, *48*:517–521 (August) 1948.

CHAPTER 18

Diseases of the
Blood-forming Tissues and Spleen

The commonest neoplastic lesion of the blood vessels is benign hemangioma (Chap. 4). This tumor is commonly found in the skin, but may occur in any part of the body; when symptoms arise from one of these they are usually the result of hemorrhage. Tumors of the cellular elements of the bone marrow (*myeloma, leukemia*) and those of the lymph nodes (*lymphosarcoma*) are not rare, however, and behave like malignant neoplasms. Hodgkin's disease resembles these neoplasms of the blood-forming tissues in its malignant clinical course, but under the microscope the lesions are also suggestive of an inflammatory disease. The true nature of Hodgkin's disease is unknown. There is little to be done for these diseases surgically, other than biopsy to establish the diagnosis. Radiation therapy has been beneficial for some of the neoplasms of lymphoid origin, causing a regression of the process, or in some instances even a cure. As a by-product of special investigation carried out during World War II, both radioactive phosphorus and nitrogen mustard have been found useful in the therapy of lymphoma and leukemia.

The spleen is not a blood-forming organ in the adult: it serves instead as a filter, removing defective or worn out red blood cells from the circulation. In a certain group of diseases known as *purpura* the chief symptom is spontaneous hemorrhage. There is a defect of some sort in the blood, and in patients with congenitally defective red cells (*hemolytic jaundice*) the spleen filters out these red cells as fast as the bone marrow can make them. Since these unfortunate patients cannot form better red cells, and since the defective ones serve well enough to transport oxygen, these patients are improved by the removal of the spleen (*splenectomy*). Experience has shown that little improvement follows splenectomy in most types of purpura, but in one form, associated with a diminution in circulating blood platelets (*thrombocytopenia*), splenectomy is often helpful. After operation, the number of platelets in the blood increases rapidly and the blood-clotting returns to normal.

The spleen is often involved in tumors arising from the bone marrow or lymphoid tissue, but true tumors of the spleen itself are rare. In severe abdominal injuries, rupture or laceration of the spleen is common. Removal of the spleen is usually necessary to control hemorrhage.

Nursing Care Following Splenectomy. The careful preparation of the patient with a disease involving the spleen permits ample time for the nurse to learn to know him. This is in contrast to the patient who enters the emergency room following severe injury and who is admitted to the ward following splenectomy. The immediate preparation is similar to that for abdominal surgery. A Levin tube is usually inserted into the stomach before operation.

Following operation, the care depends upon the type of incision which may be either abdominal or thoraco-abdominal. When the spleen is removed by the latter approach, a chest catheter is usually in place. The principles of care are those described (p. 118) for chest surgery and for abdominal surgery (p. 233).

The most frequent complications are atelectasis, hemorrhage, thrombosis, and infection. Careful observations of the vital signs are essential to allow early detection of any abnormality. Urging the patient to cough and breathe deeply helps prevent atelectasis. Antibiotics are ordered to prevent infection. When hemorrhage occurs, it will be treated by the administration of blood; when thrombosis occurs, anticoagulants may be given.

The time when the patient may be gotten up depends largely on his condition; the patient with splenectomy following injury usually gets up two or three days after surgery and may be expected to make a more rapid recovery than patients who have had splenectomy for purpuric disease.

SUGGESTED READING

1. Dunphy, J. E.: Splenectomy for Trauma, Practical Points in Surgical Technic. Am. J. Surg., 71:450–460 (April) 1946.
2. Giannini, Albert P.: Splenectomy for Essential Thrombocytopenic Purpura. Surg., Gynec. & Obst., 94:229–236 (February) 1952.
3. Lahey, Frank H., and Norcross, J. W.: Splenectomy, When Is It Indicated? Ann. Surg., 128:363–377 (September) 1948.
4. Proudfit, Fairfax T., and Robinson, Corinne Hogden: Nutrition and Diet Therapy. 10th Ed. New York, The Macmillan Co., 1951, pp. 295–305.

Unit IV. NURSING IN SURGERY OF THE ALIMENTARY TRACT

CHAPTER 19

Introduction

Anatomy and Physiology. It will be helpful to the student to think of the alimentary tract as a long tube extending from the mouth to the anus. It serves primarily to convert into the chemicals needed by the living cells of the body that portion of the food eaten which is suitable and to excrete that portion which cannot be utilized. In some of the more primitive forms of animal life the alimentary tract is indeed a simple, straight tube; but in the human being the tract is many times longer than the body, there are considerable differences in the structure and function of its various portions, and a number of important large glands are derived from it. Throughout its entire length the tube is lined by epithelial cells, and the wall of the tube is muscular.

Mouth and Esophagus. The entrance to the uppermost portion of the alimentary tract, the mouth (*oral cavity*), is guarded by the lips. Within the mouth are the tongue and the teeth, and into

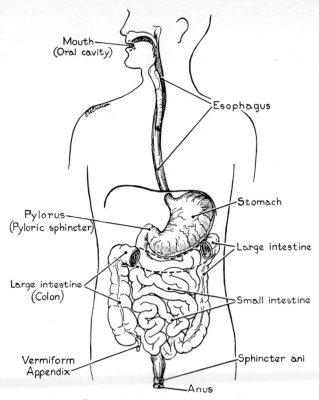

Mouth (Oral cavity)

Esophagus

Pylorus (Pyloric sphincter)

Stomach

Large intestine

Large intestine (Colon)

Small intestine

Vermiform Appendix

Sphincter ani

Anus

FIGURE 64. The alimentary tract.

the mouth empty the ducts leading from the paired saliva-producing glands (*parotid* and *submaxillary* glands). The back of the mouth opens into the esophagus; this relatively straight component of the tract runs down the neck immediately behind the trachea and similarly extends through the thoracic cavity, lying on the bodies of the thoracic vertebrae; it finally passes through the diaphragm, and empties into the stomach.

Stomach. The stomach and all of the remaining portions of the tract, except the anus, are situated within the abdominal cavity. Located anteriorly beneath the dome of the left diaphragm, the stomach is an easily distended, baglike structure, open at both ends. The wall of the stomach is thickly muscled, and at the distal opening (*pylorus*) there is an especially strong ring of muscle fibers (*pyloric sphincter*) that controls the empty-ing of the stomach.

Small Intestine. The next portion of the tract is the small in-testine. This tortuous tube is by far the longest part, and is di-vided into three sections: the duodenum, jejunum, and ileum. Bile from the liver and the digestive ferments from the pancreas are poured into the duodenum. The terminal portion of the ileum empties into the cecum, which is the first section of the large intestine (*colon*). To the cecum is attached the wormlike (*vermiform*) appendix.

Large Intestine. The large intestine is composed of the cecum and ascending right colon, the transverse colon, the descending left colon, the sigmoid colon, and the rectum. The outlet of the tract is the external orifice (*anus*) located in the middle of the perineum; it is guarded by a strong ring of muscle (*sphincter ani*) that keeps the anus closed except during the expulsion of feces or flatus.

It is obvious that the largest part of the alimentary tract lies within the abdominal cavity, and therefore most of the surgery of this tract is abdominal surgery.

Infection. The food we eat, the utensils we place in our mouths, while usually clean, are seldom sterile. It is, therefore, essential in all surgery of the alimentary tract to realize that every part of the tract may and usually does contain bacteria, many of them pathogenic. The continuous sheet of epithelial cells forming the lining membrane (*mucosa*) of the tract affords the same pro-tection from these bacteria as does the epithelium of the skin, but it must be remembered that any break in continuity, whether accidental or surgical, can serve as a portal of entry for bacterial invasion (Chap. 3).

CHAPTER 20

Nursing in Oral Surgery

CLEFTS OF LIP AND PALATE

Cleft palate and cleft lip (*harelip*) result from a failure of the developing lateral portions of the face and mouth in the fetus to unite in the midline as they do normally. These defects occur alone or in combination, and there is considerable variation in the degree of deformity of the upper lip, nostrils, alveolar process (*upper jaw*), and palate. The cleft is said to be complete when there is direct communication between the cavities of the nose and mouth and the exterior. Obviously, this deformity interferes with the nutrition of the infant, since nursing and bottle feeding are impossible. If such deformity is not corrected, moreover, a characteristic speech disturbance will be present in addition to the unfortunate appearance of the child.

Treatment. The cure of cleft lip and palate can be accomplished by surgical measures, and in favorable cases correctly treated there is perfect function and the operative scar can scarcely be detected. The operation for harelip should be undertaken within the first few weeks of life. Successful early operation improves the infant's ability to feed and enables the mother to exhibit the child without distress. Even more important, when a combined defect is present, is the pull exerted by the closed lip upon the cleft palate which approximates the separated alveolar processes and thus creates more favorable conditions for closure. These advantages far outweigh the hazard of operating upon a very young infant and the difficulty encountered in dealing with its miniature anatomy. After repair of the lip, closure of the cleft palate may be deferred until the child is 18 months old.

Repair of harelip demands both knowledge and skill, for success depends upon the accurate recognition of the misplaced portion of the vermilion border, skin, and lip muscle and the utilization of all available tissue. The opposing portions of the vermilion border must be approximated exactly to prevent notching of the lip margin. In this work infection is disastrous, for not only does the repair break down, but much-needed tissue is lost

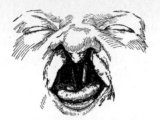

FIGURE 65. Harelip and cleft palate.

and the hope of success in a future attempt is lessened. Penicillin is administered until healing is complete.

The best procedure for closing a cleft palate is a plastic operation which utilizes relaxation incisions in the mucous membrane of the roof of the mouth. Small flaps of the membrane are elevated and are shifted so as to come together over the cleft without tension, thus closing it.

Nursing Care. Good nursing is essential; the repair may be skillfully performed and the result may be impaired by poor nursing care. The patient is always photographed before operation. He is given the preparation which is routine for patients who are to have a general anesthesia.

The regular postoperative unit is prepared. In addition, suction, sandbags and restraints should be at hand. Sandbags are placed on either side of the patient's head to prevent him from rolling on the suture line.

In the case of a baby, elbow restraints should be used constantly until the suture line is completely healed and the sutures have been removed. Wrist and ankle restraints may be used for older children depending on their age, cooperation, and advice of the surgeon.

A free airway should be maintained. The most frequent obstruction in this type of case is caused by suction of the lower lip against the upper. This may be remedied by traction downward of the lower lip with a bit of adhesive tape.

The prevention of strain on the suture line seems to be most difficult in babies. Sedation should be given to prevent crying, especially during the first forty-eight hours when the food intake may not be sufficient to prevent hunger. When this does not suffice, picking the infant up, walking with him, or rocking him may prevent crying.

The older child also demands much attention, especially during the postoperative days. Many of them are very understanding and will not disturb the suture line but others pick at the suture line and cry, remaining quiet only when the nurse holds them or amuses them. After the first day, the child will usually take part in directed play activity.

Infants should be fed by a medicine dropper fitted with a rubber tip, the dropper directed along the cheek away from the affected side. If the repair is bilateral, the dropper should be introduced centrally or along one side of the mouth at the point of least strain. The formula should be fed drop by drop to prevent regurgitation of the feeding through the nose. Milk forms a crust or film on the suture line and 5 cc. of sterile water should be given by dropper after meals to clean the mouth. In some clinics, sterile diet is ordered for all patients with repair, but in others, clean dishes and food are considered adequate. The baby should be bubbled while held in the nurse's lap rather than by the more usual over-the-shoulder method, in order to prevent trauma to the repaired lip. A nipple should not be used for feeding until the suture line is completely healed because the sucking action may be sufficiently forceful to break down the suture line. The older child may be fed with a sterile, rubber-tipped Chetwood syringe or, using a sterile medicine glass the liquids are poured, a little at a time, into the mouth. Sucking must be guarded against.

The surgeon leaves definite orders for the care of the lip. It is sometimes ordered that the suture line be kept clean of crusts and serum by wiping with toothpick swabs wet with hydrogen peroxide every half hour for the first twenty-four hours after operation and moistened with sterile oil every four hours. When no orders are left to cleanse the suture line, then the under lip and tongue should be kept in a moist condition by applying sterile white oil after cleansing with toothpick swabs dipped in sterile water or aqueous Zephiran.

Some surgeons use the Logan bow to take tension off the suture line. This is attached by adhesive tape. If the tape becomes loose, the surgeon should be notified immediately so that new tape may be applied.

Before discharge, when the patient is an infant, the mother should be asked to come to the hospital to feed the child several times under the supervision of the nurse. The mother is naturally anxious about feeding the baby and can be put at ease by proper instruction in the procedure to be followed. Older children will be able to eat a soft diet satisfactorily. The nurse should be sure that the parents know when they are to return to the surgeon. Most surgeons want a photograph made of the patient just before discharge.

After-Care. Speech training is usually necessary to prevent the otherwise inevitable nasal tone. Since the child learns to talk by imitation it is important that those associated with him understand that correct enunciation is the basis of good speech training. There should be a regular weekly practice period of one half to one hour, depending upon the age of the child. Simple words which have consonants that are defective in the child's speech should be practiced. Direct attention should not be called to defective speech at other times. There is danger that the child may become sensitive, frustrated and unhappy if he feels that he is being "pushed." Proper phonation will be acquired with patient and tactful teaching. It has been found invaluable to organize a speech clinic so that a regular teaching program can be conducted by trained workers.

TONGUE-TIE

This common deformity results from undue forward prolongation of the *frenum,* a fold of mucous membrane connecting the base of the tongue to the floor of the mouth. Causing a considerable speech defect, tongue-tie is easily cured by snipping the membrane with a scissors. Care must be taken to avoid the large blood vessels which lie beneath the tongue.

INFECTIONS OF THE MOUTH

In addition to its effective defense against bacterial invasion, the mucous membrane of the mouth possesses remarkable power of repair. Thus not only do tiny abrasions and scratches incident to the wear and tear of ordinary eating heal rapidly, but also accidental and surgical wounds heal quickly even in the face of constant bacterial contamination. It seems likely that tissues which are continually exposed to bacteria develop an increased local resistance. The deeper tissues about the mouth, however, do not possess such qualities, and are susceptible to infection. Moreover, this region is rich in lymphatics, and the inflammatory process soon spreads to the many lymph nodes beneath the floor of the mouth and in the neck. Cervical lymphadenitis is thus a common complication of all oral infections.

Stomatitis. Damaged or neglected teeth are the commonest source of infection of the tissues about the mouth. Continued lack of dental hygiene, with consequent irritation and inflammation of the mucosa of the gums by the accumulation of decaying food, prepares the way for invasion of the alveolar tissues. A very acute ulcerative inflammation of the mouth (*stomatitis*), known also as trench mouth and Vincent's angina, often develops in such a neglected mouth. The causative microbe of this disease is a spirochete. The mouth and gums are ulcerated and painful, and the infectious process may spread to the deeper tissues, sometimes with very serious consequences. If treated early and vigorously, however, the stomatitis clears up promptly. Correct treatment includes regular frequent cleansing of the teeth and massaging of the gums with sodium perborate. In severe cases it may be necessary to use penicillin, administered just as in the treatment of syphilis.

Infection of the Deeper Tissues. Bacteria commonly enter the deeper tissues through a broken tooth, or through one that is decayed (*carious*) or devitalized. Toothache is the first warning; later, the gum becomes painful and swollen. A gumboil (*alveolar abscess*) may form; this may rupture spontaneously or may be drained by surgical incision. In other instances, however, the inflammatory process spreads to involve the jaw (*mandible*) and adjoining tissues. Such a patient has severe, throbbing pain in the whole side of the mouth and face, and there is swelling of the involved jaw, extending to the cheek and neck, with inability to open the mouth freely (*trismus*). The degree of bone infection (*osteomyelitis*) varies; suppuration often occurs, and both cervical lymphadenitis and cellulitis of the tissues of the floor of the mouth (*Ludwig's angina*) are frequent complications.

Treatment. The best treatment of infections of dental origin is prevention. This means regular visits to a competent dentist in addition to proper hygiene in the home.

GENERAL MEASURES. Treatment must include rest in bed, sedatives, a mildly antiseptic mouthwash, and antibiotic therapy. Some surgeons prefer the local application of heat, while others prefer cold. In the acute stage of the disease no attempt to extract the affected tooth should be made, for the trauma incident to extraction would open up new avenues of spread for the invading bacteria and would, by devitalizing additional tissue, reduce the local resistance to bacterial growth.

INCISION AND DRAINAGE. Sometimes the acute inflammatory

process subsides without suppuration; when this occurs it is the signal to treat the original cause of the infection, otherwise there will soon be a recurrence of the trouble. In other instances the acute cellulitis is followed by pus formation, indicated usually by a softening of the central portion of the indurated tissues or by frank fluctuation. Surgical incision and drainage are then indicated, and the necessary incisions are located with careful attention to such considerations as providing free and dependent drainage without interference to blood supply, without injury to nerves or other important structures, and at the same time minimizing facial disfigurement. Warm antiseptic mouthwashes should be administered at least every two hours during the patient's waking hours, until swelling subsides. The patient should be encouraged to expectorate the pus. A sputum cup should be kept at the bedside. In many cases, free and early surgical drainage suffices to cure osteomielitis of the mandible, but at times it is necessary to remove small portions of necrotic bone.

Cellulitis; Mediastinitis. Acute infections of dental origin usually spread to the upper cervical lymph nodes on the affected side, but occasionally the process extends medially, involving the tissues of the floor of the mouth. Cellulitis in this region is attended by great swelling and induration, and since these tissues are beneath a covering of dense fascia there is likely to be compression of the structures within the upper neck. Difficulty in swallowing (*dysphagia*) and respiratory obstruction may occur. At the same time the infectious process may extend rapidly downward beneath the deep cervical fascia. Inflammation of the tissues of the mediastinum (*mediastinitis*), a highly fatal complication, may thus follow failure to recognize and properly treat cellulitis of the floor of the mouth.

Treatment. Formerly it was considered best to treat cellulitis of the floor of the mouth (*Ludwig's angina*) conservatively, but surgeons now realize the importance of early incision with division of the deep cervical fascia, thus at one stroke both relieving the compression of the deep structures of the neck and, by providing free access to the exterior, lessening the likelihood of extension of the infection down the neck into the mediastinum. Even so, there is sometimes so much edema of the inflamed tissues that respiratory obstruction occurs. A rapid increase in swelling, noisy respirations, and cyanosis are signs of repiratory obstruction. An emergency tracheotomy may be required, and the necessary instruments, therefore, must always be available and in condition for immediate use. Antibiotic therapy is, of course, begun at once.

SALIVARY GLAND DISTURBANCES

There are four salivary glands; one of these is situated immediately in front of and below each ear (*parotid glands*), and one is located on each side of the midline just beneath the floor of the mouth (*submaxillary glands*). The parotid duct on either side pierces the muscles of the cheek after leaving the gland; the opening into the mouth is lateral to the upper first molar tooth. The branches of the facial nerve, essential to the function of the facial muscles, pass beneath or through the parotid gland, an anatomic fact of great consequence to the surgeon. The submaxillary ducts open into the floor of the mouth close to the midline, on either side of the frenum of the tongue. These four openings are large enough to be seen with the naked eye, although the ducts are quite small. During the act of chewing (*mastication*) saliva flows out freely, at other times more slowly.

Stones. Small stones (*concretions*) occasionally form in any of these ducts, perhaps more commonly in the submaxillary ducts because of their more dependent position. Concretions are also formed within the much smaller tributary ducts which lie within the glands themselves. A salivary concretion is symptomless until it is of sufficient size to obstruct the duct in which it lies. When obstruction occurs the characteristic symptoms are pain, tenderness, and swelling of the affected gland, all rendered more severe during the act of eating. Examination shows a tender, swollen gland, with no discharge of saliva from its duct. Most of these stones contain calcium and, even though tiny, can be demonstrated by roentgenography.

Treatment. Small as they are, salivary stones are troublesome to treat. In favorable cases the stone may be dislodged by probing or by surgical exploration of the duct. In other instances acute infection may be present, necessitating different therapy; finally, it is often necessary to remove the affected gland in order to relieve the patient permanently.

Inflammation. Acute inflammation of the parotid gland is not uncommon, and is differentiated with some difficulty from mumps (*acute epidemic parotitis*). In the former, however, there is either an absence of secretion from the duct, or there is a purulent secretion. The symptoms are much the same as in obstruction without infection, but are usually more severe, with fever and other systemic symptoms added. Acute parotitis is sometimes a terminal complication in patients who are much debilitated by other disease, and is probably due to drying of the oral mucous membrane with consequent lowering of its resistance to bacterial invasion.

Treatment. The proper treatment for acute parotitis consists in general measures such as rest in bed, increased fluid intake, and the administration of sedatives. Antibiotic therapy is given. Local treatment includes hot or cold applications depending on the surgeon's preference; some authorities advocate x-ray therapy. If actual suppuration occurs, surgical incision and drainage are required. A mouthwash and other measures to promote oral cleanliness are essential. Acute inflammation of the submaxillary glands also occurs, but is less common than acute parotitis; there is no difference in the treatment of the two.

Neoplasms. Both benign and malignant tumors occur in the salivary glands, more often in the parotid than in the sub-maxillary glands. Parotid tumors are usually slow in growth and readily curable by excision if treated early. Occasionally the facial nerve must be sacrificed.

TUMORS OF THE MOUTH, TONGUE AND JAW

The oral cavity is a common site of neoplastic disease. The frequency of injury to the mucous membrane, the constant presence of bacteria, and the conditions arising from the growth and maintenance of the teeth are undoubtedly contributing factors. The use of tobacco may also be a possible factor.

Cancers arising from the lip, tongue, and oral mucous membrane grow more rapidly than similar tumors of the skin, and metastasis to the neighboring lymph nodes in the neck occurs relatively early. Cure is therefore less likely, and is made even less satisfactory because of the mutilation which is caused by extensive resection of the lips, tongue, or mouth. The relative merits of the surgical removal of these tumors and their treatment by roentgen-ray or radium will not be discussed here; many patients have been cured by excision and/or radiation. The presence of a small, persistent ulcer, usually but not always painless, constitutes the signal for immediate diagnosis and treatment while there is still a chance for cure.

The tumors which arise from bone elsewhere occur in the jaws (*mandible* and *maxilla*) as well. In addition, there are certain other neoplasms found in the jaws and not elsewhere which are

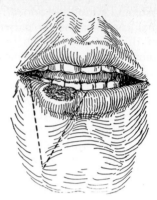

FIGURE 66. Cancer of the lip. The dotted line outlines the portion of lip which must be excised.

due to the presence of tooth-forming tissues. Dental root cysts and tooth-bearing (*dentigerous*) cysts are benign growths, cured by local removal. The adamantinoma, however, is a malignant neoplasm arising from the epithelial cells of the *adamantine glands* (enamel-forming glands), and is cured only by complete resection. The diagnosis is suggested by swelling of the jaw, with or without pain; x-ray examination usually shows a characteristic picture, but biopsy may be necessary. Dental infection and osteomyelitis of the jaw must be distinguished from neoplastic disease.

The term *epulis* refers to any tumor arising from the gums, but is usually applied to a tumor of connective tissue origin which is characterized by large, multinucleated giant cells. It is a benign lesion.

Retention cysts of the mucous glands are not uncommon, and an occasional large cyst forms from an obstructed duct located in the floor of the mouth beneath the tongue (*ranula*). These are cured by excision.

Nursing Care. The extensive operative procedures often needed in the treatment of cancer of the oral cavity are the source of much discomfort and disability. The same may be said with respect to the widespread destruction of tissues occurring in advanced inoperable cancer. The important features of the nursing care of such patients are procedures designed to increase the patient's comfort and to aid healing.

On admission, the surgeon usually orders antibiotics, vitamins and a high caloric diet in preparation for operation. The patient is photographed, necessary x-rays are taken and, when the surgeon anticipates the need for a prosthetic appliance, a mold is made. This will help restore maximum function and normal appearance. Infected teeth may have to be extracted before the major operation is performed. The usual immediate preoperative preparation for general anesthesia is given. Oral hygiene is especially essential.

In addition to the usual postoperative unit, suction should be available. Equipment necessary for tracheotomy care (p. 500) should be provided when a tracheotomy is to be done. Suction catheters should have only one hole and this should be in the end.

Following operation, the unconscious patient is placed in bed on his abdomen with his head turned face down, or on the side opposite operation. Sometimes the surgeon prefers to place the patient in bed with the head elevated in order to reduce venous pressure.

Before the nurse assumes the responsibility for the care of the patient, she should understand what has been done at operation and, if packs were inserted, she should know their location and points of attachment. She should also know whether the tracheotomy is temporary or permanent.

The nursing responsibilities immediately following surgery include: keeping the airway open, observing the patient's color, taking the blood pressure, temperature, and pulse, counting the respirations, and administering fluids and medications as ordered, including antibiotics.

The dressings applied to the neck and face of the patient usually consist of huge amounts of mechanics' waste held in place by tight bandages. This pressure dressing obliterates dead space and aids healing by preventing edema, supporting venous return, and splinting the part. When the patient has an endotracheal tube in place, the lumen must be kept open by the use of suction with a catheter inserted into and through the entire length of the tube to insure the removal of secretions. Suction should be used as often as there is audible congestion. Coughing is encouraged and, when ordered, is stimulated by passing the catheter down into the trachea. The mouth should be emptied by suction of saliva and blood because the patient will be unable to expectorate and swallowing may be difficult for several days. The endotracheal tube is removed by the surgeon or anesthetist when there is no longer danger of tracheal obstruction, usually after the patient is conscious.

Respiratory embarrassment or obstruction may be caused by packs, by the collection of excessive secretions or by bleeding. When there is a tracheotomy, care should be taken to prevent obstruction of the airway by the careless placing of blankets and sheets. By removing the packs or clots, and by sucking away the secretions, relief is immediately obtained.

When the patient has a tracheotomy, care is given in the manner described on page 500.

Pain is controlled by the use of narcotics which should be given cautiously because these agents depress respirations and the cough reflex. If the surgeon has ordered a narcotic to be given whenever necessary, the nurse should watch the depth and rate of the respirations before giving the drug. Respirations should always be above 14 per minute when a narcotic is administered unless the surgeon orders otherwise. If the patient is restless, it may be an early sign of respiratory obstruction rather than an indication of pain.

After operation the patient is fed a high caloric, high protein, fluid mixture through a Levin tube passed through the nose into the lower esophagus. Actual swallowing is not encouraged at first because of intraoral sutures, packs and/or skin grafts. As soon as sufficient time for healing has elapsed, swallowing is encouraged. The Levin tube is left in place because at first the patient will be unable to drink enough fluids to meet the daily food requirements. Milk and orange juice are avoided when there are packs in the mouth because of the tendency to ferment. Swallowing is difficult because of the anesthesia of the operative site and the loss of muscle power. The patient will be frightened in his first attempts to swallow because the fluids may run down his larynx and be expectorated through his tracheotomy tube. The nurse should understand this so that she can patiently reassure and encourage him to keep trying to swallow. Coughing from such efforts is exhausting; too much insistence on trying will tire the patient. Swallowing should be learned gradually and only water is used until the patient learns to protect his trachea. Usually by the fifth to the ninth postoperative day the Levin tube may be removed. The tube is a continual source of annoyance to the patient and the removal at the earliest feasible time will make him more comfortable and assure him that his progress is satisfactory.

Talking is usually possible but very difficult. The patient should be encouraged to communicate by writing. A large number of sheets of paper and a pencil attached to a chart back should be given him; a pad covered with plastic, from which the writing is erased by lifting the plastic material, is excellent for this purpose. A scratch pad and pencil suffice but the patient will write more freely and with less restraint when a larger amount of paper is provided.

Teaching the patient self-care by explaining his care as soon as possible (usually the second postoperative day) is advisable. Encouraging him during subsequent days is important to build up his morale. Early teaching gives the patient more security and at this time there is greater willingness to learn. The nurse must safeguard him from feeling pushed; his activity in learning should proceed according to his adaptations. Care must be taken in this area lest the patient learn self-care to win approval.

During convalescence there is often an apparent depression of spirits. Talking to the patient, encouraging him to communicate, caring for him gently, patiently, tactfully and sympathetically give him security and help lessen mental distress.

The dressings are usually removed on the fifth or sixth day, at which time sutures are partially removed and the drain is shortened. Usually after the first or second dressing the patient will use a mirror to see himself. The patient will know what to expect and will be able to accept this according to his preparation for this by the surgeon and his adaptation to living before operation. The nurse should be alert to relay the patient's reaction. She should encourage him to withdraw his attention from himself by thoughtfully making him associate with other ambulatory patients and engage in diversional therapy of some sort.

Such a patient may be discharged from the hospital after two to three weeks. Explanations of the return visits to the surgeon should be clearly defined and a written appointment slip provided. Every effort to instruct the patient's relatives during convalescence will prepare them for his return home; if they have been informed throughout his stay, they will understand his care. Dietary care should be planned during convalescence to provide for it adequately.

When a laryngectomy has been carried out, the speech therapist usually is able to begin his instruction of esophageal speech four to six weeks after operation. When a prosthetic device is recommended, it is usually made after the patient is discharged and may not be worn until complete healing has taken place.

SUMMARY

The common lesion of the oral cavity in infancy is harelip with cleft palate. Infections occur in young and old. Cancer takes its toll of the middle-aged and older individuals. The nursing care following surgery about the oral cavity is particularly concerned with assistance in breathing, swallowing, and speaking; in addition, these patients have a hard adjustment to make to the mutilation which may result.

VOCABULARY REVIEW

harelip	*Ludwig's angina*	*epulis*
stomatitis	*mandible*	*tracheotomy*
parotid	*maxilla*	*ranula*
trismus		

SUGGESTED READING

1. Cooper, Lenna, Barber, Edith M., and Mitchell, Helen S.: Nutrition in Health and Disease. 11th Ed. Philadelphia, J. B. Lippincott Co., 1950, p. 389.
2. Martin, Hayes: Cancer of the Head and Neck. J.A.M.A. *137*:1366–1376 (August 14) 1948
3. Ward, Grant E., and Hendrick, James W.: Tumors of the Head and Neck. Baltimore, Williams & Wilkins Co., 1951.
4. Ward, Grant E., and Robben, J. O.: A Composite Operation for Radical Neck Dissection and Removal of Cancer of the Mouth. Cancer, *4*:98–109 (January) 1951.
5. Welborn, Joseph F., and Waters, Mary H.: Nursing Care for the Patient Having Oral Surgery. Am. J. Nursing, *51*:74–77 (February) 1951.
6. Post, Grace C., and Mason, Katherine N.: Nursing Care in Cleft Lip Repair. Am. J. Nursing, *48*:768–770 (Dec.) 1948.

CHAPTER 21

Nursing in
Surgery of the Esophagus

Until quite recent times surgical treatment of esophageal lesions was both uncommon and not often successful. There are many reasons for this. Bacteria of all sort may be found in the esophagus. The wall of this portion of the alimentary tract is composed of smooth muscle fibers which form, it is true, a thick coat, but it is well known that muscle neither holds sutures nor heals well; this organ has no strong, fibrous sheath like the submucosa of the remainder of the tract, nor is the external surface covered with a serous coat like the peritoneum which adheres and heals so quickly. Then, too, although the cervical portion of the esophagus is readily accessible, the largest part of this tube lies within the thorax; surgical approach to it was not safe before the recent extensive developments in the field of thoracic surgery. It is also a fact that lesions of the esophagus, except those of an accidental or traumatic origin, do not produce symptoms early; the esophagus is a remarkably silent organ, and, notwithstanding the constant use that is made of it, regurgitation of food is the chief symptom of esophageal disease, and is caused only by some form of obstruction.

Regurgitation must be carefully distinguished from vomiting. The latter is the more or less forceful discharge of the contents of the stomach, whereas regurgitation is not forceful, and the material so returned to the mouth is in the same state as it was upon being swallowed, since it has not been exposed to the digestive action of the gastric juice. Chewed but undigested food is easily recognized, and no gastric juice is present.

WOUNDS OF THE ESOPHAGUS

The esophagus, because of its well-protected position, is not often injured. It may, however, be penetrated in gunshot and stab wounds of the neck, and is occasionally lacerated in a suicidal or homicidal throat-cutting. Such wounds of the esophagus show a remarkable tendency to heal spontaneously. It is important to keep the neck wound open widely so that healing will take place from the bottom upward, because any wound that communicates with the lumen of the esophagus is certain to be an infected wound, and if the wound does not have free external drainage the infectious process may extend down the neck into the mediastinum. Healing is further aided by feeding the patient through a soft rubber tube that is passed through the mouth into the stomach, and by urging him to expectorate rather than swallow his saliva. In this way the wound is kept cleaner and dryer.

An intrathoracic wound of the esophagus uncomplicated by a fatal wound of the heart or great vessels is rare, so closely together do these structures lie in the mediastinum.

BENIGN ESOPHAGEAL STRICTURE

It seems incredible, yet it is a fact, that in many American homes today there is under the kitchen sink, or elsewhere within the reach of some curious but unsuspecting child, an easily opened container of lye, one of the most caustic of all poisons. One mouthful is enough to disillusion the unfortunate child, but it is also enough to cause severe burns of the mouth and esophagus. Burns caused by lye usually heal readily without much treatment of any sort, but in healing scar tissue is produced. Scar tissue tends to contract: thus if the esophageal burn has been circumferential in nature, a circular constriction of the esophagus is the end-result.

Treatment. If the patient receives adequate care soon after the burn is incurred, much can be done to prevent serious constriction. By passing bougies frequently during the healing period and thereafter, the esophagus can be kept open so that a lumen of useful size remains. If, however, this aspect of the treatment is neglected, symptoms of progressive obstruction will appear in a few weeks. An occasional patient does not come under proper care until actual starvation and dehydration occur.

Gastrostomy. In treating patients who have already developed esophageal obstruction to a degree that renders adequate fluid and food intake difficult or impossible, the first step is to provide some other route by which the patient's nutrition can be maintained. This is done by an operation in which the surgeon creates an artificial opening into the stomach through the abdominal wall (*gastrostomy*). This procedure can be carried out under local anesthesia upon even the most debilitated of patients.

Determination of Patency. As soon as the patient's condition permits, examination of the esophagus is undertaken to determine the course of further treatment. Three methods are available, all of which are useful. The lumen of the esophagus may be inspected directly by means of the esophagoscope, an electrically illuminated tube almost exactly like the bronchoscope. It is usually impossible to pass the instrument below the constriction, but the examiner may at least view the upper margin of the contricted portion of the esophagus, and may determine with accuracy the nature of the lesion causing the obstruction. The remainder of the esophagus may be explored by means of soft rubber bougies of different sizes, but even better is the visualization of the lumen by means of fluoroscopy during the swallowing of small amounts of barium.

If the lumen is at all patent, attempts are made to enlarge it. This is sometimes possible through the use of bougies; another method is to have the patient swallow one end of a string. This end is later recovered from the stomach through the gastrostomy by carefully fishing it out with a blunt hooked instrument. Both ends of the string are then secured, and beads of graduated sizes are attached and are carefully drawn through the constricted esophagus until, after many months, the desired lumen is present. During this period, all or most of the patient's fluids and food intake must be supplied through the gastrostomy; full details of this are given in the section on surgery of the stomach.

Reconstructive Surgery. Very occasionally there is complete closure (*stenosis*) of the esophagus following a lye burn. For even such an unfortunate individual there is hope. Cases have been recorded in which there has been successful, complete construction of a new esophagus, thus rehabilitating victims otherwise restricted for the remainder of their lives to feeding by gastrostomy.

Nursing Care. The resultant stricture of the esophagus of the child or adult may be the same, but the manner in which the accident occurred may differ greatly. While lye is the usual causative agent in the child, any caustic, even hair dye, may be taken by the adult. The child was curious when he tasted the lye, but the adult usually got his burn from attempting suicide. Evaluation of the socio-economic and emotional status of either is important and guidance in care should be sought.

Preparation for treatment with bougie consists of witholding fluids for six hours. Since the surgeon usually anesthetizes the throat, the patient could easily aspirate vomitus unless his stomach is empty. It is also necessary to permit no fluids following the procedure to prevent such a complication.

The immediate preoperative and postoperative care of the patient with a gastrostomy is like that for routine surgery. Intravenous fluids are given before, if necessary, and afterward to maintain fluid balance. After twelve to twenty-four hours, the surgeon usually orders liquids to be given directly into the stomach through the gastrostomy tube. At first, water is usually alternated with 200 cc. of tube feeding (p. 50) every two hours, but later, when there is no longer danger of nausea, tube feeding is given every two to four hours depending on the amount the patient is able to take without discomfort. Some patients complain when more than 200 cc. of fluid is placed in the stomach. Such patients require frequent feedings to insure both adequate fluids and nutrition. Water must be given the patient in addition to the feeding to supply him with the 3000 cc. necessary daily requirement.

The adult should be taught within the first few days after gastrostomy to feed himself. Attaching an Asepto syringe and introducing the feeding before releasing the clamp on the tube prevents air from entering the stomach. Water should always be added, following tube feeding, to wash down the mixture. The Asepto syringe should not be removed until the clamp has been reapplied, thus preventing back flow.

Occasionally the surgeon advises patients to utilize a regular diet. The patient is taught to chew the food, and then expectorate it into a funnel which is attached to the end of the gastrostomy tube. This allows for mixture with the salivary juices and also helps preserve the teeth. If this is done in the hospital, the nurse must insure the privacy of the patient; other patients on the ward should not be subjected to this unesthetic manner of eating. Whether the patient takes tube feeding or a regular diet, it is the nurse's responsibility to see that he knows the contents of each. In addition, he should know the amount of water that he is to take daily.

Once healing has occurred and the tissues are no longer tight about the tube, an unavoidable complication of gastrostomy is the leakage of small amounts of gastric contents out onto the abdominal wall. This is disagreeable in two ways, for not only does the material have the unpleasant odor of vomitus but also it is wet and irritating to the skin. Successful placing and construction of the opening reduce leakage to a minimum, but do not completely obviate it. If the patient can lie down after meals until the stomach is nearly empty, the leakage is less. The use of soft and absorbent material for a dressing around the opening is very helpful; frequent change of dressing is advisable. A sanitary napkin cut half way through its length can be fitted around the tube and is a suitable and convenient form of dressing.

While the patient is in the hospital he should be taught to clean the area around the tube thoroughly and to apply the dressing. For the first few days, cleaning the area with sponges soaked in benzalkonium chloride solution 1:1000 is advisable. Later the use of soap and water is encouraged. There is considerable variation among individuals with respect to the tolerance of the skin to the acid gastric juice, and some have no trouble at all. Irritation can be kept at a minimum if the area is cleaned as often as necessary. A mild ointment such as zinc oxide, lanolin or castor oil may be advisable in some cases. Heavy pastes should be avoided; they are hard to remove and, therefore, there is greater chance that the essential cleansing with soap and water will be neglected. The care for each patient should be outlined according to his individual need. When the hospital stay has been too short to insure adequate learning, then the nurse should refer him either to a nurse of his own choice or to the public health nurse for further instruction.

In many instances, the care of a patient, especially a child, with a lye stricture is a long-term problem. There may be repeated hospitalizations and operative procedures. During this period efforts must be made to prevent the patient from becoming a chronic invalid. Regular education must not be neglected, and family relationships and responsibilities must be somehow continued.

TRACHEOESOPHAGEAL FISTULA

This condition, in which there is an open communication between the trachea and the esophagus, is usually congenital and produces serious symptoms in the newborn infant. Occasionally the lesion occurs later in life as a complication of tuberculosis, cancer, or trauma. As soon as the newborn infant begins swallowing, usually on the occasion of the first feeding, the milk runs into the trachea. Coughing, cyanosis, aspiration pneumonia, and even asphyxia may result. Death is inevitable unless the communication can be successfully closed by operation. Needless to say, the intrathoracic operative procedure which must be done is very hazardous in the case of a newborn infant, and the mortality rate is high. Gastrostomy is routinely performed for feeding.

Nursing Care. The nursing care of the infant is directed toward preparation for operation by prevention of any further aspiration of mucus and fluid and, at the same time, to treat the existing pneumonitis and atelectasis. Fluids by mouth are withheld. Antibiotics are administered and oxygen therapy is provided. Dehydration is overcome by the use of parenteral fluid.

Prevention of aspirating mucus from the accumulation in the mouth and pharynx is accomplished by adequate sucking of the mucus from the mouth by means of a suction device. A catheter (No. 8 French), attached to the suction apparatus, is introduced into the pharynx as often as necessary. In some patients, constant suction is applied. The suction should not be too strong. The baby must never be left alone. Choking and cyanosis must be prevented. The treatment is continued until the surgeon feels that the condition of the baby is such that he may operate.

Following operation either constant or intermittent hypopharyngeal suction is used, depending upon the amount of secretions present. The baby is given oxygen for at least twenty-four hours and antibiotics are administered as ordered.

About six or eight hours after operation, gastrostomy feedings are begun by giving the baby small amounts of water and then increased amounts of formula are given as ordered. To feed through the gastrostomy, the nurse inserts an Asepto syringe in the end of the gastrostomy tube, and adds the water or formula before releasing the clamp on the tube so as to prevent air from entering. After the formula is introduced, a small amount of water should always be added so that all of the formula will be delivered into the stomach. Before removing the Asepto syringe the clamp is reapplied to the gastrostomy tube. The baby should be observed for distention following the feeding. This may be prevented by holding him upright after each feeding. The dressing around the tube should be inspected frequently and changed when it is wet. The skin surrounding the tube may become irritated from the gastric juices. This may be prevented by daily, thorough cleansing of the skin with aqueous Zephiran solution 1:1000 followed by the application of a soothing ointment. A satisfactory ointment for this purpose may be made by mixing castor oil 150 gm.; zinc oxide, 30 gm.; starch, 65 gm.; and petrolatum, 125 gm.

Feedings by mouth are begun when the esophageal closure is healed, usually about the seventh postoperative day. Boiled water or 5 per cent glucose is usually ordered. The nurse must guard against permitting the baby to take the feeding too rapidly and close observation should be made of the ease with which the baby swallows. Any coughing, choking or regurgitation should be reported immediately. Holding the baby in a semi-sitting position, while feeding him, makes swallowing easier than in the recumbent position.

Constant observation by a nurse is essential until the baby is able to take his feedings in the normal manner and take the amount required for an infant of his age and weight.

Before the baby goes home his family must be warned that any difficulty arising when the baby swallows should be reported to the surgeon.

ESOPHAGEAL DIVERTICULA

The term diverticulum means a little outpouching. Diverticula are common lesions of the alimentary tract, occurring at any point; esophageal diverticula are second in frequency only to those of the large intestine (*colon*). Diverticula occur wherever the muscular coat is thin normally, or when it is thinned out by wear and tear or disease; a tiny opening permits a small pocket of mucosa to protrude just as the inner tube of a tire might herniate through a hole in the casing. As the result of the gradual accumulation of food, fluid, and gas, the diverticulum gradually enlarges; pressure of the enlarging diverticulum produces either regurgitation or progressive obstruction, or both.

Diagnosis is based upon those symptoms, and is confirmed by observation of the orifice of the diverticulum by means of the esophagoscope and by demonstration of the diverticulum on the roentgen film after a swallow of barium. A sizable diverticulum of the cervical esophagus may, if filled, be actually seen and felt in the neck by the examiner.

Treatment. The only successful treatment is surgical removal. There is little risk associated with the surgical removal of a diverticulum of the cervical esophagus, but, as might be expected, the risk is greater when dealing with a diverticulum of

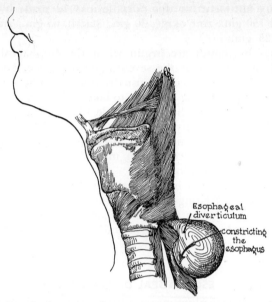

FIGURE 67. Diverticulum of esophagus. Observe how expansion of the diverticulum may cause compression of the esophagus.

the intrathoracic portion. Breakdown of the surgical closure of the esophagus, with consequent fistula formation and infection of the mediastinum, is likely to be disastrous.

Nursing Care. In contrast to all other patients with esophageal disease, the person with a diverticulum of the esophagus appears to be in good health. He has not lost weight and he is not dehydrated.

When the patient is ordered to have an esophagoscopic examination, the preparation and care following are like that described for bronchoscopy (p. 115).

Preoperative care is given in the routine manner.

Preparation to receive the patient following operation includes the regular postoperative unit. It is advisable to have suction equipment at hand to remove excess secretions in the throat.

Observing the patient's pulse, rate of respiration, temperature and blood pressure are essential. The dressings should be observed for bleeding. Oozing of serosanguineous fluid may occur through the opening left in the incision by means of a drain.

Turning the patient and making him cough every hour for at least twelve hours help prevent atelectasis.

As soon as the patient is well oriented he should be told that he should not drink or eat anything and that he should expectorate mucus and excess saliva. Fluids are usually withheld about four days, then tap water is cautiously administered. Clear liquids are given about the sixth day, soft diet on the eighth day and a regular diet on the tenth day.

The patient is usually permitted out of bed on the second postoperative day, and may be discharged as early as the seventh day. Instruction from the nurse and dietitian concerning diet should be reinforced with a diet list printed or written out for the patient. His return visit is usually only a few days after discharge. A return slip and instructions as to the time and day he should return to his doctor are given the patient so that good follow-up care may be given.

ACHALASIA OF THE ESOPHAGUS

In this relatively uncommon condition, also known as cardiospasm, there is progressive obstruction to the passage of food and fluid at the junction of the esophagus and the stomach. The cause of this peculiar malady is not known. Regurgitation of increasing severity occurs, and malnutrition to the point of actual starvation follows. The enormous enlargement of the lower esophagus is readily demonstrated by roentgenography. Some patients are successfully treated by the passing of bougies which stretch the narrowed lumen, others may be cured by operation.

TUMORS OF THE ESOPHAGUS

The recent progress which has been made in the treatment of esophageal neoplasms is one of the more encouraging developments in cancer therapy. Most of this recent progress is a by-product of the development of the field of thoracic surgery. The esophagus is lined by epithelial cells that resemble those of the skin and oral cavity, and, therefore, the commonest neoplasm is a squamous cell epithelioma.

The symptoms of increasing difficulty in swallowing solid food and loss of weight in a person over 45 should suggest cancer of the esophagus to the examiner. Diagnosis is confirmed by direct inspection of the esophagus by means of the esophagoscope and tissue for microscopic examination is taken from any suspected area. In more advanced lesions, when the symptoms of obstruction are more outspoken, the extent of the lesion and the degree of obstruction can be studied by roentgenography.

Treatment. The operative procedure to be used depends upon the location of the tumor. In the cervical portion of the esophagus, which is most accessible to the surgeon, cancer is very rare. Tumors are commonly found in all portions of the intrathoracic esophagus. The esophagus does not stretch readily, and has a rather poor blood supply. Following removal of the portion of the esophagus bearing the tumor it is usually necessary to resort to one of several devices to reestablish continuity of the alimentary tract. One method involves the pulling of the stomach up into the chest, joining it to the resected end of the esophagus (*esophagogastrostomy*). This works well for the lower esophageal lesions. Another method is to substitute a length of small intestine for the esophagus, either in the chest or under the skin of the chest (*extrathoracic esophagoplasty*). More recently success has followed the use of a plastic tube placed in the chest to which both ends of the resected esophagus are attached.

Resection of the esophagus is carried out through a thoracotomy incision, with all the necessary precautions incident to thoracic surgery.

Surgery of such magnitude as this carries with it a considerable mortality. Without operation, however, every patient who has carcinoma of the esophagus would soon die, and die most miserably. With increasing experience the mortality rate of this type of surgery will become reasonably low.

Nursing Care. The interval between the onset of symptoms and admission to the hospital varies, but it is usually long enough to cause emaciation and sometimes severe dehydration. Immediate care is directed toward building up the nutritional status. When only liquids can be swallowed, a high vitamin, high protein and high caloric diet should be given; frequently the nutrition is supplemented with parenteral fluids. Esophagoscopy is usually ordered; the care of the patient is like that described for bronchoscopy (p. 115).

The immediate preoperative preparation is given in the routine manner. Emotional support should be given according to the needs of the patient; all need kind and sincere reassurance.

Since the operation is done through the chest and abdomen. the patient usually will return from surgery with a chest catheter and Levin tube. Oxygen is usually administered until the patient becomes accustomed to the alteration of the chest contents brought about by the stomach or jejunal and esophageal anastomosis. Oxygen therapy and Levin tube suction are frequently discontinued the second day. Tap water in small amounts (30 cc.) is ordered on the second or third day and clear liquids alternating with tap water may be ordered up to 45 or 60 cc. by the third or fourth day. When the patient complains of fullness he should not be urged to take the fluids and this should be reported. He will be able to take fluids better when sitting up than when lying flat. Regurgitation sometimes occurs when he lies flat in bed. Food is given sparingly until the seventh to tenth day when healing of the suture line has taken place.

The patient should be taught the value of good nutrition, and how to arrange a high caloric intake in small amounts. Large amounts of liquids will cause fullness and should not be taken at the expense of small amounts of food with a high protein, carbohydrate and fat content. The difficulty the patient may have in maintaining his weight may be lessened if he knows how to handle his dietary problem in the most effective manner. Regurgitation may be prevented if the patient knows that he should not lie down for two hours after a meal.

Some patients are operated upon for palliation only; this permits them to eat in the normal manner for the rest of their lives, and allows association with family and friends at the table, a very important factor for morale building. Follow-up care is necessary to evaluate the status and to permit help from the surgeon if any difficulties arise.

SUMMARY

The esophagus is no longer an inaccessible organ and surgeons can now repair, remove, and replace this structure. Care of patients undergoing esophageal surgery always involves attention to respiration and nutrition. The results of the treatment of esophageal cancer are discouraging, largely because patients seek treatment late in the disease.

VOCABULARY REVIEW

stricture	*diverticulum*	*esophagoplasty*
gastrostomy	*achalasia*	*tracheoesophageal*
bougie	*esophagogastrostomy*	*fistula*

SUGGESTED READING

1. Battersby, J. S., and Greve, Mary L.: Modern Treatment of Atresia of Esophagus. Am. J. Nursing, *50*:158–161 (March) 1950.

2. Edgerton, Milton T.: One Stage Reconstruction of the Cervical Esophagus or Trachea. Surgery, *31*:239–250, 1952.
3. Diller, Doris: Nursing Care in Esophageal Conditions. Am. J. Nursing, *47*: 811–813 (December) 1947.
4. Garlock, J. H.: The Re-establishment of Esophagogastric Continuity Following Resection of Esophagus for Carcinoma of the Middle Third. Surg., Gynec. & Obst., *78*:23–28 (January) 1944.
5. Haight, Cameron: Congenital Atresia of the Esophagus and Tracheo-esophageal Fistula. Surg., Gynec. & Obst., *84*:504–506 (April) 1947.
6. Longmire, Wm. P.: Esophageal Conditions and Their Treatment. Am. J. Nursing, *47*:807–811 (December) 1947.
7. Loveland, Dorothy: Endoscopy. Am. J. Nursing, *47*:732–734 (November) 1947.

CHAPTER 22

Nursing in Abdominal Surgery

Since the major portion of the alimentary tract and its associated organs lies within the abdominal cavity, it follows that most of the surgery performed upon the tract is included in the field of abdominal surgery. The operative procedure of opening the abdominal cavity is called laparotomy. Well-trained surgeons know many ways of entering the abdominal cavity and a great variety of operations upon the viscera inside the cavity; success depends in large part upon skill in selecting and carrying out the proper one. It is a fact, nevertheless, that there are certain principles common to all of these operations; surgeons have them constantly in mind, and nurses function far more capably if they too know them.

Anatomy of the Abdominal Wall. The abdominal cavity is sheathed in a thick, muscular wall that is supported from above by the ribs, posteriorly by the spinal column, and below by the bony pelvis. On each side, attached to the lower ribs, to the tough, fascial covering of the spinal muscles, and to the crest of the pelvis are three muscles, overlying one another. The fibers of the outermost (external oblique) run from the side down toward the midline; the fibers of the middle one (internal oblique) run from the side up toward the midline, at right angles to the first; and the fibers of the inner muscle (transversalis) run horizontally across the abdomen. Each of these three muscles is attached to its mate from the opposite side of the abdomen by means of a tough, fibrous fascia which also serves as a sheath for the fourth set of abdominal muscles. This last set (rectus abdominis) runs in a vertical direction, from the sternum and lower ribs down to the pubic bone on either side of the midline; these are the muscles which are readily seen in persons of an athletic build. These sets of muscles constitute a wonderfully strong arrangement, for there is a muscle to meet a pull or a stress in any direction. All of them are activated by the spinal nerves, a fact of much importance, for division of a nerve is followed by paralysis of a corresponding segment of muscle.

The size and tone of these muscles vary from person to person. A young, athletic individual usually has heavy, strong muscles, whereas a thin, middle-aged woman who has borne many children is likely to have a relaxed, flabby abdominal wall. The effect of the position of a patient is worthy of consideration. One might think that the abdominal muscles would be most relaxed when the distance between ribs and pelvis is the shortest, as in the semi-sitting (Fowler's) position; actually this is not the case, as a little self-study will show. The abdominal muscles are best relaxed when the patient is lying flat on his back with the thighs flexed and supported by means of a pillow beneath the knees.

Anatomy and Physiology of the Peritoneum. This glistening, smooth membrane resembles the pleura and the pericardium and, like them, is composed of endothelial cells. The peritoneum lines the abdominal cavity and also forms the outer covering of the viscera which lie within the peritoneal sac. The peritoneal sac corresponds roughly to the abdominal cavity, but is not identical with it, since there are several important organs which, although in the abdomen, lie wholly outside of the peritoneal sac and do not have any peritoneal covering. There are other structures which lie beneath the peritoneum but are covered in part. The chief function of the peritoneum is to provide a smooth, slippery surface so that the movements produced by the contractions of the muscular walls of the different portions of the alimentary tube (*peristalsis*) may be frictionless and unimpeded. There is, actually, no free space in the peritoneal cavity under normal conditions, for the viscera are closely packed together, the peritoneal surfaces are in contact, and one portion of the alimentary tract expands in size only at the expense of another, or as the whole abdomen expands. Anyone who has ever eaten a hearty meal can attest to this last fact.

The peritoneum is endowed with great reparative power, and the speed with which it heals helps to make intestinal surgery safe. If, following an incision, the peritoneal edges are carefully approximated, the line of closure will be watertight and airtight within a few hours. Under such conditions healing is probably complete in about eighteen hours, and the healed peritoneum cannot be distinguished from the original since this membrane heals by regeneration and not by scar formation. Interestingly enough, this same remarkable power of rapid agglutination and healing may be a menace as well as a help, for small or large portions of the peritoneum, damaged by disease or trauma, may become adherent on contact, thus forming the justly dreaded adhesions.

Lymphatics are richly distributed throughout the peritoneum, and absorption of soluble material is rapid. The inflammatory response (*peritonitis*) to infection or other irritants is both prompt and effective. The parietal peritoneum is well supplied with sensory nerve endings; the visceral peritoneum is less sensitive, but pulling (*traction*) upon any part of the peritoneum causes severe pain and may even produce shock.

Anatomy of the Abdominal Viscera. It will aid in understanding the various folds of the peritoneum and the attachments (*mesenteries*) of the stomach and intestines if one recalls that early in the embryologic development of the human being all of the organs lie behind the peritoneal sac. During growth, some of them, notably the stomach, intestine, and liver, push forward, so that they become covered by peritoneum on all surfaces except where they are attached posteriorly to the large blood vessels. The small and large intestines, however, continue to elongate, and this can be accomplished only by the production of loops or coils. Thus the small intestine, which is many times longer than the abdominal cavity, comes to lie in loops or coils which are practically free in the cavity, being attached only by their blood vessels. As these coils have pushed out into the peritoneal cavity, their covering of peritoneum has come along with them, so that the intestine and its vessels are entirely sheathed by the membrane. The fanlike attachment of the bowel, composed of the vessels with peritoneum on both sides, is the mesentery of the small intestine. The large intestine is not so long, and instead of being thrown up into coils, it is rotated into a loop that

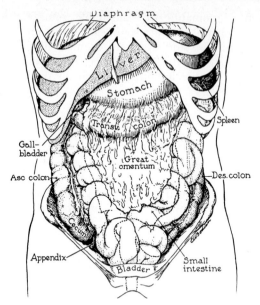

FIGURE 68. The abdominal viscera, seen from the front.

travels once around the periphery of the abdominal cavity. This portion of the bowel is not thrust completely forward into the cavity; therefore the anterior half only is covered by peritoneum, with two exceptions: the transverse colon is pushed down into the cavity by the stomach, and the lower descending colon (*sigmoid*) is elongated, so that both of these portions have well-developed mesenteries and are almost completely sheathed in peritoneum.

The surface of the liver, except the portion attached to the diaphragm, is covered by the peritoneum. The pancreas and kidneys, however, remain entirely behind the peritoneum, as do also the adrenals, the ureters, and the great vessels. The spleen, in reality an oversized and modified lymph node with no known digestive function, lies free in the peritoneal cavity save for its pedicle of blood vessels.

Anomalies. It is not surprising, considering the complicated arrangements of the viscera, that abnormalities due to maldevelopment are common. The different organs may be out of place, poorly or incompletely developed, or even absent. Some of these developmental anomalies are remediable, some are not; others are of interest only as they are significant in the understanding of abdominal symptoms and signs. An example of this last is *situs inversus,* in which all the positions of the organs are reversed, the liver being on the left, the stomach on the right, and the appendix on the left.

ABDOMINAL DIAGNOSIS

How does the surgeon know when to operate, and how does he know where to make his incision? These decisions are based upon his interpretation of the patient's symptoms, the signs observed upon physical examination, and the results of laboratory studies and certain special examinations. In gathering and evaluating these facts, all who come into contact with the patient can be helpful to the surgeon; the greater the nurse's understanding, the greater her usefulness.

Symptoms. The commonest complaint is pain. There is probably no one who has not had some kind of an abdominal pain at one time or another. Much is to be learned, however, from careful investigation of the complaint: what kind of a pain is it, where is it felt, does it stay in one location or radiate, how long has it been present, is it continuous or intermittent? Clinical experience has shown that certain types of pain are characteristic of certain conditions. Thus, cramplike pain indicates violent muscular contraction; excruciatingly sharp, continuous pain usually is caused by the sudden distention of a hollow viscus; continuous abdominal pain that is aggravated by the least motion of the abdomen points to peritoneal inflammation (*peritonitis*). Since the peritoneum and the abdominal viscera are served by sensory fibers derived from the lower spinal nerves, the location of the pain gives a clue to the organ involved. It must be remembered, however, that more than one organ may derive its sensation from the same intercostal nerve. In general, upper abdominal pain is produced by abnormalities of the stomach, liver, gallbladder and bile ducts, spleen, and pancreas. Pain in the region just above the umbilicus suggests trouble in the small intestine, whereas pain around the umbilicus or below it is likely to be caused by lesions in the large intestine, including the appendix.

There is an important group of symptoms related to abnormal function of different portions of the alimentary tract, including belching (*eructation*), vomiting, passage of gas by rectum (*flatulence*), constipation, diarrhea, loss of appetite (*anorexia*), and a vague disturbance that the patient usually speaks of as "indigestion." Each of these calls for special analysis: thus vomiting may be occasional or frequent, it may occur immediately after meals or later, and the character and amount of the vomitus are significant.

Much can be learned by investigation of bleeding from the alimentary tract when that occurs. The amount of blood, the frequency of its passage, and whether it is fresh, clotted, old, or chemically altered are all observable facts which can shed much light on the position and nature of the source of the hemorrhage. Gross amounts of blood that has been partially digested before passage render the feces black or tarry in appearance; minute traces of such changed blood can be detected by the sensitive chemical reaction to benzidine or guaiac.

Signs. Inspection is the first step in carrying out the physical examination of the abdomen. The presence or absence of normal breathing, distention, visible peristalsis, and localized protuberance may be observed. Next comes gentle palpation, from which information may be derived concerning the tone of the abdominal musculature, the location of tenderness (pain elicited upon pressure), and the presence or absence of tumor masses or free fluid in the cavity. Under some conditions various organs may be felt, wholly or in part, but normally this is not the case. Deeper, heavier palpation may disclose tenderness not felt on gentler pressure, and the sudden release of the pressure may cause a sudden spasm of pain, known as rebound tenderness, due to the sudden jarring of the neighboring viscera. Rebound tenderness is present only when there is inflammation of the peritoneal surfaces. Care is also taken to investigate the umbilicus and the inguinal and femoral rings, lest an unsuspected hernia be overlooked. As a final step in examining the abdomen a digital rectal examination is performed, by which means further information is gained concerning the viscera situated in the pelvic portion of the abdominal cavity.

Laboratory Studies. Specimens of vomitus and feces are studied in the laboratory, and chemical, microscopic, and bacteriologic procedures are matters of routine. Various tests have been devised to study the functions of the different organs, and these are described in detail subsequently under the discussion on the surgery of each organ. By having the patient swallow a radiopaque substance such as barium, and by injecting it into the rectum (*barium enema*), the roentgenologist can visualize the lumen of the entire alimentary tube, a diagnostic aid of the greatest value. The lumen of the rectum and lower sigmoid can be directly inspected by means of a lighted tube (*sigmoidoscope*), and a flexible instrument has been devised which can be passed into the stomach. Through this instrument (*gastroscope*) a large part of the interior of the stomach can be directly observed. Indeed, a considerable portion of the peritoneal cavity itself can be inspected through a special instrument (*peritoneoscope*) which is introduced into the cavity through a tiny incision.

Decision to Operate. The surgeon is ready to operate when evidence sufficient to make a diagnosis has been gathered. Often the information obtained from the history and physical examination is enough; sometimes, however, a positive diagnosis cannot be made, even after exhaustive studies have been carried out. Nevertheless, the surgeon is justified in performing an exploratory operation upon such a patient if there is a possibility that the patient may have a lesion which can be treated surgically. This is particularl true in the case of patients who have the so-called acute or surgical abdomen. It is, in fact, far more important for the surgeon to know when to operate than it is for him to know the exact diagnosis.

ABDOMINAL INCISIONS

In choosing an incision the surgeon's first consideration is to secure satisfactory exposure of the region containing the structures that are to be operated upon. Next in importance is consideration of those factors which bear upon the healing of the wound. Nerve and blood supplies must be conserved, and undue tension or stress avoided. Thought must be given to the prevention of painful scars or disabling contractures. Finally, the cosmetic appearance should be considered.

Midline, Transverse, and Rectus Incisions. In order to expose the upper abdominal viscera three different incisions are commonly used, midline, transverse or subcostal, and rectus. For operating upon the stomach or transverse colon, the midline incision is ideal: exposure is good, no important nerves or blood vessels are divided, and there is little or no strain on the wound after operation. For exposure of the pelvic organs a low midline incision is best, and the exposure is further improved by the use of the Trendelenburg position (Fig. 70).

The midline incision does not afford easy access to the struc-

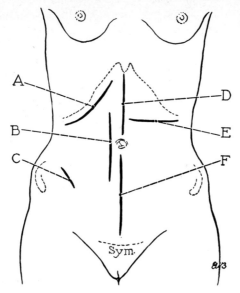

FIGURE 69. Abdominal incisions. *A,* Subcostal; *B,* paramedian; *C,* McBurney; *D,* high midline; *E,* transverse; *F,* low midline.

tures on either side, however; for procedures on the biliary tract, a right transverse incision, and, for approach to the spleen, a left transverse incision, are better. In the transverse incision the belly of the rectus abdominis muscle is divided transversely, but care is taken not to injure the nerve supply. The muscle receives its blood supply from both ends, so that division of the vessels at the incision does not impair the blood supply. This incision heals well, and the eventual scar is the least conspicuous of any.

The rectus incision is made parallel to the long axis of the muscle, and, since it can be made as long as desired, good exposure is obtainable. The direction of the incision, however, makes it impossible to prevent the division of the nerves supplying the fibers between the incision and the midline, and this fact explains the relatively high incidence of hernias that follows rectus incisions, for there is likely to be a permanent weakness wherever the muscle fibers are paralyzed. A modification of the rectus incision has been devised which overcomes this objection. The rectus sheath is divided near the midline, but instead of dividing the muscle fibers, the whole muscle belly is retracted laterally, exposing the posterior sheath and peritoneum. This is

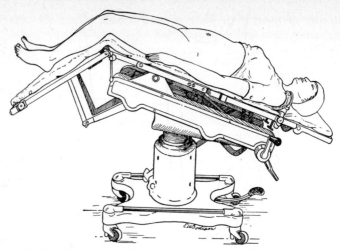

FIGURE 70. Trendelenburg position. Note use of shoulder braces to prevent slipping of patient.

known as a paramedian incision, and it is useful in the mid and lower abdomen, too.

McBurney Incision. An excellent incision that has a wide range of usefulness is the muscle-splitting (McBurney) incision. This is used for the approach to structures in the mid and lower lateral portions of the abdomen, notably for the exposure of the appendix, the ureters, and the sympathetic ganglia. The skin is incised in an oblique direction, parallel to the fibers of the external oblique muscle. The fibers of this muscle are split, not divided, exposing the internal oblique muscle; its fibers, in turn, are split, exposing the transversalis; the fibers of this innermost muscle are likewise split, and the peritoneum is exposed. There is no damage done to muscles, nerves, or blood vessels, and when the retractors are withdrawn the muscles fall back into their normal positions, each covering the opening in a different direction and thus affording a very strong closure, for the contraction of the muscles tightly closes the wound.

Closure. The closure of abdominal incisions is commonly accomplished in layers: the peritoneal edges are approximated first, then the muscles, the fascia, and finally the skin. Some surgeons prefer to use sutures of catgut, others prefer sutures of silk, cotton or stainless steel wire; good results are obtainable with any of these if they are properly used. When the surgeon anticipates the collection of blood or serum in the wound, or wishes to provide for the escape of pus, a drain is left in the wound.

POSTOPERATIVE NURSING CARE OF LAPAROTOMY PATIENTS
Dressings

A clean wound that has been tightly closed without drainage need not be dressed until the fifth or sixth postoperative day, at which time the surgeon will usually remove the skin sutures. The nurse must have ready and sterilized, in addition to the proper dressings, adhesive tape, and solutions, dressing forceps without teeth, and sharp-pointed scissors. Stay sutures, if used, are generally removed on the tenth to fourteenth postoperative day. As a rule, all dressings over the healed wound can be discontinued two or three days after the last sutures have been removed.

Wounds which are open and draining pus, bile, or other material need frequent dressing, daily at least, and often every few hours. When a wound must be dressed daily or oftener the nurse usually does it, and she will do well to have the surgeon show her exactly what he wishes done. It is convenient to have an individual tray set up for such a patient, with a sterile clamp, sterile sponges in a jar of aqueous benzalkonium chloride 1:1000 solution, sterile dry sponges, and suitable dressings. After the soiled dressing has been removed, the incision and the area around it are cleaned by sponging, dried, and a fresh dressing applied. Since frequent removal and replacement of adhesive tape are hard on the patient as well as uneconomical, other methods of holding the dressings in place are more suitable. If Montgomery straps are used, the adhesive tape, when soiled, should be changed. After it is removed, there is often some adhesive substance left on the skin. Benzine or ether may be used to clean this off the skin, but the area should be washed with soap and water before adhesive tape is again applied. A convenient type of drainage dressing is shown in Figure 50.

Various types of drains, packs, and tubes are used in abdominal wounds, depending on the nature of the surgery performed. The nurse should ask for and receive specific instructions as to the care and handling of these. Mention will be made of some of these later.

Measures Which May Prevent Complications

Although a great variety of surgical procedures are carried out within the abdominal cavity, there are many complications common to all laparotomies. The incidence of many of these complications can be reduced by proper nursing care and their treatment rendered more successful by the promptness with which the nurse recognizes and reports these complications to the surgeon.

The need for special observation of postanesthetic patients has already been discussed in Chapter 8.

The patient is grateful for a good back rub, smooth sheets, and a fresh pillow. The pressure of tight or heavy bedclothes upon the patient's feet is avoided by the use of a frame or a pillow beneath the covers at the foot of the bed.

Slight elevation of the head of the bed often makes the patient more comfortable, but Fowler's position should not be used unless specifically prescribed by the surgeon. The elevation of the knees and flexing of the thighs incident to Fowler's position tend to bring about stasis of the blood stream, especially in the popliteal and pelvic vessels. It has been postulated that this might increase the incidence of postoperative thrombosis, and therefore many surgeons prefer their patients to be flat in bed after laparotomy.

Relief of Pain. Every patient is going to have pain, really severe pain, during the first day or two. Hypodermic injections of morphine or other narcotics should be given every four to six hours during the first twenty-four hours after operation, as it is to the patient's advantage to rest quietly and comfortably during that period. In ordinary cases, after the second or third day, smaller doses or less strong narcotics are used and then only when necessary.

Change of Position. A simple measure which may accomplish much is the frequent shifting of the patient's position. In this way no single portion of the lungs remains dependent for long, a fact which helps to prevent atelectasis or pulmonary infections, or both. At the same time the return flow of blood from the extremities and lower abdomen is facilitated, as a result of which there is less chance of thrombosis in the large veins and the incidence of embolism is lowered. There is a favorable effect upon intestinal tone and upon the expulsion of flatus. Finally, by avoiding long periods of pressure upon the skin that overlies the bony prominences, bedsores (*decubitus ulcers*) are prevented. A sick patient needs help in moving about, particularly if movement is painful, as it nearly always is during the first two or three days after laparotomy. He should be encouraged to move slowly and carefully, and to allow others to help him change his position. These patients should be helped on and off the bedpan with particular care.

Prevention of Atelectasis. A patient who has a sore abdomen is not going to take a deep breath if he can help it, but such restriction of the respiratory excursion of the lungs favors the production of atelectasis. Such patients can and should be made to expand the lungs fully at intervals. To effect this the surgeon usually orders the patient to be turned and required to cough and breathe deeply at hourly intervals for the first twelve to eighteen hours after operation.

Common Postlaparotomy Complications

Vomiting. During the period of recovery from anesthesia vomiting is probably the commonest complication. Aspiration of the vomitus must not be permitted. The vomitus must be inspected for blood and measured so that the effect upon fluid balance can be determined. When postoperative vomiting persists beyond the first day some cause other than the effect of the anesthetic agent must be suspected and found. Vomiting should be suppressed as much as possible, for the violent straining incident to it is harmful to wound healing, and is likely to start up fresh bleeding in the operative region. Sedatives, quiet, inhalation of carbon dioxide, strong suggestion, and gastric suction aid in controlling vomiting.

Hiccough. Hiccough (*singultus*) can be an extremely distressing complication and, if persistent, severely taxes the strength of the patient and jeopardizes the healing of the wound. Any of the measures used in controlling vomiting will, at times, control hiccoughing; of these, gastric suction is the most successful. The appearance of persistent uncontrollable hiccoughing, although its cause is not understood, is generally regarded as an ominous sign so far as the prognosis of the illness is concerned.

Bleeding. The dressings are to be inspected often so that *bleeding* or other drainage may be promptly discovered and reported. Internal bleeding is suspected if blood is passed by rectum, or is vomited, or if there is a significant change in the rate or quality of the pulse.

Wound Disruption. The role of infection in preventing wound healing has been discussed in an earlier chapter; occasionally, however, even in the absence of demonstrable infection, an abdominal wound fails to heal as it should. The reasons for this are still obscure, but probably include too much motion of the abdomen and longstanding dietary deficiency. The sudden appearance of a considerable amount of straw-colored serous drainage from a wound which was apparently healed should lead the nurse to suspect a breaking down of the wound (*disruption, dehiscence*). This often occurs shortly after the removal of the skin sutures, and is usually precipitated by coughing or other strenuous exertion. A quick look beneath the dressing discloses the wound disruption; in some instances omentum or loops of intestine are extruded (*evisceration*). The wound and viscera should be quickly covered with sterile towels moistened with sterile physiologic saline solution, after which the patient must be taken to the operating room for reclosure of the wound. Contrary to what one might expect, such wounds, when resutured, usually heal promptly, and most of these patients eventually recover.

Difficulty in Voiding. This is another usual complication. It is understandable: some of the muscles involved in the act are apt to be painful; there is little or, at best, precarious privacy in a hospital; and nearly everyone, from the earliest infancy, has become accustomed to voiding in the upright position. Tactful handling and a few simple procedures are successful in getting the majority of patients to void after operation, but some require catheterization. The patient's worries and fears should be allayed, and he should be given as much privacy as possible. Warming the urinal or bedpan, applying a hot water bottle to the pubic region, or the application of warm water to the genitalia is often helpful. When not contraindicated by the nature of the operative procedure, a small-sized warm enema (not over 112° F.) or the administration of a parasympathetic stimulant such as Prostigmin is usually successful. Male patients, when possible, should be permitted to stand. Once the patient has gotten started he is not likely to have further trouble. It is interesting that the patient most apt to have difficulty is the one who is certain before operation that he will have trouble; those who do not give it a thought are seldom unable to void.

Unless the patient has taken large amounts of fluids or is extremely uncomfortable it is generally safe to allow eighteen or twenty-four hours to elapse after operation before resorting to catheterization; a longer period is likely to result in dangerous dilatation of the bladder.

Distention. A common complaint of many patients after a laparotomy is "gas pains." This symptom occurs during the first two or three days after operation; and the nature of its cause is discussed on page 242. The distention and pain incident thereto are relieved by changes in position, the use of the rectal tube, and by enemas when the latter are not contraindicated by the nature of the operation which has been performed. Continuous gastric suction drainage prevents "gas pains," and early ambulation appear also to have a beneficial effect.

Convalescent Care

Convalescent care[1] is based upon the surgery performed, and upon the reaction of the individual to it. Consideration of his needs and progress will determine the diet, the time for ambulation and guidance necessary to prepare him for discharge. The value of early ambulation has been mentioned previously (page 96).

Food. It is better, in general, to increase the diet gradually. Unless the type of operation performed requires a special program, liquid diet the first day, soft diet the second, and diet as desired thereafter are satisfactory. During the first few days, the patient should not be urged to eat more than he desires; fluid balance should be kept up with parenteral therapy if necessary. Permitting him to choose his diet is advisable; too often it is taken for granted that the patient has a poor appetite, whereas questioning might reveal that he merely has a dislike for the particular diet offered. Encouraging the patient to voice his opinion concerning his diet is often very helpful in promoting proper nutrition and also offers the nurse an opportunity to begin explaining the essentials of well-balanced meals. Finding out what the patient ate at home is essential. A patient may be well informed about the daily requirements for good nutrition but, by and large, explanation concerning the components of a well-balanced diet is advisable. In addition, planning should include substitutions for the foods the patient dislikes. A knowledge of how food costs may be reduced by utilizing alternative substances is practical and often important for the management of

[1] See Brown, pages 36–58.

an adequate diet in the home. The nurse and patient should plan together but a feeling of independence should be developed in the patient.

Planning Total Care. During the days following operation, the nurse must learn from her patient the factors important for continuity of care. The patient's general condition, his problems and his relation with his family are aspects of prime importance in guiding him to meet his needs. How he will be cared for when he goes home is a vital part of total care. Dressings to be changed, special medications to be given and plans for the return visits are some of the aspects of care which should be considered before the moment of the discharge order. Planning with the patient and his family will encourage independence and alleviate anxiety. Sometimes treatments may require additional help in the home. In such a case the doctor, nurse and patient plan for their execution. The doctor may wish that the treatments be given by a professional or practical nurse. The nurse should then arrange with the help of the family and doctor to provide such care, but, if the treatments are to be carried on by a member of the family, the nurse should undertake the necessary instructions and demonstrations to insure proper care.

SUMMARY

In any general hospital a large proportion of the major surgery is within the field of abdominal surgery. In rendering care the nurse is greatly aided by a knowledge of the anatomy of the abdomen and the physiology of the gastrointestinal tract. Good nursing prevents complications and minimizes unpleasant symptoms. A vital part of the nursing function is aiding with the plan for total care.

VOCABULARY REVIEW

peritoneum	*eructation*	*Trendelenburg*
laparotomy	*flatulence*	*position*
viscera	*anorexia*	*hiccough*
mesentery		*distention*

SUGGESTED READING

1. Christian, Theresa: Nursing Care in Abdominal Surgery. Am. J. Nursing, *50*:797–798 (December) 1950.
2. Cooper, Lenna F., Barber, Edith M., and Mitchell, Helen S.: Nutrition in Health and Disease. 11th Ed. Philadelphia, J. B. Lippincott Co., 1950, pp. 383–385.

3. Palumbo, Louis T.: Some Recent Advances in Surgery. Am. J. Nursing, *50:* 658–661 (October) 1950.

4. Sheldon, Nola S., and Blodgett, James: Early Rising in Postoperative Care. Am. J. Nursing, *46:*377–378 (June) 1946.

CHAPTER 23

Peritonitis and Ileus

PERITONITIS

A little more than fifty years ago, peritonitis was a word to cause grave head-shaking among physicians and to strike terror to the hearts of patients' families. The onset of fever, the quickening of the pulse, the rigid, painful abdomen, and the flushed, drawn face were signs well known to Hippocrates, but it remained for Lister to show surgeons how to operate safely within the abdomen; it remained for Reginald Fitz and John B. Murphy to demonstrate that many cases of peritonitis were due to the perforation of an inflamed appendix and could be prevented by early removal of that appendix; and for present-day surgeons to show how the concomitant intestinal obstruction (*ileus*) due to the inflammation of the intestine could be successfully combated, and how chemotherapy could be successfully used against the infection itself.

Abundantly supplied with lymphatics, the peritoneum presents a vast surface capable of rapid absorption. One result of this is the prompt systemic reaction to toxins or other deleterious agents produced by the bacterial invaders. High fever, rapid pulse, and prostration occur in acute suppurative peritonitis. An equally serious feature is the loss of the tone and contractility of the intestinal musculature. A form of intestinal obstruction (paralytic ileus) is the result of this paralysis of intestinal activity; intestinal contents accumulate just as though there were an actual barrier to their passage; distention follows and may lead to necrosis of the bowel wall with perforation. Paralytic ileus introduces the further complications of vomiting, fluid loss, electrolyte imbalance, and starvation. It is not hard to see why untreated peritonitis is a highly fatal disease.

Inflammation of the peritoneum (*peritonitis*) is caused by a wide variety of agents, including pathogenic bacteria, certain viruses, chemical irritants, and free blood. Since none of these is found in the peritoneal cavity under normal conditions, it fol-lows that peritonitis must always be the result of either an injury or a disease that provides a portal for the entry of the etiologic agent.

Pathology. The peritoneum quickly loses its smooth glistening appearance, becoming dull or even red and swollen. There is exudation of fluid containing fibrin and leukocytes. In a rapidly spreading infection of overwhelming virulence (*generalized peritonitis*) there may be frank pus everywhere in the peritoneal cavity, but in less severe cases natural barriers to the spread of the infection are interposed. This walling-off process is accomplished by the adhesion of opposed inflamed surfaces, and by the mar-velous protective action of the omentum—an apronlike structure of fat and blood vessels sheathed in peritoneum and hanging down from the transverse colon—which has the property of mov-ing into and enveloping an area of inflammation. Thus the peritonitis may be restricted, or localized, assuming more or less the characteristics of an abscess.

Even recovery from peritonitis is fraught with danger, for in the healing process one or more localized abscesses sometimes de-velop, and loops of intestine may become permanently adherent, leading in some instances to the development of mechanical in-testinal obstruction. Often, however, healing is so complete that afterward no trace of the inflammation can be found.

Prevention. The importance of preventing peritonitis is ob-vious. Little need be said about the necessity for the strict ob-servance of aseptic technic in performing abdominal operations: that is a sine qua non. There is still great need, however, for further and continued education so that persons with appendici-tis or other illnesses that may lead to peritonitis will early seek and obtain adequate treatment.

Treatment. The clinical diagnosis of acute peritonitis is easily made; it is more difficult to ascertain the cause, yet this is most important since proper therapy depends on it. The program for treatment is fourfold: (1) eradicate the source of the infec-tion; (2) combat such infection as has already developed; (3) combat the paralytic ileus; (4) restore and maintain the pa-tient's fluid and electrolyte balance and nutrition. Ideally, all of these things should be done simultaneously, but practically, in very ill patients, the last three items must take precedence over surgical procedures until the condition of the patient has been improved sufficiently to enabled him to withstand operation. Thus, while the surgeon still seeks to discover the cause of the peritonitis, he may begin treatment by administering intravenous fluids and antibiotic agents, and may also begin decompression of the distended alimentary tract by the use of continuous suction with an indwelling gastric or duodenal tube, introduced through the nose. Usually within a few hours there is great improvement in the patient's condition, and the operation to remove a perforated appendix or whatever is necessary may be safely undertaken.

When the peritonitis begins very suddenly, however, as the result of an acute perforation of a gastric or duodenal ulcer, or in a case of a penetrating wound of the abdomen, the patient is usually not too ill to undergo operation at once. In fact, it may be stated as a general rule that every patient having a perforation of an intra-abdominal viscus must be operated upon and the perforation closed as soon as possible.

When peritonitis is not the result of perforation of the alimentary tract, there may be no need for abdominal surgery. Gonococcal or tubercular peritonitis is properly treated by antibiotics, drugs and general measures, as is also the occasional blood-borne pneumococcal or streptococcal peritonitis that complicates an infection which has originally started elsewhere in the body. Similarly, no operative treatment is needed for the transient peritonitis due to small hemorrhages incident to the rupture of an ovarian follicle. Often, however, a diagnosis cannot be made with certainty, and in such instances exploratory laparotomy may be necessary.

Postoperative Position. For many years surgeons have advocated the use of Fowler's position in the treatment of peritonitis, believing that the gravitation of the pus into the lower abdomen (*pelvis*) aided in recovery, since accumulations of pus (*abscesses*) could be more readily found and more safely evacuated (*drained*). Lately there has been less accord on this method, and some surgeons prefer to have their patients flat; others, indeed, advocate having the patient lie upon his abdomen.

Outcome. Successful treatment of the peritonitis is followed by return of the tone of the intestinal muscle and of peristalsis, usually within forty-eight to seventy-two hours. The onset of improvement is marked by diminished output through the suction tube, and by the passage of increasing amounts of flatus and stool per rectum.

ILEUS

In the performance of any laparotomy, even though asepsis is complete and the utmost precautions are used in the gentle handling of the abdominal viscera, there is bound to be some slight trauma to the delicate peritoneum. Varying degrees of paralytic ileus are therefore a common complication of laparotomy. The slight distention and the uncomfortable gas pains of the first postoperative day or two are a mild form of this disorder. The extent and the severity of the peritoneal inflammation depend upon many factors, such as the nature of the causative agent, the amount of peritoneum involved, the rapidity with which the process spreads, and the interval between onset and treatment.

There is need for differentiating between intestinal obstruction that is the result of an actual blocking of the lumen of the tract (*mechanical ileus*) and that which results from the loss of intestinal contractility (*paralytic ileus*). In the first instance the mechanical barrier must be removed, the occluded lumen must be re-opened. As a rule, surgical procedures are necessary.

Paralytic Ileus. In paralytic ileus the intestines become distended because of the loss of muscle tone and from the accumulation of intestinal contents. The sources of the contents of the distended bowel are food, fluid, ingested air and the secretions of the alimentary mucosa and associated glands. There is nothing abnormal about these sources: only their accumulation is wrong. As the distention increases not only is the muscular wall overstretched, thus delaying the return of peristalsis, but there is an additional danger in that the circulation of the bowel wall is reduced by the pressure upon it, leading to ultimate necrosis of the tissues and perforation. If untreated, distention progresses rapidly, and soon the upper intestinal tract and stomach are filled, vomiting of large amounts of foul-smelling fluid begins, and the whole vicious cycle is under way.

Treatment. In paralytic ileus, surgery does not help; it may even be harmful. In mild cases, and particularly in those where intestinal tone returns in a day or two, it is often sufficient merely to restrict or prohibit the intake of fluid and food by mouth. In general, the tone of the intestinal musculature will return as the peritoneal inflammation subsides, so that treatment must be primarily directed toward the cure of the peritonitis. While this is being done, however, several measures can be taken which will protect the intestinal wall and hasten the return of peristalsis. These include enemas, hot applications to the abdomen (*stupes*), and the administration of such drugs as Pitressin and Prostigmin. Experience has shown, however, that these are of little use until the intestinal contractility begins to return. A simple and useful procedure, and one often overlooked, is the frequent turning and moving of the patient, which has the effect of pouring the intestinal contents from one loop to the next, sometimes with great success. The most effective measure, however, is the use of continuous withdrawal by suction of the intestinal contents. By this means the distended alimentary tract can be decompressed, and recurrence of the distention prevented.

TECHNIC OF DECOMPRESSION. If the distention is progressive, or if vomiting has begun, continuous decompression is the proper treatment.

One of several types of tubes made of rubber or plastic material may be introduced through the nose into the stomach. The tubes used most frequently are: the Levin (No. 14 or 16 French), the Miller-Abbott and the Cantor. The Levin tube is used when the contents of the stomach are to be aspirated. The double-lumen Miller-Abbott tube has a rubber balloon at the tip inflated with air; the Cantor has a mercury-weighted bag at the tip. These devices aid in carrying the tube beyond the stomach, but are useful only if there is motility of the stomach and intestine.

Before passage of the tube is begun, the nurse should explain to the patient what the necessary treatment will be to enlist his cooperation and allay fear. She should be sensitive to any anxiety and try to encourage him to voice any apprehension he may have. The necessary equipment includes: mouth wipes, curved basin, lubricating jelly, glass of water, adhesive tape and the type of tube the doctor has ordered.

The tube may be inserted while the patient is in the sitting position with head forward, or in the recumbent position, with head hyperextended. The latter position seems desirable when the Cantor tube is passed. After the surgeon has introduced the tube into the nasopharynx, the patient should take a few swallows of water to help carry the tube into the stomach. If intubation of the intestine is desired, the position of the patient is then changed every two hours as follows: (1) He is placed on the right side in Trendelenburg position while enough tube is inserted to bring the tip to the pylorus; (2) he is placed on his

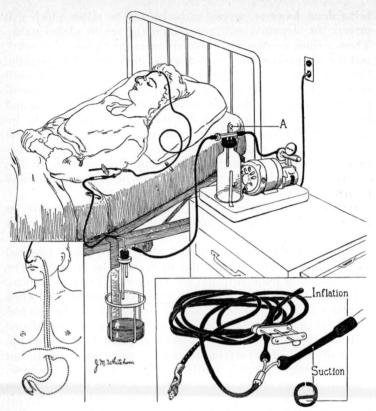

FIGURE 71. Treatment of distention by suction. The degree of negative pressure is regulated by the thumb-screw on the valve at *A*. Insert at lower right shows Miller-Abbott double-lumen tube. Insert at lower left shows tube entering duodenum. Suction may also be obtained from apparatus as shown in Figure 51, or by the water siphon method of Wangensteen.

back in Fowler's position while 2 inches more tubing is inserted, which should bring the tube into the duodenum; and (3) on his left side with the bed flat while another 2 inches of the tube is inserted. The tube is then secured to the cheek with adhesive. X-ray or fluoroscopic examination is made to determine the position of the tube.

The tube is then connected to an apparatus that furnishes constant but gentle suction (Fig 71). Negative pressure equal to 2 feet of water is sufficient to withdraw fluid and air. Care must be taken that the negative pressure does not exceed 5 feet of water. Excessive negative pressure may cause the tube to adhere to the intestinal wall by sucking the mucosa into the small openings of the tube. The surgeon usually orders irrigations of the tube, using either tap water or normal saline. Instilling a measured amount of fluid (usually 30 cc.) by means of an Asepto syringe, waiting two minutes and then withdrawing the fluid with the syringe is a means of keeping the holes of the tube open. Whenever it is not possible to withdraw the fluid, it is obvious that the holes are clogged and therefore no fluid will be drained off when the tube is attached to the suction machine. This should be reported to the surgeon. Overfilling of the stomach (*gastric dilatation*) is a very serious complication and must not be permitted to occur. Vomiting around the tube is an indication that the suction is ineffective. In general, whenever the nurse instills fluid into the tube, she should assume that the fluid should be withdrawn and when there is no withdrawal help should be sought from the surgeon.

The effect of continuous suction drainage is little short of miraculous. The tube is well tolerated by most patients, and can be left undisturbed for several days, if necessary.

It has been stated before that the maintenance of fluid and electrolyte balance is an important factor in combating ileus. In addition to parenteral fluids, medications which are frequently ordered are vitamins B and C. Solutions of glucose, sodium chloride, potassium chloride and protein are regularly used to maintain fluid and chemical balance. An accurate record of intake and output is essential. An output of 1100 to 1200 cc. of urine in twenty-four hours is usually a good indication of adequate fluid intake.

The patient needs much attention and encouragement during this time. He may complain of soreness of his throat from the tube. Good mouth care, lozenges and instillation of drops into the nasal passages are measures which can be used. The surgeon sometimes advises the patient to chew gum to stimulate the flow of saliva to prevent parotitis.

Intravenous feedings are unpleasant for the patient because moving about is restricted. Too often the patient lies in one position overlong because the nurse has not encouraged him to turn. Care in turning will prevent the needle from becoming dislodged.

Consideration should also be given the family when they visit the patient. The hospital personnel are accustomed to the equipment necessary to care for the patient but this frequently is very alarming to the visitors. Explaining it to them will relieve them of their anxiety.

SUMMARY

Peritonitis and its regular sequel, paralytic ileus, are still dangerous, potentially lethal manifestations of disease. The means are at hand to deal with these conditions. Surgery, antibiotics, gastrointestinal intubation and decompression, the restoration and maintenance of fluid and chemical balance, and good nursing care are needed.

VOCABULARY REVIEW

ileus	*Levin*	*Cantor*
peritonitis	*Miller-Abbott*	*double-lumen*
intubation		

SUGGESTED READING

1. Blodgett, James B., and Sheldon, Nola Smith: Intestinal Suction. Am. J. Nursing, *46*:90–92 (February) 1946.
2. Abbott, W. O.: Indications for Use for Miller-Abbott Tube. New England J. Med., *255*:641–646 (October) 1941.

CHAPTER 24

Nursing in Gastric Surgery

The alimentary tract may be compared to the assembly line of a modern factory. The raw material, the food that is eaten, is fed into the mouth where it is mechanically processed into a pulp by chewing. In the mouth, too, the first step is taken in effecting the chemical breakdown of the raw materials, for saliva contains a starch-splitting *enzyme*. The material is then moved along into the stomach, where preparations have already been made for further processing. There is a wonderful communications system in the human body, quite as good as that in any factory, and each processing plant in the digestive system is notified well in advance of the need for its activity. The arrival of the habitual time for eating or the very sight of food serves as a sufficient stimulus to initiate gastric activity. The secretory phase of gastric activity is controlled by the vagus nerves which originate in the brain and travel down along the esophagus to the stomach.

The stomach completes the job of mechanical processing, and introduces a new step in the chemical processing of the raw material. The glands of the mucous membrane that lines the stomach secrete, in addition to mucus, both hydrochloric acid and pepsin. Pepsin is a protein-splitting (*proteolytic*) enzyme and, in combination with the hydrochloric acid, powerfully attacks the protein part of the food eaten, breaking it down into less complex and more soluble compounds. The question may well be asked, why does not the gastric juice digest away the stomach itself? The answer is that it would do so if the stomach were not protected by the mucus-secreting membrane, and wherever the continuity of the mucous membrane is broken the potent gastric juice can and does eat away the wall of the stomach, as will be seen later, in the discussion of ulcers of the stomach.

The discharge of the pulpy, fluid mass that is the end-product of gastric digestion from the stomach into the next portion of the tract is controlled by a powerful circular muscle (*sphincter*) which surrounds the stomach outlet (*pylorus*). From time to time the pyloric sphincter relaxes, permitting the passage of a jet of gastric contents into the duodenum. The control mechanism of the pylorus is not fully understood, but great variation in activity has been observed under normal conditions in the same and in different persons. Usually, after an ordinary meal, emptying of the stomach begins in a few minutes, and within forty minutes to an hour the stomach has finished its work and all of the ingested material has been passed along. The emptying mechanism is extremely sensitive, however, and gastric function is often deranged by any acute illness that a person may contract, as well as by intrinsic disease of the stomach. This is particularly true of children: it is common knowledge that almost every illness in childhood begins with an "upset stomach."

The final phase in the chemical breakdown of the food eaten is begun in the duodenum. The secretions of the duodenal glands, the pancreatic juice, and the bile from the liver are all poured into the lumen of the duodenum. Bile is strongly alkaline, and one of its functions is to neutralize any hydrochloric acid that may come through the pylorus. Moreover, the several

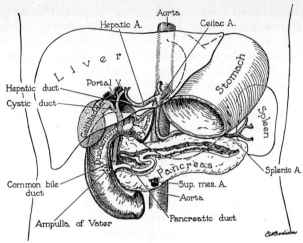

FIGURE 72. Diagrammatic sketch to show intimate anatomic relations of stomach, duodenum, biliary tract, and pancreas. Part of the stomach and the anterior wall of the duodenum have been removed for the sake of clarity.

enzymes secreted by the pancreas and the intestine are efficient in an alkaline medium, and possess the ability to split protein, starch and other carbohydrates, and fats.

Not only are the stomach, the duodenum, the biliary tract, and the pancreas closely integrated as a functional unit: they are also most intimately related anatomically. One branch of the aorta, the celiac axis, furnishes the arterial blood supply of all of these structures, and the venous blood from all of them passes by way of the portal vein into the liver. A glance at Figure 72 will further emphasize the contiguity of these organs. It is not surprising, then, that diseases of one of these may involve others, that the symptoms arising from such diseases are often confusing and difficult to interpret, and that surgical procedures upon these organs must be designed so that there is no crippling disturbance of function. In the past, failure to observe properly this last principle has often led to trouble worse than the disease for which the surgery was originally undertaken.

PYLORIC STENOSIS IN INFANTS

Vomiting that begins in the first few weeks of life and becomes progressively more severe until the baby is vomiting all or more than the quantity of fluid taken by mouth, is characteristic of hypertrophic pyloric stenosis. In babies so afflicted the pyloric sphincter muscle is greatly enlarged and thickened, so that relaxation with proper opening of the pylorus is impaired or even impossible. The cause of this condition is not known. Frequent regurgitation of part or all of a feeding is the rule rather than the exception in nearly every newborn baby, but persistent vomiting should lead the attending physician to suspect pyloric stenosis. Diagnosis may be confirmed by the observation of an enlarged stomach, visible through the abdominal wall; by palpation of the hypertrophied pylorus; and by the introduction of a small quantity of barium into the stomach, so that the obstruction may be visualized under the fluoroscope. Surgery affords the only hope of cure, and in the hands of well-trained operators the mortality is surprisingly low.

Preoperative Care. The preoperative preparation of these tiny starved infants is fully as important as the actual operation. Unless the diagnosis is made promptly and the infant is in a relatively good state of nutrition and hydration, it is necessary to postpone surgery for a week or ten days. During this period strenuous efforts are made to improve the status of the infant's nutrition by means of parenteral therapy. Gastric lavage, one or more times daily, helps to reduce the size of the stomach, and occasionally will relieve the obstruction somewhat, permitting the ingestion of small amounts of nutritive fluid which may succeed in passing the constricted pylorus.

Fredet-Ramstedt Pyloroplasty. The most successful and widely used procedure is the Fredet-Ramstedt pyloroplasty, named for the two surgeons who first described it. The operation may be performed under local anesthesia, but a light ether anesthesia is preferable because it is helpful to the surgeon if the infant can be prevented from crying or otherwise straining during the procedure. The enlarged pyloric muscle is exposed through a small upper right abdominal incision, and an incision made which splits the muscle bundle parallel to the long axis of the lumen of the pylorus. Care is taken to make the incision only sufficiently deep to expose the submucous layer (*submucosa*), so that the actual lumen is not entered. There is thus no chance for leakage of stomach contents and for infection. The edges of the muscle bundle are gently spread apart, and nothing further need be done; the obstruction is relieved, the infant at once starts to gain and grow normally, and in later years pyloric function remains normal.

Nursing Care. In preparing to take care of the baby following operation, it is advisable to have oxygen and an electric aspirator ready for use. If the baby had general anesthesia, it is judicious to place the baby in a crib with the foot elevated; this helps to prevent aspiration in the event of vomiting. If no anesthesia was used, it is helpful to raise the head of the crib one notch to prevent vomiting. In some clinics, the head is raised higher than this, necessitating some device to keep the infant in this position. Small sandbags placed under the arms prevent the baby from sliding down. Another means which has proven helpful is by placing the buttocks of the baby in a little hammock made of diapers which are secured to each side of the crib.

Parenteral fluids are administered for the first twenty-four hours or until fluid intake by mouth is adequate. Fluids should be given slowly, which means between 8 to 15 drops per minute.

Feedings are usually begun eight to twenty-four hours after operation. The general principle is to start with small amounts, increasing gradually. If the baby vomits, the surgeon is notified. One method of feeding begins with a 4 cc. feeding eight to twelve hours after operation, with 4 cc. increments every two hours. As the volume increases to ordinary amounts, the interval between feeding is lengthened. One-half strength formula or breast milk is given; full strength is more difficult to digest because the emptying time of the stomach is prolonged when a high fat content formula is administered.

The baby is fed by eye dropper until amounts over 30 cc. are reached. Very little air is swallowed by this technic. After this, the baby should always be picked up to be fed from the bottle and the head of the bed is elevated for at least twenty minutes thereafter. By the time the infant leaves the hospital, on approximately the seventh postoperative day, he usually has been placed on a four hour feeding schedule.

It is helpful when the mother is present to feed the baby in the hospital before discharge. To find out if she has any apprehension or questions concerning the care of the infant is the responsibility of the nurse. It is not usual for a tiny baby to have such an operation and, therefore, the nurse should give explanations according to the needs. These needs are only discovered by conversation, with interest directed to the care of the infant.

ULCERS OF THE STOMACH AND DUODENUM

Acute or chronic ulceration of the stomach or duodenum is an exceedingly common lesion. It is of frequent occurrence in men of all ages, much less frequent in women, and rare in children. Despite much study over a period of many years, the cause remains unknown.

Although ulcers of the stomach and duodenum (the so-called peptic ulcers) produce a variety of symptoms and signs due to differences in location, activity, and chronicity, there is one symptom that is so characteristic as to be pathognomonic. This symptom is hunger pain. It is a boring, severe type of pain felt commonly in the epigastrium, to one or the other side of the midline, and often radiating straight through to the back on the same side. This pain characteristically occurs when the stomach is empty, usually two to four hours after a meal, and is relieved by eating or by taking bicarbonate of soda. Many of the patients who have this kind of pain will volunteer the information that a glass of milk or other food or a dose of soda relieves the pain. Hunger pain is particularly common in the chronic form of the disease.

Of the many patients who have ulcers, the largest proportion are a rather characteristic type: the tense, restless or irritable individuals, who are apt to be heavy tobacco consumers. No explanation of this observation has been advanced; there are plenty of restless people and chain smokers who do not have ulcers and, indeed, the existence of an ulcer is sufficient to render the most placid person irritable or to drive him to worse habits than smoking.

The acute ulcer may take many courses. One of these is acute perforation. As has been stated, the basis for the original ulceration is not understood, but it is easy to see how the powerful gastric secretions can digest away the wall of the stomach once the break in continuity of the mucous membrane has been established. If the perforation occurs in a portion of the stomach, or duodenum that is anatomically in contact with another structure, a localized inflammatory lesion is the result; but if the perforation takes place into the free peritoneal cavity an acute peritonitis is the result. Another and frequent course taken by an acute ulcer is erosion of a blood vessel in the wall of the stomach with consequent massive hemorrhage, or repeated hemorrhages. A third possibility is that the acute ulcer will progress very slowly, with much concomitant inflammation and scarring, resulting in pain, recurrent small hemorrhages, and deformity of the stomach or duodenum, often complicated by obstruction. A fourth possibility, and perhaps the commonest one, is that the acute ulcer will heal without having given rise to the serious complications just mentioned. Since this is so, the largest proportion of patients who have a peptic ulcer can be treated successfully by medical means and should not be operated upon. Many patients suffer from recurrences of their ulcer, however, and in some the ulcer persists continuously as a chronic ulcer; the patients of this last group are the ones for whom surgery is most often necessary.

Diagnosis of Peptic Ulcer

Symptoms. Pain of the "hunger" type, epigastric distress with frequent sour eructation, or the vomiting of blood (*hematemesis*) are among the commoner symptoms which cause the patient to seek medical aid. In many instances the patient will have had similar symptoms months or years before. An occasional patient has an exsanguinating hemorrhage as the first symptom; such a patient may suddenly collapse on the street or elsewhere. Large amounts of blood may be passed per rectum unnoticed by the patient, or he may have noted the passage of a large tarry stool. Still other patients, especially those whose symptoms have not been sufficiently troublesome to cause them to seek medical advice, may not come to the physician until late in the disease, at which time the chief complaint is likely to be vomiting with inability to retain enough food to maintain nutrition. Physical examination may reveal the signs of anemia if there has been repeated loss of blood, or of starvation and dehydration if the patient has been vomiting; in many patients, however, no abnormal physical signs are to be found.

Perforation. The perforation of a peptic ulcer into the peritoneal cavity is not difficult to diagnose. The abrupt onset of excruciating upper abdominal pain, followed quickly by generalized abdominal pain, weakness, and discomfort in breathing, is accompanied by the physical signs of acute generalized peritonitis, including rigidity of the abdominal wall, grunting respiration, acute tenderness, fever, leukocytosis, and shock.

Gastric Acidity Test. Valuable information is gained from examination of the secretory activity of the stomach. In nearly every normal person the gastric juice is slightly acid when fasting; following the stimulus of eating there is an increase in the amount of hydrochloric acid secreted. In the case of the patient with a peptic ulcer, however, there is nearly always a higher than normal concentration of acid in the fasting stomach, and after stimulation the acidity of the gastric juice increases rapidly. The usual procedure is to introduce a small tube into the stomach

TABLE 2.

Results of Gastric Analyses in Typical Patients

(Expressed in Degrees of Free Hydrochloric Acid)

	FASTING (UNITS)	AFTER HISTAMINE (UNITS)
Normal	5	25
Peptic ulcer	20	70
Gastric cancer	0	0

early in the morning before the patient has eaten breakfast. A sample of gastric juice is withdrawn, but the tube is left in place. Gastric secretion is then stimulated by one of various methods, such as: (1) having the patient eat two slices of bread; (2) introducing a small quantity of alcohol through the tube; or (3) administering a small dose of histamine intramuscularly. Further samples of gastric juice are withdrawn at intervals; later these are analyzed for their acid content and a comparison with normal standards is thus obtained. It is customary to express gastric acidity in degrees which represent the equivalent of the number of cubic centimeters of one-tenth normal hydrochloric acid per 100 cc. of gastric juice.

The samples are also examined for the presence of blood. Delayed emptying of the stomach may be suspected if the sample contains many bacteria or particles of undigested food.

Roentgenography. Easily the most important and valuable diagnostic procedure, however, is roentgenography. A competent roentgenologist, observing the stomach and duodenum under the fluoroscope as the patient swallows a mixture containing barium sulfate, can often see the ulcer. Even when the ulcer is in such a position as to be obscured, it can be diagnosed by the accompanying deformity of the stomach or by the associated alteration in the motility of the gastric muscles. It is important that the patient be properly prepared for fluoroscopy. The stomach should be empty; breakfast must therefore be deferred until after the examination. An enema should be given so as to eliminate as much of the gas in the large intestine as possible. In certain persons the stomach tone and motility are greater than average although no ulcer is present, and in these the hypermotility seen in the first examination may be suppressed or abolished by a few days of rest and by the administration of tincture of belladonna (atropine). Roentgenography also affords a means of observing the effect of therapy, since examinations carried out at intervals shows whether the ulcer is healing or not.

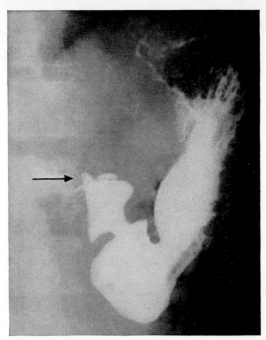

FIGURE 73. X-ray film showing a duodenal ulcer outlined by barium. Arrow points to crater of ulcer.

Benzidine Test. There is usually blood in the stool of the ulcer patient, and the nature and amount of this blood depend upon the amount and rate of bleeding and upon the motility of the intestinal tract. Following a large hemorrhage there is usually gross blood in the stool, although it is very dark red or black as a result of digestion while passing through the tract. Small amounts of blood may be detected only by chemical test (benzidine), for the cells are digested. Since meat eaten by the patient can give a falsely positive test, a positive benzidine test on the stool is of value only if the patient has been on a meat-free diet for three or four days previously.

Gastroscopy. A relatively new diagnostic method is the direct observation of the stomach mucosa through the gastroscope. Since it is not yet possible to examine the pyloric portion because of the limitations of the instrument, the majority of gastric ulcers cannot be visualized. Some ulcers may be seen, however, and the experts in this field believe that they can detect in many cases an

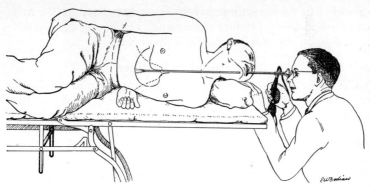

FIGURE 74. Examination of the stomach through the gastroscope. Note position of patient.

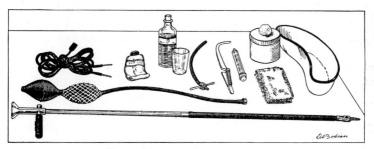

FIGURE 75. Set-up for gastroscopy.

alteration in the appearance of the mucosa which indicates an ulcer that is beyond the view of the gastroscope.

Nursing Care. It is desirable that the patient be instructed not to eat or drink anything for at least eight hours before gastroscopy. When the patient is known to have retention in his stomach, a lavage is done to prevent regurgitation of fluids with the danger of subsequent aspiration into the lungs. The general preparation is similar to that described for bronchoscopy on page 115.

After treatment, the patient should be made comfortable and should be instructed not to swallow anything from two to four hours. The hazard of aspirating food or fluid into the trachea should be carefully explained. This is especially important for the outpatient who leaves the hospital before the anesthesia has worn off. He should also be told that a sore throat is not unusual

but this will be transitory. A rest period is advisable, for most
patients find this procedure exhausting. The length of time will
depend upon the reaction of the individual.

Treatment of Peptic Ulcer

The greater portion of all ulcers of the stomach and duodenum
will respond to and may be cured by a program of treatment that
includes rest, special diet, and medication. Sippy, an American
physician, was responsible for the popularization of this regimen,
and his standard diets for the treatment of ulcers, though now
somewhat modified to meet the requirements of modern knowledge of dietary deficiencies, are still commonly used. Rest in bed,
freedom from business cares or other worries, and abstention
from tobacco and alcoholic beverages are enforced in the first
period of the treatment. The most important principles to be
observed in the diet are that the feedings shall be small and frequent, served at regular short intervals, and that the diet should
contain no mechanically harsh material and should lack none of
the essential vitamins. Medication includes an antispasmodic,
usually tincture of belladonna, mild sedatives if the patient is
restless, and alkali to neutralize the high acidity of the gastric
juice. The carbonates of bismuth, calcium, and sodium were
most commonly used until recently; at present it seems that the
colloidal suspension of the mildly alkaline aluminum hydroxide,
administered at frequent intervals by mouth, or continually by
means of an inlying tube, is a more effective agent in combating
the hyperacidity. Another extremely useful medication is Ban-
thine, one of a group of drugs which have the ability to block
the action of the vagus nerve. This drug can be tolerated by
most individuals and, if taken regularly, will reduce secretion of
hydrochloric acid to the vanishing point.

If therapy is successful, the patient's symptoms disappear, and
the ulcer can be seen to be healing when studied by roentgenography. Under these conditions the patient is permitted very gradually to resume his former activities and to return to a full,
ordinary diet. The medication is discontinued. This whole program, however, must be spread over a period of three to six
months or longer.

Operative Treatment of Complications

It is generally accepted that surgical treatment for peptic ulcer
is indicated when symptoms persist despite thorough medical

Sippy Diet (Modified)

The basic feeding is three ounces (90 cc.) of milk (half cream), given every hour from 6 a.m. to 10 p.m. inclusive, and on any hour during the night if the patient is awake. The basic feeding is supplemented as follows:

DAY	7 A.M.	10 A.M.	1 P.M.	4 P.M.	6 P.M.	9 P.M.
2	3 oz. sieved cereal 2 tsp. sugar 1 soft-cooked egg 2 saltines	3 oz. sieved cereal 2 tsp. sugar			1 soft-cooked egg 2 saltines 3 oz. sieved cereal 2 tsp. sugar	
3	3 oz. sieved cereal 2 tsp. sugar		custard			
4	3 oz. sieved cereal 2 tsp. sugar	custard	milk toast (1 slice) 1 sq. butter		cream soup 1 soft-cooked egg 4 saltines	
5	3 oz. sieved cereal 2 tsp. sugar	milk toast (1 slice) 1 sq. butter	1 soft-cooked egg 2 saltines	custard	cream soup 3 oz. steamed rice 1 sq. butter	4 cookies
6	1 soft-cooked egg 4 saltines	3 oz. sieved cereal 2 tsp. sugar	cream soup 2 saltines 3 oz. sieved cereal 2 tsp. sugar	3 oz. sieved cereal 2 tsp. sugar	1 soft-cooked egg 2 saltines	dessert
7	1 soft-cooked egg 1 slice toast 1 sq. butter	1 oz. cottage cheese 4 saltines 1½ oz. orange juice		dessert	cream soup 1 soft-cooked egg 1 slice toast 1 sq. butter	4 cookies
8–14	3 oz. sieved cereal 2 tsp. sugar 1 soft-cooked egg 1 slice toast 1 sq. butter	dessert 1½ oz. orange juice	½ c. mashed potatoes 1 sq. butter dessert	2 saltines 1 tbsp. jelly	1 soft-cooked egg 3 oz. steamed rice 1 slice toast 1 sq. butter	dessert

14–21 Soft diet without meat, including intermediate nourishment three times a day of 6 oz. of milk (half cream) with crackers.
Hourly milk is discontinued.

21–28 Same as on days 14–21 with addition of ground meat.

Meulengracht Diet

The Meulengracht diet is a soft diet with the following modifications:
1. Amount of food................ad libitum, especially milk (no coffee or tea until ordered by physician)
2. Intermediate feeding, 10 a.m., 3 p.m., 9 p.m., of 8 oz. of milk (half cream)
3. At least three soft foods to be included in each meal
4. Liver to be given at least twice a week

treatment, or when complications arise that are not amenable to medical therapy. It is not always easy to differentiate between a gastric ulcer and gastric cancer; furthermore, a cancer not infrequently arises from an ulcer. For these reasons it is wise to operate upon any gastric ulcer that does not show evidence of healing after a proper course of medical treatment. This indication does not apply to duodenal ulcers, because cancer of the duodenum is an extremely rare disease.

Perforation. The most dramatic complication is the sudden perforation of the wall of the stomach or duodenum into the free peritoneal cavity. Well recognized as an urgent surgical emergency, a perforated peptic ulcer is best treated by early laparotomy with simple closure of the perforation by means of sutures. This treatment is highly successful: the mortality is low if the procedure is carried out within the first few hours after perforation has occurred; on the other hand, it rises very rapidly if more than eighteen hours has elapsed, and few patients are saved if treatment is not undertaken within the first twenty-four hours after perforation. That is because a rapidly fulminating bacterial peritonitis develops on top of the highly irritating chemical peritonitis which results from the discharge of the gastric juice into the peritoneal cavity.

Hemorrhage. Another common complication of peptic ulcer which may require emergency treatment is sudden massive hemorrhage. There is some bleeding with all peptic ulcers but this usually subsides as the ulcer heals. In the more chronic type of ulcer, however, particularly when there is considerable scar tissue in the base of the ulcer, a large vessel may become eroded. From such a source an exsanguinating hemorrhage sometimes occurs because the scar tissue prevents the natural retraction and contraction of the walls of the opened blood vessel.

Conservative therapy, including elevation of the foot of the bed, quiet, the administration of morphine, and an ice cap to the abdomen, should be tried first; nothing is permitted by mouth, and both transfusions and intravenous fluids are given with extreme caution and slowness, so as to maintain the blood pressure at as low a level as is safe in order to facilitate clotting of the blood at the bleeding point. If the bleeding persists, or if it occurs again after a short interval, operation should be undertaken with the purpose of exposing the bleeding point and controlling the hemorrhage. Surgical treatment should be carried out earlier in older patients because they do not withstand the acute loss of blood so well as younger persons. Large amounts of blood should be on hand to give to the patient during and after the operation.

Lumen Obstruction. Some degree of obstruction of the pyloric lumen is a frequent complication of peptic ulcer. Sometimes the obstruction is caused by the edema which is a part of the inflammatory reaction about the acute ulcer, and in such cases the blockage usually is relieved by conservative treatment. When the lumen in the pyloric region is narrowed as a result of the formation of scar tissue, however, the obstruction persists and surgical intervention is necessary. Equally important as the operation is the preoperative preparation, for many of these patients suffer from extreme malnutrition and dehydration which must be treated before operation is undertaken.

Pain. The persistence of severe pain despite medical therapy is another indication for operation. In such instances it is common to find that the ulcer is a penetrating one, often invading the pancreas. If possible, such an ulcer should be eradicated.

NEOPLASMS OF THE STOMACH AND DUODENUM

Benign tumors of the stomach and duodenum are rare. Occasionally a polyp (*epithelial papilloma*) of the mucosa develops, and makes its presence known by bleeding. Simple excision is curative. Benign fibroma is sometimes found in the wall of the stomach, but is usually not productive of symptoms.

Carcinoma of the stomach, on the other hand, is one of the commonest forms of human cancer, and is one in which treatment, up to the present time, has proved least satisfactory. One of the many puzzling features about it is the difference in its rate of occurrence in males and in females. If one excepts all forms of skin cancer, gastric cancer is the commonest form of cancer in men, but it is far less often observed in women. The ratio is about five to one. Another remarkable fact is the rarity of carcinoma arising from the adjacent and contiguous duodenal mucosa. Probably the worst feature of cancer of the stomach is the absence of symptoms early in the disease, so that the great majority of the victims of this malignant tumor have no warning that might lead them to seek medical aid while the tumor is still in the early, curable stage. It is a disease of middle age and beyond, being fairly uncommon in those under 40 years of age.

Diagnosis of Carcinoma of the Stomach

Until a better method of treatment is evolved, only those patients in whom the tumor has not spread beyond the walls of the stomach can be cured; thus early diagnosis is imperative. The occurrence in men over 40 of any vague complaint which might be referable to the stomach should be followed by a thorough investigation and by careful observation thereafter if the diagnostic studies are inconclusive.

Symptoms. One of the commonest early symptoms is a change in the individual's appetite, either a gradual loss of appetite (*anorexia*) or a distaste for certain foods that formerly were eaten with enjoyment. There may be some upper abdominal discomfort which the patient refers to as "indigestion," or a heavy feeling, or a pressing weight. Eventually, as the tumor grows and metastasizes, the afflicted person loses weight and strength and becomes severely anemic, and symptoms of obstruction appear, with regurgitation of undigested food. Actual pain is a very late symptom. In an occasional case, when the tumor is situated at or very near the pylorus, obstruction occurs early in the disease, so that the patient is forced to seek medical advice while there is still a chance for cure. Hemorrhage is the rule, although the bleeding is usually slight until the final stages.

Gastroscopy and Roentgenography. There are no diagnostic physical signs of gastric cancer while it is still in the curable stage; by the time the physician can palpate the tumor mass through the abdominal wall, cure is unlikely. Accurate early diagnosis is based upon gastroscopy and roentgenography. By these means the tumor, or its deforming effect on the gastric outline and motility, is observed.

Gastric Acidity. Reduction in the acidity of the gastric juice is a characteristic phenomenon. Commonly there is complete absence of free acid (*achlorhydria*); this is in striking contrast to the high acidity found in peptic ulcer (Table 2, p. 253), but it must be borne in mind that exceptions are frequent.

Treatment of Carcinoma of the Stomach

Cure may be accomplished surgically by complete removal of the growth; this involves the removal of a part or all of the stomach. Since it is usually not possible to tell before operation whether or not the tumor has spread beyond the confines of the stomach, many patients are found at operation to have an incurable lesion. For some of these, procedures are carried out which are palliative though not curative, such as removing some of the tumor-bearing stomach to prevent further hemorrhage, and short-circuiting procedures to relieve obstruction. These palliative operations make life more bearable for the victims, and in some instances add an appreciable period of comfort and usefulness to the life of the patient. Therapy by means of radium or by deep roentgen irradiation has not been successful.

The rate of permanent cure of patients who have cancer of the stomach is still very low, probably less than 10 per cent for the country as a whole. While a continuous effort is being made to find a better method of treatment, the main hope, as in most other forms of cancer, still lies in early diagnosis and prompt treatment.

OPERATIONS ON THE STOMACH AND DUODENUM

Preoperative Care. It must be reemphasized that many of the patients who need operation have, as a preoperative complication of their illness, either dehydration or starvation or both to some degree. The parenteral methods of treating these conditions have been discussed in Chapter 5, page 49. Another preparatory measure of great importance is gastric suction drainage (p. 243). In patients who have had pyloric obstruction the stomach is likely to be much enlarged, with edema and weakening of the stomach wall as a consequence of the prolonged dilatation, so that the tissues are in poor condition for healing. Finally, it is immensely important that the stomach be emptied immediately before operation, so as to prevent the spilling of a large amount of infective material into the peritoneal cavity if it should prove necessary to open the stomach during operation. This is usually accomplished by placing a Levin tube in the stomach. The patient should be prepared for what is to happen in a manner that he will understand. He should be told that it is essential for him to have an empty stomach before operation and that the tube will remain in the stomach for a short time after operation. Understanding what will be done to insure the best care not only enlists the cooperation of the patient but also gives him a sense of security.

Before the tube is inserted into the nostril, the tip may be dipped into isotonic saline solution to provide for easy passage.

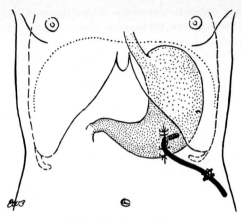

FIGURE 76. Gastrostomy.

After the tube is inserted, the stomach contents are then with-drawn either with a syringe or by attaching the tube to suction equal to 2 to 5 feet of water. The tube should be secured to the cheek and/or forehead with adhesive tape, so that motion will not be transmitted to the sensitive nasal mucosa.

Gastrostomy

All operative procedures upon the stomach and duodenum come under the heading of laparotomies, so that all that has been said (p. 224) is applicable. Occasionally it is necessary to open the stomach for the purpose of removing a foreign body; simple opening of the stomach, followed by closure, is called *gastrotomy*. To be differentiated from this last is *gastrostomy*, already men-tioned in connection with disease of the esophagus. Gastrostomy has for its purpose the creation of a permanent opening through the abdominal wall into the lumen of the stomach so that the patient may be fed. Through a small upper left abdominal in-cision the anterior wall of the stomach is exposed, drawn for-ward, and sutured to the anterior abdominal wall about the in-cision. A small opening is made into the lumen of the stomach through which a catheter is introduced; this opening is sutured tightly about the catheter so that no leakage will occur, and the catheter is firmly fixed by suture or adhesive tape to the ab-dominal wall so that it will not slip out. This operation may be easily performed under local anesthesia, a considerable advan-tage when dealing with very ill patients.

Nursing Care. Within a very few hours the peritoneum of the stomach and that of the abdominal wall become adherent and sufficiently leakage-proof so that water and nutritive fluids may be cautiously introduced through the tube; after seventy-two hours it is usually possible to feed the patient an adequate diet through the tube. An adequate formula for tube feeding has been previously listed on page 50. The technic for instilling the formula and the care of the surrounding wound have also been described (p. 216).

Healing of the tract is complete after ten days, and it is then possible to remove and replace the tube as desired for cleaning purposes. If, however, the tube is not replaced immediately, there may be contraction or even complete healing of the opening; but as a rule it is necessary to operate in order to close the gastrostomy when it is no longer needed.

Gastroenterostomy

Preoperative Care. The importance of careful preoperative preparation in this operation is obvious, for these patients who have had pyloric obstruction are starved and dehydrated, and have large, atonic, and bacteria-laden stomachs.

Operative Technic. The short-circuiting operation to relieve pyloric obstruction is gastroenterostomy, meaning, literally, the construction of an opening between the stomach and the intestine. There are two ways of doing this: in one, the posterior gastroenterostomy, the opening (*anastomosis*) is made between the posterior wall of the stomach and the first loop of the jejunum, this loop being brought up adjacent to the stomach through an opening which is made in the mesentery of the transverse colon, so that the loop of jejunum passes behind the transverse colon. This is the most satisfactory method, but sometimes it cannot be performed. The other method is the anterior gastroenterostomy, in which the loop of jejunum is brought up over the front of the transverse colon, and the anastomosis is performed between the jejunum and the anterior wall of the stomach. In either case, stomach contents may then pass through this new opening directly into the jejunum, by-passing the pylorus and the duodenum, as shown in Figure 77. Under modern conditions this operation is performed with very little risk to life, and, if used in properly selected patients, the results are highly successful. In most clinics inhalation anesthesia is commonly used for this procedure.

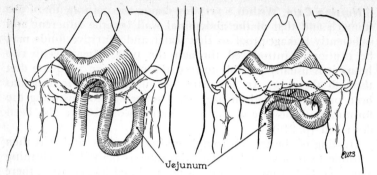

FIGURE 77. Gastroenterostomy. *A*, Anterior (antecolic) ; *B*, posterior (retrocolic) .

Nursing Care. The preparation, in general, of patients for surgery of the stomach is adequate hydration and withdrawal of the contents through a Levin tube connected to suction. Sometimes a lavage is carried out, if there is evidence of pyloric obstruction. Careful measurement of intake and output cannot be overemphasized. The character of the drainage should also be observed and charted. The general aspects of care necessary for all patients who anticipate surgery as described previously should be carried out to insure the optimum physical and mental comfort.

After operation these patients are treated essentially the same as any laparotomy patients, but with special attention to the Levin tube siphonage and diet. The Levin tube is usually connected to suction for about twenty-four hours to keep the stomach empty and to promote healing. The drainage should be observed frequently to determine the color, consistency and amount. The drainage may be bright red for a half hour or so immediately after surgery, but thereafter it should be dark red or brown. If it continues to be bright red, the surgeon should be told because it signifies active bleeding. The drainage should be measured and recorded at least every twelve hours. The surgeon usually orders irrigations of the tube which may be carried out as described on page 245.

The diet after gastroenterostomy or resection depends upon the patient and surgeon. Usually, after the tube is removed, tap water is given in small amounts (30 cc.) every hour for the first day, then a liquid diet increased to 60 or 90 cc. is usually offered.

Frequently the patient may progress more rapidly than this, up to soft diet in limited portions on the fourth day. However, each patient is given food according to his tolerance, preventing a set rule for a dietary regimen. It is important to try to supply adequate fluids and solid food but not to urge eating or drinking if there is a complaint of fullness. The soft diet given in six small feedings is gradually increased to a normal diet in six small feedings.

In learning about his diet, the patient should be encouraged to assume responsibility for the planning of his diet. The factors which should be emphasized as the nurse plans with him are the importance of adequate fluid and food intake and the maintenance of weight.

In the postoperative feeding schedule complete withholding of fluid is unnecessary because one can be sure that there will be fluid in the stomach anyway, since the gastric mucosa is going to continue to secrete just as before operation; and if this fluid does not leak through the new suture line, it is unlikely that a little water given by mouth will do so. On the other hand, it is entirely conceivable that a large amount of fluid might, by its very weight, cause tearing and consequent leakage; it is wise, therefore, to limit the amount of fluid or other material in the stomach to small, safe amounts until the suture line is healed. This limitation applies not only to fluid given by mouth, but also to fluid which might accumulate in the stomach as the result of gastric secretion plus some failure of the new anastomosis to function well, and it is thus extremely important to observe the patient carefully, so that the stomach can be aspirated at any time that it shows a tendency to fill up.

Vomiting, and especially the repeated regurgitation of small amounts of stomach contents, should lead at once to the suspicion of an increasing accumulation of fluid or gas, or both, in the stomach. Diagnosis of this complication is confirmed by percussion of the stomach, and by the aspiration of a large quantity of fluid upon the passage of a stomach tube, and should be followed immediately by the introduction of an inlying tube to which is applied the Wangensteen continuous suction apparatus. This complication is not at all uncommon after gastroenterostomy, particularly at first when the immediate swelling of the recently incised tissues is present; many surgeons prefer to introduce the inlying tube during or directly after operation.

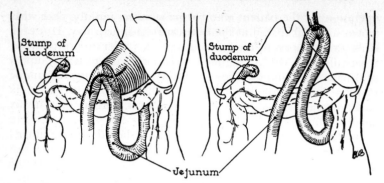

Figure 78. *A,* Partial gastrectomy (Polya antecolic end-to-side gastrojejunos-tomy). *B,* Total gastrectomy.

Vagectomy

Since the secretion in the stomach of hydrochloric acid is controlled by impulses traveling down the vagus nerves from the brain, it is possible to reduce remarkably the secretion of acid by dividing the vagus nerves (*vagectomy*). Both nerves must be cut; this can be done through an incision in the chest or through an abdominal incision. Because cutting the nerves interferes with the motility of the stomach, delaying the emptying, it has been found best to combine gastroenterostomy with vagectomy in the treatment of duodenal ulcers.

The postoperative care of a patient who has had this procedure is the same as after gastroenterostomy. It may be necessary to employ suction drainage longer than when vagectomy is not done, and Urecholine may be used to improve gastric motility and muscle tone.

Gastrectomy

The term gastrectomy is used to designate the operations in which some or all of the stomach is removed. In a partial gastrectomy a portion of the stomach is removed, in a subtotal gastrectomy nearly all of the stomach is removed, and in a total gastrectomy the entire stomach is removed.

Gastrectomy, although first successfully performed more than half a century ago, until quite recently has been associated with a formidable mortality. Modern methods of building up the patient before operation, and modern knowledge of diet after operation for the patient who has no stomach left, together with modern technical skill at the operating table, are now successful in bringing through five out of every six patients who undergo removal of the entire stomach. Furthermore, if a small portion of the stomach can be spared, the mortality is scarcely higher now than that after simple gastroenterostomy.

In partial gastrectomy the feeding plan is the same as that in gastroenterostomy (p. 264). A commonly used regimen for the feeding of the total gastrectomy patient is as follows:

DAY	HOUR	AMOUNT	FOOD
1–4			Nothing by mouth
5	6 a.m.–10 p.m. every hour	15 cc.	Tap water
6	6 a.m.–10 p.m. every hour	30 cc.	Tap water
7	6 a.m.–10 p.m. every hour	45 cc.	Tap water
8	6 a.m.–10 p.m. every hour	60 cc.	Tap water alternating with broth three times a day
9	6 a.m.–10 p.m. every hour	75 cc.	Tap water alternating with broth as desired
10	6 a.m.–10 p.m. every hour	90 cc.	Tap water alternating with broth, fruit juice, and milk
11	6 a.m.–10 p.m. every hour	120 cc.	Tap water alternating with broth, fruit juice, and milk
12 and thereafter	8 a.m., 10 a.m., 12 N., 3 p.m., 6 p.m., 8 p.m.	Fluids ad lib.	Soft diet six in small feedings

The diet is usually increased to six small feedings as outlined and remains so in the majority of cases. When this regimen is to begin, it is necessary to consider the personality of the patient in order to select the type of diet. If he is one who has good teeth, is careful to chew his food and eats fairly slowly, a regularly prepared diet, high in calories, seems to be tolerated without untoward effects. However, if the patient has poor teeth and/or eats rapidly, it is advisable that he eat a finely chopped and soft texture diet. A fair appetite is usual, but a small amount of food satisfies and the slight discomfort which may follow causes him to limit his intake. His weight may be maintained with good effort but he will not get fat after a total gastrectomy. Discomfort after eating may be relieved or averted if the patient lies down for a few minutes after each meal. Cold foods should be avoided because they tend to bring about distress. Untoward symptoms following a meal include excessive fullness, weakness, nausea, palpitation and sweating.

The nurse should begin explaining the essentials of good nutrition, the components of his diet, and their preparation when the patient is well enough to be interested. In order to make this applicable to daily living, the nurse must find out what the patient likes and dislikes. It is of little value to make out a menu and discuss preparation of foods which are not acceptable to the patient. Much explanation on the part of the nurse may cause resistance; it is better to try to encourage the patient to assume responsibility. Progress is evidenced by questions, and later by assurance that he can cope with this important aspect of self-care.

The patient will be requested to return to his surgeon for check-ups. It must be kept in mind that the majority of these patients were operated upon because they had cancer of the stomach. The nurse should try to do all she can to make him understand that his surgeon will wish him to return even though he feels perfectly well.

Outcome. Many persons, following removal of a large portion of their stomach may, after a due period of convalescence, resume a normal life, including their former eating habits. This is not true, however, of those patients who have had total gastrectomy; in these the ingested food passes directly from the esophagus into the jejunum, and is not subjected to any of the digestive processes normally encountered in the stomach. Furthermore, the small intestine cannot receive the quantity at one feeding that the stomach can. For these reasons, the gastrectomy patient must necessarily eat small amounts, must eat often, and must eat foods which are predigested or which do not require much processing in order to become assimilable. The removal of the stomach also affects the proper formation of the red blood cells, so that anemia similar to primary anemia develops unless the necessary factors are supplied to the patient afterward.

If, however, only a small portion of the stomach has been removed, all these elaborate precautions are unnecessary, for such a patient needs only the same postoperative care as that afforded the patient who has had a gastroenterostomy, and will, like the latter, eventually return to a nearly normal mode of existence.

Complications of Gastroenterostomy and Gastrectomy

Unfortunately there are some special complications of gastroenterostomy and gastrectomy which occur with sufficient frequency to warrant further consideration.

Marginal Ulcer. First and commonest of these is the so-called marginal ulcer. This is an ulcer which develops along the line of junction between the gastric and jejunal mucous membranes at the site of the gastroenterostomy, and which is due, presumably, to the action of the acid gastric juice upon the jejunal mucosa, which ordinarily is exposed only to alkaline secretions. Why this type of ulcer should occur in only a small fraction of all such anastomoses is not known. The symptoms are much like those of peptic ulcer, and the complications are likewise similar. Perforation and peritonitis may occur, as also may perforation into the transverse colon, with resulting gastrocolic fistula. Medical treatment is unsatisfactory; surgical treatment is difficult and dangerous and is followed by a high incidence of recurrences. Some surgeons recommend vagectomy as the best treatment for marginal ulcer. It is intriguing, however, to note that marginal ulcer occurs as a complication of the combined vagectomy and gastroenterostomy procedure.

Duodenal Fistula. A less common complication of gastrectomy is leakage of the closed stump of the duodenum, with formation —if the patient survives—of a duodenal fistula. This complication also follows certain operations upon the common biliary duct, particularly when reconstruction, or reimplantation of the duct into the duodenum is attempted. It is a dangerous complication because: (1) there is excessive loss of fluid and electrolytes with consequent imbalance and loss of enzymes necessary for adequate digestion; and (2) the powerful secretions rapidly digest away the tissues of the abdominal wall and wound.

Nursing Care. The vital signs are those associated with a very ill patient. A fever, rapid pulse, low blood pressure, great prostration and severe abdominal pain are signs and symptoms that the nurse may observe in a patient with duodenal leakage.

The fluid lost through the fistula is comprised of gastric, duodenal, pancreatic and biliary secretions; up to 7 liters a day may be lost through this opening even when no fluids are taken by mouth. The maintenance of fluid, electrolyte and nutritional balance necessitates strenuous intravenous therapy. In addition, large amounts of vitamins are also given to aid healing. It is not uncommon for the patient to receive over 5000 cc. of intravenous

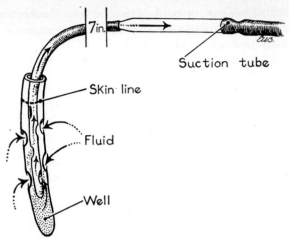

FIGURE 79. Sump drain. The outer tube holds the tissues of the wound away
from the suction tube.

fluid in a twenty-four hour period. It is desirable to achieve a
urinary output of between 1500 and 2000 cc. Careful and prompt
recording of all intake and output permits accurate appraisal of
the therapy. The nurse should also observe the flow of the intravenous fluids frequently to maintain the rate desired. Usually
no more than 45 drops per minute are ordered; this permits
utilization of proteins and prevents fever, vomiting and overflow
through the kidneys.

The surgeon frequently orders the collected fistula drainage
to be re-fed when the patient has an inlying stomach tube. When
this is not done, bile salts are given.

Vitamin intake during the time of copious drainage consists
of ascorbic acid, 1000 mg.; thiamine, 50 mg.; riboflavin, 50 mg.;
nicotinic acid, 500 mg.; and liver extract, 2 cc. daily. Vitamin K
is given when there is hypoprothrombinemia, or it is sometimes
given to prevent it.

The very active and abundant digestive ferments found in the
upper portion of the gastrointestinal tract cause rapid excoriation of the skin as they seep over the abdominal wall. Within a
few hours after the secretions flow out of the fistula, the skin is
digested; it appears fiery red and oozes plasma similar to skin
which has been burned. The ingredient most responsible for this
is trypsin from the pancreas.

Various methods have been devised to prevent the contact of secretions with the skin. One method of protecting the skin from secretions is to employ suction with a sump drain in the fistula (Fig. 79). The bedclothes are held off the area by a cradle which is placed over the patient. In addition, medications may be ordered to be placed on the skin around the tube where the inevitable seepage occurs. Ten per cent tannic acid, Kaolin, and aluminum hydroxide gel are preparations which have been used to neutralize the secretions. Also sponges soaked in beef extract or egg white have been placed around the tube in an attempt to divert the trypsin. Ointments seem to be of little value because the secretions tend to burrow through or seep under them.

Frequent cleansing of the entire area is important and it has been observed that when this is done every hour, followed by re-application of whatever medication is ordered, digestion of the skin can be kept at a minimum. Sponging the area with aqueous benzalkonium chloride solution is satisfactory for cleansing the area; at times plain castile soap and water are used.

Another method, used less frequently, consists of placing the patient on a Bradford frame in the prone position. The stream of secretions may then be collected in a basin. This, however, seems rather uncomfortable for the patient and prevents frequent turning, but is applicable when other means are not available.

As the patient improves, it is often possible to get him to do his own cleansing by conveniently arranging a tray with necessary supplies. The time that such a suggestion can be made depends entirely on the individual patient, but rarely does he feel well enough for a week or ten days after the discovery of the fistula.

Convalescent care following such an episode is regulated upon the individual needs of the patient. Sometimes it is followed by an operation to close the fistula, but usually the fistula closes spontaneously.

SUMMARY

Benign ulcer and carcinoma are the common lesions of the stomach; ulcer frequently occurs in the duodenum. Surgery is performed for the serious complications of ulcer, and for cancer. Operative mortality is kept low by proper hydration of patients and drainage of the stomach before and after operation. The patient's well-being after operation depends largely upon how successfully he can maintain his nutrition.

VOCABULARY REVIEW

pyloroplasty	*sump drain*	*marginal ulcer*
gastroscope	*gastroenterostomy*	*duodenal fistula*
vagectomy	*gastrectomy*	*trypsin*
hyperacidity		

SUGGESTED READING

1. Albright, Hollis L., and Leonard, Field C.: Duodenal Fistula—Problems in Management. Ann. Surg., *132:*49–63 (July) 1950.
2. Dragstedt, Lester: Gastric Vagotomy. Am. J. Nursing, *48:*278–281 (May) 1948.
3. Fletcher, Archibald G.: The Present Status of Total Gastrectomy in the Treatment of Gastric Cancer. Surgery, *30:*403–433 (August) 1951.
4. Grimes, Orville H., Bell, H. Glenn, and Olney, Mary B.: Congenital Hypertrophic Pyloric Stenosis. J. Pediatrics, *37:*522–529 (October) 1950.
5. Heger, Catherine: Surgical Nursing Care of Patients with Duodenal Ulcer. Am. J. Nursing, *52:*861–862 (July) 1952.
6. Krause, Marie V.: Nutrition and Diet Therapy. Philadelphia, W. B. Saunders Co., 1952, pp. 164–168.
7. Palumbo, Louis T.: Surgical Treatment of Duodenal Ulcer. Am. J. Nursing, *52:*857–860 (July) 1952.
8. Scott, H. W., Jr., and Longmire, W. P., Jr.: Total Gastrectomy; Report of 63 Cases. Surgery, *26:*488–498 (September) 1949.
9. Wilson, Helen A.: Nursing Care in Gastric Vagotomy, Am. J. Nursing, *48:* 282 (May) 1948.

CHAPTER 25

Surgery of the Liver, Biliary Tract, and Pancreas

Anatomy and Physiology. The liver is the largest and heaviest organ in the body, and the multiplicity of its functions is even now not completely understood. From the standpoint of the surgeon, the most important function of the liver is the secretion of the bile, which is, among other things, essential to proper digestion. The bile is collected in the liver into the vast system of biliary ducts which finally drain into the main biliary ducts of the right and left lobes of the liver. These unite into a common hepatic duct just at the hilum of the liver. A short distance below this junction a smaller duct joins the hepatic duct. This is the cystic duct, and it leads into the gallbladder, a pear-shaped, saclike organ situated along the posterior inferior margin of the right lobe of the liver.

The gallbladder has a double function, serving both as a reservoir for bile and as a concentrating mechanism, for some of the water is absorbed, so that the bile which remains for a time in the gallbladder becomes more concentrated than that secreted by the liver. The secretion of bile is continuous, but the rate may be increased by certain stimuli, including the eating of a meal, particularly one high in fats, and by certain drugs such as magnesium sulfate. These stimuli, in addition to increasing the rate of secretion of the bile, cause the emptying of the bile from the gallbladder. Bile passes down the cystic and hepatic ducts into their common prolongation, known as the common biliary duct, which enters the posterior wall of the duodenum, adjacent to the head of the pancreas, through the ampulla of Vater. Just before opening into the lumen of the duodenum, the common duct is joined by the main pancreatic duct, so that the bile and the pancreatic juice enter the duodenum together. This is important, for, although there are usually accessory openings of other little pancreatic ducts into the duodenum, an obstruction to the opening in the ampulla of Vater blocks the passage of all of the bile and most of the pancreatic juice, preventing these most important digestive juices from reaching the food upon which they are supposed to act.

The pancreas (sweetbread) is a fish-shaped organ that lies behind the peritoneum, directly back of the duodenum, lower border of the stomach, and transverse colon. It serves both as a gland of digestion, secreting the pancreatic juice into the duodenum, and as an endocrine gland, the pancreatic islands of Langerhans secreting insulin directly into the blood stream.

To the left, just lateral to the tail of the pancreas, lies the spleen. This organ, although anatomically in the closest of relations to the other organs of digestion, plays no known role in the function of the alimentary tract.

The anatomic location and relationships of these organs is best appreciated by studying Figure 72. Note that the arteries which supply the liver, the spleen, the pancreas, the stomach, and the duodenum are all derived from the same branch of the aorta, and that the blood from all of these organs is carried to the liver through the tributary branches of the portal vein.

JAUNDICE

This condition, in which the skin becomes yellow, is so common that almost everyone knows something about it. In order to appreciate the significance of jaundice, however, the student must know the facts about the remarkable cycle in which the blood and bile pigments are interrelated. When a red blood cell becomes too old to function efficiently it is removed from the circulating blood by the reticuloendothelial cells of the body which are in the spleen, liver and bone marrow. The worn-out cell is taken apart, and the hemoglobin, that brilliant red chemical compound which has the ability to transport oxygen, is changed into the bile pigments by the reticuloendothelial cells. The bile pigments travel in the circulating blood to the liver, where they are taken out of the blood by the liver cells. The bile pigments are called bilirubin and biliverdin, and are responsible for the yellowish green color of the bile. The bile passes from the liver, by way of the extrahepatic biliary ducts previously described, into the duodenum, becoming mixed there with the other intestinal contents. In the intestinal tract nearly all of the bile pigment is absorbed, and is carried by the circulating blood to the bone marrow, where the hemoglobin is resynthesized. The absorption is not complete, however, and enough bile pigment is lost with the feces to color these, which accounts for the normal light brown of the stool. In the ordinary course of events, the amount of bile pigment free in the circulating blood is small, so that the concentration of it is too low to color the blood plasma visibly. In certain pathologic conditions, however, the amount of bile pigment in the circulating blood is increased sufficiently to stain the plasma and to stain all the tissues of the body; it is this which constitutes jaundice.

Jaundice may be produced in a number of ways. In the first place, there may be excessive destruction of red blood cells, liberating a great amount of altered hemoglobin. This is what happens in congenital hemolytic icterus and in severe reactions following the transfusion of mismatched blood. Another cause of jaundice is severe disease of the liver, in which case the liver may be so damaged that it is unable to remove the pigment completely from the blood. This occurs when the liver is seriously damaged by cancer, or by infectious hepatitis or the virus of homologous serum jaundice. A third common cause of jaundice, and this is the one in which surgeons are chiefly interested, is obstruction to the extrahepatic biliary ducts, which prevents the discharge of bile from the liver and results in the regurgitation of the liver bile back into the blood vessels in the liver. Thus it is apparent that jaundice may be the sign of several quite different diseases.

It is usually easy to recognize jaundice clinically, for the bright yellow tinting of the sclerae is striking. The skin is yellow, and itching (*pruritus*) is common and often very distressing. The urine is stained a deep brown, and can be tested to show the presence of the bile chemicals. If no bile is reaching the intestinal tract, the stool color is altered, and the feces become putty or light gray in color. It must be remembered, however, that jaundice may not be recognized if the patient is examined by ordinary artificial light, even though the jaundice is severe. Daylight or a blue light must be used. The relative degree of jaundice is measured in the laboratory by tests on the patient's blood. One of these, the van den Bergh test, measures the amount of bilirubin in the blood plasma.

DISEASES OF THE LIVER

It is not remarkable that such a large and important organ as the liver is frequently the site of serious disease; unfortunately, however, only a few of these diseases are amenable to surgical treatment. Chronic degenerative disease, generalized inflammatory disease, and carcinoma of the liver—both primary and secondary—are common, but there is no surgical treatment which is successful in these conditions. An occasional benign tumor, usually a hemangioma, occurs and is cured by operative removal. On the other hand, the injury caused the liver by obstruction or disease of the extrahepatic biliary ducts and the gallbladder can be remedied by the adequate treatment of the causative condition. Liver abscess is about the only intrinsic disease of the liver which can be benefited by surgery.

Pyogenic Abscess. Acute pyogenic abscess of the liver is usually the result of the spread of infection from somewhere in the intestinal tract, as from an inflamed appendix, often by way of the portal vein. The portal vein, or a tributary, may be infected (pylephlebitis). The onset of this condition is usually marked by chills and a high spiking type of fever. The patient is acutely ill, bacteria are often cultured from the blood stream, and jaundice develops. There are commonly multiple abscesses in the liver in association with pylephlebitis, and it is not practicable to drain them surgically, as they are small and too numerous to find. The treatment consists in removal of the original cause of the infection if possible, supplemented by transfusions, antibiotics, and other supportive therapy. The mortality rate is high.

Occasionally, however, there is only a large, single liver abscess. This may develop quite insidiously, and may be suspected in a patient who has fever, leukocytosis, and vague complaints of pain or discomfort referable to the upper abdomen. Examination may reveal some enlargement of and tenderness over the liver. Diagnosis is made certain by aspiration of purulent material with a needle. The proper treatment is surgical drainage, performed in such a way as to prevent contamination of the peritoneal cavity.

Amebic Abscess. One of the more serious complications of amebic dysentery is the occurrence of abscess of the liver due to amebae. This is to be suspected when pain, enlargement of the liver, and fever occur in one who has amebae in his stools, or in one who has lived in a region where amebic dysentery is common. It is important to differentiate this type of abscess from the ordinary pyogenic variety because surgical drainage of an amebic abscess only results in severe secondary infection and few cures. Such abscesses are more properly treated by aspiration and by the introduction of emetine or other antimony compounds directly into the abscess cavity. Antibiotic therapy has been found useful, too.

CHOLECYSTITIS

Inflammatory disease of the gallbladder is called cholecystitis. There are two varieties: an acute inflammation which is similar to acute appendicitis or to any acute inflammation with all the characteristic pathologic changes, and a chronic type of inflammation, and with all shades of gradation between these two. It is commonly a disease of young adult and middle-aged women, but can affect either sex and people of all ages. Inflammatory disease of the gallbladder may occur with or without the formation of gallstones, although it is more common for the two conditions to be associated. No satisfactory explanation of the cause of disease of the gallbladder has been advanced.

Symptoms. The onset of acute cholecystitis is usually rather abrupt. The patient feels ill; nausea and vomiting are common. There are increasingly severe pain and tenderness in the right upper abdomen, just beneath the margin of the ribs. The patient is found to have fever, leukocytosis, and slightly elevated pulse and respiratory rates; it is often observed that respiratory movements are somewhat restricted, so as to avoid motion of the right upper part of the abdomen. There is definite tenderness in the right upper abdomen, and usually there is spasm of the abdominal muscles in that region; in some patients a tense, enlarged, tender gallbladder may be palpated. The history of a previous similar attack which subsided after a few days of illness is often given by the patient.

The symptoms and signs of chronic cholecystitis are less dramatic, but may be just as distressing to the patient. There is usually the story of recurrent attacks similar to the type in acute cholecystitis, but probably less severe and shorter in duration. Such patients also complain of epigastric distress and eructation (*belching*) occurring after meals, especially fatty meals, and call this complaint "indigestion." They will admit that they have learned to avoid fried foods, fats, and eggs. Often these patients suffer in addition from gallstone colic (see Cholelithiasis), for stones are frequently found in association with chronic gallbladder disease.

Complications. There are several complications of cholecystitis. During an acute attack the gallbladder may become filled with pus (*empyema of the gallbladder*), the wall of the gallbladder may become gangrenous, and perforation may occur. At times peritonitis is the sequel to this latter complication, or the perforation may take place into a sealed space, giving rise to an abscess. Another type of complication is cholangitis, the spread of inflammation to the bile ducts both inside and outside of the liver; this may lead to serious damage to the liver. A third variety of complication sometimes follows repeated attacks, with resultant scar formation, causing constriction which results in obstruction of the duct leading from the gallbladder (cystic duct) or of the adjacent common duct.

Treatment. The treatment of cholecystitis is surgical, and consists in the removal, whenever possible, of the offending gallbladder. Surgeons are not yet in full agreement as to the proper time for the removal of the gallbladder, some surgeons feeling that it is better and safer to let an acute attack subside before they operate, others believing that the safest course is to operate at once in order to forestall the development of complications. The general condition of the patient naturally affects the decision as to the time for operation, and the type of operation performed depends largely on the conditions found when the abdomen is opened.

CHOLELITHIASIS

The presence of stones in the biliary tract is called cholelithiasis. Gallstones are composed largely of cholesterin crystals (cholesterin is present in large amounts in bile) and some of them have a high calcium content. Cholesterin stones are soft and are not radiopaque, whereas calcium stones are hard and throw a shadow on the roentgen film. Why these stones should form in the gallbladder and biliary ducts is not known. Stone formation is commonly associated with cholecystitis (p. 277). Gallstones often give rise to symptoms for mechanical reasons, too, even though there be no associated inflammation of the gallbladder or ducts. It is also a fact that during the performance of routine postmortem examinations, gallstones are frequently found which had never given rise to any symptoms. Gallstones vary greatly in size and in number. There may be one or two very large stones, there may be two or three dozen small stones, or there may be myriads of tiny concretions resembling sand. As might seem likely, the size of the stones does have some bearing upon the course and nature of the disease.

Symptoms. The most characteristic symptom of cholelithiasis is gallstone colic, one of the severest kinds of pain to which mankind is heir. The pain is caused by the passage, or attempted passage, of a stone from the gallbladder through the cystic duct or the common duct. The pain is excruciating, it is usually felt in the right upper quadrant of the abdomen just beneath the costal margin, and commonly there is radiation of the pain to the lower tip of the right scapula. This radiation of pain is felt characteristically around the surface of the right chest wall, rather than going straight through the body. Nausea and vomiting usually accompany the colic. Fever, if present at all, is slight, and there is no evidence of acute inflammation of the peritoneal surfaces as in acute cholecystitis. The pain may last a few minutes or several hours, and generally can be relieved only by large doses of morphine. Following the subsidence of the pain (usually due to the successful passage of the stone) the patient rapidly recovers, although there may be slight persistent soreness in the right upper abdomen.

Complications. Often enough a medium sized or large stone does not successfully pass through the common duct: this gives rise to obstruction which, in turn, results in jaundice. Occasionally a stone too large to pass through the ducts causes ulceration and pressure necrosis of the wall of the gallbladder or duct at the point where it is lodged. This may result in perforation with abscess formation, or sometimes in the formation of a false communication between the biliary tract and the intestinal tract. Occasionally a stone lodges squarely in the ampulla of Vater, obstructing not only the biliary system but the pancreatic duct as well.

Treatment. The treatment of gallstones is surgical. When the stones are formed in the gallbladder and at no other point the removal of that organ will cure the disease. When, however, the stones are formed in the hepatic or common ducts, those structures are opened and the stones removed; the ducts must obviously be preserved, and, therefore, there is always the possibility of recurrence of the stone formation. Fortunately, the incidence of recurrence in such cases is not high.

NEOPLASTIC DISEASE

Carcinoma arises from any portion of the biliary tract. It is natural that the onset should be occult and insidious; jaundice is the usual first symptom. Until very recently, carcinoma arising in the liver, gallbladder, or bile ducts was regarded as hopeless, but more radical technics are now in use which may result in cures in some cases. There is one lesion which is somewhat more amenable: this is the small cancer which arises from the ampulla of Vater. The strategic location of this tumor results in the rapid development of jaundice, leading to early diagnosis. A radical operation can be performed with expectation of permanent cure in favorable cases.

DIAGNOSIS OF BILIARY TRACT DISEASE

In the majority of instances, disease of the biliary tract can be diagnosed by the characteristic symptoms and signs of the disease, but in some patients the symptoms and signs are vague and atypical. There are, in addition, a great many other conditions

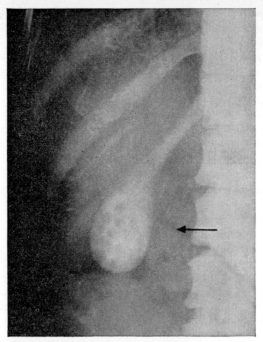

FIGURE 80. Cholelithiasis. The nonopaque cholesterin stones appear as holes in the gallbladder as outlined by tetraiodophenolphthalein on the x-ray film.

of the upper abdomen which may be easily confused with biliary tract disease, including peptic ulcer, pancreatitis, liver abscess, kidney disease, and a number of less common conditions.

The diagnostician has available, however, an excellent method of examining the function of the biliary tract, the gallbladder dye test devised by Graham and Cole. This test is based upon the fact that tetraiodophenolphthalein, a radiopaque chemical, is excreted from the blood into the bile by the liver. In the same way that the gallbladder concentrates bile it concentrates the radiopaque dye in the normal gallbladder sufficiently to throw a shadow outlining the gallbladder upon the x-ray film. The value of this test depends largely upon the care with which the patient is prepared and the method by which the dye is administered. When the dye is given by mouth it is obvious that the amount which can be secreted in the bile depends upon the efficiency of the absorption of the dye from the intestinal tract.

If the gallbladder is outlined by this test, it is safe to assume that the function of the biliary tract is not far from normal. In such a gallbladder, however, the presence of nonopaque cholesterin stones may be demonstrated. These stones will appear as holes in the gallbladder shadow. Calcium stones are visible in the plain x-ray film. If the gallbladder cannot be visualized it is safe to assume that there is altered function of the gallbladder, a definite evidence of a diseased biliary tract. If, in such cases, the same result follows the administration of a double dose of the dye, the evidence for biliary tract disease is a little more conclusive.

A synthetic drug called Priodax (β[4-hydroxy-3,5-diiodophenyl]-α-phenyl-propionic acid) has been introduced. It is much pleasanter to take and causes less gastrointestinal irritability than tetraiodophenolphthalein.

Nursing Care. Preparation of the patient for cholecystography begins by giving the patient a fat-free supper, followed by six tablets, 0.5 gm. each, of iodoalphionic acid (Priodax). Explanation should be made to the patient that no eggs, cream, butter or other fats should be eaten. Black coffee, clear tea and water are permitted. No purgatives, food or drink other than the liquids mentioned may be offered after supper. The nurse should find out what the patient knows about this painless procedure, and should explain that it will include two x-rays in the morning and one after a fatty meal at noon. Apprehension which precedes the unknown is minimized by a simple and straightforward explanation.

To enhance visualization, an enema is given in the morning about a half hour or an hour before the first x-ray. In some clinics, two enemas are ordered, given one-half hour apart. The second enema is given to further insure the evacuation of gas which, when present, prevents good visualization.

The nurse should be aware that complaints of slight nausea may occur after taking the dye in about 25 per cent of the patients. The drug is ultimately excreted in the urine; it causes pain on urination in about 5 per cent of the cases.

OPERATIONS ON THE GALLBLADDER AND BILIARY DUCTS

Cholecystectomy. The most frequently performed operation is the removal of the gallbladder, termed cholecystectomy. The gallbladder is easily exposed through an incision in the upper right abdominal wall. Care is taken to identify the common duct,

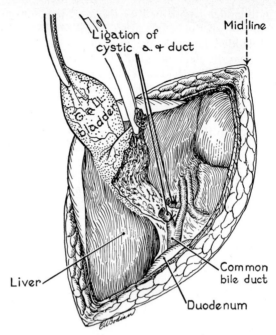

FIGURE 81. Cholecystectomy.

the cystic duct, and the cystic blood vessels which are branches of the hepatic artery and portal vein. The cystic duct and vessels are divided and ligated, after which it is easy to remove the gallbladder. Most surgeons place a cigarette drain in the wound, the inner end of the drain being near the stump of the cystic duct. This is done so that if leakage occurs the bile will escape from the wound rather than spread over the entire peritoneal cavity. This drain is generally left in place for five or six days, at the end of which time it may be safely assumed that the danger of leakage is over.

Cholecystotomy. The simple opening of the gallbladder, cholecystotomy, for the purpose of drainage of the bile or the removal of stones, is less frequently performed than it was a few decades ago. This procedure is at best only palliative, and must be followed later, in order to cure the patient, by cholecystectomy. Cholecystotomy is valuable, however, as an emergency procedure in a debilitated patient who would be a poor operative risk for a more extensive operation.

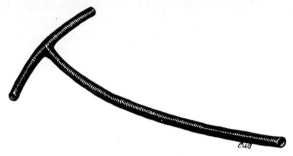

FIGURE 82. T tube.

Other Operations. Occasionally it is necessary to open and explore the common duct. This procedure is called *choledochotomy;* if this is done for the removal of stone it is called *choledocholithotomy.* Stricture of the common duct, a most serious condition, is sometimes present as a congenital anomaly and sometimes is the result of disease or improper surgery. Plastic operations are undertaken upon the common duct for the relief of these conditions.

In certain cases when there is an obstruction in the terminal portion of the common duct, as in cancer of the head of the pancreas, or when some operative procedure has necessitated removal of this terminal portion of the duct, it becomes necessary to make a new connection (anastomosis) between the biliary and alimentary tracts. One method is to anastomose the gallbladder to the stomach (*cholecystgastrostomy*); a more satisfactory method when possible is to reimplant the common duct into the duodenum (*choledochoduodenostomy*), or jejunum (*choledochojejunostomy*). Many surgeons use a T tube in operations on the common duct. By this means, the passage of bile from the liver to the intestine can be made certain. Furthermore, radiopaque solutions may be introduced into the ducts, so that residual stones or obstructions can be visualized (*cholangiography*).

Nursing Care. In general, the nursing care of patients who have had operations upon the gallbladder or bile ducts is the same as for other patients who have undergone a laparotomy (p. 233). It should be remembered, in addition, that operative procedures carried out in the upper part of the abdomen are particularly likely to be followed by restriction of respiratory movements incident to the pain and muscle spasm in the operative area. Distention, too, is almost always more severe following biliary tract surgery than it is in other uncomplicated laparotomies. Extra effort must be made, therefore, to encourage the patient to breathe fully and to cough. Frequent turning of these patients is also an aid in keeping the lungs expanded; turning helps to stimulate peristalsis as well, and thus aids in the control of distention.

Synthetic vitamin K is routinely administered to jaundiced patients before and after operation; 4.8 mg. injected intramuscularly each day is adequate therapy. It is important to supply vitamin K because this substance is essential to the production of prothrombin, a vital element of the coagulating mechanism of blood. Vitamin K is ordinarily absorbed in the alimentary tract from the diet, but is not absorbed when bile does not reach the tract.

There are no special precautions to be taken with respect to the postoperative feeding of these patients but, as a rule, fluids and food are not readily taken during the first two or three days. The jaundiced patient is a difficult problem for the nurse and dietitian because he has no appetite or even has a positive distaste for food. The same is usually true of patients having a biliary fistula. The loss of all or a large part of the bile from the digestive tract causes considerable disturbance in digestion as well as loss of appetite; improvement may follow the administration, usually by stomach tube, of the lost bile.

DISEASES OF THE PANCREAS

Pancreatitis. Acute pancreatitis, a fulminating and serious inflammation of the pancreas, is characterized by the abrupt onset of severe upper abdominal pain, vomiting, rapid pulse, and prostration. The cause of this disease is not known. Patients having acute pancreatitis are almost invariably subjected to laparotomy because the clinical picture of the disease so closely resembles those of acute cholecystitis and perforation of a peptic ulcer that they cannot be safely treated without exploration. The amylase test is helpful in differentiating pancreatitis from other diseases. This test depends upon the appearance in the circulating blood of abnormal amounts of amylase, the starch-splitting enzyme secreted by the pancreas. At operation the pancreas is seen to be swollen and hemorrhagic, and there are areas of necrosis in the neighboring fat as the result of the escape of the potent pancreatic enzymes. Many of these patients recover and it is likely that they would do as well if not operated upon.

Recovery from this disease may rarely be followed by diabetes mellitus or by the formation of a pancreatic cyst. Such cysts sometimes grow to large size and then require surgical treatment. Some cysts can be removed but others must be treated by making a connection between the interior of the cyst and the stomach or jejunum (*internal drainage*), or between the cyst and the external abdominal wall (*marsupialization*).

Chronic pancreatitis causes attacks of severe pain. No form of treatment has been found to affect this condition directly, but the pain can be relieved by division of the sympathetic nerves to the upper abdomen.

Resection of Pancreas for Carcinoma. Carcinoma of the pancreas is not uncommon. As in other forms of abdominal cancer, the onset is insidious: in most instances the tumor has spread beyond the point where it can be cured before symptoms occur. Such a tumor arising in the head of the pancreas commonly makes itself known by obstructing the common biliary duct, resulting in a progressive and usually painless jaundice. Surgical treatment is being used more frequently for this condition, and essentially the same operation is performed as for cancer arising in the ampulla of Vater. The surgeon removes the entire duodenum, the pancreatic end of the common bile duct, part or all of the pancreas, and sometimes the spleen. The stomach and central end of the common bile duct are anastomosed to the jejunum. Despite this extensive procedure, the patient may have little disability afterward unless total removal of the pancreas was carried out; in that event, the patient becomes a total diabetic and needs insulin and careful attention to the diet.

Nursing Care. The preparation for operation depends largely upon the condition of the patient. When the patient is jaundiced and dehydrated, parenteral fluids and vitamin K are administered. There has usually been a loss of weight and the appetite is below normal. The nurse should try to encourage the patient to eat food which is high in calories, protein and vitamins.

The nurse should give this patient and his family emotional support: first, by winning their confidence with a careful explanation of the happenings on the ward, and second, by answering questions, to reinforce their confidence in the surgeon and staff. Making the patient feel as secure as possible by kind and patient attention is the way to minimize anxiety.

The patient with a total or partial resection of the pancreas is usually rather unhappy during his convalescence. The many urine and blood tests required to determine his diabetic status and the regulation of diet are new to him and do not add to his comfort. His appetite is poor and he feels weak. He sometimes shows resentment, often focusing upon the diet. Patience and much kindness is necessary to encourage him to eat; repeated assurance that he is doing well is advisable.

During his stay in the hospital the essentials of food and nutrition should be taught. When he is a diabetic and he is to receive insulin when he goes home, the same careful instructions given to all diabetic patients must also be given to him.[1] The need for follow-up care should be carefully understood by patient and family before discharge.

SUMMARY

Surgeons deal successfully with inflammation and stones in the ducts of the liver, in the gallbladder, and in the common duct. Neoplastic disease presents greater difficulties. The causes of stone and inflammation are not known although removal of the gallbladder for these conditions is one of the most commonly performed and completely curative procedures in surgery. The causes of pancreatic inflammation are likewise obscure, and their treatment about as unsatisfactory as the treatment of cancer in that organ.

VOCABULARY REVIEW

ampulla of Vater	*cholecystectomy*	*cholecyst-*
jaundice	*T tube*	*jejunostomy*
cholecystitis	*cholesterin*	*pancreatitis*
cholelithiasis	*cholangiography*	

SUGGESTED READING

1. Buckley, Marie, and Crenshaw, Virginia P.: Nursing Care of a Patient with Cholecystitis. Am. J. Nursing, *46*:812–815 (December) 1946.
2. Christopher, Frederick: A Textbook of Surgery. 5th Ed. Philadelphia, W. B. Saunders Co., 1949.
3. Diffenbaugh, Willis G., and McArthur, Selim W.: Mortality and Morbidity in Surgery of the Biliary Tract. Arch. Surg., *59*:1070–1076 (November) 1949.
4. Kirklin, B. R., and O'Donnell, D. B.: Present-Day Cholecystography. J.A.M.A., *151*:261–265 (January 24) 1953.
5. McGowan, John M.: Dynamics of Biliary Drainage. Surgery, *18*:470–478 (October) 1945.

[1] See Brown, pages 650–695.

6. Proudfit, Fairfax T., and Robinson, Corrinne Hogden: Nutrition and Diet Therapy. 10th Ed. New York, The Macmillan Co., 1951.
7. Whipple, A. O., Parsons, W. B., and Mullins, C. R.: Treatment of Carcinoma of Ampulla of Vater. Ann. Surg., *102:*763–779 (October) 1935.

CHAPTER 26

Surgery of the
Small Intestine and Appendix

The final digestion and absorption of the nutritive material contained in food are accomplished in the small intestine. The fluid, pulpy material which is finally emptied into the large intestine (colon) contains little but water, mucus, indigestible fibers of vegetable origin, and cellular debris. On the average, this end-result of digestion reaches the colon three to five hours after mealtime. The chief function of the colon is the reabsorption of the considerable amount of water, another example of the remarkable efficiency of the human body in the conservation of needed materials. By the time the intestinal content reaches the lower end of the colon, the rectum, it has been converted into the familiar semisolid feces. One or more times daily this material is finally evacuated from the body during the act of defecation.

THE ILEUM AND JEJUNUM

The uppermost portion of the small intestine, the duodenum, is but 12 inches in length. The remainder of the small intestine is about 20 feet in length, of which the upper portion is jejunum and the lower part is ileum. There is not much difference in the appearance of the jejunum and the ileum, although the latter is somewhat thinner walled and smaller in caliber. The chief difference is in the type and function of the digestive glands which line these two portions of the small intestine. One of the most remarkable things about the small intestine is the paucity of diseases which affect it despite its great length and the constant wear and tear to which it is subjected.

Inflammatory Lesions

Perforation of the Ileum. At the present time, because of the splendid efforts of physicians and public health officials, typhoid is a rare disease; perforation of the ileum is, however, a common complication. Diagnosis is difficult because the patient is already so ill that the onset of peritonitis may be obscured. For this reason it is common practice for the surgeon to palpate the abdomen of each typhoid patient every day, so that the slightest change is more likely to be noted. The treatment consists in simple closure of the perforation, which obviously must be carried out within the first few hours in order to save the patient's life.

Regional Enteritis. There is a little understood, chronic, granulomatous lesion of the small intestine which is called regional enteritis. This may affect any portion of the small intestine, but is most likely to occur in the terminal ileum, in which case it is called terminal ileitis. The cause is not known. In the early stages of the disease the clinical picture includes crampy abdominal pain, fever, and diarrhea. Very often a mistaken diagnosis of appendicitis is made and appendectomy is performed. Later in the disease the symptoms may be less acute and the cramps and diarrhea occur intermittently. Blood can always be detected in the stool. Careful fluoroscopic observation of barium passing through the small intestine may show abnormal intestinal patterns or actual deformity of the bowel which confirms the diagnosis. Because of the frequency of widespread involvement of the intestine, patients with this disease should be operated upon only if such complications as ileus or the formation of fistulas occur. Antibiotic therapy is helpful but not curative.

Tuberculosis. The small intestine is not infrequently the site of tuberculosis. This is nearly always but one manifestation of a generalized tuberculous infection. Unless obstruction occurs, the treatment is the same as that given other forms of tuberculosis, namely, rest, antibiotic therapy, and other measures undertaken to increase the patient's resistance to the infection.

Subcutaneous Injuries to the Abdomen

Nearly everyone is familiar with the damage inflicted upon the abdominal organs by penetrating wounds of the abdomen. The need for prompt surgical exploration in order to arrest hemorrhage and close perforations of the alimentary tract is well understood.

It is not so commonly known that a hard blow upon the abdomen, which need not damage the abdominal wall in any way, may produce rupture of the liver or spleen, or may tear the intestinal wall. Such injuries are caused by the sudden displacement within the abdomen of the abdominal contents; where these viscera and contents are relatively fixed in position and cannot quickly adjust themselves to meet the applied force, damage is likely to occur. An example of this is the upper end of the jejunum which is firmly fixed to the posterior abdominal wall by the ligament of Treitz.

Any patient who has received a kick or other hard blow in the abdomen, or who has received a crushing injury to the abdomen, should be carefully observed for several hours. If there is persistent pain, or if the signs of internal bleeding or of peritoneal irritation appear, the abdomen should be explored so that the internal injury can be repaired.

Neoplasms of the Small Intestine

Tumors of the small bowel are rare. This fact is difficult to explain, particularly since tumors of the alimentary tract just above and just below the small intestine are fairly common. Benign papillomas and hemangiomas of the mucous membrane of the small intestine are occasionally found, and make their presence known by the occurrence of hemorrhage. Fluoroscopic studies may reveal the presence of these small tumors. Cure is effected by surgical removal. Malignant tumors are extremely rare, and can seldom be diagnosed sufficiently early to be cured.

OPERATIONS ON THE SMALL INTESTINE

Jejunostomy. Under some circumstances it is desirable to have an opening into the upper portion of the small intestine through which the patient may be fed. This opening (*jejunostomy*) is usually made into the uppermost segment of the jejunum and is carried out in exactly the same manner as is a gastrostomy.

Ileostomy. For very different reasons, an entirely similar procedure (*ileostomy*) is carried out on the lowermost segment of the ileum: here the purpose is to afford an outlet to the alimentary tract when, for some reason, it seems desirable not to utilize the colon. This operation is commonly performed in the treatment of chronic ulcerative colitis, and the details of ileostomy care are given in the section on that disease (page 302).

Resection. It is occasionally necessary to remove segments of the bowel (intestinal resection). The continuity of the alimentary

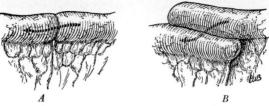

A   *B*

FIGURE 83. Intestinal anastomosis. *A*, End-to-end; *B*, side-to-side (lateral).

tract can be reestablished in several ways, by joining together the remaining ends of the intestine (*end-to-end anastomosis*), by closing one end and joining the other end to the side of the first (*end to-side anastomosis*), or by closing both of the remaining ends and creating a new opening between the sides of the two segments of bowel (*side-to-side* or *lateral anastomosis*), as illustrated in Figure 83.

MECHANICAL ILEUS

One type of intestinal obstruction, paralytic ileus, has already been discussed in connection with peritonitis (Chap. 23). Intestinal obstruction is also commonly produced by mechanical causes. Some of the more frequently encountered causes of mechanical ileus are strangulated hernia, bands of adhesions after peritonitis, rotation or twisting of the bowel (*volvulus*), telescoping of the bowel within itself (*intussusception*), and tumors which occlude the lumen of the intestine either by growth inside of the intestine or by pressure from without. Mechanical ileus is a serious condition and results in the death of the patient unless the obstruction is promptly and effectively relieved. Because of the variety of conditions that can cause this disease, persons of all ages and both sexes are affected.

Symptoms. The four cardinal symptoms of mechanical ileus are cramplike abdominal pain, vomiting, distention, and constipation. Of these, in acute obstructions, the cramps are the earliest and most important symptom. The onset of vomiting may be within a few minutes, or may be delayed. The progression and severity of the symptoms depend upon the degree of obstruction and the anatomic position at which it occurs. When the block is in the upper portion of the small intestine the symptoms develop quickly and are violent; when the terminal portion of the small bowel or the colon is obstructed the onset of symptoms may

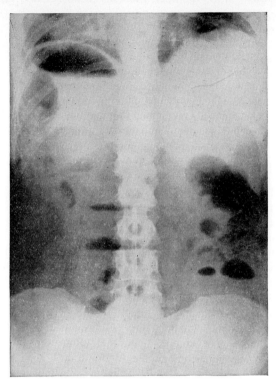

FIGURE 84. X-ray film of abdomen taken in upright position. Distended loops of small intestine containing gas and fluid are visible, but no gas is seen in large intestine. This patient had mechanical ileus.

be more insidious. In the latter case, particularly if the colon is involved, constipation and slowly developing distention of the abdomen are likely to be the first symptoms.

It is obvious that the patient who has intestinal obstruction quickly develops dehydration and disturbance of his chemical balance. There is also grave danger that, just as in paralytic ileus, overdistention of the bowel will result in necrosis and perforation of the intestinal wall, leading to peritonitis. It is also thought by some that the absorption of toxic substances from the intestinal contents takes place, and that this absorption, which does not occur when the bowel wall is normal, is responsible for the severe prostration which is part of the clinical picture.

Diagnosis. One of the most difficult problems in surgery is the differential diagnosis between mechanical and paralytic ileus. It is essential for the surgeon to know with which of these conditions he is dealing, because the treatment of the one is nearly the opposite to that of the other. Considerable light is thrown upon this subject by the history of the illness; in the absence of those conditions which are known to cause paralytic ileus (e.g., peritonitis or recent laparotomy), symptoms of ileus point to a mechanical cause. If, however, the peritonitis or laparotomy occurred several weeks or longer before symptoms of ileus presented, the possibility of an obstructing band of adhesions must be considered. When the ileus is caused by the strangulation of a hernia, the correct diagnosis is readily made by examination of the patient and recognition of the hernia. In general, severe and persistent cramping pain is characteristic of mechanical ileus, for the pain is due to the violent peristaltic action of the intestine above the obstruction as it attempts to overcome the block. Usually this pain does not occur in paralytic ileus, for in this condition the bowel wall is atonic. An x-ray film of the abdomen taken in the upright position is often of great diagnostic aid. The loops of intestine above the point of obstruction, being filled with gas and fluid, are readily visible and of characteristic appearance. Finally, the abrupt onset of the symptoms of ileus in a patient not previously ill is strong evidence for the presumptive diagnosis of mechanical obstruction.

Treatment of Mechanical Ileus

The conservative nature of the treatment of paralytic ileus has already been mentioned (Chap. 23). This treatment might be successful in certain instances of mechanical obstruction, particularly in those cases in which the circulation of the obstructed bowel is not impaired. Unfortunately, however, there is no safe way of determining the status of that circulation other than by exploratory operation. All of the therapeutic measures used in the treatment of paralytic ileus are employed in mechanical obstruction and for the same reasons, but the most important measure is the relief of the mechanical block. This usually necessitates laparotomy. The need for intravenous fluids is obvious. Antibiotic agents, especially penicillin, have proved to be beneficial and should be administered at once.

Decompression. Distention is combated by the use of an inlying nasal tube to which is attached a constant suction apparatus (Fig. 71, p. 244). The Miller-Abbott tube, a long double-lumen tube to the lower end of which is attached an inflatable rubber balloon, is especially useful in such cases. By having the patient lie on his right side the end of the tube is more easily passed through the pylorus. When this has been accomplished, as adjudged by the changing character of the fluid obtained from the tube or by its position as seen under the fluoroscope, the balloon is partially inflated. The peristaltic contractions of the small intestine seize this balloon and propel it down the alimentary tract, dragging the tube along with it. The loops of intestine are thus successively decompressed, and the tube may reach the point of obstruction. This procedure, by virtue of the decompression accomplished, may actually relieve the obstruction; unless this takes place in a very few hours after the onset, however, the treatment is not safe because of the danger of circulatory impairment already mentioned. Some surgeons prefer the Cantor tube, a single lumen tube to the end of which is attached a balloon containing a small amount of liquid mercury.

Choice of Operation. Operation should be undertaken as soon as the diagnosis has been established and the condition of the patient rendered more favorable. As a general rule, the best results follow operative procedures which deal directly with the cause of the obstruction; palliative procedures such as enterostomy above the obstruction or short-circuiting anastomoses around the obstruction are occasionally life-saving but are usually unsatisfactory. In cases where the circulation of the obstructed loop has been impaired, as in strangulated hernia, constricting bands of adhesions, or volvulus, the appearance of the bowel is carefully observed for ten or fifteen minutes after the constriction has been relieved; in many instances the loop of bowel is obviously so badly damaged because of the lack of circulation that it must be removed. These patients are seriously ill, however, and stand operation poorly; only such procedure as is absolutely necessary should be carried out.

Nursing Care. The patient is usually admitted as an emergency. Dehydration, poor color and great pain, frequently accompanied by listlessness, are the signs and symptoms that are seen. The patient may be apprehensive about his illness and what has to be done if he is alert, but also gives evidence of great relief in being admitted because he knows that something will be done to relieve his excruciating pain. The nurse will have to judge according to his condition how much explanation can be given toward emotional support. Suffice it to say that it is good to explain simply and specifically what procedure is going to be done; more than this is often not understood.

The principles of care are those used for the patient with paralytic ileus (p. 242), namely withdrawal of the fluid and air from the intestines, antibiotics and parenteral fluids. As soon as the drainage of fluid and air is established, the pain produced by the forceful peristalsis begins to decrease. Accurate measurement of intake and output are essential. If an immediate operation is to be done, drainage of the stomach is usually done by means of a Levine tube and the tube is left in place. The immediate preoperative preparation consists only of shaving the abdomen and administering the preoperative medication.

Following operation, suction drainage is continued. Parenteral fluids and antibiotics are given. Electrolyte balance is often difficult to achieve and is estimated from determinations of the blood chemistry and the urinary output. The drainage from the tube will decrease as the patient improves; the output of urine will be 1000 cc. or more. The general care of any patient with abdominal surgery is applied. Each patient is treated individually according to his need. When recovery seems assured, it is time for the nurse to begin health teaching regarding nutrition, cleanliness, and follow-up care.

THE APPENDIX

The vermiform appendix, so called because of its resemblance to a worm, is attached to the first portion (*cecum*) of the large intestine, close to the junction of the cecum and terminal ileum (*ileocecal junction*). This vestigial organ serves no known function in the human being. The structure of the appendix is like that of the intestinal tube in general, and its mucous membrane resembles that of the cecum with which it is continuous. At the base of the appendix its lumen communicates with that of the cecum; at the other end the lumen ends blindly, a fact which is undoubtedly responsible, in part, for the frequent inflammation of this organ. Although it is usually about the size and shape of a little finger, the appendix in different patients may vary greatly in length (3 to 20 cm.) and in position. It may lie freely in the peritoneal cavity, it may hang down into the pelvis, it may lie along the lateral border of the cecum, or it may be located behind the cecum (*retrocecal*).

Acute Appendicitis

Acute appendicitis is a common disease, affecting people of all ages. It is a most treacherous disease, and the proper treatment is the prompt removal of the appendix (*appendectomy*). The importance of making an early diagnosis, therefore, cannot be over-emphasized. Every patient who complains of spontaneous and persistent lower abdominal pain and who has recognizable tenderness in the region of the appendix must be suspected of having appendicitis and must be treated for it unless some other cause of his symptoms can be satisfactorily demonstrated. The recent decrease in the death rate from this disease is largely attributable to the extensive efforts which have been made to inform the public about these facts. There is no place for home remedies in the treatment of appendicitis.

Symptoms. The first symptom is usually cramplike abdominal pain, ordinarily in the region of the umbilicus. Within a few hours this pain increases in severity, becomes more constant, and gradually shifts to the right lower quadrant of the abdomen. Nausea and vomiting commonly occur, and the patient at this time has fever and protective spasm of the muscles of the right lower abdomen.

Diagnosis. Palpation of the lower right abdomen causes pain: the point of greatest tenderness is usually found midway between the umbilicus and the anterior superior spine of the right ilium (McBurney's point). In addition, there is an increase in the number of white blood cells (*leukocytosis*).

In many persons, however, the symptoms and signs of this disease are less typical and there is often difficulty in making a correct diagnosis. There are, in addition, many other diseases which give rise to symptoms and signs so similar to those of appendicitis that mistakes in diagnosis are difficult to avoid. Among the diseases which must be considered in the differential diagnosis are acute pyelitis, renal or ureteral colic, food poisoning, gallbladder disease, and, in females, lesions of the ovary and tube.

Complications. The complications of improperly treated or untreated acute appendicitis are dangerous. The inflammation of the appendix is often fulminating and within a few hours to two or three days, the wall of the appendix may become gangrenous;

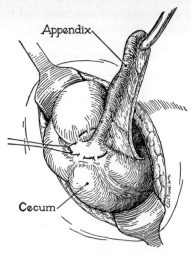

Appendix

Cecum

FIGURE 85. Appendectomy. Following division and ligation of the appendix and its mesentery the appendical stump will be inverted into the cecum beneath the purse-string suture which has already been placed in the cecal wall.

perforation often occurs. Depending upon the position of the appendix within the abdomen, and upon the speed of the inflammatory process, either generalized peritonitis or a local abscess may result from perforation. The gravity and complications of peritonitis are discussed in Chapter 23. Mechanical ileus sometimes occurs later as the result of inflammatory adhesions caused by appendicitis. Not infrequently during the course of appendicitis bacteria enter the veins of the appendix. Since these are tributaries of the portal venous system, pylephlebitis may occur with subsequent formation of multiple abscesses in the liver. All of these complications are prevented by the removal of the appendix early in the attack. It is significant that the mortality rate from acute appendicitis treated by appendectomy before perforation of the appendix had occurred was less than 0.1 of 1 per cent in several large series of patients treated in large metropolitan hospitals. On the other hand, in these same clinics the mortality from acute appendicitis in which perforation did occur was about 10 per cent, prior to the introduction of antibiotic agents. The mortality rate has fallen much below this figure as a result of the use of antibiotics; nevertheless, the best therapy of these dangerous complications lies in their prevention.

Unfortunately, there are still too many patients who do not seek medical aid until after perforation of the inflamed appendix has occurred. The treatment of these patients depends upon their condition and upon the nature of such complications as have developed. Dehydration, chemical imbalance, and paralytic ileus must be promptly and strenuously treated when they occur. Surgeons do not yet agree as to the proper time for appendectomy under such conditions and each case must be judged according to circumstances. Spreading infection is combated by the use of antibiotic agents and by the removal of the cause of the infection as soon as the patient's condition warrants the operative procedure. If a localized abscess has formed, this is drained, and appendectomy may be postponed until a later date. The formation of intraperitoneal abscess is a common complication of perforative appendicitis; such abscesses usually form in the pelvis, but occasionally are found beneath the diaphragm (*subphrenic abscesses*). Abscess formation is to be suspected by the onset of fever, pain, and leukocytosis in a patient apparently making a satisfactory convalescence. Pelvic abscess can be diagnosed by palpation of the abdomen and by rectal examination; subphrenic abscess is more difficult to diagnose and can be detected only when the physical signs appear or x-ray evidence is demonstrated by displacement of the liver or elevation of the diaphragm. In suspected cases the diagnosis may be confirmed by introduction of a needle and aspiration of pus.

Nursing Care. Since the patient with acute appendicitis is usually admitted as an emergency, the first contact the nurse may have is when the patient returns from the operating room. She may learn from his chart if he has ever been in a hospital, what his previous illnesses have been and information concerning his family. These facts will aid her in formulating ideas about an appropriate approach to him and his family.

Good nursing care postoperatively is first directed toward the prevention of complications which may result from the use of anesthesia. Vital signs must be carefully observed. The patient is encouraged to breathe deeply, to cough, and to turn each hour after he awakens. The patient is permitted up according to the individual surgeon's plan, usually the day following operation. He may have diet as tolerated. This operation is now considered one of the less traumatic ones but the nurse should bear in mind that any hospital experience may have a severe psychologic impact upon the patient. In uncomplicated cases, the patient leaves the hospital in three or four days and may return to full activity in a week.

The patient with appendicitis and his family often afford a fine teaching opportunity to the nurse. It has been stated that about 90 per cent of the patients who have appendical perforation have taken a cathartic at the onset of the disease. Because of this cathartics are contraindicated whenever a patient has a pain in the abdomen, especially if the patient is a child. The best nursing care for the patient, until the doctor is available, is to put the patient to bed, keep him quiet and permit him to have only a liquid diet.

The nursing care when the patient has appendicitis with perforation varies according to the treatment which, in turn, depends on the severity of condition. An intestinal tube is inserted when needed to deal with paralytic ileus. Repeated enemas are given if distention develops. Antibiotics are given to combat the existing infection.

The nurse observes the vital signs carefully for there is usually an increase in the pulse rate, followed in a few hours by a temperature rise, when there is abscess formation. When such an incident occurs, it should be reported. The position of the patient in bed should be in accordance with the doctor's order; sometimes, the patient is kept flat while, at other times, the head of the bed is elevated in an effort to encourage the infection to gravitate into the pelvis.

Additional points of nursing care include those described in Chapter 23, page 240.

MECKEL'S DIVERTICULUM

Meckel's diverticulum is a blind pouch arising from the wall of the ileum, usually 1 to 2 feet above the ileocecal valve. This pouch is the remnant of the duct which connects the intestine and the yolk sac during the first few weeks of fetal life; in most people this duct is completely obliterated prior to birth, but in 1 or 2 per cent a part of it persists and forms this diverticulum. Although many persons have this congenital anomaly all their lives, symptoms are produced only if the diverticulum becomes the seat of a pathologic process. Acute inflammation (*diverticulitis*) does occur and its symptoms and signs are indistinguishable from those of acute appendicitis. Since this is so, where surgeons find an uninflamed appendix when operating upon a patient suspected of appendicitis, they should always inspect the lower ileum in order that an acutely inflamed Meckel's diverticulum be not overlooked. The proper treatment for lesions of Meckel's diverticulum is removal *(diverticulectomy)*.

Occasionally an interesting lesion of Meckel's diverticulum is responsible for intestinal hemorrhage. This occurs when a typical peptic ulcer develops in the gastric type of mucous membrane which frequently lines the diverticulum.

SUMMARY

Despite the great length and importance of the small intestine, it is seldom the primary site of disease, and is only operated upon when damaged by injury or involved in disease of adjacent viscera. Mechanical ileus is a common affliction and requires accurate recognition and prompt, strenuous treatment. Acute appendicitis is of very frequent occurrence; when recognized early and treated by appendectomy, the results are uniformly good; the complications of neglected appendicitis can be lethal.

VOCABULARY REVIEW

ileum	*jejunostomy*	*resection*
ileus	*appendectomy*	*regional*
jejunum	*McBurney*	*enteritis*

SUGGESTED READING

1. Christopher, Frederick: A Textbook of Surgery, 5th Ed. Philadelphia, W. B. Saunders Co., 1949, pp. 1027–1038.
2. Ladd, William E., and Gross, Robert E.: Abdominal Surgery in Infancy and Childhood. Philadelphia, W. B. Saunders Co., 1941, pp. 155–164.
3. Mullins, Elise: Ruptured Appendix with Peritonitis. Am. J. Nursing, *49:* 672, 1949.
4. Stafford, Edward S., and Scott, H. William: The Mortality of Appendical Perforation. South. Med. J., *41:*834 (September) 1948.
5. Wangensteen, Owen H.: Intestinal Obstruction. Springfield, Ill., Charles C Thomas, 1942. pp. 3–261.
6. Waples, Genevieve, and Thompson, Bernice: Colostomy Care: I. The Use of the Lamson Appliance; II. The Use of the Buikley Colostomy Irrigator. Am. J. Nursing, *48:*233–235 (April) 1948.
7. Wolff, William I., and Hindman, Robert: Acute Appendicitis in the Aged. Surg., Gynec. & Obst., *94:*239–247 (February) 1952.

CHAPTER 27

Nursing in Colon Surgery

The large intestine is composed of the thin-walled cecum and ascending colon, which occupy the right lateral portion of the abdominal cavity, the transverse colon which crosses the upper abdomen and from which depends the apronlike omentum, the thick-walled descending colon which lies along the left lateral margin of the abdomen and, finally, the sigmoid colon, so named for its S-shaped curve, which becomes the rectum as it passes through the lower border of the abdominal cavity. It is interesting that these portions of the colon differ not in their anatomic locations alone: the structure, the nature of their blood supply, and the nature of the pathologic processes which affect them are different.

INFLAMMATORY LESIONS OF THE COLON

Food Poisoning. Probably the commonest form of colitis is that encountered in acute food poisoning. It is hardly necessary to point out that the treatment of this condition is not surgical, but unfortunately the symptoms may easily be and often are mistaken for those of acute appendicitis.

Chronic Ulcerative Colitis. A much more formidable disease, although far less common, is chronic ulcerative colitis.[1] The cause of this condition is not known. Young adults of both sexes may be affected. As the name implies, the mucous membrane of the colon becomes ulcerated; characteristically involving only the sigmoid and rectal portions of the large intestine in the early stages, the disease may progress to involve the entire colon.

Symptoms. At first the symptoms are mild, and the patient notices only a slight increase in the frequency of evacuation of his bowel; later the patient complains of severe lower abdominal cramps, frequent diarrheal stools containing blood and pus, loss of weight, and weakness. This disease is characterized by spontaneous remissions so that a patient, apparently very ill, may suddenly improve and recover completely. In many cases, however, the course of the disease is less favorable.

Treatment. As in other inflammations, the most beneficial

[1] See Brown, pages 528–532.

therapeutic principle is that of rest. To accomplish this, all food and fluid by mouth are withheld, and the patient is maintained in metabolic balance by total intravenous alimentation, including vitamins. Antibiotic agents are administered to combat the bacteria always present in the colon.

ILEOSTOMY. In patients who do not respond sufficiently to such treatment, the colon may be put to rest surgically; this is accomplished by the performance of an ileostomy, done in such a way that all of the intestinal content is expelled from the ileostomy and none is permitted to enter the colon. Following this operation many of the patients do very well and are able to resume their usual activity. The colon appears to heal, but careful examination often reveals persistence of the inflammation despite the fact that the colon is functionless. It is only in an occasional patient that the ileostomy can be closed and the normal activity of the colon is resumed.

COLECTOMY. Other patients who undergo ileostomy for acute ulcerative colitis either do not improve or actually continue to become more ill, and die unless further operative procedures are undertaken. For these patients relief from symptoms can be secured by removal of the inflamed bowel; since the entire colon is so commonly involved a total colectomy is necessary. The removal of the entire large intestine is a formidable and hazardous operation, but good results follow careful preparation of the patient and judicious division of the procedure into two more stages. Sometimes the rectum can be spared, and at a later date an anastomosis carried out between the lower small intestine and the rectum; usually this is not possible and the patient must face the future with a permanent ileostomy. Because carcinoma not infrequently arises in the colon of patients who have had ulcerative colitis for a long time, total colectomy is performed more often than formerly.

Nursing Care. The surgical nursing care of the patient should continue without interruption the general supportive care begun on the medical service. As quickly as possible, the nursing staff must learn to know the patient and his response to care. The personality of the usual patient with ulcerative colitis is apt to deviate considerably from the norm.

If the patient is permitted to eat he is put on a low residue diet because this minimizes mechanical irritation of the colon. Small, frequent feedings are usually more easily tolerated. Local heat to the abdomen may be indicated. The doctor frequently orders phenobarbital to combat restlessness and iron for secondary anemia. In addition, antibiotics are usually ordered to reduce the bacterial growth in the intestinal tract. A Cantor tube is passed eighteen hours before operation for intubation of the small intestine. All regular preoperative measures for abdominal surgery are carried out.

Total Care of the Ileostomy Patient. Proper indoctrination of the patient should begin before operation, especially if the patient has not yet had his ileostomy. If he already has it, he is acquainted with the problems, although he may yet cherish the wish that it is temporary and will be depressed at the loss of this last hope. It is a grave error to minimize to the patient the difficulties involved in living with an ileostomy. The proper way to present the subject is as a challenge to the individual. Do not suggest that all will be easy, but tell the patient that management of an ileostomy is a difficult, life-long job and indicate to him that his surgeon and nurse believe that he has the ability and courage to handle the situation. Tell him of others who have surmounted this obstacle and arrange to have the patient, after his own operation is over, meet one or more individuals who are taking good care of their ileostomies. It is also useful to tell the patient that all of the good ideas about ileostomy management have been developed by patients who have ileostomies. The student nurse will note later in this chapter that a different view is taken of colostomy management; that is because the management of a colostomy is child's play compared to the constant and harassing nature of ileostomy management.

After operation, the plan for physical care follows that of any postoperative surgical patient. Intravenous fluids are given as needed to maintain adequate intake. Limiting the intake of fluids by mouth will inhibit the tendency of the ileostomy to discharge excessive amounts of intestinal content. Tap water is given to test the tolerance of the patient. If this goes well, a low residue diet is offered. The patient is taught that progression of diet toward normal will depend to some extent upon himself. Many foods are tolerated by some without difficulty, while in others they may cause severe diarrhea.

The discharge from the ileostomy is at first thin, green and watery, but later it becomes semisolid in favorable cases. In all patients, there is a difficult problem of skin care. The abdominal wall must be protected from the irritating intestinal juices. Absolute cleanliness is the first step. Every effort should be made to

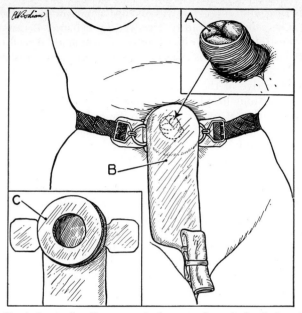

FIGURE 86. *A,* Protruding ileostomy; *B,* ileostomy bag; *C,* fitted ring which is cemented to skin.

keep the patient's dressings clean and dry. This necessitates changing the dressings frequently, often every hour, but at least every two hours, depending entirely upon the individual case. Each time the dressings are changed the patient's abdomen should be thoroughly washed with soap and warm water and dried. After the skin is cleansed, tincture of benzoin may be applied to insure complete dryness and protection. Often the application of a medicament such as mentioned on page 271 (duodenal fistula) will help protect the skin. The patient should be taught to change his own dressings as soon as his physical condition permits. He should be instructed carefully and should be helped many times before making the attempt to change his own dressings.

As soon as possible he should be fitted with a bag which is cemented to the skin and which provides a receptacle for the collection of feces. There are several types of bag available at present. Probably the one most commonly recommended is the "Rutzen" bag. There is a flat ring, made to fit closely about the ileostomy, which is cemented to the skin. The bag is cemented to this ring and further supported by a narrow belt about the waist. The cement is readily dissolved by benzine. Because there is no possibility for intestinal juices to come in direct contact with the skin, this bag is especially helpful in preventing excoriation.

The objective of the nurse during care is to help prepare the patient to resume his place in his family and community. To curb excessive attention to the ileostomy by encouraging him to take part in some diversional or occupational therapy is essential. To guide him in establishing the essential principles of good health habits requires patience and tact. The nurse must learn to give untiringly of her time and effort during this period. Questions are often beyond the responsibility of the nurse; the doctor should be informed about these. The many complexities in the personality and the great emotional instability which is often present bring forth problems which will tax the ability of all.

Before discharge of this patient, the complete plan of care at home should be understood by patient and family. Supportive after-care from the social worker or nurse should be provided or continued according to his need.

OTHER INFECTIONS

Tuberculosis and lymphopathia venereum also cause inflammatory lesions of the large bowel. Treatment of these is primarily medical, but occasionally complications arise, such as perforation or obstruction, which must be dealt with surgically.

Diverticulitis. A common disease of the colon which is not primarily inflammatory in nature is diverticulitis. This disease usually occurs in patients past middle age. The chronic form is characterized by bouts of griping lower abdominal pain associated with severe constipation, whereas the more acute form may simulate acute appendicitis. Serious hemorrhage can also occur. In some persons, multiple little outpouchings (*diverticula*) are found in the wall of the colon, particularly the descending and sigmoid portions; whether these diverticula develop as the result of a congenital defect or as the result of the stress and strain to which the wall is put, is not known. The occurrence of acute or chronic inflammation in these structures is favored by the irritation caused by the collection of fecal material in them.

Most patients are successfully relieved of their symptoms by medical means, but occasionally perforation occurs. Peritonitis or a localized abscess follows perforation, depending upon the

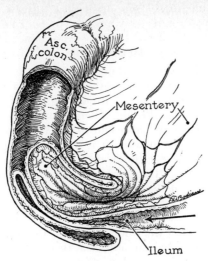

FIGURE 87. Intussusception.

anatomic position of the diverticulum. Since this disease usually occurs in elderly patients who are not good risks for major surgery, operation in cases of diverticulitis is undertaken only when all other measures have failed.

INTUSSUSCEPTION

Intussusception is a telescoping of the bowel. One segment or loop of intestine becomes invaginated in the next portion, the process being initiated and continued by waves of peristaltic contraction. The commonest site of this mishap is at the junction of the terminal ileum and the cecum. The ileum is sucked up into the large bowel until it can go no farther because of the pull on the mesentery. Since the intestinal mesentery is proportionately shorter in adults than in infants and young children, adults seldom present this condition. The symptoms are like those of acute mechanical ileus; in addition, the intussuscepted bowel may form a palpable abdominal tumor, and there is usually passage of a bloody stool. Gangrene of the involved intestine quickly develops, and intestinal resection may be necessary unless surgical exploration is undertaken within a few hours after the symptoms begin. Frequently the early, mild case may be cured by reducing the intussusception by means of an enema, the fluid entering the colon from below pushing the invaginated bowel back and out.

MEGACOLON

An occasional infant or young child may develop intractable constipation with progressive swelling of the abdomen. Roentgenologic examination, after introducing a barium enema, will disclose a hugely dilated colon. There is probably more than one cause of this condition (also known as Hirschsprung's disease), but in some patients, at least, it is due to a congenital absence of some of the nerve cells of the colon, so that peristalsis is absent or ineffective. Treatment consists in the removal of the abnormal portion of the colon.

VOLVULUS

The last portion of the colon, known as the sigmoid because of its S-shaped turns, has in adults a relatively long mesentery. Occasionally this loop of colon, when overfilled or under other abnormal circumstances, may turn or be pulled out of position, with a resulting twisting of its attached mesentery. This twisting or rotation of the mesentery causes occlusion of the mesenteric blood vessels, just as twisting a segment of a rubber tube occludes the lumen. As a result gangrene of the bowel develops. The symptoms again are like those of acute mechanical ileus. This condition is called volvulus. Obviously, early surgical intervention is necessary to save the circulation of the bowel and the life of the patient.

POLYPOSIS OF THE COLON

A polyp of the colon is a benign papillary adenoma of the mucosa. Varying in size from the head of a pin up to a marble, this neoplasm may occur anywhere in the large bowel. The delicate epithelial covering of the surface of this tassel-like tumor is easily ulcerated, with subsequent bleeding, which is the nature of the patient's complaint. Polyps may be seen directly on sigmoidoscopic examination, or may be outlined in the x-ray film by a barium enema. Often there are dozens or even hundreds of these tumors in the same individual, producing bloody diarrhea and severe secondary anemia. The most serious aspect of multiple polyposis of the colon is the fact that there is frequently malignant degeneration of one or more of the polyps, resulting in cancer of the colon. Surgical removal of the involved portion of the colon is advisable, and sometimes it is necessary to remove the entire colon and rectum in order to cure the patient.

CANCER OF THE COLON

Affecting men and women of middle age and older, malignant tumors arising from the epithelium of the lining of the colon are a moderately common type of cancer. These neoplasms may occur at any point from the ileocecal valve to the rectum, and are characterized, like other forms of cancer, by an insidious, painless onset. The symptoms are progressive constipation, abdominal distention, loss of weight, and passage of small or large amounts of blood in the stool. Sometimes the tumor can be palpated through the abdominal wall, or observed through a sigmoidoscope. The diagnosis is usually made, however, by x-ray examination during the administration of a barium enema.

It is fortunate that many cancers of the colon are relatively slow to metastasize, so that surgical cure can be accomplished. These tumors do not respond well to radiation therapy, and the modern method of treating them is to excise the portion of bowel containing the tumor, together with the adjacent portion of the mesentery. Whenever possible, the continuity of the colon is restored, but in many instances this is not feasible, so that the patient must be left with a colonic opening in the abdominal wall (*colostomy*). Since the colon always contains a large population of pathogenic bacteria, operations upon it are attended by serious danger of infection. Recent advances in preoperative preparation, chemotherapy, antibiotic therapy, and surgical technic have combined to lessen this danger, so that an encouraging number of cures are now being accomplished.

PREOPERATIVE CARE

Enema Administration. Almost every patient who is thought to have disease of the colon is subjected to x-ray visualization of the colon; many are directly examined by means of a sigmoidoscope. Proper results can be obtained from these methods only if the bowel has been as thoroughly emptied as possible, for gas and feces distort the x-ray picture and interfere with visual examination. Prior to these examinations the patient should be prepared by the administration of a soapy enema the night before, and again early in the morning.

Many of these patients have some degree of mechanical obstruction; the colon above the tumor is apt to be distended and filled with fecal material. This can sometimes be successfully treated by the use of mild saline cathartics and daily enemas for a period of several days; in other instances it may be necessary for the surgeon to establish an opening into the bowel above the obstruction. This is done not only to relieve the obstruction, but also to permit the colon to return to a more normal size and state of health, a most important consideration in the carrying out of the necessary surgical procedures.

Diet. It is also of great help to place the patient on a low-residue diet, thus reducing the bulk of the feces. A sample menu follows:

BREAKFAST	LUNCH	SUPPER
Fruit juice (100 cc.)	Strained soup	Broiled steak
Soft boiled egg	Baked fish	Rice
Toast (1 slice with butter)	Baked potato	Sieved beets
Cereal with milk and sugar	Sieved peas	Bread (1 slice with butter)
Coffee or tea	Bread (1 slice with butter)	Milk (200 cc.)
	Milk (200 cc.)	Canned peaches
	Ice cream	

Meat should be lean but need not be ground. Eggs may be served any style except fried. Liver should be given at least once a week. Milk should be boiled three minutes, and the total amount should not exceed one pint in twenty-four hours. Fruits are limited to small amounts of juices, canned pears and peaches, and ripe bananas. All vegetables are sieved. Only white or plain rye bread is used. Refined or sieved cereals are used. Pudding, ice cream, gelatin, cake, and custard are satisfactory, provided they do not contain fruit or nuts.

Antibiotic and Drug Therapy. The number of pathogenic bacteria in the feces may be remarkably lowered by the use of antibiotic agents (streptomycin, aureomycin, Terramycin, neomycin) or drugs (Sulfasuxadine, Sulfathaladine). When possible, one of these agents should be given to the patient prior to colon surgery in order to lessen the danger of postoperative infection. Neomycin is the most rapidly acting of these agents, and will even be effective when instilled into the open bowel during operation.

Intestinal Intubation. Preoperative intestinal intubation and deflation facilitate the performance of colon surgery and completely avert postoperative distention and "gas pains." Twelve to eighteen hours before operation, a Miller-Abbott or a Cantor tube is introduced into the stomach through the nostril, and encouraged to pass the pylorus and travel down the small intestine. When the tube has progressed nearly to the cecum, it is prevented from further movement by fastening with adhesive

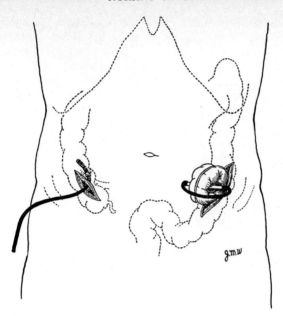

FIGURE 88. *Left,* Cecostomy; *right,* colostomy.

strapping to the cheek. Gentle suction is then begun. The tube is irritating to the nose and pharynx, but patients readily put up with this mild annoyance when they are told that the tube will not only make the operation more safe but will also prevent much postoperative discomfort.

OPERATIONS ON THE LARGE INTESTINE

Colostomy. Colostomy, the establishment of an opening of the bowel through the abdominal wall, is carried out at nearly any point along the colon; the common sites, however, are the cecum (*cecostomy*), the transverse colon, and the upper portion of the sigmoid colon. The desired portion of the bowel is delivered through a small wound, and is held out on the surface of the abdomen by means of a gauze sponge, a cigarette drain, or a clamp, no sutures being placed in the bowel. As there are multitudes of pathogenic bacteria in the lumen of the large intestine, the bowel is not opened for forty-eight to seventy-two hours; this delay permits the wound about the colon to become sealed off and thus prevents infection of the deeper tissues and peritoneal

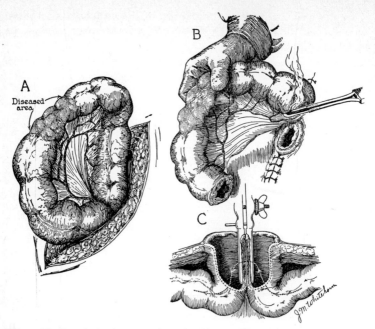

FIGURE 89. Exteriorization resection of colon. *A,* The diseased segment is exteriorized. *B,* Resection of the exteriorized segment, using the actual cautery. *C,* Reestablishment of continuity by crushing the spur between the approximated ends of the colon (side view).

cavity. An opening is then made with scissors or cautery while the patient is in the ward; no anesthesia is necessary. If the patient is unable to withstand obstruction for this period, a tube may be inserted earlier, and flatus allowed to escape.

Resection. The operative removal (*resection*) of the different parts of the large intestine is carried out according to certain rules which have been established by surgical experience. It has been found safer to remove the entire cecum and ascending colon (*right colectomy*), even though the lesion may involve only a small portion of those structures; the continuity of the intestinal tract is reestablished by performing an anastomosis between the terminal ileum and the transverse colon (*ileocolostomy*). In dealing with the transverse and descending colon, however, it is technically feasible to resect only the involved segment; when this segment is not too long, it is often possible to reestablish continuity by direct anastomosis of the remaining ends of the bowel.

In the past, because of the danger of infection, an alternative technic was devised which made use of the principle of exteriorization. At operation the diseased segment of intestine with its mesentery was mobilized, brought through the wound, and placed outside the abdominal wall, the efferent and afferent loops of bowel being carefully approximated as they passed through the wound (see Fig. 89). Two or three days later the exteriorized segment of bowel was resected, leaving two open ends of bowel at the skin edge of the wound. At a later date the resultant colostomy could be closed. This type of resection is still employed when the patient's condition or the nature of the lesion so requires.

Total Colectomy. Total colectomy is usually performed in two or three stages. At the first operation a permanent ileostomy is established and, if the patient's condition permits, the right half of the colon is resected. The second operation, two to six weeks later, consists in removal of the transverse and descending portions of the colon. At a third sitting, after a suitable interval, the sigmoid colon and rectum are removed in the manner to be described under the treatment of cancer of the rectum (*abdominoperineal resection*).

NURSING CARE AFTER OPERATION

All that has previously been stated with regard to the general postoperative care of patients who have undergone laparotomy applies to those who have had surgery of the colon. There are also certain additional features. Suction drainage through the inlying tube is continued until active peristalsis is restablished, as evidenced by audible bowel sounds and the passage of flatus. Following the removal of the Miller-Abbott or Cantor tube the patient should be kept on a liquid or a low residue diet until healing is complete. Laxatives and cathartics are forbidden, but mineral oil is used when encouragement of defecation becomes desirable. The use of enemas is not permitted at first, but after healing has progressed well, small enemas may be used to induce defecation. If the anastomosis is well above the rectum, the rectal tube may be used to aid in passage of flatus; often, when the suture line is near the rectum, a tube is placed through the anastomosis from the rectum in order to permit constant escape of flatus. Should the tube become dislodged, however, it must be replaced only by the surgeon.

Care of Patient with Colostomy

Before the nurse accepts the responsibility for the nursing care of a patient with a colostomy, it is desirable that she have some understanding of the physical and psychologic aspects of the condition. She must develop the proper attitude herself before she can be of real help to a patient.

It has frequently been stated that the patient's abhorrence of a colostomy may be readily overcome. This seems, however, not to be as easy as once was advocated. It has been found that there are numerous factors which enter into the physical and psychologic adjustment. The manner in which the patient will react to his entire hospital experience will depend on his fear of operation, death, incapacitation following operation and subsequent social rejection. His reaction will depend to a great extent on the adaptations he has made to living before the onset of his illness. His reaction to this severe stress brings forth many of his fundamental emotional convictions. It is at the time of the onset of symptoms that most patients begin to experience fear; this gradually progresses until a crisis is reached. The greatest stress seems to be evident around the time of surgery.

The following recommendations are directed toward helping the nurse care for a colostomy patient and are based on objectives which are fundamentally positive in orientation. They are:

1. The nurse must know the details of the plan of care.
2. She must establish good rapport. Confidence generated by an understanding interest in the patient and his family is essential.
3. The nurse who is best known to the patient should accompany him to the operating room.
4. She should accept without argument any expressions of resentment by the patient. They give evidence of his desire to live and resume his place. If the patient is permitted to express his resentments, resolution will be more apt to take place.
5. The patient should be encouraged to talk, and when the nurse becomes aware of fears or anxiety these should be noted and reported to the surgeon as soon as possible.
6. When instruction for irrigating the colostomy begins, all members of the team should know exactly what is going to be done, and what progress is being made. This plan of care should be outlined and recorded. Any inconsistencies

or uncertainties are very detrimental to acceptance and learning on the part of the patient. The nurse assumes the responsibility for teaching the patient; she should be aware that teaching and telling are not the same.

7. She should be aware of the great variance in ability to learn on the part of different patients; that the first look at the colostomy by the patient is a shocking experience to him. Refusal to learn, which is often exhibited, may not be willful but can be evidence of anxiety and depression. Understanding, patience and kindness are the important attributes which are significantly helpful in resolving his worries.

8. The nurse must have a positive attitude toward cleanliness, feces and disfigurement. The attitude of the patient concerning these must not be permitted to reflect negative feelings on the part of the nurse. A negative attitude will not only retard learning but will actually be destructive to the ability of the patient to function in all areas of living. It may be stated that gesture and tone often reveal the nurse's attitude as much as or more than her words.

9. The nurse should encourage the patient to have a part in the plan of procedure of irrigations. However, a tendency for him to focus too much attention upon the procedure is a warning signal. She should direct his thinking to prevent this treatment from becoming the focal point of all his activity.

10. She should encourage the patient to accept the support of his family. His ability to talk to them freely will encourage the rapport that was in existence before he became ill. If the nurse has the continued confidence of the family she is in good position to influence their acceptance of the patient.

11. When the patient goes home, it is highly desirable that someone besides the patient understands his care and aids him in bridging the gap between hospital and home. The person for this may be a nurse or a member of the family. If it is a nurse who has not known the patient previously, she should get the information on the details of care before she goes into the home. These would include what the patient knows about his illness as well as what self-care he has been able to carry out in the hospital. When it is a

member of the family who is to help, instructions and demonstrations in the care of the patient should have been carried out in the hospital.

12. Lastly, the nurse should rehearse with the patient the plan of follow-up care which the surgeon has planned and, in addition, strengthen his security by assuring him of the willingness of the surgeon to see him if he has any questions or worries.

The type of colostomy referred to here is a permanent one, usually established in the sigmoid colon; regular evacuation of the feces from the bowel is initiated by irrigation. The aim in treatment is to create a "dry" colostomy: one where spillage does not occur during the interval between the daily mechanical cleansing of the bowel.

In considering the patient with a temporary colostomy, everything that has been said also applies but there is usually less severe emotional stress because the patient has the hope, from the onset, of the closure of the colostomy with subsequent normal bowel function. However, if such a patient did not know how to care for himself in the best possible manner, the colostomy would become a barrier between him and his family and society. It is this type of patient who frequently denounces the colostomy to his friends and relatives because of his inability to function in his former areas of living.

Whenever the patient has a colostomy which is a palliative measure for an incurable cancer, he is usually in the terminal stage of his illness. This time may vary from a few months to years, depending on the virulence of the malignancy and the extent of the growth. The colostomy in such patients is often in the transverse colon; in this location irrigations are not entirely successful in preventing accidents. It is this variety of patient who needs much physical care as well as emotional support in order to make him as comfortable as possible.

When a colostomy has been performed, the dressing of the primary abdominal wound is usually sealed with collodion or Whitehead's varnish. Sterile petrolatum gauze is placed on the skin and around the colostomy loop, which is then covered with gauze dressings held in place with adhesive plaster or a scultetus binder.

When the colostomy is opened by the surgeon, on the second or third day after operation, there is often an evacuation of liquid stool. Additional preparations must therefore be made. A rubber sheet covered with a towel should be placed crosswise between the patient and the draw sheet. A curved basin is placed against the side of the patient for collection of the feces.

The surgeon orders irrigations once or twice daily The amount of solution varies from 250 to 1000 cc. depending upon the length of colon remaining. The purpose of the irrigation is to cleanse the intestinal tract of feces, gas and mucus, to prevent intestinal obstruction, and to establish regularity of evacuation. In many clinics nurses carry out this treatment.

The time selected to carry out the procedure depends on when it is convenient, but should be about the same time each day. However, this does not mean that this is the time when the patient must carry out the procedure when he returns home; he should plan to do it when it is most convenient at home. Each day there should be a demonstration with careful explanation and teaching suited to the ability and acceptance of the patient. Refusal to look at the colostomy at first should be accepted; too much explanation should not be made lest the patient feel he is being forced. Each patient must be carefully evaluated. Individuals do not react the same, they do not learn with the same rapidity and the nurse each day must accept her patient according to his changing ability. The nurse must guard against the fact that sometimes the patient will carry out the procedure because he wishes to win her approval rather than a desire for independent and free self-care.

The equipment suggested for an irrigation is the same as that used in giving an enema. In addition, several curved basins, a dressing basin lined with newspaper, dry and boric acid sponges and gauze dressings are necessary. The solution used may be tap water, normal saline solution, or soap, heated to 108° F. The irrigation pail is adjusted so that the fluid is 18 inches above the colostomy opening. After the dressings have been removed and placed in the newspaper in the basin, the colostomy area should be cleansed with boric sponges if the skin is soiled. A curved basin is then placed against the side of the patient to collect the return fluid. The rectal tube should be gently inserted 6 to 8 inches; the solution is allowed to run in ahead of the tube to distend the colon. Occasionally after the introduction of the tube it seems to meet a temporary obstruction: this is a natural contraction of the intestine which will relax in time. Another curved basin may be held over the opening to direct any sudden gush of fluid. Complete emptying of the bowel requires from twenty to fifty minutes. Slow evacuation of feces and gas may be hastened by turning the patient from one side to the other. This may always be resorted to when the patient is uncomfortable because of distention.

There is other, more elaborate equipment which can be obtained for colostomy irrigation. The patient should be encouraged to try various types of irrigators until he discovers which permits easy administration of an irrigation. Another aspect of care which can be varied is the amount of solution used. The patient is often told that he may use as much solution as is needed until he feels that all feces have been evacuated. This statement should be qualified by the explanation that there is no advantage to excessive irrigation; it is undesirable for a patient to focus too much attention upon the irrigation and develop a compulsive practice. There is a difference between an enema and an irrigation; in the enema the solution is placed into the gut and peristalsis then causes evacuation, whereas in the irrigation the fecal material is washed out by means of large amounts of solution and peristalsis.

Some patients, following permanent sigmoid colostomy, are able to evacuate feces daily through their colostomy without irrigation or enema. The colostomy in these is situated at the lower end of the midline laparotomy incision. They sit on an ordinary toilet, lean slightly forward and evacuate their feces directly into the bowl. Usually these patients learn quite by accident, after receiving the usual instruction and after carrying out the enema procedure, that peristalsis and evacuation are possible without an introduction of solution into the intestine. It seems apparent that the psychologic aspects are extremely closely allied to the physical functioning.

Sometimes the colostomy consists of two openings, that of the proximal and that of the distal segment of colon. At times it is necessary to clean the distal bowel because of the accumulation of mucus. This may be done immediately after the irrigation of the proximal loop. After the patient has been placed on a bedpan, the ordered solution should be introduced into the distal loop through a rectal tube. When there is an obstruction the fluid should be siphoned off. In such an instance, the bowel below the obstruction may be cleansed by giving a small enema through the anal canal.

Following the irrigation the colostomy area should be washed with soap and water. An appropriate dressing is then applied to protect the colostomy and to collect any fluid or feces. The first few days after the colostomy has been opened, fecal material often flows freely so that the soiling and the odor are offensive. Changing the dressings according to the need and washing the area will make the patient, and all those around him, more comfortable; this also protects the skin against any excoriation which may occur if the fluid is permitted to remain on the abdominal wall.

Following operation, the patient is usually continued on suction drainage through the Cantor tube so that oral feeding is not possible. After removal of the tube, the patient is given liquid diet, and this is increased as tolerated with the emphasis on constipating foods. In some clinics, a rigid constipating diet is given while, in others, the patient is advised to eat according to his own wishes. The patients often have strong feelings concerning foods. They believe that some cause diarrhea and increase the danger of spillage. The important things for the nurse to teach to the patient are the components in foods which are essential, and the various foods which contain these within the limits of his diet.

After ten or twelve days the colostomy is usually regulated fairly well. Some surgeons order a colostomy bag to be worn until the patient feels secure without one. Others believe that the patient should not be given a bag because it might weaken his faith in the colostomy regulation. It may be said that when a patient has an "unfavorable" colostomy, as in terminal cancer, it is often very desirable for the patient to wear a bag because it permits him to be out of bed without the apprehension of soiling his clothes. There are various types of bags, some made of disposable synthetic materials, which are placed over the colostomy and fit snugly against the abdomen when the straps are adjusted.

Before the patient leaves the hospital he should be able to care for himself fairly well unless he has a terminal illness. Instructions, as was stated before, are begun as soon as possible and proceed at the rate the patient can accept them. Repetition in teaching is the rule, not the exception. Equipment for home care should be like that used in the hospital. It is helpful to furnish patients with printed instructions. It is advisable that someone who knows how to carry out the procedure be in the home with a patient when the latter first irrigates himself. If the nurse who is going to do this can visit the patient in the hospital, the carry-over of teaching and the confidence and security of the patient are reinforced. If it is a member of the family, they should have had patient and thorough instructions during which they have evidenced a sincere desire to help the patient in a positive, unpitying manner. The satisfaction of sending a patient home who is able to care for himself and who believes he can resume his former activities in his home and society is rewarding to all those who have had a part in helping him in the adjustment.

SUMMARY

Lesions of the colon, especially cancer, are common and are often amenable to surgical therapy. Decompression of the intestines by intubation and suction, and the reduction of the bacterial content of the colon by modern antibiotic therapy make colon surgery safe. Ileostomy and colostomy are frequent sequels of colon surgery; ileostomy care is a constant challenge to the patient and nurse, whereas colostomy care is relatively simple.

VOCABULARY REVIEW

colectomy	megacolon	ileocolostomy
diverticulitis	cecostomy	polyposis
intussusception	irrigation	
volvulus	peristalsis	

SUGGESTED READING

1. Cancer Nursing. National Cancer Institute and N. Y. Dept. of Health, 1950, pp. 44–47.
2. Dennis, Clarence: Ileostomy and Colectomy in Chronic Ulcerative Colitis. Surgery, 18:435–451 (October) 1945.
3. Lahey, Frank H.: Indications for Surgical Intervention in Ulcerative Colitis. Ann. Surg., 133:726–741 (May) 1951.
4. Presman, D.: A New Method of Skin Protection for Ileostomies and Colostomies. Surgery, 13:322 (February) 1943.
5. Friedman, M. H. F.: Aluminum Hydroxide Gel for Erosions in Patients with Bowel Fistulas. J.A.M.A., 131:520–521 (June 8) 1946.
6. Sutherland, Arthur: The Psychological Impact of Cancer and Cancer Surgery. Cancer, 5:857–872 (September) 1952.

CHAPTER 28

Nursing in Proctologic Surgery

The special field of proctology includes the diagnosis and treatment of lesions of the rectum, anus, and perineum.

Anatomy and Physiology. The rectum, the terminal segment of the alimentary tract, lies wholly outside the peritoneal cavity, and is in intimate relationship with the bladder, seminal tract, and prostate gland in the male, and with the posterior wall of the vagina in the female. The muscular coat is thicker than that of the remainder of the large intestine. The anus is the outlet of the tract; except during defecation and expulsion of flatus, it is kept tightly closed by the action of the strong, circular muscles of the anal sphincter. The rectum and anus are supported by the muscles of the perineum as well. The glandular epithelial lining of the rectum (*rectal mucosa*) is replaced, just within the anus, by the squamous epithelium of the skin, which is continuous with that of the perineum.

Distention of the rectum by feces or flatus produces the normal desire to defecate, and defecation is accomplished by expulsive constriction of the rectum occurring simultaneously with relaxation of the anal sphincter. The expulsive effort is aided by contraction of the abdominal and perineal muscles, thus increasing the intra-abdominal pressure. The act of eating stimulates intestinal peristalsis; this, in turn, acts to propel feces and gas into the rectum, and, as a result, the desire to defecate usually follows the ingestion of a meal. Anything that irritates the rectal mucosa also produces the desire for defecation; included in this category are irritating chemicals, fluid stools, and any type of ulceration of the rectal mucosa. The desire to go to stool, felt urgently and frequently (*tenesmus*), is a symptom of rectal irritation.

Constipation, which can be defined as inadequate emptying of the bowel, is largely a medical problem, but has many surgical aspects nonetheless. Obviously, mechanical obstructions produce constipation; it is important to know, however, that often very minor inflammatory lesions of the rectum or anus can sufficiently interfere with the normal function of these structures to produce constipation, or to greatly increase habitual constipation.

319

Methods of Examination. The patient may be placed in the lithotomy position, in the Sims' lateral position, or in the knee-chest position; the first two are more comfortable for the patient, but the knee-chest position permits the most adequate examination of the perineum, anus, and rectum. Following inspection of the perineum and anus, a digital rectal examination is made. For this a rubber glove or a rubber finger cot, coated with petrolatum or lubricating jelly, is used.

Proctoscopy. Additional information is gained from direct inspection of the rectal mucosa by means of a proctoscope. This is a short tube of suitable caliber, fitted with a blunt stylet which is removed as soon as the instrument has been passed beyond the sphincter. The proctoscope must be well lubricated, and should be warm. Some instruments are fitted with electric illumination, which is more satisfactory than a flashlight or head mirror. The proctoscope is passed upward under direct vision. Under ideal conditions it is possible to examine by this means, or by using a longer tube (sigmoidoscope), the lower 10 or 12 inches of the alimentary tract. A satisfactory examination of this sort can be made only if the bowel contains no feces, and therefore these patients must be prepared shortly before examination by the administration of a cleansing enema.

Fluoroscopy. An additional means of examining the rectum and lower sigmoid colon is by use of the barium enema. The patient is previously prepared by cleansing enemas. He is then placed on the fluoroscopic table and a barium solution is carefully injected into the rectum; the filling of the bowel is visualized on the fluoroscopic screen or by means of x-ray films.

FECAL IMPACTION

An occasionally overlooked but simple cause of constipation is a mechanical obstruction of the lumen of the rectum due to the accumulation of hard, dry feces. This occurs in infants, and sometimes in adults who have been careless about elimination. Diagnosis is made by the discovery of the hard mass of impacted feces on digital examination of the rectum. A soap or an oil enema may soften the feces sufficiently to permit expulsion, but at times it is necessary for the surgeon to break up the impacted feces with the finger. This condition is also a complication of injury or disease of the central nervous system; thus, paralyzed patients, who have lost the ability to move the bowels readily, develop impactions unless cleansing enemas are regularly administered.

FISSURE IN ANO

Rectal fissures are in reality small ulcers of the rectum, occurring at the mucocutaneous junction. This lesion is one of the most painful of rectal complaints, the pain characteristically occurring during and immediately after defecation. The cause of anal fissures is not known. The ulcer tends to become chronic, and usually surgical excision is necessary to accomplish healing and cure. Sometimes local applications, the use of mineral oil to soften the feces, and digital dilation of the sphincter suffice to bring about healing.

ANAL PRURITUS

Another extremely distressing rectal complaint is intractable itching of the anus and adjoining skin. This is caused at times by a fissure, or by eversion of the rectal mucosa with consequent secretion of mucus, but more often no pathologic condition of the anus is apparent. The incessant itching usually leads to irritation and excoriation of the perineal skin because the patient cannot refrain from scratching; indeed, many of the patients have been observed to scratch during sleep. The cure is accomplished by remedying any pathologic condition of the rectum that can be found, and by local measures designed to decrease the itching and hence the scratching, thus permitting the irritated skin to heal. The application of alcohol, the use of cold baths, and keeping the perineum shaved and dry will alleviate the milder cases, but often it is necessary to anesthetize the perineal skin temporarily. This is accomplished by the careful subcutaneous injection of minute amounts of 95 per cent alcohol.

HEMORRHOIDS

The rectum is richly supplied with veins (*hemorrhoidal veins*), and, as a result of man's upright position and the increased pressure incident to straining during defecation, dilatation of these veins is common. A hemorrhoid is a dilated vein, situated immediately beneath the rectal mucosa or skin of the anus, and is comparable to a varicose vein in the leg. External hemorrhoids are those occurring outside the sphincter, beneath the anal skin; internal hemorrhoids are those occurring within the rectum.

Symptoms. There is scarcely a person who goes through life without experiencing in some degree the symptoms of hemorrhoids. These symptoms are bleeding, pain, and protrusion, occurring singly or in all possible combinations. Of course constipation usually accompanies hemorrhoids when defecation is painful or when it is feared that the act may cause pain, and naturally constipation, by increasing the difficulty of defecation, aggravates the hemorrhoidal condition; thus a vicious cycle is initiated.

External Hemorrhoids. The common symptom is the sudden appearance of a painful little mass just at the anus, due to the thrombosis of the involved branch of the hemorrhoidal vein.

Internal Hemorrhoids. The common symptom of these is bleeding, which may range from a few drops seen on the toilet paper to 50 or 100 cc. of blood lost with every defecation. Pain does not commonly occur with internal hemorrhoids, but protrusion through the sphincter is frequent. In severe cases large internal hemorrhoidal masses may become ulcerated, the veins may thrombose, and the whole swollen mass may prolapse through the sphincter, causing severe pain.

Diagnosis. External hemorrhoids are diagnosed upon inspection of the anus, but internal hemorrhoids, unless prolapsed, can be seen only on proctoscopic examination. Since there are many causes of rectal bleeding, careful direct examination of the rectum must be made in every case in which bleeding is a symptom.

Treatment. *External Hemorrhoids.* The pain and swelling due to thrombosis of an external hemorrhoid subsides in three or four days, so that treatment is necessary only to make the patient more comfortable. Local application of anesthetic drugs (*anodynes*), mineral oil, and warm sitz baths are useful; also the patient will feel better if he restricts his activity, avoiding lifting or other strenuous work.

Internal Hemorrhoids. These, however, usually require more aggressive treatment. In mild cases the use of mineral oil by mouth and the local application of suppositories or ointments which contain astringents to shrink the rectal mucosa, suffice to relieve the patient's symptoms. When there is persistent bleeding, or when prolapse and ulceration occur, surgical treatment is required. Some surgeons prefer to treat hemorrhoids by the injection of sclerosing solutions, as in treating varicosities of the legs. Others prefer to excise the hemorrhoids (*hemorrhoidectomy*).

ISCHIORECTAL ABSCESS

In view of the nature of the contents of the rectum it is not surprising that inflammation and ulceration of the rectal mucosa sometimes occur, and at times virulent bacteria penetrate through the rectal wall into the tissues outside. There is considerable fat and loose connective tissue in the ischiorectal spaces, permitting the formation of large abscesses.

Symptoms. Such an abscess is situated deeply at first, and there may be little in the way of external signs. The patient complains of severe, throbbing pain about the rectum, and cannot sit comfortably; later there is increasing constipation and the usual systemic accompaniments of infection, including fever, malaise, and leukocytosis. The perineum overlying the abscess is tender, and late in the disease redness and induration occur. Rectal examination may be impossible before the patient is anesthetized, owing to the exquisite tenderness, but when such examination is made the abscess can be palpated.

Treatment. An ischiorectal abscess must be incised and drained as soon as possible to prevent further spread of the infection. It is essential to secure adequate drainage and, therefore, good exposure and relaxation are needed, usually requiring general anesthesia. The abscess cavity is often large, containing much foul-smelling pus. Following drainage the patient improves very rapidly, and is quite comfortable within a day or two.

FISTULA IN ANO

Sometimes complete healing follows the prompt drainage of an ischiorectal abscess, but more commonly healing progresses until only a small draining sinus remains. Such a persistent draining sinus, which communicates with the old abscess cavity and hence with the lumen of the rectum, is a fistula in ano. This is a chronic lesion, and over many months or years it will not only fail to heal, but is likely to spread, forming other intercommunicating openings. Eventually multiple openings may form all around the rectum and perineum, each draining small amounts of pus; this is called a "watering-pot" perineum. One may wonder why a patient will permit such a lesion to go on and on; actually there is little pain or discomfort, and the drainage seems not to be very annoying to the less fastidious. It is the communication with the rectum which causes the fistula to persist, because a little flatus or fecal material is squeezed into the infected tract from time to time.

Treatment. In order to cure a rectal fistula it is necessary to lay the tract wide open into the rectum, dividing the sphincter. The large shallow wound resulting from this maneuver is permitted to heal from the bottom up, care being taken to prevent the skin edges from coming together until the deeper tissues have filled in. The patient is temporarily incontinent of feces after division of the sphincter, but if the sphincter is divided in only one place it nearly always heals with complete return of function. When multiple fistulous tracts are present it is usually not possible to remove them all at one sitting, as the resultant defects might lead to permanent incontinence. Such patients are best treated by excision of the fistulous tracts in two or more stages, which permits the sphincter muscle to heal and regain its function between each operation.

RECTAL INCONTINENCE; IMPERFORATE ANUS

Congenital maldevelopment of the rectal sphincter, or severe damage to this important muscle caused by disease or injury, permits the anus to remain open with consequent uncontrollable discharge of feces, flatus, and mucus. A plastic operation, in which a sling of fascia that can be controlled by contraction of the gluteal muscles is placed about the rectum, has been successful in restoring anal control to many patients who have had this most distressing condition. An occasional infant, on the other hand, is born without an anal opening. This, of course, constitutes an acute surgical emergency to relieve the complete mechanical obstruction. In some instances it is only necessary to puncture a diaphragm of skin, but in others the lower portion of the rectum and the sphincter are absent or poorly developed, making the establishment of a normal anus often difficult or impossible.

LYMPHOPATHIA VENEREA

The close anatomic relationship and the lymphatic drainage of the vagina and rectum result in frequent involvement of the rectum in lymphopathia venerea. This venereal disease is caused by a virus and is contracted during sexual intercourse with an infected person. It occurs chiefly in Negro women. The infection produces a chronic, granulomatous lesion, with ulceration during the acute stage; later, when healing occurs, there is formation of heavy scar tissue. Scar tissue always has the tendency to contract, and the result of this process in the rectum is a gradual progressive constriction of the lumen (*rectal stricture*).

Symptoms and Diagnosis. Lymphopathia of the rectum causes rectal pain and bleeding, discharge of pus, and progressive constipation. Diagnosis is established by the clinical appearance of the rectum, and by a positive reaction to the intracutaneous injection of the Frei antigen.

Treatment. No specific therapy has yet been developed for this disease. Antibiotic therapy (aureomycin) is useful in the acute stage as it helps to reduce the amount of secondary bacterial infection. A useful rectal lumen can usually be maintained by means of regular dilation with soft rubber dilators (*bougies*). This must be done very carefully, and for long periods. In severe cases, however, a colostomy may be necessary in order to relieve the obstruction.

NURSING CARE IN RECTAL SURGERY

General Measures. In general, the nursing care of patients who have undergone rectal surgery is much the same, no matter which condition has been treated. Despite the contamination of the wound with feces, healing proceeds very well, perhaps an indication of the local tissue resistance to the bacteria which are habitually present. Immediately after operation, of course, the patient is observed for signs of hemorrhage; this is especially important after hemorrhoidectomy. Most patients have severe pain after rectal surgery, and large doses of morphine or other opiates are necessary during the first twenty-four hours.

Preparation for Defecation. The patient is encouraged to refrain from defecation for forty-eight to seventy-two hours after operation, in order to lessen to some extent the bacterial contamination as well as to avoid undue strain on the wound. Mineral oil by mouth and liquid or other low residue diet are given to minimize the difficulty of defecation. On the third evening after operation it is the custom of many surgeons to order a rectal instillation of mineral oil which is to be retained if possible. This is followed the next morning by the administration of a cathartic (magnesium sulfate or Rochelle salts); defecation is then initiated since the stool has been made as soft as possible. After the bowels have moved well the patient is permitted to have a regular diet. Digital dilation of the rectum relieves painful spasm and prevents the formation of postoperative stricture.

Moist Heat. The most helpful therapy, however, is the application of moist heat, including compresses, irrigations, and sitz baths. These have the effect of cleansing the region and relaxing spasm, thus reducing both the degree of infection and the severity of pain.

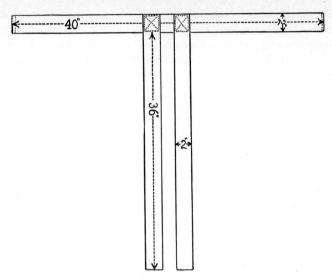

FIGURE 90. Pattern for modified T binder for perineal dressings.

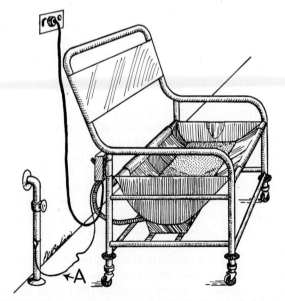

FIGURE 91. Chair for sitz bath; note that the chair is grounded (wire at *A*) to prevent electrical hazard from faulty heating unit.

COMPRESSES. Hot moist dressings may be applied after the compresses or gauze dressings have been wrung out of the ordered solution heated to 125° F. The moisture and heat will be retained when they are protected with a piece of plastic material. They may be held in place with a modified T binder.

IRRIGATIONS. Convenient equipment to administer perineal irrigations consists of a sterile bottle containing an Asepto syringe. The irrigations usually are given twice daily and after defecation. Excess moisture after the treatment may be sponged off with gauze or cotton.

SITZ BATHS. The sitz bath, which derives its name from the German word meaning seat, is taken in a sitting position. In many clinics a specially constructed tub is available to seat the patient so that only the hips are immersed in water; however, an ordinary bathtub half full of water is suitable for the treatment. The temperature of the water is gradually increased from 110 to 120° F. Care must be taken that the temperature does not exceed this last because a burn would result. The patient sits in the water from ten to fifteen minutes. The treatment should be terminated if the patient becomes exhausted before the prescribed period of time is ended. The application of a cold compress to the forehead adds to the comfort of the patient.

NEOPLASTIC DISEASE OF THE RECTUM
Rectal Polyposis

The benign adenoma of the rectal mucosa (*rectal polyp*) is a common lesion. The symptoms of rectal polyposis include bleeding, mucoid discharge, and sometimes protrusion of the polyp through the anus. Polyps may be single or multiple, and may be on a pedicle (*stalk*) or may have a broad base. Their size varies from pinhead to that of a small lemon. A rectal polyp may be removed by excision or by fulguration with electrocautery. There is, however, a high incidence of malignant degeneration in these polyps, so that microscopic examination of the polyp should always be made.

Carcinoma of the Rectum

The rectum is one of the more common sites of cancer. It is fortunate that this lesion produces symptoms relatively early, and that metastasis as a rule occurs but slowly, so that many patients can be cured. Although more common in men of middle age, cancer of the rectum occurs in both sexes and in both young and old.

Symptoms. The appearance of blood in the feces should lead to prompt examination of the rectum. In most instances the cause of such bleeding will be found to be due to hemorrhoids, but cancer should always be suspected and searched for. Later in the disease tenesmus and constipation occur, and finally anemia, loss of weight, weakness, and progressive intestinal obstruction. Pain is not apt to be a symptom until invasion of structures outside the rectum has taken place.

Treatment. Many operations have been devised for the cure of rectal cancer; of these the most satisfactory at present is the abdominoperineal resection (Miles operation). This operation is used in the treatment of lesions of the lower sigmoid colon as well. The patient is prepared for operation in the manner already described in connection with surgery of the colon (p. 307).

Technic of Miles Operation. Through a low midline abdominal wound the abdomen is explored to determine the operability of the lesion. The next step is division of the sigmoid colon. The upper end of this divided colon is brought out onto the abdominal wall, forming the terminal colostomy which will be a permanent one. The lower portion of the sigmoid colon is freed from all its attachments, as is the rectum; these structures are left beneath the peritoneum of the pelvic floor and the abdominal wound is closed. The patient is placed in either the lithotomy or Sims' lateral position, depending on the surgeon's preference. A circular incision is made around the anus, and the anus and rectum are freed from their attachments to the perineal muscles. When this has been done the whole segment including the rectum, the tumor and the lower sigmoid is readily drawn through the perineal wound.

The chief disadvantage of this operation is that the patient is left with a permanent colostomy. A number of surgeons are now attempting a new procedure which is designed to leave the rectal sphincter intact; the sigmoid colon is brought down through the sphincter, and thus a new and functioning anus is established. The substitution of this operation for the Miles operation will depend on the number of actual cures obtained.

Nursing Care. The postoperative care of patients who have undergone a Miles operation not only includes that described for patients with extensive abdominal surgery (p. 233) and a colostomy (p. 312), but also the care of the perineal wound. These patients have usually been intubated for decompression of the intestinal tract prior to operation, and gentle suction is continued afterward. Difficulty in urination is so regular a temporary complication of this operation that an indwelling bladder catheter is inserted immediately before operation. On return to the ward this is connected to straight drainage. The urinary output is regularly measured and recorded every six hours. Antibiotic therapy is routine.

Immediately following operation the nurse should observe the perineal dressings frequently in order to detect bleeding. Sterile gauze dressings and a cotton pad are placed over the wound; the dressings may be held in place with a modified T binder. It is essential that the wound be kept as clean as possible and that the bits of fibrin come off to promote quick healing. A urinal should be used by female patients to prevent soiling during urination. If the dressing has become wet it must be changed immediately. Should the perineal wound become infected, as it occasionally does, the enzymes streptokinase and streptodornase are extremely useful in liquefying the discharge and promoting healing. As soon as the abdominal wound has healed, sitz baths can be given; these are very effective in cleaning up the perineal wound and in adding to the patient's comfort.

Surgeons differ in their views on early ambulation following abdominoperineal resection of the rectum. The author prefers to permit his patients to remain in bed until the colostomy is functioning and the Cantor tube out. This will usually be at least seventy-two hours after operation. At this time the indwelling bladder catheter may be removed and the patient allowed to try voiding. Should he be unsuccessful after a few hours, the catheter is reinserted.

Instructions in colostomy care are given as outlined in the preceding chapter. Included in the plan for total care are the details for care after discharge from the hospital.

SUMMARY

Rectal disease is extremely common, and ranges from minor annoyance to potentially lethal carcinoma. Diagnosis of these diseases is not difficult, requiring only that the patient take his complaint to a doctor who will examine the rectum. Bleeding from the rectum is a warning which should be heeded. Because the rectum ordinarily contains pathogenic bacteria, rectal wounds are not expected to heal without infection; nevertheless, the results of rectal surgery are remarkably satisfactory.

VOCABULARY REVIEW

impaction	*hemorrhoids*	*incontinence*
fissure	*ischiorectal abscess*	*sitz bath*
pruritus	*fistula*	

SUGGESTED READING

1. Agnew, James W.: Abdomino-perineal Resection. Am. J. Nursing, *51*:225–226 (April) 1951.
2. Carmel, A. Gerson: Proctologic Nursing. Am. J. Nursing, *48*:626–629 (October) 1948.
3. Dericks, Virginia C., and Robeson, Kathryn: Problems of Colostomy Patients. Pub. Health Nursing, *41*:16–27 (January) 1949.
4. No One Knows I Have a Colostomy: Am. J. Nursing, *51*:703–704 (December) 1951.
5. Patterson, Mary G.: The Care of the Patient with Cancer. Pub. Health Nursing, *42*:377–383 (July) 1950.
6. Streuben, Ethel M.: Nursing Care for the Patient with an Abdomino-perineal Resection. Am. J. Nursing, *51*:226–228 (April) 1951.

CHAPTER 29

Nursing in Urologic Surgery

Anatomy and Physiology. The urinary tract is composed of the paired kidneys and ureters, the urinary bladder, and the urethra.

Kidneys. The kidneys are located in the upper posterior part of the abdomen on each side of the vertebral column, behind the peritoneal cavity. They are well protected from external injury by fat, the lower ribs, and the thick lumbar muscles. Each kidney receives a large branch (*renal artery*) from the aorta and returns a large tributary (*renal vein*) to the vena cava, so that a considerable volume of blood constantly circulates through these organs. The product of the kidney, urine, is processed from the blood by the highly specialized epithelial cells of the glomeruli and tubules in the renal cortex; it then passes down the collecting tubules into the kidney pelvis, an epithelial-lined cavity in the hilum of the kidney. The renal pelvis funnels into the ureter, through which the urine is conducted into the bladder.

Ureters. The ureters are about half the diameter of a lead

331

pencil; they are lined with epithelium, and have a strong coat of smooth muscle fibers which undergo contraction waves for the propulsion of the urine, similar to the peristalsis of the intestinal tract. On each side the ureter courses downward from the kidney pelvis, passes behind the peritoneum, crosses over the iliac vessels at the pelvic brim, lies to either side of the sigmoid colon in the pelvis, and crosses the floor of the pelvis to reach the base of the urinary bladder. The terminal portions of the ureters pass obliquely through the muscle of the bladder wall; the openings *(ureteral orifices)* are at either end of the base of the trigone, a triangle of which the vesical orifice (beginning of the urethra) forms the apex.

Urinary Bladder. The urinary bladder lies immediately beneath the symphysis pubis outside the peritoneal cavity in the anterior and lowermost portion of the abdomen. It has an epithelial lining and a heavy coat of smooth muscle fibers. Collapsing completely when empty, the bladder in the adult has a normal capacity of 300 or 400 cc.

Normal kidneys secrete urine continuously, although the rate of secretion depends upon numerous factors, and the urine is transmitted to the bladder by the ureters; this is an intermittent process, however, and urine enters the bladder from the ureteral orifices in tiny gushes or jets. The urine accumulates in the bladder, gradually distending it, and as the distention approaches the bladder capacity the desire for micturition becomes increasingly appreciated. Voiding results in relief and an empty bladder.

Urethra. The bladder outlet *(vesical orifice)* opens into the urethra, and in the bladder wall in this region are the sphincter muscle and its nerves, which have the important function of controlling the discharge of urine through the urethra, the act of voiding *(micturition)*. The male urethra passes through the prostate *(prostatic urethra)*, beneath the skin of the perineum *(membranous urethra)*, and along the length of the penis *(penile urethra)*, terminating at the external opening *(external urinary meatus)* at the tip of the penis. The female urethra is very short; it is generally believed that this fact accounts for the greater incidence of cystitis and pyelitis in females, as it is mechanically much easier for bacteria to gain entrance to the female bladder.

METHODS OF EXAMINING THE URINARY TRACT

As in every branch of medicine and surgery, the first and most important steps are the taking of a careful history of the patient's illness and the performance of an exacting physical examination. Much additional confirmatory and even essential information, however, is gained from special examinations, including urinalysis, renal function tests, cystoscopy, and roentgen visualization. The preparation of the patient for these examinations, the performance of some of the tests, and the collection of specimens are a part of surgical nursing. It must be emphasized that the results of these special examinations are reliable only when the examination is conducted according to established standard conditions. This is particularly true of renal function tests.

Examination of the Urine. Proper collection and examination of the urine show the amount secreted during the period of collection, the nature and concentration of the constituent chemicals, and the presence or absence of abnormal substances, cells, or bacteria. Preliminary examination is made of a specimen freshly voided into a clean container. The volume and specific gravity are measured and the appearance is noted. Small samples are then tested for reaction (acid or alkaline), for albumin, and for sugar. A portion is centrifuged and the sediment is examined microscopically to determine the nature of such crystals, casts, bacteria or cells as may be found. Normal urine does not contain albumin or sugar, and there should be no bacteria or cells except an occasional epithelial cell from the lining of the urinary tract. If the specimen cannot be examined as soon as voided it should be placed in a refrigerator; even so, the results of study will be less reliable, as cells sometimes break up and disappear.

In the care of the urologic patient it is a routine procedure to measure and record on a twenty-four hour basis the volume of all urine, as the daily total output has much significance.

Two-Glass Test. A convenient way of determining the origin of pus (leukocytes) in male urine is to have the patient divide a voiding into two glasses. The first specimen washes out the penile urethra, whereas the second specimen contains practically pure bladder urine. Pus in the first glass, therefore, indicates an inflammation of the penile urethra only *(anterior urethritis)*, while pus in both glasses indicates inflammation in the bladder *(cystitis)* or higher in the urinary tract.

Urine Cultures. In infection of the urinary tract it is important to identify the causative bacteria; stained smears of the sediment of centrifuged urine are helpful, but usually a culture is necessary for positive identification. An essential part of this test is to obtain urine without contamination from outside sources. In the male, unless the patient has urethritis, sufficiently uncontaminated cultures may be obtained by cleaning the end of the penis (*glans*) with 70 per cent alcohol or tincture of Zephiran, following which the patient voids directly into a sterile culture tube. If it is necessary, however, to know which kidney may be harboring bacteria, the specimen for culture must be taken directly from the kidney pelvis or ureter during cystoscopy. It is usual to obtain a specimen by catheter from females for culture and microscopic examination.

Phenolsulfonphthalein Test. This commonly used test of renal function, usually called the "phthalein test," is a convenient and accurate method of measuring renal function. Phenolsulfonphthalein, a nontoxic dye, is injected intravenously; it is eliminated rapidly from the circulating blood by the kidneys, appearing in the urine within two to five minutes after injection. If the kidneys are functioning normally, 60 to 80 per cent of the dye is excreted within two hours after injection.

The routine procedure for the two-hour total phthalein excretion is as follows: The patient is given 400 cc. of water; he then empties his bladder as completely as possible, immediately after which he is given 1 cc. of phenolsulfonphthalein intravenously. The patient voids one hour and two hours after the injection, emptying his bladder each time. The two specimens are collected separately, properly labeled, and sent to the laboratory. Phthalein is colorless in acid solutions, bright red in alkaline. In the laboratory the output of phthalein is measured by adding sodium hydroxide for alkalinization, diluting the specimen up to 1 liter by adding water, and comparing a sample against samples of known concentration in a colorimeter. A variation of this test is carried out during cystoscopy when one ureter is catheterized. In this modified phthalein (differential) test the appearance time can be noted, and the function of the two kidneys measured separately as the bladder urine comes from the ureter which is not catheterized.

Cystoscopy. Although there are several varieties of cystoscope, the purpose of all is the same and that is to visualize the interior of the bladder. Because of the length and the narrow diameter of the male urethra, water cystoscopy is used in male patients. The instrument is in essence a large-bore metal catheter, carrying a telescope, an electric bulb for illumination of the bladder, and a tube to permit withdrawal or insertion of fluid, and through which ureteral catheters or small instruments are introduced

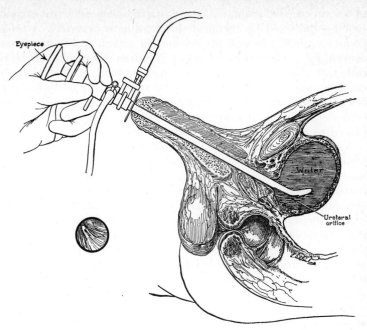

FIGURE 92. Water cystoscopy. Inset shows view of ureteral orifice as seen through cystoscope.

and manipulated. Cystoscopy is carried out under rigid aseptic precautions, and some form of anesthesia is necessary. The operator scrubs as for any surgical procedure. The penis is cleaned with aqueous solution of Zephiran.

Anesthesia. Adequate anesthesia for cystoscopy is usually obtained by the instillation of xylocaine 1 per cent into the urethra and bladder, but in difficult cases sacral or spinal anesthesia may be necessary. For children or very nervous persons general anesthesia is advisable. The patient is prepared beforehand as for a laparotomy. An enema is given in order to help eliminate as much intestinal gas as possible so that roentgen examinations will be more satisfactory. Shortly before cystoscopy the patient is given 400 cc. of water to ensure an adequate urinary output during the examination, particularly if a differential phthalein test is to be made. Morphine is usually given when the treatment is begun.

Care of Instruments. Since the materials and the construction of a cystoscope do not withstand sterilization by heat, careful cleaning followed by chemical sterilization is necessary. A satisfactory method is to soak the instrument (taken apart) in a basin containing a solution of 1:1000 of Zephiran (aqueous). Ureteral catheters are sterilized in the same manner. Rubber kidney catheters are available which may be sterilized by boiling. After removal from the boiling water, they should be dropped into cold sterile water at once to stiffen them. They may then be placed in a sterile glass tube and labeled.

Nursing Care Following Cystoscopy. Introduction of the cystoscope causes irritation of the smooth muscle fibers which is manifested by painful contractions, and following the examination there is discomfort as soon as the anesthesia wears off. Many surgeons order opiates; some order scopolamine or atropine, depending on the amount of pain the patient seems to have. Most patients feel well after twenty-four hours of rest in bed, forced fluids, and application of a hot water bottle to the lower abdomen. Sitz baths also are helpful in alleviating pain. The total intake of fluids for the twenty-four hours after a cystoscopy should be 5 liters.

Roentgen Visualization of the Urinary Tract. Calculi (*stones*) of the urinary tract may be seen in plain x-ray films of the abdomen. Two additional methods of visualization are commonly used: intravenous pyelography and retrograde pyelography.

Intravenous Pyelography. This is accomplished by the intravenous injection of an iodine-containing compound which is eliminated from the blood by the kidney in sufficient concentration to render the urine temporarily more radiopaque than the adjacent soft tissues; a film made at this time will outline the renal pelves, ureters, and bladder, provided renal function is not too much impaired by disease. The solution commonly used is Urokon. The patient is prepared by administering an enema and withholding food and fluids for at least eight hours before the examination, for a high concentration is desired. A plain roentgen film is taken first; then the dye is injected intravenously. X-ray films are made five, fifteen, and thirty minutes after the injection. As might be expected, intravenous pyelography is most satisfactory when there is no disease of the urinary tract.

Retrograde Pyelography. The most accurate and satisfactory roentgen visualization of the tract is accomplished by retrograde pyelography. The chief disadvantage of this method is that it requires cystoscopy and ureteral catheterization. With the ure-

teral catheter inserted up to the kidney pelvis, 3 to 8 cc. of radiopaque solution is injected into the pelvis through the catheter
and a roentgenogram immediately made without moving the
patient. The catheter is then withdrawn part way and a second
film taken, showing the ureter.

Some urologists prefer not to catheterize both ureters at the
same sitting because there is occasionally a temporary renal shutdown following ureteral catheterization, which is not serious if
only one kidney is involved. This means that two cystoscopies
are necessary for retrograde pyelograms of both kidneys, which is
an added drawback.

Air Cystoscopy. This technic, in which a straight open-bore
tube is used, is possible in women because of the shortness of the
urethra and because of the ease with which it can be dilated.
The advantages of this method over water cystoscopy include
greater simplicity of equipment, direct view of the bladder, and
the ability to use ureteral bougies and catheters with a larger bore.
A real disadvantage, however, is that the examiner cannot visualize the entire bladder, whereas the arrangement of lenses of the
water cystoscope permits visualization of virtually all of it.

Technic. The patient is prepared first as for water cystoscopy.
She is draped for pelvic examination (Chap. 48); the bladder is
catheterized and xylocaine is instilled into the urethra. Pelvic
examination is then made, following which the patient is shifted
to the knee-chest position and made as comfortable as possible.
The perineum and external genitalia are cleaned with aqueous
Zephiran. The urethra is gently dilated with a series of smooth
metal (Hegar) dilators up to 11 F. The Kelly cystoscope is
passed into the bladder and its obturator removed; as this is done
there is always a rush of air into the bladder which is opened by
the pull of gravity upon the dependent abdomen. The operator
wears a head mirror which reflects a narrow beam of light
through the cystoscope into the bladder.

All details of technic are the same as in water cystoscopy with
the exception of the use of wax bulbs. Because of the larger bore
of the air cystoscope, it is possible to apply a wax bulb to the tip
of the ureteral catheter. The wax bulb is made just before use by
melting a bit of sterile beeswax, dropping it onto the tip of the
catheter, and molding this drop until it has the desired thickness.
The wax bulb can be made larger or smaller as needed, and it
furnishes an accurate method of estimating the diameter of the
ureteral lumen, and of judging the results of the dilatation of

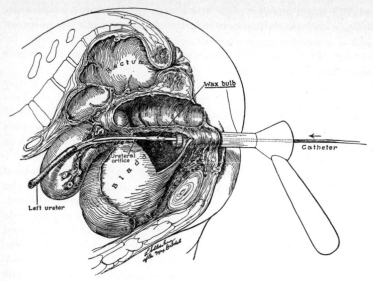

FIGURE 93. Air cystoscopy.

ureteral strictures. An additional advantage of the wax bulb is
that the wax will be scratched if it passes over a calculus; thus
a scratch on the wax bulb seen after withdrawal of the catheter
indicates the presence of a calculus. Indeed, an occasional small
stone becomes adherent to the wax and in this way is delivered
from the ureter.

PREPARATION OF INSTRUMENTS. The Kelly cystoscope is all metal
and is sterilized by boiling.

The ureteral catheters used in air cystoscopy are stiffened by
wire stylets. The catheters and the stylets are sterilized separately
either by soaking in 1:1000 oxycyanide of mercury or by boiling
for ten minutes, according to their composition. Then a nurse,
scrubbed just as though ready for an operation and in sterile
gown and gloves, inserts the stylets into the catheters. Small
sterile rubber shields are placed on the ends of the catheters and
then they are put into long sterile glass tubes which are plugged
with sterile cotton and labeled with the date of sterilization and
the size of the catheter.

There are two types of ureteral catheters. The catheter which
is used for collecting specimens and lavaging the kidneys is the
plain renal catheter. The other type is permeated with bismuth

so that when an x-ray film is made it will be seen in the x-ray film. This type may also be employed for the same purposes for which the plain renal catheter is used.

NURSING CARE. Following air cystoscopy the nursing care is the same as after water cystoscopy (p. 336).

CONGENITAL DEFORMITIES

Exstrophy. In this unusual and serious anomaly of the new-born the urinary bladder lies out on the lower abdominal wall and is open. The infant is obviously incontinent; the ureteral orifices are in plain sight. Infection of the tract soon occurs. Plastic surgery offers hope of cure by closing the bladder, but unfortunately these little patients often have other and less remediable deformities as well.

Reduplications. Double ureter, double renal pelvis, and even double kidneys occasionally occur; more rarely, these conditions are bilateral. Function is usually unimpaired and no treatment is necessary.

Other Renal Anomalies. Occasionally there is total absence of one kidney; it is always essential, therefore, before contemplating the removal of a kidney, to make sure that there is a normally functioning kidney on the opposite side. Misplaced (*ectopic*) kidneys are not uncommon; they are usually asymptomatic, but unless the mass can be positively identified in some other way, the discovery of an asymptomatic mass in the midabdomen or pelvis calls for roentgen visualization of the upper urinary tract. Another uncommon renal anomaly is a fusion of the two kidneys across the posterior abdomen, forming the so-called *horseshoe* kidney. Multiple cysts of the kidney (*polycystic kidney*) occur and may replace much of the renal cortex, resulting in loss of kidney function. Pain, increasing size, or infection may necessitate the removal of such a kidney.

DISEASES OF THE BLADDER

Cystitis. Inflammation of the lining of the bladder results from the introduction of pathogenic bacteria from without by way of the urethra, or by descent of bacteria in the urine from an infected kidney.

Symptoms. The patient complains of pain in the lower abdomen, of increased frequency and urgency of urination, and of burning during urination. There is often fever, and examination of the urine shows pus, that is, large numbers of white blood cells.

Treatment. Unless there is an obstruction which prevents the complete emptying of the bladder, or unless bacteria continue to come into the bladder from the kidneys, cystitis responds readily to treatment which includes the forcing of fluids and appropriate antibiotic and drug therapy. Cultures are always taken so that therapy may be specifically directed at the causative bacteria. If the cystitis does not clear up promptly following the use of these simple therapeutic measures, the patient should have a cystoscopic examination as the inflammation may be due to the presence of a stone (*calculus*) or an ulcer.

Retention. Retention of urine in the bladder may be acute or chronic. The causes in general are three: mechanical obstructions, such as urethral stricture or prostatic enlargement in the male; acute inflammatory disease adjacent to the lower tract, such as perirectal abscess; and neurologic disease or injury which disables the control mechanism of the nervous system.

Symptoms. The patient complains first of difficulty in initiating micturition, and later is unable to empty the bladder completely, so that there is constantly some residual urine, a condition favoring the persistence of infection. The bladder muscle, working against obstruction, becomes hypertrophied, but occasionally a weak spot develops which leads to the formation of a diverticulum. In acute retention there is complete inability to void, but when the bladder becomes overdistended (the capacity may reach 1500 cc. or more) there is often continual or intermittent seepage through the urethra; this is known as *paradoxical incontinence.*

Treatment. The treatment of retention depends upon the cause, but obviously one important feature is to establish urinary drainage promptly. This may be accomplished by the insertion of an indwelling catheter, by repeated catheterization, or, if passage of a catheter is not possible, by making an operative opening into the bladder through the abdominal wall (*cystostomy*). The emptying of an overdistended bladder should be accomplished gradually, as too sudden release of the pressure may cause renal hemorrhages and failure.

Complication. If the retention is due to injury or disease of the central nervous system it is likely that the paralysis of the bladder control mechanism will be of long duration or permanent. The long continued use of an indwelling catheter will certainly result in urinary tract infection, an often fatal complication in such cases. Fortunately in these patients an auto-

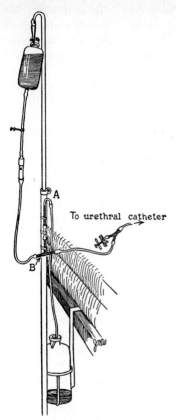

To urethral catheter

FIGURE 94. Apparatus for intermittent bladder irrigation and drainge. Irrigating fluid drips slowly into the bladder through the T tube until the pressure inside the bladder is sufficient to raise fluid level in side arm of T tube up to A. When this occurs the fluid running over at A initiates a siphon into the drainage bottle which produces enough suction to empty the bladder. This cycle is then repeated, and its duration depends upon the rate of inflow of the irrigating fluid.

matic bladder may develop, so called because it empties itself involuntarily when full. When infection does occur in a neurologic bladder the most useful method of handling the problem is by the use of the intermittent bladder irrigator apparatus, combined with chemotherapy.

Incontinence. Accidental trauma may damage the bladder sphincter or control mechanism so that there is continual leakage of urine from the urethra. In males this incontinence may be controlled by a specially designed clamp worn on the penis. Incontinence in females usually is a late complication of childbearing, and is apt to be of the stress variety, occurring chiefly when coughing, laughing or straining. This can be treated by an operation in which the sphincter is tightened.

Neoplasms. Carcinoma not infrequently arises from the epithelium which lines the bladder. The appearance of blood in the voided urine is the symptom which usually causes the patient to seek aid. Unfortunately, bleeding from a tumor does not occur until the tumor is large enough to become ulcerated. A smaller tumor may be discovered earlier only if it is located near the ureteral orifice or vesical orifice, where it can cause the symptoms of obstruction. Diagnosis is made by cystoscopic examination and biopsy. Fulguration or radiation of bladder cancers has not proved very satisfactory. Total removal of the bladder (*cystectomy*) offers more hope of a permanent cure.

Cystectomy

Surgical removal of the bladder necessitates the transplantation of the lower ends of the ureters in order to provide for the excretion of urine. Ureteral transplantation is a formidable procedure, and the greatest success has followed a method by which the ureters are implanted successively in stages into the sigmoid colon preliminary to cystectomy. This means that the urine is excreted through the rectum. As might be expected, there is some diarrhea at first, but it is amazing how well the patient with a successful transplantation gets along. The ureter must be implanted in the bowel in such a way that no leakage occurs, that the chance for bacteria to enter the ureter from the colon is minimal, and that there is no constriction of the ureter which might cause obstruction to the outflow of urine with consequent dilatation of the ureter (*hydro-ureter*) and kidney (*hydronephrosis*). At the first operation one ureter is transplanted; as soon as healing has occurred and satisfactory function is ascertained, the second operation, which includes transplantation of the remaining ureter and total removal of the bladder, is carried out.

Complications. In addition to all the ordinary complications of any laparotomy, there are the possibilities of peritonitis from leakage of the wound in the colon, urinary leakage into the peritoneum, and infection with or without obstruction of the upper urinary tract. Probably a certain amount of infection of the upper tract always occurs; but since the advent of chemotherapy and antibiotics this complication is not so serious as formerly provided there is no obstruction to urinary outflow into the bowel.

Nursing Care. Preparation for cystectomy includes establishing good nutrition, adequate hydration and antibiotic therapy. Cancer of the bladder is treated the same in either sex, but occurs about four times more often in men.

The thought that the bladder must be removed and that the urinary excretion will be transferred to the intestinal tract is certainly not a happy one for the patient. The reassurance and kindness which the nurse offers are very helpful to the patient and are necessary to give him some security.

Immediately before operation a Levine tube is usually placed in the stomach. The general preoperative and postoperative care is the same as that for laparotomy. In addition, the immediate postoperative care is aimed to facilitate the excretion of urine and maintain the electrolyte balance of the patient. A large colon tube is usually kept in the rectum to drain the urine and feces until healing and renal function seem satisfactory; this is usually five to seven days. Irrigating the rectal tube with normal saline to insure patency by removing any fecal material is necessary. Following the removal of the tube, the nurse should learn from the surgeon the frequency he advises the patient to empty his bowel. It has been found when urine remains in the bowel, sodium chloride in the urine is partially reabsorbed by the bowel. To prevent this the bowel must be emptied frequently, usually every two to four hours. When excretion takes place this often it may lower the potassium content of the blood. To combat or prevent these disturbances the patient may be given a low chloride diet, supplemented with potassium salts. When the electrolyte balance becomes disturbed the patient may exhibit some degree of acidosis characterized by nausea, vomiting, fatigue, weakness and loss of weight.

Good nutrition is emphasized; a low residue, high caloric diet is frequently ordered as soon as the patient can take food. When sodium is limited, the proteins must obviously be decreased in the diet. While the patient is in the hospital blood studies are done frequently and the patient may be expected to receive whole blood and other fluids to maintain a normal blood level.

When the patient has a colostomy or when the urine is excreted through cutaneous openings in the abdomen, as after pelvic exenteration, some type of bag must be worn to allow for the collection of urine. The bag or cup used for the cutaneous opening or colostomy may be the type cemented to the skin. The patient must be taught how to apply and remove the bag and how to clean the skin area. Skin cement is removed with benzine or ether. The skin is then thoroughly washed with mild soap and water, and dried well before the cement is reapplied. The surgeon and nurse should work out a complete plan of care for such a patient so that day by day instructions may be given in an assured and unhesitating manner.

The onset of electrolyte imbalance may not occur until months after surgery. In preparing the patient to go home, it is important that the nurse emphasize follow-up care to permit a periodic checkup to evaluate his status so that he may be aided according to his need.

DISEASES OF THE KIDNEY AND URETER

Renal Trauma. The kidney is well protected from external violence, but penetrating wounds or severe blows upon the abdomen or crushing wounds sometimes cause laceration of the renal cortex. Severe pain and tenderness over the kidney are accompanied by gross blood in the urine (*hematuria*). Ordinarily the bleeding stops and the kidney heals with remarkably little loss of function. Occasionally, however, the damage is so great that the bleeding is dangerous and an immediate nephrectomy is necessary to save life.

Pyelitis. The commonest cause of inflammation of the lining of the kidney pelvis is infection with the colon bacillus or other pathogenic bacteria found in the large bowel. The explanation of this is obvious in patients who have had ureteral transplantation, but there has been no satisfactory explanation of those infections which often occur in patients who have had no operation. Pyelitis is not so common in men as in women. Whether the infection is an ascending one to the kidney by way of the urethra, bladder, and ureter, or whether the infection is blood-borne is a matter of controversy; very likely it occurs in both ways.

Symptoms and Diagnosis. The symptoms of pyelitis are aching pain in the flank and lumbar region, increased frequency and burning urination, and, occasionally, chills. The patient has fever and leukocytosis and feels badly, and examination of the urine shows large numbers of pus cells (*leukocytes*). Urine culture is done to identify the causative bacteria. It is important to cure pyelitis because continued infection eventually leads to infection and destruction of the renal substance, which, in turn, finally causes renal failure.

Treatment. Many patients with pyelitis respond rapidly to therapy which includes rest in bed, adequate fluids, and chemotherapy. Other patients, in whom the offending bacteria are not susceptible to such chemotherapeutic and antibiotic agents as are now known, tend to develop a chronic infection which is very intractable. Of course, in any patient who has an associated obstruction of the urinary tract the infection will not respond well to ordinary therapy until the obstruction is treated and relieved.

Renal and Perirenal Abscesses. As the result of a blood-borne infection, usually staphylococcal or streptococcal, a large abscess forms in the kidney substance or in the fat about the kidney.

Symptoms and Diagnosis. The symptoms are pain in the flank or back and the usual systemic symptoms of an acute infection. Often the diagnosis is difficult to establish as there may be at first no symptoms or signs of involvement of the urinary tract. Later there is tenderness in the region of the kidney, and pus cells appear in the urine. Pyelograms show distortion of the renal pelvis or displacement of the kidney. Renal function becomes impaired only if there is considerable destruction of the kidney cortex.

Treatment. Treatment consists in incision and drainage of the abscess together with antibiotic therapy. The prognosis is good unless the patient has abscesses elsewhere in the body, as often happens in blood-borne infections of this sort.

Tuberculosis of the Kidney and Urinary Tract. Tubercle bacilli enter the kidney substance from the blood stream; the primary site of the tuberculosis is always in the lungs. As the disease progresses, sooner or later a tubercle ruptures into the collecting tubules or renal pelvis, thus distributing the tubercle bacilli into the ureter and bladder, in which the typical lesions of the tuberculosis then develop.

Symptoms. Renal tuberculosis is an insidious disease, and is likely to have progressed far before causing symptoms. The first complaints are usually loss of weight, persistent unexplained fever, or the appearance of blood and pus cells in the urine.

Diagnosis. Diagnosis is established by the characteristic appearance of the pyelogram, which shows irregular ulceration of the border of the calices of the pelvis, and by the identification of tubercle bacilli in the urine, which is done by examining stained smears and by making special cultures.

Treatment. Careful examination must be made of the urine and function of each kidney, for if there is bilateral involvement the patient cannot be cured by surgery. If, however, only one kidney is infected and no tubercles are seen in the bladder, the surgical removal of the tubercular kidney is curative in the majority of cases. These patients need, in addition to nephrectomy, the usual supportive and hygienic measures used routinely for all patients who have tuberculosis in any of its numerous manifestations. Antibiotic and drug therapy is used.

Urinary Tract Calculi. Stones form in the kidneys, ureters and bladder, and vary in size from pinhead to large stag-horn calculi which fill the entire renal pelvis. The formation of stones cannot always be satisfactorily explained, but they are composed of the crystals of the various chemicals found in urine, and almost always contain calcium, carbonates, and phosphates, as well as other crystalloids. One known cause of the formation of stone is the excessive excretion of calcium which occurs in hyperparathyroidism; the finding of repeated urinary calculi in a patient should lead to examination for a parathyroid adenoma. Stones in the kidney may produce no symptoms, but if urinary tract infection occurs, the stone may be discovered in the search to find a reason for the persistence of infection. Often, however, stones cause obstruction, and one of the most severe varieties of pain, i.e., renal and ureteral colic, is caused by the passage or attempted passage of small calculi from the renal pelvis through the ureter to the bladder.

Symptoms. The characteristic clinical picture of nephrolithiasis or ureterolithiasis is an attack of excruciating, cramplike pain in the flank, lower abdomen, and groin. Accompanying this are urinary frequency and the appearance of gross blood in the urine, caused by the abrasive action of the stone as it is passed.

Diagnosis. Following subsidence of the acute colic, the urologist attempts to locate the stone. All urine is collected and strained so that a stone may not be passed per urethram undetected. Plain roentgenograms and pyelograms are usually necessary.

Treatment. Large doses of morphine are necessary to relieve the pain. If the stone is lodged in the ureter, it may sometimes be dislodged and passed following the passage of a ureteral catheter or bougie. A stone in the renal pelvis or one firmly fixed in the ureter must be removed surgically (*nephrolithotomy* or *uretero-*

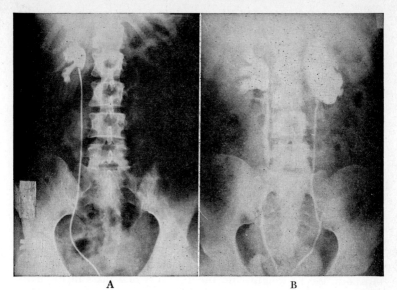

A   B

FIGURE 95. Retrograde pyelograms. *A,* Normal; *B,* bilateral hydronephrosis.

lithotomy); otherwise there may be permanent damage to the kidney and loss of renal function consequent to the obstruction.

Hydronephrosis. A gradual or partial obstruction to the outflow of urine from the kidney produces progressive dilatation of the renal pelvis, which may become very large, with consequent destruction of the renal cortex. In an advanced hydronephrosis the kidney is little more than a hollow shell containing a large pelvis. Obviously the most important result of this condition is the progressive loss of renal function. If the obstruction is relieved early, the kidney shows a considerable ability to regain normal function and may do so completely; but if the hydronephrosis is large and of long duration the function is permanently lost. A sudden complete obstruction, on the other hand, usually results in renal shutdown followed by rapid and permanent atrophy of the kidney. There are many causes of hydronephrosis, including congenital valves or kinks in the ureter, aberrant blood vesels which obstruct the renal pelvis at its junction with the ureter, calculi, swelling due to infection, obstruction to the outflow of urine from the bladder, and neoplasms.

Symptoms. Hydronephrosis may be asymptomatic, but at times there is dull pain in the flank, and if the hydronephrosis is large, a mass is felt in the kidney region. If infection is present the systemic symptoms and signs are apt to be severe.

Diagnosis. Diagnosis is made on the basis of pyelography, which readily demonstrates the enlarged renal pelvis.

Treatment. Treatment depends upon the cause, the amount of renal function remaining, and the severity of the infection if present. An attempt is made to clear up the infection by ureteral catheterization and drainage together with chemotherapy, but if ureteral drainage is not feasible a direct operative opening is made into the kidney (*nephrostomy*) for drainage. If the obstruction is amenable to surgery, the necessary procedures are done. In cases in which there is infection plus permanent severe loss of renal function, however, removal of the kidney is the procedure of choice.

Neoplastic Disease. Renal tumors are of common occurrence and most of them are malignant. Unfortunately, symptoms appear late, often too late for cure, as the first symptom may be the pain in bones due to metastases. Bloody urine (*hematuria*) without pain, loss of weight, and the discovery of a mass in the flank are the usual signs of a renal tumor. The diagnosis is established by pyelography, which shows a characteristic deformity of the renal pelvis. If the tumor has not spread beyond the kidney capsule, cure is effected by nephrectomy.

Kidney tumors which occur in children differ from those seen in adults. Arising from tissues of nervous origin, they are quite radiosensitive. Nephrectomy combined with deep x-ray therapy results in some cures.

Operations on the Kidney

Removal of a stone through an incision in the kidney cortex is called *nephrolithotomy;* if the incision is made in the kidney pelvis for extraction of a stone it is called *pyelolithotomy.* A simple opening into which a tube is inserted for drainage is called *nephrostomy.*

Nephrectomy and other procedures are not undertaken until there is complete information as to the condition and function of the opposite kidney as well as of the diseased one. The patient is prepared as for any abdominal operation. Spinal anesthesia is somewhat more satisfactory than inhalation anesthesia, as complete muscular relaxation is important for proper exposure of the kidney. Approach to the kidney is made through an incision parallel with the lowermost rib in the flank. The posterior

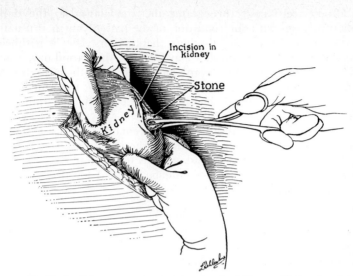

FIGURE 96. Nephrolithotomy. The incision in the kidney will be closed by sutures.

peritoneum is retracted and the peritoneal cavity is not entered. Removal of the kidney is a difficult operation because of the shortness of the large renal vessels which must be divided and ligated. Serious loss of blood is not uncommon, and transfusion is a routine matter. The wound is sutured but drains are always employed. Except in the case of nephrectomy, there are copious amounts of drainage, largely urine, so that the dressings need frequent changing. The postoperative complications are the same as in a patient who has had a laparotomy.

Nursing Care. Preparation to receive the patient is like that after a laparotomy. After plastic repairs and nephrectomy the patient is turned from his back to the side of operation for the first forty-eight hours, but after this period turning from side to side is encouraged. All other patients are turned from side to side so that pulmonary complications and distention may be prevented. When a catheter has been inserted into the kidney it is usually connected to sterile rubber tubing which drains into a bottle at the bedside. Unless the drainage from this catheter leading from the kidney is more than 5 cc. per hour, the surgeon must be notified at once. It is important that all voided specimens as well as the drainage be accurately measured and recorded.

Fluids are forced throughout the convalescence; the daily amount varies with the condition of the patient but it is usually no less than 3 liters and no more than 5 liters. Diet is withheld for the first day; a liquid diet may be given the second day, a soft diet the third day, and a regular diet on the fifth or sixth day.

The dressings are changed whenever necessary; the wound and surrounding skin should be thoroughly cleaned each time that the dressings are changed.

The length of time that the patient remains in bed varies with the condition of the patient; at times he is gotten up as early as the fifth day, but the twelfth day seems to be more common.

Lifting of heavy weights should be avoided for three months following operation.

SUMMARY

Although the urinary tract is but a small part of the human body, the diagnosis and treatment of urologic infections, obstructions, and neoplasms require special technics and equipment. The only significant difference between the male and female urinary tract is the length of the urethra. The continuous excretion of urine is essential to life, and the maintenance of this function is the aim of urology.

VOCABULARY REVIEW

ureter	*phenolsulfon-*	*cystectomy*
urethra	*phthalein*	*hydronephrosis*
micturition	*pyelography*	*nephrolithotomy*
cystoscope	*exstrophy*	

SUGGESTED READING

1. Christopher, Frederick: Textbook of Surgery. 5th Ed. Philadelphia, W. B. Saunders Co., 1949, pp. 1225–1287.
2. Davis, D. M., and Strong, G. M.: Urological Nursing. 5th Ed. Philadelphia, W. B. Saunders Co., 1953.
3. Fleming, Elizabeth C.: Kidney Stone. Am. J. Nursing, *49*:568–570 (September) 1949.
4. Korenberg, Morton: The Electrolyte Disturbance in Ureterocolostomy. J. Urol., *66*:686–687 (November) 1951.
5. McLester, James S.: Nutrition and Diet in Health and Disease. Philadelphia, W. B. Saunders Co., 1949, pp. 452–484.
6. Newton, Kathleen: Urologic Nursing. Am. J. Nursing, *50*:167–170 (March) 1950.
7. Rusche Carl: Preparation, Operative Technique and Postoperative Management of Uretero-intestinal Anastomosis. J. Urol., *65*:550–552 (April) 1951.

8. Daut, Richard V.: Urologic Conditions in Women. Am. J. Nursing, *50:*479–482 (August) 1950.

9. Everett, Houston S.: Urology in the Female. Am. J. Surgery, *52:*521–659 (June) 1941.

10. Wharton, Lawrence R.: Gynecology Including Female Urology. Philadelphia, W. B. Saunders Co., 1943, pp. 769–962.

11. Lowsley, Oswald Swinney, and Thomas Joseph Kirwin: Clinical Urology. 2nd Ed. Baltimore, Williams and Wilkins Co., 1944, pp. 1102–1205.

CHAPTER 30

Nursing in Plastic Surgery

Plastic surgery is the operative correction of congenital or acquired deformities for the purpose of restoring function and improving appearance. The scope of the subject is broad: indeed all surgery is plastic surgery, in that the careful surgeon always tries to avoid unsightly scars and interference with proper function.

The art of plastic surgery is ancient. As early as 800 B.C. Hindu physicians were familiar with skin shifting operations and had developed a technic for reconstructing the nose with a flap shaped from the forehead and hinged downward. Essentially the same operation is often utilized today. Plastic procedures were employed and described in the first century A.D. by Celsus, a Roman, and the writings of Galen, who lived in the second century, contain references to plastic operations. In the fifteenth century a Sicilian named Branca repaired and reconstructed noses by

transferring flaps of skin from the arm. Despite this early progress, interest in the subject lagged until the middle of the nine-
teenth century, since which time the development and perfection of anesthesia, asepsis, and operating methods have provided
surgeons with the means for greater accomplishments. The mu-
tilations resulting from the two world wars gave further impetus.

GENERAL PRINCIPLES

Of utmost importance in plastic surgery are gentleness and
care in the handling of tissues. Avoidance of bruising, the most
rigid aseptic technic, careful and delicate hemostasis, and scrupulous regard for detail are necessary for satisfactory results, for
contused and infected tissues heal with unsightly scars. Operators
must use the finest instruments, the slenderest needles, and the
most delicate suture materials. Surface stitches are removed as
soon as safety permits to avoid additional skin markings. Dead
spaces must be eliminated, and tension on tissues must be
avoided. The placing of incisions along natural skin lines makes
the scars less noticeable.

Selection of Grafts. In the transplantation of tissues and in the
transfer of grafts the surgeon utilizes his knowledge of different
methods to select the one most suitable for the purpose. Transplanted tissues should resemble in texture and color the surfaces
to which they are to be transferred. Good results can be accomplished by careful selection as the body provides a variety of skin
colors, thicknesses, and textures. For example, the skin of the
neck and that which lies behind the ear is thin, soft and pliable.
As a rule it presents gradation in pigmentation, and it can readily
be transferred to the face. Skin from the inner surface of the
upper arm or thigh is also delicate but paler. Skin from the back
and shoulders is thick and heavy and in general less useful for
full-thickness grafting although it provides adequate material for
the split-thickness graft. Technics have been developed whereby
grafted skin can be tattooed and impregnated with harmless pigment to blend closely with the skin of the face or lip or the hair-
bearing cheek. Alterations of the nose for cosmetic reasons demand careful study and frequently the construction of a cast of
the face in plaster before surgery is undertaken. Grafts which are
transferred from distant parts of the body are not elevated until
thorough study has determined the safest and simplest method
and the most favorable donor site. In such instances the preserva-

tion of the blood supply is of great importance and at times assures the success of the procedure.

Anesthesia. Operative procedures about the face present problems in anesthesia and frequently necessitate intratracheal intubation and the administration of "anesthesia at a distance." Local or regional block anesthesia with xylocaine is especially useful.

Preoperative and Postoperative Care. Prophylaxis against potential infection by means of antibiotic therapy, the correction of anemia and hypoproteinemia before operation, and consideration of possible avitaminoses are all invaluable aids in securing satisfactory wound healing. Conscientious postoperative care is often the deciding factor in a successful operation.

Closure of Defects

Defects of varying sizes in the skin and underlying tissues resulting from the excision of tumors or from accidental wounds can frequently be repaired and made inconspicuous by the local readjustment of tissues. The inherent property of elasticity in the skin permits it to be stretched and extended after proper and sufficient undermining. Triangular defects may be closed in a Y; oval defects are convertible into a T; rectangular ones may be made into an ellipse and sutured in a straight line, or the borders of the rectangle may be extended and undermined and the flaps thus formed sutured in the fashion of an H. Additional incisions or excisions may be made adjacent to a defect to permit the rotation of skin to cover the denuded area.

Repair of Scars

All incisions and wounds, no matter how acquired, leave scars upon healing. The cosmetic result is dependent upon a number of factors, such as tension, infection, loss of substance, careful handling, and the like. Unsightly scars can frequently be excised and replaced by more presentable ones. Depressed scars resulting from the loss of deep structures are corrected by thorough excision and repair which unites these deep tissues to form a proper support for the skin. Such scars commonly occur in the healing of carbuncles and deep infections which have resulted in extensive destruction of tissue.

Repair of Keloids

Certain persons, especially Negroes, have a tendency to produce thick, weltlike scars (keloids); masses of connective tissue are

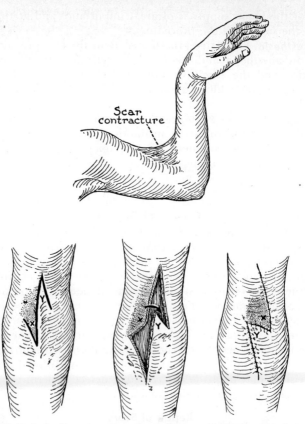

FIGURE 97. Z-plasty for relaxation of contracture. Following the Z incision
(*A*), flaps X and Y are elevated (*B*), and transposed (*C*).

found in keloids, as though the proliferative process in wound
healing failed to stop at the proper time. The removal of such
heaped-up and deforming scars can often be satisfactorily effected
surgically, and the prevention of further keloid growth can be
accomplished by careful x-ray therapy.

Repair of Contractures

One of the characteristics of scar tissue is its tendency to contract. Scars which cross joints, therefore, even though they may
heal by first intention, are apt to produce contractures which
limit or prevent motion. Relaxation and free motion can often

be restored by the simple Z-plasty. In this procedure two triangular flaps of equal size are elevated adjacent to the line of contracture. The excised contracted scar forms the middle bar of the Z. The flaps are then rotated so that their apices cross the line of contracture, increasing its length by about 50 per cent. This simple procedure finds application in the relief of contractures of the fingers and thumb, the wrist and elbow, and even large surfaces such as the neck, the axilla, the knee, and the thigh. Wide scars, however, must be treated by more elaborate methods.

Pilonidal Cyst and Sinus

In the skin of the posterior midline of the body, over the lower sacrum, are occasionally found small epithelial-lined cysts, which may communicate by means of small pores with the exterior. The lining of these cysts or sinuses is usually hair-bearing, which explains the name *pilonidal* (nest of hair). Pilonidal cyst and sinus are congenital defects, more common in males than in females, and do not cause symptoms unless infection occurs. The symptoms and signs are similar to those of any acute localized infection, and the immediate treatment consists in the application of heat and later, if necessary, surgical drainage. If the patient has repeated attacks of inflammation it is necessary to excise the cyst or sinus in order to accomplish a permanent cure.

SKIN GRAFTING

The procedure of transferring a portion of skin from one area to another area in the same individual is called an *autograft,* whereas the transfer of a graft from one individual to another of the same species is called a *homograft.* Autografts are generally successful, and the graft in its new site becomes a permanent feature. Homografts, on the other hand, as a rule are not successful, except in certain special instances. Although it would be desirable to be able to use skin from one individual for another, as in severe burns, the results do not justify such a procedure.

Small Deep Grafts. The simplest type of skin graft is the free graft. Segments of skin are cut from one portion of the body (*donor area*) and transferred to the site where needed (*recipient area*). This principle was used by Reverdin, who found that small superficial pieces of epithelium would survive and grow when transplanted to granulating surfaces. A further and more useful application of this principle was developed by Davis in the small

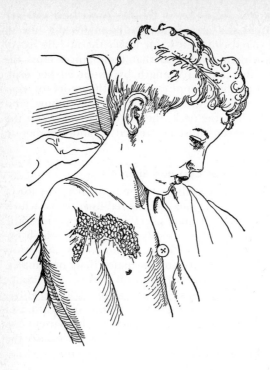

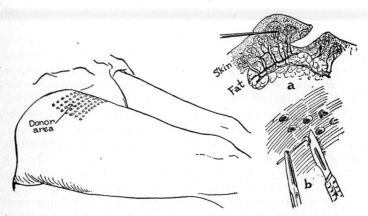

FIGURE 98. Small deep grafts. Depth of graft and method of cutting are shown at *a* and *b*.

deep graft which, although only 5 to 7 millimeters in diameter, contains in its central portion the full thickness of the skin and provides a thicker and healthier type of covering. Hundreds of these grafts can be cut from the thigh or any other desired site and can be seeded on large granulating areas to form islands of epithelium which grow out in all directions to coalesce and cover the defect. This type of graft has been especially useful to cover extensively burned areas which have become infected. They also provide durable covering in chronic ulcers of the leg. Useful as they are, there is, however, one major objection, for the resulting epithelialization is spotty and presents a less attractive cosmetic result than whole-thickness or split-thickness grafts which have an unbroken surface. Small deep grafts are easily cut under local anesthesia, even in small children, and their care is relatively simple. Both donor and recipient areas are usually dressed with a layer of petrolatum or xeroform gauze under a little pressure. The donor area is not disturbed for ten days, at which time it is usually found to be healed. The grafted area is dressed in four or five days. Occasionally, when the surface is heavily infected, the dry dressing may be replaced by saline compresses which are changed frequently. The addition of penicillin to the salt solution is often beneficial.

Free Full-thickness Graft. Small defects can be covered by full-thickness skin excised from the neck or the inner surface of the arm or thigh and transferred to the area to be repaired as free grafts. The donor area is usually closed immediately. The size of the graft is limited, for these grafts depend for their viability upon the rapid establishment of nutrition from the new base, and their early life is precarious. Small areas about the face can be covered satisfactorily by this method. The cosmetic effect in these relatively minor procedures is usually pleasing, but the conditions for success are exacting. Viability in free full-thickness grafts is usually evident after four or five days. There may be some superficial and harmless desquamation.

Split-thickness Graft. This graft has been growing in popularity and usefulness in recent years. It is cut either by free hand or with a mechanical device, and consists in a sheet of epithelium which is only a portion of the full thickness of the skin. Regeneration and healing take place rapidly on the donor site with minimal scarring.

The first of these grafts was described by Ollier and Thiersch. They were usually cut free-hand with a long-bladed knife from

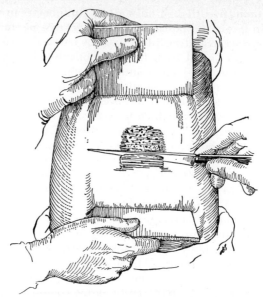

FIGURE 99. Split-thickness graft. It is difficult to cut uniform grafts freehand; the use of the mechanical dermatome gives excellent uniform results.

the skin of the thigh, which was held taut by boards or suction boxes. More recently the combined ingenuity of surgeons and instrument makers has produced a variety of instruments designed to provide perfect grafts of uniform thickness in large sheets. The most popular of these is the Padgett-Hood dermatome, a half circle drum provided with a cutting blade which is moved back and forth at a calibrated distance from the surface of the drum, to which the skin adheres.

Split-thickness grafts furnish ideal covering for a great variety of defects and are particularly useful in burns. Here they are planted in continuous sheets or are cut into small squares and seeded on granulations after the fashion of small deep grafts. In a study carried out during World War II, furthermore, it was found that a split graft could be made to grow on the granulations in osteomyelitic bone cavities. These "skin dressings" greatly hastened healing and the control of infection.

Pedicle Graft. Occasion frequently presents for the transplantation of large portions of skin with the underlying fat and supporting connective tissues. Such grafts cannot at any time be isolated from the blood supply. In order to accomplish this transfer the operation must be carried out in stages which permit a new blood supply to be established from a new source before the original one is severed. Such operations may assume great complexity depending upon the demands of a particular plastic problem. For example, when tissues are torn from the dorsum of the hand and the extensor tendons lie bare and exposed, the viability of those tendons and the function of the hand can be preserved only by early covering with full thickness skin and fat. A large defect of the forearm may demand the same type of covering before a necessary bone graft or muscle transplant can be done. In many extensive wounds large areas of scar tissue must be replaced by healthy normal skin before additional operations can safely be performed on the deeper structures. In a wide variety of such lesions successful covering is obtained through the use of the single pedicle flap. The skin and fat of such a flap are elevated on the abdominal wall or elsewhere; it is essential to preserve a portion of its attachment through which pass the blood vessels nourishing the flap. The free portion is sutured to the recipient area but remains temporarily dependent on the existing blood supply through the pedicle. After two or three weeks new vascular channels will have become established between the flap and the new structures to which it has been sutured, permitting the severance of the pedicle. This division is carried out in stages or in a single procedure, depending upon the size and shape of the flap and the condition of the tissues. The stump of the pedicle is sutured back into its bed. If the flap thus elevated is reasonably narrow, the donor defect can sometimes be closed immediately by undermining the surrounding skin and taking advantage of its elasticity. Larger donor areas must be covered by split-thickness grafts.

Tubular Pedicle Grafts. These are among the safest and most useful of grafts and are especially dependable when full-thickness skin and fat must be transplanted to a distance from the donor site. They have an advantage over the simpler forms of pedicle flaps in that at no time during their transfer is any open area exposed. These tubed pedicles are usually constructed on the abdomen, although they are sometimes made on the flank or on the back, and smaller ones may be built from the skin of the arm or leg if these tissues are sufficiently relaxed. There are several methods by which they are constructed. All are variations of the

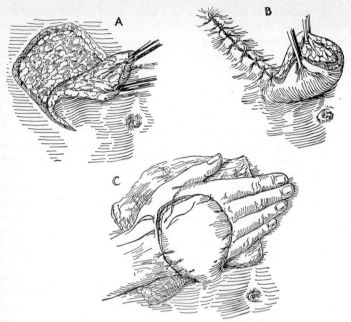

FIGURE 100. Pedicled flap graft. *A*, A flap of skin and subcutaneous tissue are
elevated; *B*, the resulting defect is closed; *C*, the flap is sutured in
position where needed, in this instance on the back of a hand.

original method in which staggered parallel incisions are made,
the intervening flap is elevated, and the surrounding tissues are
widely undercut. The lateral margins of skin are then sutured
together beneath the central flap; the flap forms a roll or tube of
skin and its edges are sewed together. The resulting graft resembles a satchel handle with circulation supplied from both
ends. After twelve to twenty days one end or the other can be
closed off with a rubber tourniquet to test the adequacy of the
circulation passing through the opposite pedicle. When it is
ascertained that the flap remains of good color and is viable
throughout, the end closed by the tourniquet can be severed and
reimplanted at any desired site. Such a flap may be transferred
directly to the recipient area or may be moved anywhere in the
body, moving first one end and then the other. A convenient
method attaches one end of the flap to the hand or wrist, from
which it can be carried elsewhere for ultimate implantation.
Segments of healthy skin measuring 10 by 25 centimeters are

readily available from the average adult, and much larger flaps have been constructed.

Postoperative Care

From the standpoint of nursing and postoperative care, plastic procedures necessitating skin grafting are apt to be exacting. Pedicle flaps must be protected against pressure and must be watched for signs of impending *ischemia* (scarcity of blood) and necrosis. Frequently the adjustment of a dressing or the removal of a few constricting sutures will save a threatened flap. Serum or pus gathering beneath a split graft separates it from its nutritive base and must be removed. Flaps in the process of transfer must be watched for strangulation. Infection must always be guarded against, and prophylactic measures using sulfonamides or penicillin are recommended. All dressings are done aseptically with the surgeon and assistants masked. Grafts are often helped in their struggle for survival by the use of sterile compresses moistened in warm normal saline solution.

THE TREATMENT OF DEFORMITIES

A wide variety of deformities are correctable by plastic surgery. Many of these deformities are congenital, others are acquired as a consequence of injury or disease. Surgery for cosmetic reasons alone is frequently justifiable; the healthy person of pleasing appearance should be careful not to underestimate the effect upon another's personality of an obvious deformity, even though the deformity causes no physical disability. A child's entire social development may be improved by a single operation which converts abnormally protruding ears into close-set ones. Satisfactory technics have evolved for reconstructing noses, ears, lips, and eyebrows.

Congenital deformities of the hands and feet are common. Extra fingers or toes (*polydactylism*) are removed. Webbed fingers or toes (*syndactylism*) are treated by division of the web in such a manner as to preserve the function and skin of both digits. It is interesting that both of these conditions are hereditary.

MAXILLO-FACIAL SURGERY

The development of plastic surgery has greatly widened the scope of this field. Perhaps the most notable application has been been directed toward oral surgery for malignancy. Cancer involving the tongue and mouth raises serious problems in removal and reconstruction. The sacrifice of a portion of the mandible together with the removal of part of the floor of the mouth or a large portion of the cheek represents only the beginning. These defects must be closed, and the closure must be acceptable from a functional and from a cosmetic standpoint. Such procedures often necessitate the provision of pedicle grafts lined with epithelium to provide coverage not alone for the exterior but for the oral cavity as well. Metal splints or bone grafts are required to replace portions of the mandible or maxilla. Dentures have an important role in such reconstruction. And very often these exterior operative procedures must have added to them wide dissection of the lymph nodes on one or both sides of the neck, removing all tissues partaking in the metastatic pathways of oral cancer.

COSMETIC SURGERY

The cosmetic aspects of plastic surgery are perhaps less important in a sense than the correction of congenital defects or the excision of tumors. Even so, they may assume grave importance. The author recalls a famous actress whose career on the stage was prolonged by a "face lifting" procedure which restored her youthful appearance. Recently, technics have been developed to overcome the unsightly pitting of the skin secondary to acne. Curiously enough, such scarred and pitted skin can be rendered smooth and quite normal simply by sanding its surface much as one would smooth a roughened piece of wood. To this same category belongs mention of rhinoplasty. These are operations on the nose designed to straighten those which are crooked, to remove unsightly bumps or to build up defects in the nasal bridge with grafts of cartilage. Such defects may, of course, be congenital or acquired. In either case, this correction may have bearing not only on the appearance of an individual but on his acceptance in society, his earning capacity, and his self-esteem.

The plastic surgeon may find himself confronted with problems in urology, gynecology and orthopedics. He may have to construct a vagina which is congenitally absent, or he may have to build a urethra in a patient with hypospadias. He may be faced with a congenitally malformed or traumatized hand in which a thumb is missing and for which transference of bone, tendons, nerves and blood supply as well as skin is needed. Indeed, the potential challenges are endless, and the results are limited only by the capacity of human physiology and the ingenuity of the surgeon.

Occasionally, following trauma or as the result of an operation for cancer, a facial mutilation is too extensive for successful reconstruction. In such a case the appearance of the patient can be greatly improved by the construction of a prosthesis (mask or other artificial replacement). The skill of the prosthesis-maker is such that very close scrutiny is necessary to detect the difference between the real and the artificial.

MAMMAPLASTY

The nurse should have an appreciation of the mental and physical aspects of the patient with mammaplasty so that she may give effective nursing care.

Tremendously hypertrophied breasts, such as in virginal hypertrophy in a young girl or very large and pendulous breasts of an older woman, definitely affect the personality. Also they are a definite handicap by virtue of the excessive weight and will prevent in engagement of sports and other activities. Often there is evidence of an inferiority complex. Self-consciousness and reluctance to meet social and business obligations are probably the most obvious characteristics.

There is difficulty in fitting clothes; the young girl is not able to wear the styles in clothing that are becoming to other girls. The brassiere must be specially made to fit properly; other garments must be made to order or altered when ready-to-wear apparel is purchased.

The weight of the breasts puts added strain upon the shoulders. There is difficulty in preventing the brassiere straps from pressing deeply into the skin. Backache, poor posture and kyphosis are complications which develop when the condition is permitted to persist.

The operative procedure is usually not recommended when only an improvement in personal appearance is sought but the conditions mentioned above often make it a necessary procedure.

The nurse should be kind, pleasant and tactful in her approach so that the confidence of the patient may be won as soon as possible. The routine of the ward should be explained. She should understand that various doctors routinely examine all patients in the hospital so that when she is examined she will not think she is subjected to curious gazes. It should be remembered that she is much more sensitive than the average patient.

Preparation for operation is similar to that for general anesthesia. The operative area should be prepared in the usual manner. Skin marking with brilliant green to outline the operative site is usually done by the surgeon the day before operation.

The operative region is dressed with a large pressure dressing. Drains, when used, are removed by the surgeon after the first twenty-four hours. Signs and symptoms of hemorrhage and infection should be reported to the surgeon. The patient is usually gotten out of bed the second or third day. Several large packages of sterile mechanic's waste are the only additional supplies necessary to do the first dressing. This is done about the fifth or sixth day unless drains have been inserted at the time of operation. The surgeon usually removes the sutures about the tenth day and the patient is discharged about the twelfth day. Before the patient leaves the hospital the nurse should make certain that she understands the type of brassieres to wear. The surgeon usually advises her to wear a good supportive brassiere day and night for six months. The brassieres should be made of tightly woven material such as nylon or fine broadcloth and double thickness of material used whenever extra support is necessary. The sleeping brassiere is made in the usual manner with the additional feature of lacings under the arm so that it may be adjusted when the patient is lying down. These brassieres should be specially made, and vary in price according to the different corsetières and the choice of material. Until the brassieres are made a properly applied elasticized bandage gives the necessary support. A member of the family should be instructed, along with the patient, in the application of the bandages before the patient is ready for discharge.

The mental state of the patient seems to improve greatly after the operation; she is happy that the procedure is completed and does not seem to be worried about meeting people. The adjustment to society seems to be fairly easy because she no longer feels that she appears a "freak" to others.

NURSING CARE IN PLASTIC SURGERY

The preoperative and postoperative nursing care of these patients involves all the same principles which have already been discussed in connection with the care of patients having other types of surgery. There are, however, certain additional features which need particular attention. These are: (1) the personality problem which nearly always is present in patients who are having plastic surgery; (2) the special care of the various kinds of grafts which are employed; and (3) special care necessitated by the special region of the body involved, as in operations about the mouth and neck. Plastic surgeons are often as much artists as scientists, and each will have his special preferences as to the details of care. For that reason, it seems more appropriate to outline here only the principles involved.

Before operation the nurse must spend sufficient time with the patient to gain insight into the patient's personality, his hopes and fears, and his way of reacting to stress. At the same time the nurse must start to orient the patient's thinking toward recovery and the assumption of an active place in the world about him. This can be of more value than a successful outcome to the operation. The nurse must learn to be unaffected by the most hideous deformities, so that the patient can realize that his appearance does not prevent him from enjoying ordinary or normal relationship with other human beings.

In the case of the patient who presents a long-term problem, perhaps necessitating multiple procedures during one long or several hospital admissions, it is well for the surgeon and nurse to develop a detailed plan for the care of the patient. This should include indoctrination of the patient and his family, suitable occupational or diversional therapy, as well as the plan for rehabilitation. As an example, the case of a patient who had sustained a serious destructive injury to the hand might be considered. At first, the problem of reassurance would be paramount. Next would be the problem of keeping up the morale of the patient while he was undergoing the multiple procedures needed to construct as useful a hand as possible. Finally, would come the job of re-training the patient so as to enable him to earn a living in a new way.

There are certain basic considerations applicable to the care of all grafts. Motion is undesirable since it prevents the graft from acquiring the new blood supply it needs. Infection is disastrous since bacteria can kill the cells of the graft. Bleeding is harmful for it may separate the graft from the recipient area. The surgeon may ask the nurse to observe the circulation in a flap or pedicle graft; if she sees blanching or cyanosis, the surgeon is to be notified at once.

Most plastic procedures are surface operations, so that the patient, if he has not lost too much blood, will not be sick. There will be no impairment of his respiratory, alimentary, or urinary tract functions. This is not the case following maxillo-facial surgery, and the special care needed in this field has been outlined on page 208.

SUMMARY

Plastic surgery is concerned with the repair of surface deformities, whether these be congenital, traumatic, due to disease, or due to procedures intended to cure disease. Most of the patients will have personality problems, and many will need extensive rehabilitation. Immobilization of wounds and grafts, the control of hemorrhage, and the avoidance of infection are of the utmost importance in this field.

VOCABULARY REVIEW

keloid   *rhinoplasty*   *mammaplasty*
Z-plasty   *dermatome*   *syndactylism*
pilonidal   *pedicle graft*
split-thickness graft *maxillo-facial*

SUGGESTED READING

1. Barsky, Arthur J.: Principles and Practices of Plastic Surgery. Baltimore, Williams and Wilkins, 1950.
2. Brown, J. B., Byars, L. T., and McDowell, F.: Preoperative and Postoperative Care in Reconstructive Surgery. Arch. Surg., *40:*1192–1210 (June) 1940.
3. Brown, J. B., and Cannon, B.: Repair of Major Facial Injuries. Ann. Surg., *126:*624–632 (October) 1947.
4. Brown, James Barrett, and McDowell, Frank: Skin Grafting. 2nd Ed. Philadelphia, J. B. Lippincott Co., 1949.
5. Christopher, Frederick: Textbook of Surgery. 5th Ed. Philadelphia, W. B. Saunders Co., 1949, pp. 1403–1438.
6. Krause, Marie V.: Nutrition and Diet Therapy. Philadelphia, W. B. Saunders Co., 1952, pp. 222–228.
7. Lewis, G. Kenneth: Early Care of Traumatized Hand with Pedunculated Flaps. Am. J. Surg., *79:*660–666 (May) 1950.
8. Pearlman, Louis M.: Plastic Surgery. Am. J. Nursing, *51:*618–620 (October) 1951.

CHAPTER 31

The Care of Burns

Perhaps no single agent has been more useful or longer known
to man than fire. No doubt human burns, an undesirable by-
product of this agent, have been observed and studied from man's
earliest times. As the twentieth century progresses, the problem
grows increasingly complex. While, on the one hand, there rises
a greater understanding of the pathologic physiology of human
burns, man's ingenuity, on the other hand, devises more and
more potent means of destroying himself.

Burns are wounds resulting from exposure to heat, chemicals,
electricity or radioactive agents. They can be classified as to degree on the basis of the amount of tissue damaged or destroyed.
This involves not only an estimate of the percentage of body surface which has been burned but also of the depth of destruction
of the involved tissue. An experienced observer can make such
an estimate with reasonable accuracy from the initial appearance
of the wounds. Determinations of this nature are important in
planning therapy and in making individual prognoses. For convenience burns are divided into first, second and third degree.
First degree burns are those in which exposure has been mild. On
inspection, they present only erythema of the skin. The injury is
confined to the most superficial layers of the epithelium which
may be cast off in the healing process. Mild sunburn and wind-
burn are of this type. Second degree burns are deeper and produce blister (*bleb*) formation, but elements of the epithelium
remain undamaged beneath the surface and are capable of
growth and regeneration of the integument in the healing
process. In third degree burns there is total destruction of the
skin and, occasionally, of the deeper structures, and charring of
the tissue occurs.

All degrees of burns may result from varying amounts of exposure to any one of the necrotizing agents, and in general, most
burned patients present areas involved in at least two and sometimes in all three degrees. In addition, they commonly have
wounds of other types such as fractures or lacerations. The
respiratory system may be involved through the inhalation of

smoke or through actual burning of the lining of the trachea and bronchial tree. These added injuries serve to complicate the treatment of any given individual and, of course, may add dangerously to the gravity of the overall picture. For the purpose of clarification discussions of therapy here will be confined solely to the burn itself. With the exception of burns resulting from contact with chemical agents in which case a wound caused by an acid may be neutralized by an appropriate alkaline substance, a description of the treatment of thermal burns suffices for all types. In general, it seems wise to divide therapy into three stages: the initial period, the supportive period, and the reconstructive period.

THE INITIAL PERIOD

An extensively burned individual presents simultaneously many problems. First of all, there is the wound itself. Burn wounds are occasionally relatively clean bacteriologically; one example is that which results from scalding. More often they are prone to be grossly contaminated by fragments of clothing, oil, grease, street dirt, or by well-intentioned, but harmful, home remedies. In addition to bacteria already at the site of such a wound further contamination may come from the hands and from the nasopharynx of anyone else in contact with the patient. Ideally, the first attention to these wounds should be administered by individuals who are masked, gowned and gloved, and who are operating under the most scrupulous sterile technic. The wounds are mechanically debrided and frequently may be rendered cleaner by repeated gentle irrigations with normal saline solution. The free use of soap and water or some other detergent to the wound is often helpful.

Closed Method. Once these preliminary preparations have been made, one must choose between two general methods of caring for the wound. The first and most popular is the so-called "closed method" in which the wound is encased in sterile dressings and completely excluded from its environment. For this purpose a thin layer of fine mesh gauze impregnated with petrolatum or some similar substance is applied to the wound. This is in turn covered by an abundance of absorptive gauze, perhaps with the addition of some substance similar to mechanic's waste. The whole is then enclosed in a firm binder designed to provide an elastic type of support and compressing the involved tissues within a bulky dressing. Elastic bandages serve this purpose well. The dressings must be applied rapidly but with great care, for they are meant to be left undisturbed for a week or more. Extremities are often splinted. Burned hands and fingers should always be supported securely in a neutral position. This type of therapy is excellent for the extremities, but for the trunk, face and abdomen it is apt to be less useful.

Open Method. The face, and especially the genitalia and perineum, adjacent as they are to bacteriologically contaminated body orifices, are almost impossible to dress satisfactorily. For them, and in the hands of some surgeons for all burns, the so-called "open method" of treatment has advantages. In the open method, following mechanical cleansing, an effort is made to produce an eschar to cover the wound and to act, in a sense, as a protective dressing. Many substances have been tried. Tannic acid alone or in combination with silver nitrate, gentian violet, triple dye, and others have all had their supporters. More recently, sprays of triethanolamine and similar agents have been employed. To these have been added solutions of antibiotics for local application. The newer of these substances have the advantage of producing a thin, pliable eschar which is transparent and through which the progress of the underlying burn wound can be observed. Patients treated by the open method must lie on sterile bed linen, must be protected from contact with bedclothing, and must be kept warm. It seems to the writer that a happy solution of the problem of which of the methods to use is to be guided by circumstances and to employ either or both in response to the demands of the extent, location and character of the injury.

Burn Shock. While the wound is receiving its inital care, simultaneous attention must be afforded to other aspects of the patient's condition. Measures to control pain must be instituted at once. This is accomplished usually with morphine or one of its derivatives. These can, and frequently should, be administered intravenously in order to secure a prompt response. The problem of pain control becomes much easier once dressings have been applied or a protective eschar produced. *Burn shock* must be considered from the first. The entire mechanism of this phenomena is not known, but there are certain basic phenomena in its production which are understood. In a burn there occurs an immediate outpouring of large quantities of serum from the cir-

culating blood into the injured tissues. The walls of the capillaries undergo changes which permit this diffusion of serum into
the tissues and out of the circulating blood. There is a corresponding reduction in blood volume, and the blood which still
does circulate becomes concentrated. In this state the blood
becomes thick and viscid with a preponderance of cellular elements in a reduced fluid medium. These changes occur regularly
in burn shock and produce restlessness, tachycardia, shallow respirations, apprehension and a falling blood pressure. The failure
to excrete urine in adequate amounts often presages death. In an
effort to combat and control this shock stage, those substances
which have been lost to the circulating blood must be replaced
by intravenous therapy. For this purpose, blood plasma or one
or another of its substitutes (plasma expanders) is used generally. The volume required over the course of the first day or
two in an extensive burn may be enormous. Elaborate formulas
have been devised to predetermine the plasma requirements.
These are based on an accurate estimate of the percentage of the
body surface which has been involved in the burn. Fluid requirements may also be ascertained by hourly hematocrit determinations, which measure the changing degree of hemoconcentration
and give indication of the desired rate of plasma administration.
The intravenous administration of saline and glucose solutions
is also indicated to a limited extent in severely burned patients,
although alone these solutions are of little value in combating
shock. Fluid requirements of this sort are best met by oral intake
on the part of the patient; this is usually possible. Occasionally,
in this initial stages of therapy whole blood transfusions are indicated and desirable, although for the most part, these are more
useful at a later stage when anemia develops.

Antibiotic Therapy. Efforts to combat infection must never be
neglected. These also are measures which should be instituted at
once. While some forms of therapy are based on the inclusion of
antibiotics in the wound dressing itself, a more effective program
appears to follow the oral or intramuscular route of administration. Tetanus antitoxin, or toxoid, is given.

Disaster Teams. It will be apparent that numerous demands
in therapy must be met simultaneously in treating these patients
in the initial stages of their injuries. To meet these demands and
to facilitate rapid, gentle and efficient care many institutions have
wisely formed "burn teams" specially trained for this work. In

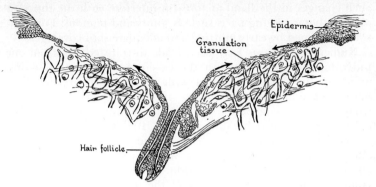

Figure 101. Regeneration of the epithelial surface of the skin after a severe burn.

the event of disaster such arrangements would be of inestimable value.

THE SUPPORTING PERIOD

This might be said to begin when the patient has survived the initial trauma and begins to recover from his injury. In this period, the wound may heal completely if it is first or light second degree in character. Second degree burns will usually manifest evidence of healing in a week or ten days. Epithelial islands rise from the depths of the skin (so-called *rete pegs*) and begin to proliferate across denuded areas. If the burn has not been too deep and if infection has destroyed additional tissue and thus interfered with the reparative process, this type of skin coverage may be entirely adequate. When the burn has been more extensive, approaching or actually third degree, skin grafting procedures become necessary. These are undertaken at the earliest possible time, often in seven to ten days, and may coincide with the first dressing of patients treated by the closed method. Of the available types of grafts, the best for this purpose are of the split thickness variety. Sheets of skin are cut, by means of a calibrated instrument (*dermatome*), from uninjured surfaces for transfer to the granulation tissue covering the burned surfaces. Delay and infection are responsible for excessive overgrowth of granulation tissue and for the development of large amounts of scar tisue. Scar deformities and constriction ensue.

Such changes in the hand or forearm interfere with the function of underlying moving parts such as joints and tendons. Function is best retained by early grafting and adequate skin coverage.

Numerous attempts have been made to transfer skin from one individual to another. With the exception of identical twins, in whom the method has met with success, such grafting procedures have always failed.

During this same period, the nutritional state of the patient must be maintained by adequate diet. It is usually felt that an intake ranging from 3000 to 3500 calories a day for the average adult is preferable to a greater intake which might result in anorexia, vomiting, and distention. Diets high in protein and vitamin content are desirable, and the oral route may be augmented by parenteral administration. Antibiotic therapy must be continued; organisms which may be resistant to those agents in use reappear, necessitating a change to another antibiotic. Fluid and electrolyte balance are watched to assure adequate urinary output without permitting edema to develop. Derangement of potassium balance, indicated by weakness, lassitude and characteristic electrocardiographic changes, occasionally necessitates the inclusion of potassium in parenteral therapy. This is also the stage in which anemia commonly appears, necessitating blood replacement by transfusion with whole blood or with washed red cells. Iron, liver and vitamin B_{12} may be utilized to hasten an individual's own hematopoietic response.

It is also in this period that the so-called "toxic state" is encountered. Here, probably because of widespread infection in an extensive burn wound and as a result of absorption of dead tissue, profound alterations may appear in the patient. Fever, tachycardia and asthenia are commonly encountered. Liver failure, sometimes associated with renal failure, is apt to prove fatal. Survival from the initial trauma may be followed by death in this second period, or this period of support may be drawn out for many months. In a sense, it extends up to the time when skin coverage of the wounds nears completion. Since homografting (from one individual to another) is not successful, the surgeon must use the patient himself as a skin donor. Ofttimes he is hard put to find sufficient and suitable sites from which skin is available for coverage. In these circumstances, partial coverage is afforded by "postage-stamp" grafts or by Davis grafts (small, deep grafts), depending on those isolated islands of skin to proliferate and coalesce. Many times warm sterile saline compresses or surgical removal of eschar or both are necessary to prepare denuded surfaces for grafting procedures.

RECOVERY PERIOD

The chain of events heretofore mentioned gradually merges into the final or *recovery period*. This is a time of convalescence and rehabilitation during which the survivors regain lost weight and strength and in which function is restored. Despite vigorous efforts aimed at their prevention, scar contractures may appear across joints, in the axilla, between the chin and thorax, and in similar locations. At this stage, the ingenuity of the plastic surgeon may be necessary to improve and correct these defects. In the instance of extensive facial burns, it may be necessary to construct portions of the nose, or of ears, or to build eyelids and eyebrows. A stenosed mouth may need opening, and lips may have to be constructed. Many of these reconstructive procedures are accomplished only through multistaged operations requiring great skill and patience on the part of both surgeon and patient. These patients may require untold aid to regain their morale before they can face the world and resume their occupations. The services of physiotherapists and occupational therapists are of importance in helping the crippled to overcome stiff finger joints or in learning to walk again. Occasionally, a severe third degree burn of a foot or leg may require amputation and necessitate the provision of a prosthesis.

Late Sequelae of Burns. Years after the trauma a burn scar may ulcerate, and the involved tissue may be found to have undergone malignant changes. This is particularly true of x-ray and radium burns. Many of the early workers in roentgenology, unaware of these dangers, fell victims to these often fatal lesions. The mechanism of metaplasia from a burn scar to epithelioma is poorly understood. It appears that the thin, scarred, and poorly nourished epithelium which regenerates to heal some burns is poorly equipped against stress, stretching, and pressure, and tends readily to break down and ulcerate. Such a process repeated over and over again is prone to become chronic, resistant to therapy, and finally malignant.

BURNS RESULTING FROM ATOMIC ENERGY

Exposure of even momentary duration to the enormous amount of heat and other forms of energy resulting from nuclear fission produces most devastating injuries. Human beings sufficiently close to an atomic explosion are lethally burned; those somewhat more remote may escape thermal burns of severity but suffer from the effects of radiant energy of shorter wavelengths. Needless to say, injuries of other varieties also occur, incident to the effect of the blast.

Specific means of therapy are lacking. In addition to the usual burn therapy, strenuous antibiotic therapy and transfusion of blood are used.

NURSING CARE OF BURNED PATIENTS

The nurse should be prepared to help the surgeon when a burned patient is admitted to the hospital by anticipating the need for morphine and supplying everyone in attendance with masks, gowns and gloves. The patient's clothing should be removed carefully, being cut wherever necessary. Rings should be removed; if edema prevents their removal they should be taken off with a ring cutter. Careful record of all fluids and treatments administered should be begun at once. After the surgeon has completed the initial dressing the patient should be placed in the kind of bed that will facilitate the best nursing care. For a severely burned patient a fracture bed, supplied with a sponge-rubber mattress, is useful, as it makes the handling of the patient and the use of the bedpan easier. All in attendance on the patient should wear masks.

Frequently there are delirium and incontinence of urine and feces. At times, when the thighs are burned or when he anticipates incontinence, the surgeon inserts an indwelling catheter to prevent soiling of the bandages and for the more accurate determination of the amount of the urinary output.

Fluids should be forced. The diet should be as high in caloric and vitamin content as the patient will tolerate.

The removal of the dressings is difficult when the burn is extensive and severe. A portable bathtub half filled with warm water or normal saline solution should be placed by the bed to provide for the immersion of the patient. In this way the dressings can be removed more quickly and with less pain.

It should be realized that it is often a healthy man, a busy housewife, or an active child who is burned. The burned patient is suddenly converted from an active individual into a bedridden one. He is fearful and emotionally upset. Since the process of healing is slow, various phases of mental depression are usually encountered. Winning his confidence and offering constant re-assurance will help to keep up his morale. Too many visitors should be guarded against; they must be prohibited if they seem to upset him. Whenever possible, and as quickly as possible, occupational therapy should be instituted. The problems of nursing care are usually solved more easily when the patient's morale is comparatively normal.

SUMMARY

A burn is a destructive wound of the skin, and sometimes of the deeper tissues, caused by heat, other forms of radiant energy, and chemicals. If more than a small portion of the body is involved, there are systemic effects of a serious nature. Large numbers of severely burned patients may be one result of a disaster; communities and their hospitals should be organized and prepared to meet such an emergency.

VOCABULARY REVIEW

hemoconcentration *contracture* *burn-shock*
eschar *blebs* *nuclear fission*

SUGGESTED READING

1. Curtis, Artz, et al: The Problem of Burns in Disaster. U. S. Armed Forces Med. Journal, *4*:39–48 (Jan.) 1953.
2. Cooper, Lenna F., and Barber, Edith M., and Mitchell, Helen S.: Nutrition in Health and Disease. Philadelphia, J. B. Lippincott Co., 1950, pp. 389–390.
3. Evans, Everett Idris: The Early Management of the Severely Burned Patient. Surg., Gynec. & Obst., *94*:273–282 (Mar.) 1952.
4. Morton, John H., Kingsley, Harry D., and Pearse; Herman E.: Studies on Flash Burns: The Protective Effects of Certain Fabrics. Surg., Gynec. & Obst., *94*:497–501 (March) 1952.
5. Peterson, Grace G.: A Method of Treating Burns. Am. J. Nursing, *50*:785–786 (December) 1950.
6. The Emergency Treatment of Burns. Am. J. Nursing, *53*:179–182 (Feb.) 1953. (Released by Federal Civil Defense Administration.)
7. Levenson, S. M., Davidson, C. S., Lund, C. C., and Taylor, F. H. L.: The Nutrition of Patients with Thermal Burns. Surg., Gynec. & Obst.. *80*:449–469 (May) 1945.

CHAPTER 32

Surgery of the Breast

Anatomy and Physiology. In order to understand the diseases of surgical interest associated with the breast it is necessary to consider briefly the normal development and physiologic changes which take place in this complex organ. The breast arises in the embryo from an epithelial thickening and bears a close relationship to sweat glands. Sexual differentiation, with stimulation to growth in the female, is accomplished in adolescence under hormonal influences. The gland rapidly achieves a high degree of specialization with pronounced physiologic variations which are responsible for many of the interesting clinical entities which are seen by the surgeon.

Grossly, the breast varies in appearance not only with sex but also in respect to age and in response to the general physiologic changes associated with puberty, menstruation, and pregnancy. Variations in position and number also occur as evidenced by the not infrequent appearance of supernumerary breasts (*polymastia*). Such accessory breasts may be found anywhere along the milk line, between the inguinal region and axilla, as in quadruped mammals. They occur as single or paired imperfect organs above or below the normal ones, and they are of no clinical significance except for the aberrant breast which sometimes appears in the axilla, where it seems especially prone to develop into carcinoma. Total absence of one or both breasts is of extreme rarity, although occasionally the nipple fails to develop or matures imperfectly. Deformities of the nipple (cleft, inverted or otherwise malformed) are significant only as they interfere with nursing.

The average breast is composed of fifteen or twenty lobes, each of which contributes a duct directed toward the nipple. These branching ducts terminate in numerous acini or glands, and the entire structure is imbedded in fat which is in turn supported by a framework of connective tissue. The nipple is a relatively tough, rubbery structure providing an exit for the major tubules formed by the confluence of the ducts arising from the lobules. Surrounding the nipple is the areola in which, as in the nipple, there is an abundance of erectile tissue. This tissue contributes to the erection of the nipple in response to the stimulation provided by the act of nursing.

The breast has a generous blood supply and is richly supplied with lymphatics, which ramify about the acini and ducts. The majority of the lymphatics drain toward the axilla along the pectoral fascia, but the upper and medial quadrants of the breast are drained along the perforating lymph vessels directly into the thorax. Other lymphatic pathways lead into the mediastinum and even cross the midline to communicate freely with those of the opposite breast. They are of extreme importance in the consideration of the proper surgical approach to carcinoma arising in the breast. It is through these channels that the malignant cells are disseminated at an early stage in the disease, and only by their radical removal together with that of the breast can there be a prospect of effecting a cure.

The breast is subject to functional change and aberration as much as any structure in the body as it responds to the hormonal stimulation secondary to puberty, menstruation and pregnancy. During adolescence the female breast grows in mass chiefly as the result of an increase in the fat and connective tissue components with slight change in the volume of the secreting mechanism. Before each menstruation a change occurs which is characterized in most women by discomfort and a sense of engorgement. There may even be a slight discharge from the nipple. These uncomfortable symptoms are the result of a temporary proliferation of epithelial components, both glandular and ductile, and they disappear with the progress of menstruation. With the onset of the menopause and the concurrent cessation of hormonal stimulation, the breast undergoes involution and atrophy.

In pregnancy the glandular elements of the organ hypertrophy in preparation for lactation. The hormone prolactin from the anterior pituitary is responsible for the production of milk following delivery. Involution of the breast takes place following the cessation of nursing, lactation ceases, and the breast again becomes subject to the changes associated with the menstrual cycle.

Aberrations from these normal functional changes form an interesting group of conditions. In this category falls the phenomenon of *witch's milk* which appears briefly in newborn infants whose breasts, under the influence of the maternal prolactin, secrete small amounts of milklike fluid. Milk may also appear briefly at puberty in either sex (*puberty mastitis*). In the male, enlargement of one or both breasts during and following puberty results in the condition known as *gynecomastia*. This enlargement often subsides spontaneously but may remain to constitute a source of embarrassment and discomfort. Surgical intervention is indicated only for cosmetic reasons. In the adolescent female the normal enlargement of the breasts may be abnormally continued to produce the so-called virginal hypertrophy. In this condition the breasts sometimes become extremely large and are uncomfortable, unwieldy and embarrassing. Severe cases are treated by the plastic surgeon (mammaplasty, page 365).

DISEASES OF THE BREAST

Diseases of the Nipple

When there are developmental defects with retraction, it is often possible during the period of lactation to draw out the nipple with a breast pump, although occasionally it may be necessary to resort to a plastic operation.

Most obstetricians direct their patients to prepare for lactation by massaging and oiling the nipples with the object of preventing maceration and cracking. Cleanliness and dryness must be maintained.

At times painful fissures follow maceration of the nipple by the mouth of the infant and provide a portal for the entrance of bacteria with resultant inflammatory disease of the breast itself. Once a fissure becomes established, the nipple may be protected in nursing by the use of a shield. The local application of bland ointments or of compound tincture of benzoin protects the breast and promotes healing.

Tumors of the nipple are rare, although occasionally the surgeon encounters a fibroepithelial growth. These are usually pedunculated; they are benign and are cured by local excision.

Paget's Disease of the Nipple. This is a carcinoma arising from the squamous epithelial cells of the nipple; it usually appears in the fourth and fifth decades of life and is rarely seen in younger women. It begins as an eczematous lesion involving the nipple, the areola, and subsequently the cutaneous surface of the breast. The tissues are moist, retracted and raw, and bleed easily. Extension to the axillary lymph nodes of this epidermoid type of carcinoma follows in due course. Adequate treatment demands radical removal of the breast, pectoral muscles and axillary contents. The prognosis is somewhat better than in carcinoma arising within the breast itself.

Diseases Caused by Trauma

Hemorrhage into the subcutaneous tissues or into the glandular substance may result from blows upon or penetrating wounds of the breast and is sometimes differentiated from true neoplasms with difficulty. The history and the appearance of superficial ecchymosis are helpful in the diagnosis.

In traumatic fat necrosis the differentiation from carcinoma can frequently be made only after microscopic study of the involved tissue. This lesion may present the same firm, painless mass with overlying skin retraction seen in malignancy. Diagnosis is further complicated by the fact that many women who have possible cancer of the breast will recall some antecedent injury.

Wounds of the breast usually offer no special problem unless the patient is lactating, in which case a fistula may occur and fail to close until lactation is terminated. The scar of a healed penetrating wound sometimes obstructs a duct; the result of this is a retention cyst. Under these circumstances, should lactation occur, a milk cyst (*galactocele*) may form.

Inflammatory Diseases

These are usually associated with pregnancy and lactation.

Mastitis. So-called "caking" is a painful condition where obstruction in the ducts interferes with drainage of the secreting glandular tissue. Swelling and engorgement appear in the affected portion of the breast, accompanied by an elevation in temperature.

The symptoms subside with the reestablishment of drainage through the duct system. However, should bacteria gain entrance to such a lesion through a wounded nipple, acute mastitis with abscess formation may result. Most acute suppurative lesions of the breast are due to Staphylococcus aureus, and many can be successfully treated in the early stages by the administration of sulfonamides or penicillin. Unless the therapeutic response is prompt and complete, it is usually necessary to terminate lactation. Abscesses lying deep within the substance of the gland tend to spread to adjacent lobules and to coalesce, with extensive destruction of the mammary tissue. Surgical drainage is often necessary when conservative measures fail. In such instances incisions into the breast should be made in a radial direction in order to avoid unnecessary severance of uninvolved duct structures.

Mastitis is occasionally seen in adolescent girls and young adult women who have acute infectious parotitis (*mumps*). The resultant inflammation and tenderness, like that seen in the ovary or testis, subside spontaneously but may leave the breast atrophic and crippled.

Chronic Suppurative Mastitis. This is at times the sequal to acute mastitis when the causative organism is of low virulence. Recurring episodes of a mild inflammatory nature mark the course of this disease and are more prone to appear during menstruation. The administration of antibiotics together with hygienic measures often suffices for treatment, although open drainage may have to be resorted to.

Tuberculous Mastitis. This is a rare disease. A tuberculous focus elsewhere in the body finds opportunity for dissemination in the actively lactating breast. Such a spread takes place through the lymphatics or through the blood stream to produce a diffuse process in the breast. Numerous cold abscesses appear and there is rarely invasion of the axillary glands. Removal of the breast may be necessary to bring about a cure.

Cystic Disease of the Breast

Retention Cyst; Galactocele. This may manifest itself in any one of several ways. The simplest of these is the retention cyst (p. 381) where material dams up behind an obstruction in a duct. A galactocele resembles this condition except that there the cyst is distended by milk. Each of these conditions is treated by simple excision of the cyst.

Chronic Cystic Mastitis. This disease is frequently encountered in women at or near the menopause, when the breasts are undergoing the involution characteristic of this stage of life, or in women in whom there is an endocrine imbalance. In general, there is an increase in the fibrous elements of the gland and atrophy of the secretory elements, and irregularities in these processes produce a wide variety of pathologic changes. Cysts of varying sizes form behind obstructed ducts or arise as the result of degeneration of glandular components. Overgrowth is not necessarily confined to the fibrous tissue stroma but occurs as well in the epithelial structure. Occasionally a cyst grows to considerable size and is referred to as a *blue dome cyst*. The result of these changes is the production of a "shotty" or "cobblestone" breast which is often tender and painful. Women with this disease are apt to complain of unusual premenstrual hypertrophy and engorgement. As a rule the progress of the disease is slow. Usually both breasts become involved.

Diagnosis. The differential diagnosis between chronic cystic mastitis and carcinoma is at times exceedingly difficult. There is statistical reason for believing that carcinoma arises slightly more often in the breast which is the seat of chronic cystic disease, and certainly, when cancer appears, its early recognition is rendered more difficult by the presence of the preexisting benign changes. The patient suffering from chronic cystic disease of the breast should submit herself for frequent examination by a competent surgeon who, in the event of the appearance of suspicious changes, should have no hesitancy in resorting to biopsy to determine beyond question the presence or absence of malignancy. In the milder forms of the disease, patients may be made comfortable by wearing a firmly supporting brassiere. Occasionally simple excision of the entire breast in older women is the procedure of choice.

Neoplastic Diseases of the Breast

The classification of tumors of the breast into benign and malignant types affords the best basis for their study and for decision as to correct treatment. New growths arise from any type of tissue found in the organ. Benign tumors are treated by local surgical excision, malignant tumors by extensive and radical operations which may be preceded or followed by deep x-ray therapy.

BENIGN TUMORS

Adenofibroma. The commonest of the benign tumors is adenofibroma (fibro-adenoma, periductile fibroma, intracanalicular fibroma) which is seen most often in young women. This is usually a solitary, firm, elastic, freely movable mass which is not tender. It grows slowly and occasionally becomes partly cystic through degeneration. Local excision is the accepted treatment.

Papillary Cystadenoma. This is a tumor encountered only occasionally. It appears when the breast is functioning. Grossly it is composed of a branching papilla growing out into a duct from a highly vascular base or stalk. The whole is encapsulated and originally benign. Attention is drawn to this lesion primarily by the discharge of blood or serosanguineous fluid from the nipple. At this stage delicate local excision with every effort to preserve intact adjacent ducts will suffice. Later, if untreated, the tumor may become malignant, assuming the clinical characteristics of adenocarcinoma. Occasionally the surgeon fails to locate the source of the bleeding when these tumors are too small to palpate or are less superficially located than is the rule. Under these circumstances simple mastectomy is justifiable in consideration of the malignant potentialities of the growth.

CARCINOMA OF THE BREAST

Carcinoma of the breast is the second most common malignant tumor in the female, only cancer of the uterus exceeding it in frequency. Most carcinomas appear in the fifth and sixth decades of life, although many are seen much earlier; occasionally such a tumor is encountered in women in the early twenties. It develops also in the male. Women who have borne and nursed children seem somewhat more prone to malignant disease, yet sterility does not preclude malignancy.

Symptoms. These tumors appear insidiously and often grow to large size before they are noticed. Perhaps a blow on the breast calls attention to a growth, or it may be found in bathing or as an incidental discovery during general physical examination by a physician. These growths are neither painful nor tender. They are hard and blend with the surrounding tissue.

Diagnosis. Of great diagnostic significance is the flattening and fixation of the overlying skin which results from lymphatic infiltration by cancer cells. Superficially placed tumors may produce a small but visible dimple. In later stages of the disease the axillary lymph nodes are invaded and are palpable as hard, nontender nodules. Extensive axillary lymphatic involvement obstructs the normal drainage from the upper extremity and produces brawny elephantiasis of the arm. Some tumors grow as a large, superficial mass; others, of the scirrhous variety, cause irregular retraction of the breast tissue which appears to shrink en masse against the thoracic wall. When the skin is invaded by the extension of the growth, it may assume the pitted appearance of orange peel (*peau d'orange*); or tiny nodules encircle the lesion and spread extensively, even to the other breast (*lenticular carcinoma, carcinoma en cuirasse*); or the skin may slough and ulcerate to present the bleeding, foul, secondarily infected surface of the tumor itself. Diagnosis is easy in the late and unfavorable stage, but is more difficult when the tumor is young and curable.

Self-examination. In recent years an effort has been made to disseminate among lay people information about cancer which is designed to familiarize them with the presenting symptoms of the disease in various organs. With respect to the breast, women are urged to partake in a *program of self-examination*. This consists of a monthly inspection. The breasts should be examined first by looking in a mirror for dimples, swellings, depressions, retraction of the nipple, and so on. Such alterations frequently are best demonstrated by raising and lowering the arms. The woman then lies upon her back and carefully and gently palpates the breast on each side with the opposite hand. In this way, an intelligent and observant woman may discover an abnormality at a very early stage. Then is the time to consult the surgeon for confirmation of the finding. The author makes it a practice to biopsy all breast tumors and to submit the tissue to the pathologist for examination. Such a schedule leaves no margin for error in diagnosis.

Prognosis. The prognosis is determined by the degree of malignancy of the tumor, by the extent of the tumor when operation is undertaken, and by the thoroughness of the operation. Statistics vary, but in general only 30 per cent of patients operated upon for cancer of the breast survive five years or longer. In the cases of patients having tumors of low malignancy and without extension to the axilla, however, more than three fourths can be permanently cured. The neglected patients, upon whom operation is performed late in the disease, rarely survive, despite the most painstaking radical surgery.

Modern efforts toward the prevention and cure of cancer by the wide dissemination of information to laymen are worthy of wholehearted support. Success in the cure of cancer is directly proportional to the early recognition and treatment of the disease. This is nowhere more true than in carcinoma of the breast.

RADICAL MASTECTOMY

The key to successful treatment of cancer of the breast lies in early and thoroughly radical removal. Such surgery is based on anatomic considerations with particular regard to the lymphatic pathways through which the cancer spreads. The skin is widely excised over the breast without regard to subsequent closure of the wound. The breast, pectoral muscles, and axillary lymph nodes and fat are removed en bloc. A skin graft may be required

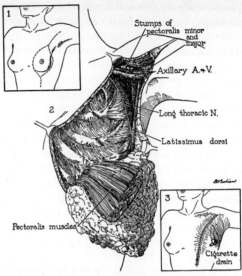

FIGURE 102. Radical mastectomy. *1*, Line of incision; *2*, the breast, pectoral muscles, and axillary nodes are almost completely removed; *3*, closure of wound.

to cover the central portion of the defect on the thoracic wall which results from wide excision of skin. The loss of function of the arm following operation is relatively slight and unimportant.

RADIATION THERAPY

Radiation therapy may temporarily heal and hold in abeyance an ulcerated growth. In some clinics it is felt that radiation therapy should be given preoperatively to help control the spread of the disease; elsewhere it is used postoperatively in an effort to kill any malignant cells disseminated during the operation or already lying beyond the limits of surgical removal. Still other surgeons feel that it is of little if any benefit and rely with some justification on radical mastectomy alone.

HORMONES AND BREAST CANCER

The relationship between ovarian activity and breast cancer has long been recognized. It has been known, for example, that cancer arising in the breast of a pregnant woman or in one who is lactating is apt to assume greater virulence than under normal circumstances, growing more rapidly and metastasizing at a faster rate. In fact, many surgeons consider such tumors inoperable.

In the treatment of metastatic spread from cancer of the breast, hormone therapy appears definitely to have a place. Never is it curative, but there is little doubt but that for a time, at least, it will arrest the growth of metastatic lesions. For this purpose the male sex hormone, testosterone, is employable and seems most helpful in bone metastases. Some investigators feel that diethylstilbestrol is more beneficial in soft tissue metastases. When testosterone is used, the voice may deepen and hair may appear excessively on the face and body, demonstrating the masculinizing potentialities of the drug. Patients receiving testosterone should be informed of these effects. Hormone therapy may be so effective as to permit pathologic fractures (at the site of a metastasis) to heal, and is often very helpful in relieving the pain associated with bone involvement.

METASTASES

Breast cancer metastasizes commonly to the brain, to the skeleton, the lung and pleura and, of course, to skin, regional lymph glands and to the opposite breast. Prior to undertaking radical surgery in the form of mastectomy, it is always our routine to secure an x-ray examination of the lungs and thoracic skeleton. Complaints of back pain draw attention to the vertebral bodies which may be involved. Needless to say, the demonstration of remote metastases precludes radical mastectomy. The careful examiner quizzes his patient in regard to metastatic involvement and eliminates the possibility of extension of the tumor before submitting a patient to operation.

NURSING CARE

There has been an increasing knowledge among the public about tumors of the breast. Through the efforts of the National Cancer Institute, The American Cancer Society, the radio, television and press, women are learning that the hope of cure lies in early recognition of the tumor followed by accurate diagnosis and adequate treatment. Women are being urged to examine themselves once monthly, at the end of the menstrual cycle, to discover any tumor in its earliest stage of growth. Fortunately, more women are now seeking treatment earlier and there is beginning to be a slight decline in the mortality rate in some areas.

It is sad that the discovery of a lump in the breast brings such terror to many women that early diagnosis and treatment is delayed. The fear of mutilation and death seems to underly their thoughts about cancer. Healthy women who have had radical mastectomies rarely tell anyone about them. The patients with lingering, hopeless conditions, where the tumor has caused ulceration with subsequent foul odor and pain from metastatic lesions, are well known.

Much has been done to educate the people in a positive way by stressing that women following radical mastectomy may lead an active life; limitation of activity need not follow the operation and a prosthetic appliance will allow clothes to fit as naturally as before operation. Whether the patient has been told that she almost certainly has a benign tumor or that she will probably have her breast removed the nurse may assume that she has been worried and concerned since the time the tumor was discovered. Apprehension, despair and resentment are usually not expressed because of the fear of rejection. Warmth, understanding and reassurance are supportive needs which the nurse can give this patient, especially at the time of admission. Treating her as a guest, making her comfortable and giving her opportunities to ask questions about anything she does not understand are essential to prevent further anxiety. Too often, the busy and impersonal environment adds to the fears of the patient.

Preoperatively, the patient should be shaved as shown in Figure 30, page 72, and prepared for general anesthesia.

When the tumor has been proved to be benign, a small dressing will be placed over the incision. Careful attention is given to the vital signs of the patient as after any surgery. The patient is usually discharged from the hospital the following day. She is given instructions to return to her surgeon for removal of the sutures, and to keep the dressing dry.

Following radical mastectomy, general supportive care is indicated. In addition, elevation of the arm, on the operative side, on pillows provides comfort and helps prevent edema. Most surgeons place a drain in a stab wound in the axilla to permit the escape of serum which accumulates beneath the extensive skin flaps. The dressings are usually large and tight in order to press the skin flaps tightly against the underlying thoracic wall until the healing process is well begun. The dressings should be inspected frequently at the back of the axilla to detect bleeding or excessive drainage. Inspection, at least every fifteen minutes, should be made for the first few hours after operation. When oozing occurs, the size and color of the stain should be noted; if it increases it should again be reported to the surgeon. Turning is difficult, and the position on the side opposite the wound is uncomfortable unless the shoulder, back and arm are supported by pillows. When a skin graft has been applied, the large pressure dressings will usually prevent it from slipping, but care must be taken that undue movement of the dressing be prevented until such time as circulation into the graft is well established. The skin graft is usually taken from the thigh; a tight bandage will be in place and is left undisturbed for about two weeks; after this interval, the area will be healed. The initial dressing of the breast area may be done on the fifth or sixth day at which time the drain is usually removed, together with the sutures.

The day after operation the surgeon encourages the patient to use her arm. A convenient and simple scheme which insures early and satisfactory function is to persuade the patient to comb her hair. Patients who have had radical mastectomy may get out of bed the day after operation. Encouraging the patient to cough and breathe deeply is essential to prevent chest complications. A diet as tolerated is usually ordered; the importance of adequate protein should be emphasized.

During the convalescent period emotional support should be given. Nearly all patients become depressed although, in most, this is brief and mild. Frequently they sleep poorly because they have dreams concerned with mutilation and loss of bodily function which frighten them. An attentive family is most essential to buoy up the spirits; if they can make the patient feel they love her and accept her she will adapt herself with greater ease. The nurse should encourage the family to show added attention since it is they who are most important in helping the patient to adapt to her former area of living.

The nurse should also find out what the patient knows about prosthetic appliances. If she is unfamiliar with them, there should be samples available to show her. A strong interest on the part of the nurse will usually bring forth many questions. Sometimes the surgeon recommends the type of appliance to be used; if not, he should always be informed about the patient's questions, to permit him to clarify any answers providing guidance to the patient and nurse. It is best when the patient can decide what she wishes to do about this aspect. The nurse's best function is to inform her. The nurse should also find out what her patient knows about breast self-examination during convalescent care; if she does not know, then she should be taught according to the plan of the surgeon, unless such practice is already accepted throughout the hospital.

Before discharge, the nurse makes certain the patient knows when to return to the surgeon.

SUMMARY

Until better means become available, the early diagnosis of and the radical operation for cancer of the breast are the best treatment for this common disease of women. Education of the public and general use of regular self-examination have already improved the cure rate and can accomplish even more. Radiation and hormone therapy also have important uses. Many lumps in the breast are not cancer, but only examination of the tissue under the microscope can make diagnosis certain.

VOCABULARY REVIEW

polymastia	*galactocele*	*mastectomy*
gynecomastia	*mastitis*	*testosterone*

SUGGESTED READING

1. A Cancer Source Book for Nurses. New York, Am. Cancer Soc., Inc., 1950, pp. 59–63.
2. Cancer Nursing. National Cancer Institute and New York State Dept. of Health, 1950.
3. Current Status of Hormone Therapy of Advanced Mammary Cancer. Council on Pharmacy and Chemistry. J.A.M.A. *146:*471–476 (June 2) 1951.
4. Newton, Michael, and Newton, Niles Rumely: Breast Abscess, A Result of Lactation Failure. Surg., Gynec. & Obst., *91:*651–655 (December) 1950.
5. Rusch, H., and Baumann, C.: Nutritional Aspects of Cancer Problems. Nutritional Review, *4:*353, 1946.
6. Smith, Genevieve W.: When a Breast Must Be Removed. Am. J. Nursing, *50:*335–339 (June) 1950.
7. Sugarbaker, Everett D., and Wilfley, Lucy E.: Cancer of the Breast. Am. J. Nursing, *50:*332–335 (June) 1950.
8. Self-Examination of the Breasts. Am. J. Nursing, *52:*441 (April) 1952.

Unit VII. DISEASES DUE TO ALLERGY

CHAPTER 33

The Role of
Surgery in Allergic Disease

Allergy has been defined as a condition of unusual or exaggerated specific susceptibility to a substance which is harmless in similar amounts for the majority of people.[1] Hay fever, hives, and asthma are some of the more common manifestations of allergy. Other less common allergic reactions include headache, circulatory collapse (*anaphylaxis*), gastrointestinal disturbances, and a variety of skin eruptions. No successful direct attack upon allergy has been made by surgery, nor is it likely that surgery will ever have a part in the direct treatment of this condition, since the allergic reaction seems to be a property of the cells of the body. Surgery is often useful, however, in attacking the causative agent of the allergy (*allergen*). Thus, the eradication of chronic bacterial infection in the paranasal sinuses is beneficial in many cases of bronchial asthma.

[1] See Brown, pages 619–637.

Anticipating Sensitivity. The surgeon, on the other hand, is often forced to deal with allergies in patients who have some other disease as well. There are persons who are hypersensitive to morphine, or to iodine, or to some other substance which the surgeon ordinarily uses in treating his patients. Again and again the value of careful history-taking is demonstrated, as the untoward effects of an allergy may usually be prevented if the surgeon is forewarned. Certain of the medicaments that a surgeon commonly uses produce hypersensitivity, or cause severe allergic reaction in previously sensitized persons; tetanus antitoxin is one of these, its ill effect being due to the horse serum from which it is prepared; penicillin is another. Patients in whom these or similar substances are to be injected should first have a skin test to determine the degree of sensitivity so that proper precautions may be taken. Epinephrine must be readily available in case serious symptoms should develop.

It is indeed fortunate that cortisone has proven so beneficial in alleviating the manifestations of serious allergic reactions.

Unit VIII. SURGERY OF THE ENDOCRINE GLANDS

THE ENDOCRINE glands of the body are the pituitary, the thyroid, the parathyroids, the thymus, the islet tissue of the pancreas, the adrenals, and the gonads (the testes in males, the ovaries in females).[1] The secretions (*hormones*) elaborated by these glands exert a powerful influence on every phase of the growth and activity of the individual, and there is a highly complicated interrelationship between the different glands. Some of these glands elaborate more than one hormone, each having a different action upon the rest of the body. Much is now known concerning the chemical structure and the nature of the action of many hormones, but there is still a great deal to be learned, particularly as to the regulatory effect of certain of the hormones upon the production or action of other hormones.

Surgery is employed in the treatment of diseases of endocrine origin, the so-called endocrinopathies, to remove overactive glands, wholly or in part, and to attempt compensation for or replacement of deficient glands. As yet the transplantation of glandular tissue from another person or from an animal has not been satisfactory, but it has been found possible to achieve much success by the implantation of slowly absorbed pellets of the active chemical principles of the hormones of some glands. In addition to this direct application of surgery to endocrinopathies, the surgeon is frequently confronted by the occurrence of all the ordinary surgical problems in patients who have also an endocrine derangement. Then, too, an endocrine derangement may be the accidental or resultant complication of a surgical procedure.

[1] See Brown, pages 638–713.

CHAPTER 34

Surgery of the Thyroid and Parathyroid Glands

THE THYROID

Anatomy and Physiology. The thyroid gland is a butterfly-shaped organ which lies in the lower part of the neck astride the trachea. There are two lateral lobes, one on each side of the trachea, which are connected by a narrow strip of thyroid tissue, the isthmus. The blood supply of the gland is rich. On the inferior surface of the thyroid lobes are the parathyroid glands, and between the inferior medial surface of the lateral lobe and the trachea on each side is located the important recurrent laryngeal nerve. Because this nerve supplies the muscles which control the vocal cords, injury to it interferes seriously with speech and proper respiration. Weakness or paralysis of the muscles permits the vocal cord to flap loosely in the lumen of the larynx.

The thyroid is one of the endocrine or ductless glands, so called because they secrete directly into the circulating blood. The secretions of endocrine glands are known as hormones. The chemical structure of the thyroid hormone, thyroxin, is well known; one of its elements is iodine. Thyroxin has a regulating effect upon the metabolism of the body. An increase in the amount of thyroxin, whether caused by disease of the thyroid gland or by therapeutic administration of the hormone, results in a speed-up of metabolism; this produces a faster breakdown of the body tissues which results in the need for more food. If the thyroid gland produces less than the normal amount of thyroxin, there is a slowing down of metabolism, usually manifested by lack of energy, diminution of activity, and gain in weight.

Basal Metabolism Test. It is important to be able to measure the rate of metabolism of the patient and a convenient test has been devised. In order to obtain the energy necessary to carry on the activities of living, the cells of the body use up protein, fat, and carbohydrate. Much of this process of utilization consists in oxidation reactions which make use of the oxygen derived from

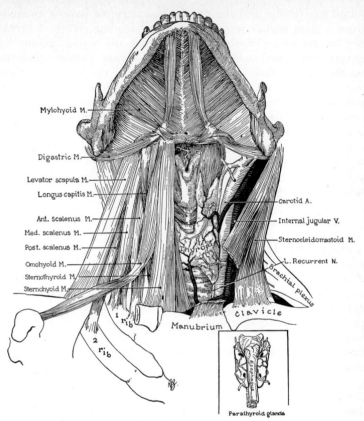

FIGURE 103. Anatomy of neck, showing relationship of thyroid to the other important structures of the neck. Insert shows the posterior aspect of the gland and the usual location of the parathyroids.

inspired air. The rate, therefore, at which metabolism proceeds can be estimated from the rate of oxygen consumption. The test is carried out by having the patient breathe for a period of time into a closed system containing a measured amount of oxygen; provision is also made in the apparatus for absorbing the exhaled carbon dioxide. The amount of oxygen consumed varies, naturally, with the activity of the patient during the test; for this reason an attempt is made to perform the test under standard conditions of minimal activity, so that the metabolism will be at the lowest rate which is normal for that patient, or basal. It has been found practicable to make the test just after the patient awakens from a good night's rest, before permitting the eating of breakfast or any other physical activity. Since the actual amount of oxygen consumed will be greater in larger persons than in smaller, tables have been made which show the average oxygen consumption under basal conditions of large numbers of individuals according to height and weight. If the patient being tested consumes the same amount of oxygen as the average normal of his size, his basal metabolic rate (B.M.R.) is reported as 0; if he consumes more oxygen than the normal average the B.M.R. is reported plus, and if less, minus. Values from $+10$ to -10 are considered within the range of normal variation and are not taken to be evidence of disease.

Disturbances of the Thyroid
THYROID DEFICIENCY

Myxedema. In adults, insufficient secretion of thyroxin produces a condition called adult myxedema. In childhood the condition is known as juvenile myxedema. It may occur spontaneously, or as a result of the removal of too much of the thyroid. Myxedema is characterized by increased deposition of fat and thickening of the subcutaneous tissue, most noticeable in the face. The voice becomes coarse. There is a loss of mental alertness and the patients seem dull. The B.M.R. is low, -15 or lower. The treatment of this condition is to make up the deficiency in thyroxin, which is done by giving small daily doses of thyroid extract. If the condition has not progressed too far, treatment brings about great improvement; therapy must be continued permanently, however.

Cretinism. In infants a congenital deficiency of thyroid hormone causes cretinism. Endemic cretinism is common in endemic goiter regions; the incidence of sporadic cretinism is not known, although it is rare in North America. There is a permanent mental deficiency in these children which is not amenable to treatment with thyroid, and there is a characteristic appearance as a result of growth abnormalities in the formative years. In addition, the signs and symptoms of myxedema are present.

GOITER

The term goiter means an enlargement of the thyroid gland. There are several varieties of goiter.

Colloid Goiter. This generalized enlargement of the entire gland usually occurs during adolescence and is more frequent in females than in males. It is the result of a deficiency of iodine in the diet, and in parts of the world where the amount of iodine in the drinking water and diet is insufficient, such as mountainous regions and the Great Lakes Basin, colloid goiter occurs with frequency. The metabolism is generally normal or slightly reduced.

Prevention and Treatment. Fortunately these goiters can generally be prevented by the addition of minute amounts of iodine to the diet, most conveniently carried out by the use of iodized table salt. The administration of iodine is seldom effective after the colloid goiter has developed, although sometimes a small dose of thyroid extract is helpful in reducing the size of the goiter. Surgical removal of the goiter is advisable for cosmetic reasons and because continued enlargement may cause pressure upon the trachea and esophagus, with resultant interference with breathing and swallowing.

Nodular Goiter. This condition is most prevalent in those geographic regions where colloid goiter is common. Irregular enlargement of part of the thyroid gland generally appears early in adult life, but may be first noticed at any age. The condition is usually progressive and the enlargement may become tremendous. Frequently the tumors compress the trachea and embarrass respiration. The goiter sometimes extends down into the thorax; this extension can best be determined by an x-ray of the chest, which should be taken in all cases of goiter. Microscopic examination of the glandular tissue shows areas of degeneration, hemorrhage, and cyst formation, with a varying amount of chronic inflammation or nonspecific thyroiditis. These goiters can be distinguished from true adenoma of the thyroid.

Treatment. The treatment is surgical removal, and this is the only method offering permanent relief. Hyperthyroidism occasionally occurs in association with nodular goiter; for this reason a basal metabolism test should always be made before undertaking operation. The treatment of nodular goiter with hyperthyroidism is essentially the same as the treatment for exophthalmic goiter.

Exophthalmic Goiter. Also known as primary hyperthyroidism and Graves' disease, this is a serious systemic disturbance. The thyroid gland is enlarged, but less so than in the colloid and adenomatous types of goiter. The enlargement is generally symmetrical, and in itself causes no symptoms. The fundamental manifestation of this disease is the production of an increased

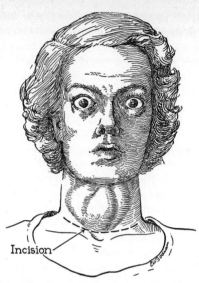

FIGURE 104. Exophthalmic goiter. Dotted line indicates location of incision for thyroidectomy.

amount of the thyroid hormone, which results in a speeding up of metabolism. Microscopic examination of the thyroid tissue shows evidence of increased activity of the cells of the gland. This disease occurs more frequently in women, generally in early adult life, but it may occur in children or in older persons.

Symptoms. Patients with hyperthyroidism complain of nervousness, trembling, increased sweating, loss of weight, increased appetite, and easy fatigability. Often they or their relatives notice a prominence of the eyes. Palpitation of the heart is a frequent complaint. In the more severe cases there may be nausea, vomiting and diarrhea.

Diagnosis. On examination the patients are found to be alert and highstrung; they are easily upset and are given to fits of anger or crying. There is evidence of considerable loss of weight. There is a pronounced trembling of the hands. The moderate diffuse enlargement of the gland is easily felt. One of the most striking signs of the disease is the exophthalmos or prominence of the eyes, which may be so great that the lids will not meet. In extreme cases of exophthalmos operative procedures upon the lids or the orbit may be necessary to save vision. Fortunately this is an uncommon complication, and the exophthalmos often **regresses** partially after the hyperthyroidism has been cured. The pulse rate is increased proportionally to the severity of the disease. The B.M.R. is always elevated and in extreme cases may be as high as +100; in moderately severe cases it ranges from +30 to +50.

Treatment. Primary hyperthyroidism is a progressive disease which usually leads to heart failure and death if not treated. Since the disease is characterized by regressions and exacerbations a temporary improvement must not be regarded as evidence of a cure.

There are several related drugs which may be used to control the manifestations of hyperthyroidism. The most widely used of these is propylthiouracil. The administration of this drug over a period of weeks or months will usually produce a complete re-mission of the disease. In fact, in a large proportion of patients, this method of treatment appears to bring about a permanent cure; since this drug has only been in use for a few years, it is not certain yet that the cures are actually permanent. Many patients, however, develop a relapse after discontinuing the drug, but it will again be effective when taken. In a very small number of pa-tients propylthiouracil is toxic to the bone marrow and results in leukopenia; obviously, it is not safe to use without regular ex-amination of the blood of each patient who is taking it. Although surgical removal of thyroid tissue has been considered during the past half century the proper treatment of exophthalmic goiter, there is now available this medical means of treating the condi-tion. It seems probable that, in the future, fewer patients with this disease will be operated upon. At present, surgical treatment is indicated for those patients who do not secure permanent re-mission after adequate medical therapy, for those who cannot tolerate the drug, for those who do not have adequate medical facilities at hand, and for those who prefer not to take the medicine.

The administration of iodine has a beneficial but temporary effect upon hyperthyroidism. Prior to the introduction of propyl-thiouracil, this was the drug of choice in preparing the patient for surgery. At the present time both propylthiouracil and iodine are used in the preoperative preparation of the hyperthyroid patient. The patient is usually given propylthiouracil until the metabolism returns to approximately normal. Following this, iodine is given for a period of about ten days or two weeks. This brings about a marked decrease in the size of the thyroid gland, decreases the blood supply and thus makes the operation less difficult. The preoperative treatment can usually be carried out on an ambulatory basis with the patient getting as much rest as possible. Whether or not the patient discontinues work during this period of treatment would depend on the severity of the disease and the type of work that was being done. A mild sedative is often useful in the treatment of hyperthyroidism. The patient should stop smoking and should avoid the use of caffeine. Because of the weight loss and the increased metabolism a diet of 4000 to 5000 calories, chiefly carbohydrates, should be given. The patient should be encouraged to take as much rest as possible.

Following adequate preoperative preparation, surgical removal of most of the thyroid gland is performed; cure of hyperthyroidism thus results from reduction in the amount of thyroxin which can be produced.

Adenoma of the Thyroid. There is a rather common tumor of the thyroid which is best called a fetal adenoma. This is not to be confused with nodular goiter. Fetal adenoma is a true tumor and is surrounded by a capsule which separates it from the remainder of the thyroid tissues. It presents as a small round nodule in the gland, which is easily palpable, and varies in size from that of a small marble to a golf ball or larger. These tumors are usually solitary, but finding more than one is not rare. Fetal adenomas have a definite tendency to undergo malignant degeneration, and about 10 per cent will in time become cancerous. This is an additional reason for the immediate removal of a thyroid nodule. It is often impossible to distinguish a small nodule of a nodular goiter or a small cyst from a fetal adenoma; therefore it is recommended that all solitary nodules of the thyroid be removed as soon as discovered.

Carcinoma of the Thyroid. Several types of carcinoma are seen in the thyroid gland, but sarcoma is rarely seen. In early carcinoma of the thyroid, when the disease appears limited to one side of the neck, total removal of the thyroid on that side, together with radical resection of the cervical lymph nodes and jugular vein of the same side, is the proper therapy. In instances of extensive malignant disease of the thyroid, cure cannot be expected from surgery; radiation therapy offers the best hope of palliation.

Thyroiditis. Because it results in firm enlargement of the gland, inflammation of the thyroid gland may be confused with carcinoma or other goiters. There are two chief varieties of this condition, Hashimoto's and Riedel's struma, but nothing is known of their causes. Often pain, tenderness, and fever occur, serving to differentiate them from cancer. Although often operated upon because of the difficulty in ruling out cancer, there is no real indication for surgical therapy in thyroiditis. Radiation and antibiotic therapy are sometimes used, but usually the condition runs its course uninfluenced by therapy.

Thyroidectomy

Inhalation anesthesia is employed by most surgeons but local anesthesia is preferred by some.

A low curved incision is made on the anterior surface of the neck, the muscles are either retracted or divided, and the gland is exposed. Removal of the desired amount of gland is then carried out, care being taken to avoid injury to the recurrent laryngeal nerves, parathyroid glands, esophagus, trachea, and structures of the carotid sheath.

COMPLICATIONS

Hemorrhage. A dramatic and serious complication of thyroidectomy is hemorrhage into the wound from one of the large thyroid arteries, usually the superior thyroid artery. The blood compresses the trachea and thus obstructs respiration; this causes the patient to have difficulty in breathing and to become cyanotic. In such cases prompt action is necessary to save the life of the patient. The dressing should immediately be removed; if there is swelling beneath the wound, this is sufficient evidence of hemorrhage, and immediate release of the pressure beneath the wound is necessary. If no doctor is available the nurse should not hesitate to open the wound and allow escape of the blood. The amount of blood lost is not important compared to the need for restoring respiration. Following the reestablishment of breathing the patient is taken to the operating room for control of hemorrhage and closure of the wound.

Thyroid Crisis. Thyroid crisis or storm is another serious postoperative complication in which the patient undergoes alarming exacerbation of the symptoms of hyperthyroidism. There is a rapid pulse, often 160 to 180 per minute, respiration is rapid, and there is high temperature. The patient is flushed, easily upset, and highly nervous. Death may occur from heart failure; therefore every effort must be made to support the patient's strength. Glucose is given intravenously along with high fluid intake. The patient is placed in an oxygen tent. Nervousness and overactivity are controlled by large doses of morphine given at regular intervals. Quiet is essential and everything possible should be done to make the patient comfortable.

Paralysis of the Vocal Cords. This follows injury to the recurrent laryngeal nerve. The clinical signs are noisy, labored respiration, and hoarseness. If the nerve has been entirely divided this will be a permanent condition, but if the nerve has only been traumatized without division, the condition will usually disappear after a few days. Following injury to both nerves there is loss of phonation and serious obstruction to respiration, which must be first treated with the administration of oxygen or of a combination of oxygen and helium; if this is not completely effective, tracheotomy is necessary as a life-saving measure.

Parathyroid Function. Removal of some or all four of the parathyroids will result in parathyroid insufficiency. If all four of the glands have been removed the condition will be permanent, but if one or more glands remain they will become hypertrophied and function will be restored to normal. This subject will be discussed further under parathyroid glands.

NURSING CARE

Postoperative Care. When the patient returns from the operating room, morphine is usually given to prevent restlessness. Special care is taken to prevent the aspiration of secretions. It is convenient to have an electric suction apparatus at the bedside to remove the excess saliva and mucus. As soon as possible the patient is placed in semi-Fowler's position in which he will feel more comfortable and will breathe more easily. The breathing and the color of the patient are watched closely so that difficult respirations and cyanosis may be instantly detected. An emergency tracheotomy set must always be kept ready for use in the ward. Increase in restlessness or in the pulse rate, or elevation of temperature must be reported to the surgeon. These are symptoms of a crisis. In addition, muscular twitching or spasm of the hands and feet should be reported so that calcium or parathyroid extract may be administered to relieve tetany.

Fluids are usually given intravenously until the intake by mouth is sufficient. Fluids by mouth may be given in large amounts as soon as nausea ceases. Coffee and tea are omitted to prevent overstimulation. The diet should be high in calories, and solid food given on the second postoperative day.

Many surgeons order oxygen in high concentration so that oxygenation of the blood can be accomplished with a minimum of effort on the part of the patient. The administration of oxygen is usually discontinued on the second day after operation.

It is desirable that the same nurse care for the patient before and after operation. Unremitting effort is made to prevent excitement, worry, mental fatigue, physical discomfort, and overexertion.

It is helpful to the patient and his family if they are made to realize that the patient's health will not be restored at once but will continue to improve for several months after discharge from the hospital.

Radioiodine

A by-product of the development of the atom bomb has been the production of many radioactive isotopes of common elements. Since the thyroid gland utilizes iodine in manufacturing thyroxin, it was logical to use radioactive iodine in studying and treating diseases of the thyroid. While radioiodine has not proven of much use in the treatment of thyroid cancer, it is definitely effective in hyperthyroidism. In many ways it would seem to be nearly ideal treatment for this condition. It is colorless and tasteless when dissolved in water, and usually only a single dose is needed. After treatment, there is a gradual return to health over a period of six to twelve weeks. If the late results are as good as preliminary results appear to be, it is probable that most patients with exophthalmic goiter will be treated in this manner in the future.

Much use is being made of radioiodine as a diagnostic tool, since a good deal can be learned about thyroid function by studying the uptake of iodine by the gland. After administering a measured amount of radioiodine, counts are taken over the gland with a Geiger counter, and the uptake calculated.

THE PARATHYROIDS

Anatomy and Physiology. The parathyroid glands are generally four in number. They are tiny bean-shaped organs of a brownish color which are situated beneath the lateral lobes of the thyroid, two on each side. There is considerable variation in their size and distribution, but the average size is about 2 millimeters. The parathyroid glands secrete a hormone which has a powerful effect upon the metabolism of calcium and phosphorus in the body and serves to stabilize the levels of calcium and phosphorus in the blood.

Disturbances of the Parathyroids

Hypoparathyroidism. Decreased function of the parathyroids is usually the result of their partial or total removal during operations upon the thyroid. This complication is more common in women than in men; why the female is predisposed is not known.

Symptoms. Hypoparathyroidism is accompanied by a decrease in the level of the calcium and an increase in the level of the phosphorus in the circulating blood. This alteration in the chemical constitution of the blood, if extensive, results clinically in tetany, a condition in which there are severe muscle spasms and even convulsions. In severe cases death may occur unless the proper treatment is begun; in the less severe cases the signs and symptoms are less striking. These patients complain of cramps in the peripheral muscles and tingling of hands and feet, and they may have spontaneous carpal spasm.

Diagnosis. There is irritability of the peripheral nerves which can be demonstrated by tapping with the finger on the cheek just in front of the external auditory meatus; this stimulates the facial nerve which causes contraction of the facial muscles (Chvostek's sign). In the normal person there is no response. Another test is to apply an ordinary blood pressure cuff to the arm and inflate it to above arterial pressure. Within two or three minutes the fingers will stiffen into a typical deformity known as "obstetrician's hand" (Trousseau's sign).

Treatment. Hypoparathyroidism can be successfully treated by injections of parathyroid extract, either alone or in conjunction with the administration of calcium. Calcium gluconate should be given intravenously for immediate relief of tetany, and daily doses of calcium chloride may be taken by mouth to maintain an adequate calcium level. In cases in which removal has been incomplete, hypertrophy of the remaining parathyroid tissue occurs and treatment is gradually discontinued.

Hyperparathyroidism. Increase in parathyroid function is usually caused by an adenoma of one of the glands, and is accompanied by an increase in the calcium and a decrease in the phosphorus in the blood. This results in removal of calcium from the

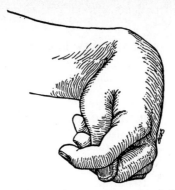

FIGURE 105. Carpal spasm (obstetrician's hand).

bones and an increase in the amount of calcium and phosphorus excreted in the urine.

Symptoms. In severe cases these patients complain of intense pain in the long bones. X-ray examination shows decalcification of the bones with cyst formation. Kidney stones are also a frequent complication as a result of the excess excretion of calcium in the urine. Hyperparathyroidism should be suspected in any patient who shows a tendency to form renal calculi. .

Treatment. Treatment consists in the surgical removal of the parathyroid adenoma. This may be located at the site of any of the normal glands or may arise from aberrant parathyroid tissue elsewhere in the neck or mediastinum. These tumors are not usually large enough to be palpable or to cause any symptoms referable to their size and are often hard to find at operation. Good results may be expected following the removal of an adenoma. The disappearance of pain in the bones is often dramatic, occurring within a few hours.

Postoperative Nursing Care. After operation these patients may temporarily develop tetany. The calcium and phosphorus levels in the blood should be followed carefully and the nurse should be alert for any signs of developing tetany.

SUMMARY

There are several varieties of goiter, and the chief reasons for surgical removal are mechanical, cosmetic, and prevention of cancer. Although the treatment of exophthalmic goiter has been one of the brilliant surgical successes of this country, it now seems probable that most patients with this disease will be treated by drugs or radioiodine.

VOCABULARY REVIEW

parathyroid	*isotope*	*propylthiouracil*
thyroxin	*myxedema*	*goiter*
tetany	*cretin*	

SUGGESTED READING

1. Cerise, Elmo J., Spears, Randall, and Ochsner, Alton: Carcinoma of the Thyroid and Nontoxic Nodular Goiter. Surg., *31*:552–561 (April) 1952.
2. Crile, George, Jr.: Treatment of Hyperthyroidism—An Editorial. Surg., Gynec. & Obst., *91*:242–244 (Aug.) 1950.
3. Christopher, Frederick: A Textbook of Surgery. 5th Ed. Philadelphia, W. B. Saunders Co., 1949, pp. 610–613.
4. Hawley, E., and Garden, G.: The Endocrines and Their Role in Nutrition. 3rd Ed. St. Louis, C. V. Mosby Co., 1949, pp. 111–119.
5. Hinton, J. W., and Lord, J. W., Jr.: Is Surgery Indicated in All Cases of Nodular Goiter, Toxic or Nontoxic? J.A.M.A., *129*:605–606 (October 27) 1945.
6. Lahey, Frank H., and Hoover, Walter B.: Tracheotomy after Thyroidectomy. Ann Surg., *133*:65–76 (January) 1951.
7. McLester, James S.: Nutrition and Diet in Health and Disease. Philadelphia, W. B. Saunders Co., 1950, pp. 668–671.

CHAPTER 35

Surgery of the Pituitary, Thymus, Pancreas, and Adrenals

THE PITUITARY

This gland, also called the hypophysis, is composed of three parts, the anterior lobe, the pars intermedia, and the posterior lobe. It is located within the cranial cavity, immediately beneath the midbrain and behind the intersection of the optic nerves (*optic chiasm*). Although the pituitary secretions, especially that of the anterior lobe, appear to be the all-important pacemakers of all endocrine activity, surgical interest centers chiefly on tumors of the gland. Pituitary tumors often cause endocrinopathy, but the main reason for treating them surgically is to relieve the mechanical pressure caused by them upon the adjacent optic nerves and midbrain.

The diagnosis and operative removal of pituitary tumors fall properly within the sphere of the neurosurgeon, and are discussed in the unit on surgery of the central nervous system (p. 423).

THE THYMUS

Situated in the chest between the sternum and the anterior surface of the great vessels and the heart, this gland is large in infancy and tends to disappear later in life. Little is known of its function or secretion. There appears to be a relationship between the activity of the thymus and a serious disease called myasthenia gravis, in which the muscles of the body tire easily. Some patients suffering from this disease have benefited by the surgical removal of the thymus.

THE PANCREAS

The endocrine portion of the pancreas, the islet tissue, secretes insulin, a hormone which is necessary for the proper utilization of carbohydrates in the metabolic processes of the body.

Diabetes. Insulin deficiency produces the clinical disease known as diabetes. The problem of the surgical patient who has diabetes is one which demands the closest cooperation between physician and surgeon. In general it may be said that the surgical problems are subordinate to the regulation of the patient's carbohydrate metabolism; once this is controlled, with continuous regulation planned, the patient may be treated like any other surgical patient.[1] Modern knowledge of diet, together with insulin and intravenous therapy, has greatly reduced the hazard of surgery for patients with diabetes.

Adenoma. A serious but fortunately uncommon disease, exactly the reverse of diabetes, is produced by a tumor (*adenoma*) of the islet tissue of the pancreas. The islet adenoma, by secreting excessive amounts of insulin, causes serious reduction in the amount of sugar in the blood (*hypoglycemia*), resulting in shock with or without convulsions, which may terminate fatally. Patients suffering from this condition learn to carry sugar or candy in their pockets, and to eat some when the symptom of faintness appears; this, of course, elevates the sugar level in the blood and temporarily prevents loss of consciousness or con-

[1] See Brown, pages 650–694.

vulsions. Suspicion of this disease warrants surgical exploration of the pancreas, for if the adenoma, often tiny, can be found and removed, a cure will result.

Nursing Care. Before operation such a patient is usually ordered additional food between meals, especially at night, to prevent weakness and convulsions. Usually, for diagnostic purposes, it is necessary for the patient to fast. Whenever this is done, it is advisable to ask the surgeon whether or not the patient should have bedside candy or orange juice. Often, during the fasting stage, it is necessary for the nurse to remain at the bedside to prevent the patient from injuring himself. These patients have been mistakenly considered to be mentally ill because of their bizarre behavior during hyperinsulinism. They need assurance of protection and help from the nurse, to make them feel as secure as possible.

After operation, the care given to a patient with resection of the pancreas may be applied. Tact, patience and kindness are required to help this patient overcome the feelings of inferiority he may have because of his insulin reactions.

THE ADRENALS

This pair of glands, also known as suprarenals from their location just at the upper pole of each kidney, secretes hormones which are essential to life, and which affect the regulation of sodium and potassium balance in the blood, carbohydrate metabolism, the activity of smooth muscle, the blood pressure, and the activity of the other endocrines, notably the gonads. Among the better known of the adrenal hormone substances are epinephrine (Adrenalin), nor-epinephrine (Levophed), cortisone and desoxycorticosterone (DOCA).

Benign Tumors. Benign tumors of the adrenal are of interest because, although of infrequent occurrence, they may produce large amounts of one or another of the adrenal hormones, with characteristic symptoms and signs. One variety of tumor causes sexual precocity in infants, or may cause virilizing effects in females. Another type, the pheochromocytoma, secretes adrenalin; the patient presents the evidence of hypertension, usually in acute crises.

Carcinomas. Malignant neoplasms of the adrenals also occur; these are less likely to produce endocrine disturbance but are more difficult to cure as they are extremely invasive, metastasizing early and without symptoms.

Addison's Disease. This grave and formerly fatal disease is due to adrenal insufficiency.[2]

Symptoms and Diagnosis. Low blood pressure, progressive weakness, and a curious bronze pigmentation of the skin are indicative. It is characteristic for the pigmentation to appear in the mucous membrane of the mouth. There are associated derangements of the blood chemistry, notably in the sodium and potassium balance.

Treatment. There is no direct surgical attack possible upon this disease, but substitution therapy has proved life-saving. Pellets of desoxycorticosterone, the active chemical principle of the adrenal cortical hormone, are implanted in the subcutaneous tissue of the back; absorption of the chemical is slow and takes place at the rate needed by the body. It is necessary to implant additional pellets at regular intervals, usually six months or longer, to control the adrenal insufficiency and maintain a normal life.

Patients with Addison's disease are especially susceptible to respiratory infections. It is always advisable for the nurse to wear a mask; even a mild cold is dangerous. The nurse should also be aware of the patient's great sensitivity to all opiates. No opiates are ordered preoperatively or after operation. More than usual tact and forbearance are called for as these patients are often irritable and difficult to handle. A special diet is used which is high in calories (5000 to 6000).

SUMMARY

Benign tumors of the pituitary, pancreas, and adrenal may produce abnormal amounts of the various hormones, resulting in serious effects upon the individual. Removal of such tumors results in cure.

VOCABULARY REVIEW

hypophysis	*hypoglycemia*	*desoxycorticosterone*
pituitary	*hyperinsulinism*	*cortisone*
thymus	*pheochromocytoma*	

SUGGESTED READING

1. Blalock, Alfred: Tumors of the Thymic Region and Myasthenia Gravis: Am. J. Surg., *54*:149–150 (October) 1941.
2. Clagett, O. Theron: Myasthenia Gravis, Medical and Surgical Treatment. Am. J. Nursing, *51*:654–655 (November) 1951.

[2] See Brown, pages 696–712.

3. Greiling, Gladys E.: Myasthenia Gravis, Nursing Care. Am. J. Nursing, *51:* 655-657 (November) 1951.
4. Krause, Marie V.: Nutrition and Diet Therapy. Philadelphia, W. B. Saunders Co., 1950, pp. 239-298.
5. Priestley, J. T., Comfort, M. W., and Sprague, R. G.: Total Pancreatectomy for Hyperinsulinism Due to Islet-Cell Adenoma: Follow-up Report 5½ Years After Operation, Including Metabolic Studies. Ann Surg., *130:* 211-217 (August) 1949.
6. Thorn, G. W., Howard, R. P., Emerson, K., Jr., and Firor, W. M.: Treatment of Addison's Disease with Pellets of Crystalline Adrenal Cortical Hormone (Synthetic Desoxycorticosterone Acetate) Implanted Subcutaneously. Bull. Johns Hopkins Hospital, *64:*339 (May) 1939

CHAPTER 36

Introduction

Anatomy and Physiology. The brain is a soft, semifluid organ, housed in a rigid case, the bony skull. In the base of the skull there are numerous small openings (*foramina*) for the passage of the cranial nerves and vessels, and one large opening (*foramen magnum*) for the spinal cord. The skull and the spinal canal are lined with a tough fibrous membrane (*dura mater*). The brain and the spinal cord are covered directly with a filmy membrane (*pia-arachnoid*) in which are blood vessels and the areas (*subaranchnoid spaces*) containing the cerebrospinal fluid, which is a clear fluid elaborated by clusters of blood vessels (*choroid plexuses*) which are situated in the cavities (*ventricles*) of the brain. The elaboration of the fluid is mainly—if not entirely—a process of filtration from the blood stream.

Within the brain there are four main cavities, constituting the ventricular system. One of these, the lateral ventricle, lies in each cerebral hemisphere and communicates with the third ventricle, which is situated in the midbrain, by means of the foramen

411

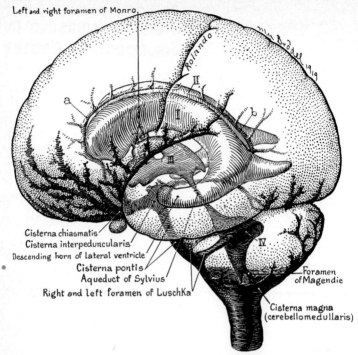

Left and right foramen of Monro

Cisterna chiasmatis
Cisterna interpeduncularis
Descending horn of lateral ventricle
Cisterna pontis
Aqueduct of Sylvius
Right and left foramen of LuschKa

Foramen of Magendie

Cisterna magna
(cerebellomedullaris)

FIGURE 106. The ventricles of the brain, and the circulation of the cerebro-spinal fluid (courtesy of Walter E. Dandy, Jr.).

of Monro. A small channel, known as the aqueduct of Sylvius, connects the third ventricle with the fourth ventricle, which is located between the medulla and the cerebellum. The spinal fluid escapes from the fourth ventricle through the openings of Luschka and Magendie into the subarachnoid spaces where it is eventually absorbed.

The arrangement of nerve cells and nerve pathways in the brain is extremely complex. Certain general features, however, must be kept constantly in mind. In general, nervous impulses from the right cerebral hemisphere are directed to the left half of the body, and those from the left hemisphere to the right half of the body. Furthermore, there is a regular representation upon the brain surface (*cerebral cortex*) of each body area: for example, a small area of the left cerebral cortex near the top of the

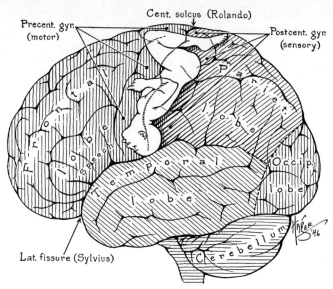

FIGURE 107. Schematic illustration of the representation of the regions of the body upon the cerebral cortex.

head controls the movements of the right leg. One of the most important of the cerebral areas is a portion of the left temporal region known as the speech center. This is unpaired, there being only one speech center, always on the left side in a right-handed person. The centers of control of automatic activity, including respiration, circulation, and metabolism, lie deeper in the midbrain and the medulla. There are twelve pairs of nerves arising from the brain itself; these are the cranial nerves. In addition to supplying impulses for ordinary sensation from the head and the motor control of the head, the cranial nerves furnish pathways for the important special senses of smell, vision, taste, equilibrium, and hearing. The spinal cord and spinal nerves serve as pathways for impulses between the brain and the rest of the body below the head.

The brain is well supplied with blood vessels, as befits so specialized and active an organ. Brain cells are delicate and die quickly (in seven minutes or less) if deprived of blood supply or oxygen. This fact is important, because (1) the many small arteries are terminal arteries, without anastomoses, and occlusion of them means loss of circulation to the area supplied by the artery; and (2) *anoxia* from any cause may result in the death of a part or all of the brain. Another characteristic of the central nervous system is the inability of this tissue to heal with restoration of function. Following injury there is loss of tissue and scar formation, but no repair of the injured or destroyed nervous cells. Loss of function due to loss of brain tissue is permanent. This is equally true of the spinal cord, and of those portions of the cranial and spinal nerves which lie inside of the skull and spinal canal.

CHAPTER 37

Intracranial Injuries

Automobile accidents, athletics, and accidental falls combine to make intracranial injuries common. The brain is well protected by its bony armor, but a blow upon the head is often of sufficient force to damage the nervous tissue, tear small blood vessels, or even fracture the skull, sometimes severely lacerating the brain itself. A violent blow upon one side of the head may cause damage to the brain opposite the side struck (*contrecoup*), just as an orange thrown forcibly against a wall may burst open on the side opposite to that striking the wall. Although bony fragments may be driven inward (as in depressed fracture) with consequent trauma to the underlying brain, severe damage to the brain sometimes results without any disturbance of the continuity of the skull. The seriousness of an injury to the head depends not upon the fracture of the skull, but upon the amount of damage to the brain. Following violence there are hemorrhage if the vessels have been torn, and swelling (*edema*) due to outpouring of tissue fluid if the brain tissue has been damaged. This resulting increase in cranial contents causes an increase in intracranial pressure. The surgeon, in treating a head injury, has therefore three problems to consider: (1) the local injury to scalp and skull; (2) the damage to the brain; (3) increased intracranial pressure. Of these three, the last is the most important consideration, since little can be done to repair actual damage to the brain.

RESULTS OF INTRACRANIAL INJURIES

Increased Intracranial Pressure. There is some variation in the intracranial pressure of normal persons, but it is usually between 120 and 180 mm. of water, as measured by a manometer connected to a needle introduced into either the spinal canal or the lateral ventricle.

Signs and Symptoms. Following an increase in the cranial contents, whether due to fluid (*edema*), hemorrhage, tumor, or other cause, symptoms and signs develop which are due to compression of the less resistant portions of the brain tissue. The brain is able to withstand gradual slow compression far better, and for a longer time, than sudden rapid increase in intracranial pressure, but a sufficient degree of either will cause irreparable and often fatal damage.

SUDDEN INCREASE. The constant and most reliable sign of sudden change in intracranial pressure is the state of consciousness of the patient. A perfectly conscious person responds well to questions, is oriented with respect to time and place, and appears alert. Unnatural drowsiness and disorientation may indicate the onset of increased pressure; wild delirium or restlessness alternating with periods of quiet may indicate the onset of coma; the completely unconscious person responds to no stimulus, breathes stertorously, and is incontinent. This sequence of events may occur with great rapidity; often it is absent when a person is rendered immediately and completely unconscious by a severe injury.

Recovery from coma presents exactly the reverse order of events. Restlessness may presage a return of consciousness; disorientation and drowsiness disappear as recovery is complete. Therefore, when a patient is observed to be restless it is extremely important to know whether he has previously been unconscious or conscious, since the restlessness may indicate either beginning recovery or progressive compression of the brain.

Other indices of acute increase in intracranial pressure are, in the order of their reliability: (1) rapid progressive elevation of body temperature, which may rise a degree or more every hour; (2) slowing of respiration (*bradypnea*); (3) slowing of pulse rate (bradycardia); (4) elevation of blood pressure. In any given patient all or none of these signs may be present, since there is the widest variation in individuals. The change in body temperature is almost as reliable a sign as the state of consciousness; the other signs are far less reliable.

GRADUAL INCREASE. Where the increase in intracranial pressure takes place over a period of many days or weeks rather than a few hours, there is a different sequence of events. Headache, dizziness, vomiting, and visual disturbance occur. Weakness or paralysis of the various cranial nerves due to continued pressure present characteristic signs. An important indication of gradual increase in intracranial pressure is *papilledema* (choked disk), which is swelling of the retinal end of the optic nerve, visible through the pupil of the eye by means of an ophthalmoscope. Retinal hemorrhages may also occur. Finally, with persistent increase in pressure the changes described in acute compression take place. Bradycardia, disorientation, and drowsiness are followed by coma and incontinence, and by death unless the compression is relieved. When the patient can no longer compensate for the slow increase in pressure the picture may become that of acute compression with startling rapidity.

Convulsions. Convulsions are probably not caused by increased intracranial pressure, but the two conditions are frequently associated since many lesions produce both. A convulsion is a vivid and terrifying demonstration of the control which the brain exerts over the body. It may be defined as an involuntary and uninhibited muscular contraction which affects a part or all of the body musculature and which results from an explosive discharge of nervous stimuli from the brain.

A convulsion is always a sign of brain abnormality. Children have a far lower convulsive threshold than adults and frequently show convulsive phenomena following minor head injuries or in toxic states. Therefore a convulsion in a child is not so indicative of severe brain abnormality as it is in an adult.

Tumors, infections, traumatic injuries, various drugs and noxious chemicals, certain alterations of the metabolic environment such as anoxemia or hypoglycemia, and congenital abnormalities—in a word, any condition which causes damage to the nervous cells of the cerebral hemispheres may produce convulsions. In addition, convulsions occur in the absence of any demonstrable cortical lesion (as in so-called idiopathic epilepsy).

Varieties. Convulsions are of two types: clonic and tonic. The tonic type, which produces tetanic spasm of muscle, is uncommon. The first or clonic type is the common variety, and is characterized by intermittent muscular contraction. Clonic convulsions are often known as epileptiform since they occur in epilepsy. Convulsions may be localized, involving only a portion of

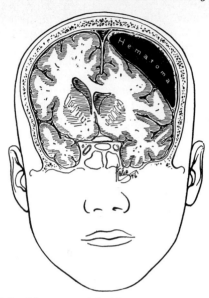

FIGURE 108. Subdural hematoma. The blood clot is compressing the brain.

the body, or they may be generalized. At times a severe seizure may begin with localized convulsions which develop into generalized convulsions. This phenomenon, if properly observed, will provide information that is useful in designating the portion of brain affected. Clonic convulsions are thought to result from stimuli arising in the cerebral hemispheres, whereas tonic convulsions result from stimuli originating in the brain stem.

Concussion. Every one speaks of concussion but no one really knows what happens to the brain in this condition. A blow or violence to the head is followed by brief loss of consciousness, then by recovery accompanied by headache, dizziness, vomiting, or brief disorientation. These symptoms may be absent or only transitory. After an interval the patient's recovery is complete. Obviously this is a mild form of head injury, and the treatment is that described on page 418.

Extradural Hemorrhage. Occasionally the middle meningeal artery is torn at the point where, leaving the skull, it enters the cranial cavity. This injury produces arterial bleeding between bone and dura, which results in rapid compression of the brain. The initial symptoms and signs are slight, but after a brief interval rapidly progressing signs appear which indicate compression of the brain. These signs often point to compression of one cerebral hemisphere. This condition demands prompt recognition in order that operative procedures designed to stop the bleeding and evacuate the blood (*hematoma*) may be undertaken in time.

Acute Subdural Hematoma (see also p. 436). One of the cerebral veins or dural sinuses may be torn with resultant bleeding into the subdural space. The signs are those of cerebral compression which, however, is much less rapid than in extradural hemorrhage where the bleeding is arterial. There is usually severe concomitant damage to the brain.

Hydroma. A similar picture is seen in subdural hydromas where a tear in the arachnoid permits escape of cerebrospinal fluid into the subdural space. These hydromas are much more frequent in children than in adults.

TREATMENT OF INTRACRANIAL INJURIES

Any person receiving a forceful injury to the head may suffer intracranial damage. The degree of violence need not be sufficient to produce immediate unconsciousness; on the other hand, loss of consciousness due to a blow upon the head should be taken as certain evidence of intracranial injury. About four fifths of the persons so injured recover with no treatment other than measures designed to protect and sustain them while unconscious. About one tenth will be so severely injured that death is inevitable. When the brain is severely damaged the patient will usually die within four hours more or less. Experience has shown that there is no form of treatment or operative procedure which can save these lives. The remaining small fraction of the whole group represents borderline cases where proper treatment may save life.

Skin wounds are dressed but not sutured, hemorrhage is checked, and fractures of long bones are splinted if necessary. Shock is treated (p. 68) but in applying heat the possibility of burning an unconscious patient must be borne in mind. Transfusions and intravenous fluids are withheld unless absolutely necessary, as it is not desirable to elevate the blood pressure in the face of possible intracranial bleeding. Nothing is permitted by mouth, to avoid aspiration of fluid.

X-ray Examination. It is unnecessary at this time to subject the patient to x-ray examination of the skull, as the treatment depends upon the damage to the brain, and not upon the condition of the skull. When it is suspected that a fragment of skull is depressed into the brain, roentgenograms should be made at the end of the observation period, if the patient's condition permits.

Spinal Puncture. Spinal puncture as a diagnostic or therapeutic procedure is the subject of an active controversy. Some authorities hold that it is dangerous and unnecessary; others consider it safe and useful. It is significant to note, however, that the results of treatment of head injuries by spinal puncture are not better than the results of treatment without that procedure.

General Measures. The patient is kept quietly in a bed with sides, and care is taken to prevent further damage from convulsive or delirious movements, from inadequate airway, or from aspiration of mucus and vomitus.

Convulsions. Since convulsions are a symptom of brain abnormality, treatment must be aimed at the correction of that abnormality. Important information as to the location of the brain abnormality may sometimes be derived from accurate observation of a convulsive seizure. The portion of the body first involved, the order of spread to other regions, the degree and duration of unconsciousness, and weakness or paralysis afterward should be noted.

During convulsions the patient must be protected from injury, such as falls, burns, biting the tongue, and aspiration. Firmly attached sides on the bed prevent the patient from falling out of bed. The insertion of a padded mouth gag between the upper and lower molars prevents biting of the tongue. When the convulsion is prolonged, turning the patient on the side and lowering the head facilitates drainage of mucus from the throat. Excess mucus may be removed by suction. If convulsions are frequent in occurrence, or are constant (*status epilepticus*), measures must be undertaken to control them lest the patient die of exhaustion. Large doses of sedatives, or even general anesthesia, may be necessary.

Observation Period. At the outset, careful and gentle examination of the patient is made, including a thorough survey to ascertain the extent of other injuries and to determine the neurologic status. This examination is repeated at intervals, to detect changing or new signs.

The degree of intracranial injury, upon which treatment is to be based, may be estimated only by observing the patient for several hours. During this observation period a careful record is kept of the state of consciousness, movements of body (including eyes), convulsions, rectal temperature, pulse, respiration, and blood pressure. Scalp wounds are closed at the end of the observation period.

Nursing Care. Nearly all those patients who show evidence of improvement during the observation period will recover with conservative treatment, consisting of rest in bed, protection from harm during unconsciousness, maintenance of water balance, and proper care of wounds and other injuries. Restlessness is at times so great that restraint of the extremities is necessary to prevent the patient from harming himself. When restraints are used, both of the arm restraints should be fastened on the side of the bed toward which the patient is turned. Pneumonia is best prevented by a frequent change of the patient's position.

Bleeding from the ear should be reported to the surgeon. The blood comes directly from the intracranial chamber through the inner and middle ear and runs out through the ruptured ear drum. No local treatment is carried out; the nurse should let it alone. There may be bleeding from the nose (*epistaxis*), and sometimes clear cerebrospinal fluid issues through the nostrils (*rhinorrhea*). The patient should be advised not to blow his nose because this may force infection into the brain. A chemotherapeutic agent is usually administered to combat or prevent infection.

After-effects. While recovery is taking place the patient often appears to be fully conscious, talking, eating, and performing other routine acts, but memory and other higher mental functions may still be disturbed. Convulsions, complaints of headache and dizziness, and other symptoms sometimes appear months after apparent recovery from injury to the brain. It is often very difficult to determine whether the symptoms constitute a real after-effect of the injury, or whether the symptoms are induced by the thought of possible monetary compensation. Both are possible.

Surgical Treatment

Of the remaining patients who have survived the observation period without improvement, some may be saved by adequate treatment. Small exploratory openings in the skull (*trephinings*) can be made without jeopardizing the patient's safety, and these may disclose beneath the skull fluid or blood which can be removed; if there is only diffuse edema of the brain, some room for expansion may be afforded by removing a portion of the skull (*decompression*). Efforts to relieve edema of the brain by dehydration are generally unsatisfactory and at best give only temporary relief. Depressed fractures of the skull should be elevated, or the bony fragments removed.

EPILEPSY

Epileptiform convulsions may be caused by many different types of brain abnormality (p. 416). The most notable advances in the study and classification of epilepsy have been made by measuring the minute electrical changes taking place across the surface of the brain (*electroencephalography*).

Persons who have convulsions in the absence of any demonstrable pathologic lesions are considered to have idiopathic epilepsy, which is the same thing as saying that they have convulsions of unknown origin. As yet no cure has been devised for this condition, which is indeed common, but the frequency of attacks may be lessened by the continued use of certain drugs, notably barbiturates and Dilantin, together with careful observance of hygienic living.

Epilepsy which is due to congenital deformities or to cerebral scars resulting from chemical or mechanical injury to the brain, is sometimes cured by the removal of the abnormal area. Unfortunately, the results of this procedure are by no means certain—in fact, epilepsy sometimes follows a cranial operation as a result of the trauma caused by the procedure.

SUMMARY

Accidental injury to the head and its contents is common. The most important index of the degree of injury is the state of consciousness. The nurse must be familiar with the signs of increasing intracranial pressure so that treatment may be undertaken before death or permanent damage to the brain occur.

VOCABULARY REVIEW

contrecoup	*epileptiform*	*rhinorrhea*
bradycardia	*concussion*	*decompression*
papilledema	*subdural*	*otorrhea*

SUGGESTED READING

1. Carini, Esta, and Robinson, Franklin: Acute Cranio-cerebral Injuries. Am. J. Nursing, *50:*423–427 (July) 1950.
2. Christopher, Frederick: A Textbook of Surgery, 5th Ed. Philadelphia, W. B. Saunders Co., 1949, pp. 446–466.

3. Everts, William and Woodhall, Barnes: The Management of Head and Spinal Cord Injuries in the Army. J.A.M.A., *126*:145–148 (Sept. 16), 1944.
4. Haynes, Walter G., and McGuire, Mary: Neurosurgical Nursing. Philadelphia, W. B. Saunders Co., 1952, pp. 73–102.
5. Gutierrez-Mahoney, C. de G., and Carini, Esta: Neurological and Neurosurgical Nursing. St. Louis, C. V. Mosby Co., 1949, pp. 26–88.
6 McLester, James S.: Nutrition and Diet in Health and Disease. Philadelphia, W. B. Saunders Co., 1950, pp. 677–686.

CHAPTER 38

Brain Tumors

(INCLUDING BRAIN ABSCESS, TUBERCULOMA, SUBDURAL HEMATOMA, AND ANEURYSMS)

The diagnosis and treatment of intracranial tumors constitute one of the most fascinating branches of surgery. The names of Horsley, Cushing, and Dandy will always bring to mind the advances in neurosurgery which have so brightened the once hopeless outlook for the many people afflicted with brain tumor. Since all intracranial space-occupying lesions produce similar symptoms and signs, it is practicable to include in the consideration of brain tumors not only neoplasms but also brain abscess, tuberculoma, and subdural hematoma.

CLASSIFICATION

Classification may be made in two ways, either by the nature of the pathologic process or by its location, both of which are important.

Gliomas. From the point of view of pathology the glioma is the commonest type, accounting for about half of all brain tumors. There are several varieties of glioma but certain features are common to all. Glial tumors arise mainly from the various types of supporting cells which are found in the brain. All glial tumors are malignant in that they are invasive, but, unlike malignant tumors arising from other tissues, they have never been known to metastasize to distant regions of the body. Contributing to the difficulty in treating these tumors surgically are: (1) the similarity in their gross appearance to that of brain tissue, so that it is hard or sometimes impossible to define the tumor boundaries; and (2) the frequent location of glial tumors in a portion of the brain essential to life. Although they are usually invasive and non-encapsulated, many gliomas grow so slowly that their recurrence and repeated removal are compatible with many years of useful life.

Meningioma; Acoustic Neurinoma. Tumors arising from the membranous covering of the brain or from the sheaths of the cranial nerves constitute the next largest group of brain tumors. These include the meningioma and the acoustic neurinoma, which are benign tumors causing symptoms and signs by pressing upon the brain.

Tumors of Pituitary and Pineal Origin. Other true tumors are those arising from the pituitary and pineal glands. These may be benign or malignant. It must also be remembered that malignant tumors arising from other parts of the body may metastasize to the brain.

Brain Abscess; Tuberculoma; Subdural Hematoma. Brain abscess and tuberculoma are not neoplastic, but are lesions of infectious origin. Subdural hematoma, the presence of blood between the dura and brain, is neither neoplastic nor infectious, but probably traumatic in origin.

SIGNS AND SYMPTOMS

Brain tumors produce symptoms and signs in three chief ways: (1) by pressing upon and damaging the adjacent portion of the brain, often giving rise to localizing signs; (2) by increasing the contents of the cranium, thus causing increase in intracranial pressure; (3) by interfering with the mechanics of the cerebrospinal fluid system, causing hydrocephalus. Increase in intracranial pressure has been discussed under intracranial injuries (p. 415). It is the slowly progressive form which is usually produced by brain tumors.

Hydrocephalus. This condition, commonly known as "water on the brain," is an integral part of any discussion of brain tumors since such tumors frequently produce hydrocephalus. Obstruction to the flow of cerebrospinal fluid from the ventricles results in dilatation of that portion of the ventricular system which is obstructed (*internal hydrocephalus*). Interference, either complete or partial, with the absorption of cerebrospinal fluid over the surface of the brain, may produce large pools of fluid on

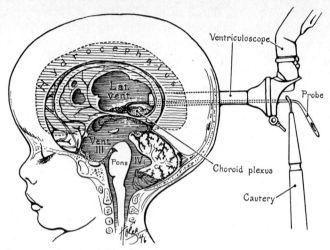

FIGURE 109. Electrocoagulation of the choroid plexus in the treatment of hydrocephalus (choroid plexectomy).

the outside of the brain (*external hydrocephalus*) as well as cause
enlargement of the ventricular system. The ventricles enlarge at
the expense of brain tissue, and if the hydrocephalus persists,
eventually the brain tissue becomes thinned out and functionless.
Hydrocephalus may be caused by tumor, congenital abnormality,
or infection (e.g., meningitis).

The removal of an obstructing tumor, if carried out before the
damage to the brain is too great, will result in the cure of hydrocephalus. Operation designed to make new openings into the ventricles (*ventriculostomy*) or to reduce the amount of fluid secreted (*choroid plexectomy*) or to create an artificial shunt of
fluid into another body cavity (*ventriculopleural, ventriculoperi-
toneal,* or *ureterosubarachnoid*) is occasionally successful in curing hydrocephalus due to congenital or infectious types of
obstruction. Frequently, however, in the congenital forms the
brain is so badly damaged, and other abnormalities so often occur
in conjunction, that little is to be expected in the way of permanent improvement.

DIAGNOSIS

Localization

The function of many portions of the brain is known, but
there are also large portions, especially of the cerebral hem-

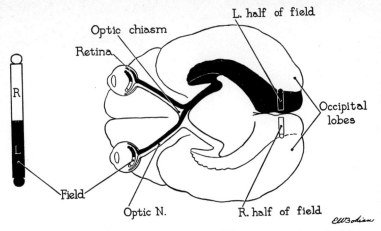

FIGURE 110. The visual pathways. The lens of the eye causes the retinal image to be inverted.

ispheres, for which no function has been definitely determined; these are the so-called silent areas. Thus the cerebral areas concerned with motor function, sensation, and vision are known, but many of the functions of the temporal and frontal portions (*lobes*) of the hemisphere are not definitely known. It is possible to remove large portions of these lobes without bringing about any measurable changes in the individual. The functions of the many long fiber tracts transmitting nerve impulses are known, as are also the functions of the cranial nerves. If a tumor is so situated as to compress or damage a portion of the brain of known function, neurologic examination of the patient reveals alteration of function. It is not often, however, that localization is so easily accomplished. Tumors may be situated in the silent areas; and even when a certain fiber tract is observed to be damaged, it is not always possible to know with certainty which portion of the long tract is affected.

Certain observations, nevertheless, are worthy of mention. Epileptiform convulsions point to a cerebral lesion, and if the convulsions are confined to or always originate in one portion of the body (*Jacksonian epilepsy*), the lesion is in the opposite cerebral hemisphere. Weakness or paralysis of a part or all of one side of the body indicates injury of the motor nerve tract leading finally to the cerebral cortex of the opposite side, but the exact point of damage must be determined by additional observations. Similarly,

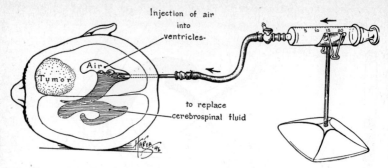

FIGURE 111. Ventriculography I. Replacing fluid in ventricle with air.

signs of partial or complete loss of sensation are useful for localization.

Tumors affecting the visual pathways can be localized accurately since the characteristic functions of the different portions of the tracts are well known. Figure 110 explains how a tumor involving one optic nerve will cause blindness of that eye, whereas a tumor in the left occipital lobe will cause loss of the right half of the visual field of both eyes (*right homonymous hemianopsia*), and a tumor at the optic chiasm (i.e., a pituitary tumor) will result in loss of the lateral half of the visual field in both eyes (*bitemporal hemianopsia*). Again, a tumor in the cerebellopontine angle characteristically causes deafness (*paralysis of the eighth nerve*) and loss of sensation and motor power over that half of the face on the same side (*paralysis of the fifth and seventh nerves*).

Unfortunately, despite the large amount of information available, only a small percentage of brain tumors can be localized with certainty by means of neurologic examination. Exact localization, nevertheless, is of vital importance to the patient, as there is grave danger in making an incorrect exposure of a brain tumor. Since the epochal discovery of ventriculography by Dandy in 1918, untold lives have been saved by the accuracy with which this method localizes nearly all brain tumors.

Ventriculography

Through an operative opening (*trephine*) made in the skull, usually in the occipital region, a needle is inserted into the posterior portion (*horn*) of one or the other lateral ventricles. In some clinics frontal or parietal openings are made. The cerebro-

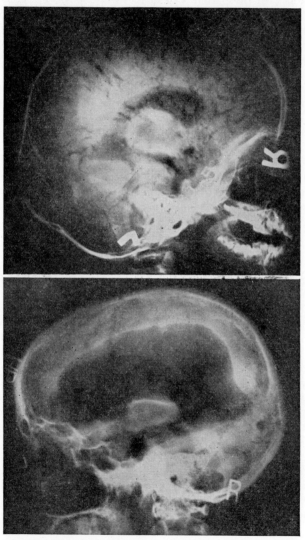

FIGURE 112. Ventriculography II. Roentgenograms. *Upper,* normal; *lower,* hydrocephalus.

spinal fluid is replaced with air, and stereoscopic roentgenograms are made with the patient's head in various positions. It is thus possible to visualize the contour of the whole ventricular system.

Tumors which occupy space within the cranium cause characteristic alteration of the normal appearance of the ventricles. For example, a large tumor compressing the cerebrum from without causes a dislocation of the lateral and third ventricles toward the opposite side, whereas a small tumor in the brain substance of the frontal lobe bulges into the anterior horn of the ventricle on that side, causing obvious alteration in the outline of that horn. A third type of abnormality is dilatation of the ventricles (*internal hydrocephalus*), resulting from obstruction to the outflow of cerebrospinal fluid.

The technic of ventriculography is difficult, and is safe only in the hands of the specially trained surgeon. The air is irritating to the brain and must be removed promptly. As in all surgical procedures, asepsis is of the utmost importance.

Pneumoencephalography

Air may also be introduced into the cerebrospinal spaces through spinal puncture but this procedure may be dangerous and should not be used in the presence of increased intracranial pressure; it is of limited value therefore in the localization of tumors and finds its chief field of usefulness in the demonstration of atrophic lesions of the brain. The subarachnoid spaces as well as the ventricles are usually filled with air in this procedure, thus enabling the surgeon to visualize to some extent the surface of the brain as well as its interior cavities. Air so injected is slowly absorbed, disappearing in about twenty-four hours. The headache which results from this procedure is less severe if the patient is kept flat in bed.

Arteriography

A radiopaque material, usually 35 per cent Diodrast (but sometimes also Thorotrast), may be injected into the carotid arteries for x-ray visualization of the major cerebral vessels. This may be done by the direct or open method in which the carotid artery is exposed in the neck and injection carried out under direct vision, or by the closed or percutaneous method in which a needle is inserted into the carotid artery through the intact skin. The latter is the simpler and more commonly used method. The technic is extremely useful in visualizing vascular abnormalities such as aneurysms, arteriovenous fistulas or arterial and

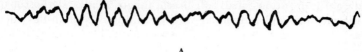

A

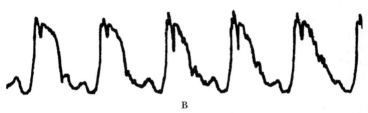

B

FIGURE 113. Electroencephalography. *A,* Normal record; *B,* record characteristic of epilepsy (petit mal type).

venous occlusions. Tumors in the frontal and temporal areas can also sometimes be accurately localized by this method.

Electroencephalography

There are definite rhythms of brain electric potentials which vary in different parts of the brain. These rhythms can be charted and abnormalities that point to a cerebral lesion studied. This field is being intensively studied and is contributing more and more to our knowledge of normal and pathologic functions of the brain.

NURSING CARE

During the admission procedure the nurse, in acquainting herself with the patient, should find out the nature and extent of his disability so that she can plan his nursing care. When the diagnosis is epilepsy, the patient usually brings to the hospital the drugs he has been taking; any information concerning these should be given to the surgeon. Patients with brain tumor sometimes have convulsions. It is advisable, when inquiring, to refer to these seizures as fainting spells, for the word convulsion or fit carries a stigma in society. The nurse should be thoroughly familiar with the care required by patients who have epilepsy.[1]

In helping the surgeon perform a physical examination, necessary equipment includes a sphygmomanometer, tuning fork,

[1] See Brown, pages 732–741.

straight pin, cotton, small soft brush, tongue blades, stethoscope, tape measure and individual vials of solutions containing vinegar, cloves, sugar, benzine and peppermint. The student is referred to a description by Brown[2] for explanation of the examination of the cranial nerves. Other diagnostic examinations frequently done are the lumbar puncture and Queckenstedt test.[3]

After the patient is undressed, his skin should be inspected. Bruises may be indicative of injury incurred by falling during a convulsion. The patient who has a diagnosis of tumor should be carefully examined about the hairline and neck for furuncles and, if any are present, the surgeon should be notified. Such an infection would necessitate postponing any intracranial operation because of the great risk of carrying infection into the brain.

Assuring the patient and the family in a warm and interested manner that all will be done for the patient that is possible is helpful in relieving some of their anxiety.

Preoperatively, the patient may have many examinations. The most common are arteriogram, ventriculogram, encephalogram, electroencephalogram and audiogram. No special physical preparation is needed for electroencephalogram or audiogram, but the patient should understand what will take place during either of these. An audiogram may be described simply as a hearing test, but when an encephalogram is ordered, the patient should be told that small wires will be placed on his scalp and that they will not cause pain. Further explanation will depend on the age and interest and anxiety of the patient. Often patients have had such examinations previously; it is always useful to find out first what experience the patient has had.

Preparation for arteriogram usually consists of withholding fluids and food several hours before the examination. Diodrast, 35 per cent, is injected into the internal carotid artery to permit visualization of the intracranial arterial system on roentgenograms. Some individuals are sensitive to this drug; one method of determining sensitivity is by placing 2 cc. of the solution under the tongue. An unfavorable reaction is evidenced by redness and swelling of the tongue. To protect the safety of each patient, a tracheotomy set must be at hand in case laryngeal edema or spasm develops.

Following the procedure, the dressing on the neck should be inspected for bleeding or swelling from a hematoma. General

[2] Op. cit., page 716.
[3] Op. cit., pages 719–720.

care will depend on whether the procedure was done under local or general anesthesia.

Infrequent sequelae are unilateral weakness and aphasia. The nurse should report these findings to the doctor, and the patient should be assured that these are transient, usually disappearing entirely in six to twelve hours.

Preparation for encephalography and ventriculography is the same as that for general anesthesia. Following either procedure, the care consists in observing the temperature, pulse, respirations, blood pressure and the state of consciousness.[4] The headache following encephalography is excruciating; usually aspirin is ordered to be given either orally or rectally, according to the condition of the patient. When nausea and vomiting occur, fluids are given sparingly. The position of the patient depends entirely on the orders of the surgeon; some surgeons prefer the patient to lie flat, others prefer to elevate the head 6 to 12 inches.

TREATMENT

Craniotomy

Any surgical exposure of the brain necessitates opening the skull, which is what the word craniotomy means. The neurosurgeon need not be endowed with skill above his brother surgeons if he is aware that small technical errors in this field are followed by large disasters. One careless motion may forever deprive the patient of the use of some portion of his body. Lack of rigid asepsis and hemostasis is fatal. The soft brain does not withstand minor trauma, bacterial invasion, or bleeding as do the other tissues of the body.

Technic. Incisions in the scalp are so placed as to be concealed beneath the hair, yet afford good exposure. Two types of opening may be made through the skull: (1) decompression, in which the bone is removed permanently, and (2) osteoplastic craniotomy, in which a flap of bone is elevated, to be replaced at the conclusion of the operation. The first type is used for very small openings, or to relieve intracranial pressure, or in the occipital (*cerebellar*) region where the heavy neck muscles will cover the defect in the skull and protect the brain. The second type is commonly used for exposing cerebral tumors.

Care is taken to avoid entering the paranasal or mastoid sinuses, as that would lead to infection. The large blood vessels must not be injured since the brain does not tolerate serious interference with its circulation. Following incision of the dura,

[4] Brown, pages 720–721.

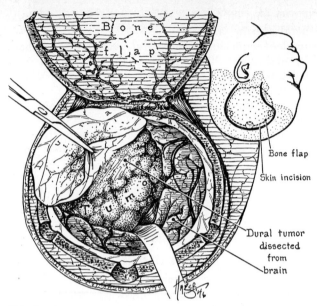

Bone flap

Skin incision

Dural tumor
dissected
from
brain

FIGURE 114. Craniotomy. Insert shows how incision in scalp is concealed beneath hair.

the brain is exposed; it must be kept moist so that the cells on the surface are not harmed. If in the course of removing a tumor a portion of the brain is also removed, the resulting defect is permanent; the space will afterward be filled with cerebrospinal fluid.

POSTOPERATIVE CARE

In addition to the usual care needed after any major operation, the neurosurgical patient requires minute observation in order that the surgeon may detect and treat increase in intracranial pressure and prevent complications which may arise as a result of the patient's state of consciousness or loss of motor function. It must be realized that any operation upon the brain, even when carried out in the most skilful manner, is a form of intracranial injury. There is always some degree of cerebral edema, outpouring of fluid, and bleeding. One of these, or at times all of them, may cause a dangerous rise in the intracranial pressure.

Relief from pressure may be afforded by aspiration of blood and cerebrospinal fluid from beneath the wound, from the cerebral defect, when there is one, or from the ventricles. At times it is necessary to remove the bone flap to make additional room for the swollen brain. Spinal puncture should be avoided, as withdrawal of fluid from the spinal canal in the presence of high intracranial pressure may allow the lower portion of the brain (*medulla*) to become compressed in the foramen magnum, with resulting injury to the vital centers.

NURSING CARE

The preoperative care of the patient with lesions of the brain depends a great deal on the signs and symptoms of the patient, which, in turn, depend on the location of the lesion. Nursing care must therefore be planned individually for the patient.

Patients may be emaciated from frequent vomiting, lack of appetite or inability to swallow. Spoon or tube feeding may be necessary and care must be taken to prevent choking and aspiration. When there is incontinence of urine and feces special efforts must be made to keep the patient clean and dry. Offering the bedpan or urinal at regular intervals may eliminate a wet bed. Enemas may need to be given if there is fecal incontinence.

Ambulatory patients with personality changes, weakness of muscles, or visual disturbances present special problems. Nursing care is directed toward protecting them from injuring themselves, from disturbing others on the ward as they walk about, and toward raising their morale. Everyone on the neurosurgical ward must help provide a safe environment for these people. They may walk aimlessly about the ward, get lost or, if furniture is misplaced, may stumble and fall. Any change in the state of consciousness, the occurrence of convulsive seizures, or the development of a very slow pulse rate must be observed and reported.

The immediate preparation for surgery is similar to that for general anesthesia. Sometimes a sedative is given the evening before but this depends on the condition of the patient. In addition to the usual postoperative unit, a suction apparatus should be available. Other necessary equipment is already available if the patient goes to the recovery room, but if he returns to the ward the essentials are: a sterile set-up for spinal tap, including manometers, ventricular needles, 50 per cent glucose, ampules of ephedrine and sodium phenobarbital.

Following operation, constant observation is necessary for at least twenty-four hours. The temperature, pulse, respirations, and blood pressure are taken every fifteen minutes for the first few hours or until the patient has fully reacted. A rising blood pressure and a slowing of the pulse and respirations are indicative of increased intracranial pressure.

The position of the patient depends upon the desire of the neurosurgeon; some order the head to be elevated 10 to 12 inches to decrease the venous pressure and thereby lessen edema, while others prefer their patients to lie flat in bed. In either case, the patient should be turned on his side to prevent the tongue from falling back, and to allow saliva and vomitus to run out. The position should be changed every hour from side to side until the patient is no longer unconscious or helpless.

Fluids are given parenterally until the patient is able to swallow. In patients unable to swallow, feeding may be by gavage, in which case the formula (p. 50) for use with the gastrostomy tube is suitable. Since there is frequently inability to evacuate the bladder or the bowel, these acts must be done for the patient. When there is incontinence the patient should be bathed after each voiding or defecation.

The state of consciousness is determined by the patient's ability to respond. When the patient is unconscious, there is no response to any stimulus; during stupor, painful stimuli will provoke a response. Sometimes there may be inability to talk because the speech center is affected, but the patient may respond by performing certain acts when requested. Asking the patient to squeeze both hands of the nurse not only tests his orientation but also demonstrates any weakness or paralysis. Observation of the movement of the face and legs should be made. Weakness or paralysis may be detected if there is asymmetry of the face when the patient is asked to show his teeth, or if he is unable to move one or both legs. Tremors, convulsions, weaknesses or paralysis should be noted. Memory and orientation are important criteria of the patient's recovery.

Following craniotomy there is frequently considerable edema of the tissues of the head which may lead to closure of both eyes. Cold compresses are then indicated to reduce swelling. The corneal reflex is tested with a wisp of cotton and when it is impaired the lids are frequently sutured shut (tarsorrhaphy), or irrigation and ointment followed by an eye shield may be ordered.

The irresponsible behavior of the semiconscious patient requires watchfulness. He may try to get out of bed, take off the head bandage, or remove the urethral catheter; his conversation may be uninhibited. Such a patient should be protected from visitors except those of the immediate family. Aphasic patients who are having difficulty either in understanding or in expressing themselves, or both, are particularly in need of help and encouragement.

As the patient progresses in his recovery, he should be encouraged to do things for himself in so far as he is able. Bathing himself should be encouraged, but if the patient is irresponsible close supervision is necessary. The patient is gotten up according to his condition, sometimes as early as the second or third day. If he has some weakness in either of his extremities, a walker is of value to lend support and confidence.

Any change in the state of consciousness, fever, blood pressure, pulse or respirations during his convalescence may be signs of severe complications. These need to be reported to the surgeon immediately because immediate attention is called for.

During the convalescent period, plans should be made as soon as possible to prepare the patient for life outside the hospital. When a large tumor has been removed, there is frequently slow progress in ability to think, remember, and to give self-care. The family or those who will be responsible for the patient must be encouraged and told that improvement may be slow but often there is greater ability to adapt at home in familiar surroundings.

Women are usually sensitive about their shaven head; an attractive turban worn until the hair grows out allows them to go about the ward and to leave the hospital without feeling conspicuous. Before the patient leaves the hospital the scalp should be cleaned with oil to remove crusts and a shampoo given.

The plans for home care of some patients require the need for further nursing care, either full-time or by a visiting nurse. The social worker can often give valuable help to the family in preparing for the care of the patient.

BRAIN ABSCESS; TUBERCULOMA

An abscess in the brain, resulting from the extension of infection from mastoiditis or sinusitis or from bacteria deposited in the brain by the blood stream, produces the symptoms and signs of brain tumor, since the abscess and surrounding inflammatory swelling occupy space within the skull. Multiple brain abscesses are almost always fatal, with death usually resulting from increased intracranial pressure. A solitary abscess may be cured by drainage or by simple tapping of the abscess. Antibiotics are used in treating brain abscesses with dramatic results. Similar inflammatory tumors are caused by tuberculosis; these tumors are usually multiple, and cure is becoming more frequent with chemotherapy and antibiotic therapy.

SUBDURAL HEMATOMA

This moderately common lesion is probably always traumatic in origin. Usually a slight blow on the head, so trivial as to be quickly forgotten, is responsible for a slow hemorrhage due to injury of a vessel on the surface of the brain. The free blood lies between the dura and the arachnoid and gives rise to signs of cerebral compression. Absorption in the subdural space is extremely poor and the hematoma may actually increase in size because of fresh hemorrhage or the high osmotic pressure of the hematoma. Subdural hematomas are bilateral in about 15 per cent of the cases and give rise to such symptoms as loss of memory, speech difficulties and dizziness. In children, particularly those with scurvy, subdural hematomas frequently develop which are usually bilateral. Accurate diagnosis is made by ventriculography, and evacuation of the subdural blood results in cure.

INTRACRANIAL ANEURYSMS

There is, in man, only one place in which an artery courses directly through a vein, and that is where the carotid artery passes through the cavernous venous sinus in the base of the skull. Not infrequently this region is damaged when the skull is fractured, and such an injury results in the formation of a carotid-cavernous arteriovenous aneurysm. Characterized by a loud cranial mummur (*bruit*) usually heard by the patient, these aneurysms cause serious interference with the circulation of the brain and face, and produce a striking pulsating exophthalmos on the same side.

Another type of arteriovenous aneurysm, the cirsoid, occurs on the surface of the brain. These aneurysms are of congenital origin, and usually cause convulsions. Small arterial aneurysms occur in the branches of the small arteries at the base of the brain. These too are usually congenital, and may cause hemorrhage of a serious nature.

The only cure for any of these aneurysmal lesions is occlusion of the vessels involved, when this is possible.

SUMMARY

Brain tumors and other space-occupying lesions within the cranium cause symptoms by compressing and/or damaging a portion of the brain. In addition to neurologic examination, special technics of examination include ventriculography, arteriography, and electroencephalography. Personality changes and other disabilities before and after operation require special nursing skill.

VOCABULARY REVIEW

glioma   *hemianopsia*   *paralysis*
meningioma   *trephine*   *aphasia*
hydrocephalus   *pneumoencephalography*   *tuberculoma*
                     craniotomy

SUGGESTED READING

1. Cecil, Russell L., and Loeb, Robert F.: A Textbook of Medicine. 8th Ed. Philadelphia, W. B. Saunders Co., 1950, pp. 1470–1482.
2. Dandy, Walter E.: Surgery of the Brain, in Lewis' Practice of Surgery. Hagerstown, W. F. Prior Co., *12:*1–682, 1932.
3. Dotter, Pamela, and Wade, Eleanor: Brain Tumor. Am. J. Nursing, *51:* 300–303 (May) 1951.
4. Krause, Marie V.: Nutrition and Diet Therapy. Philadelphia, W. B. Saunders Co., 1950, pp. 333–341.
5. Penfield, W., and Steelman, H.: The Treatment of Focal Epilepsy by Cortical Excision. Ann. Surg., *126:*740–762 (Nov.) 1947.
6. Pilcher, Cobb: Preoperative and Postoperative Care in Neurosurgical Procedures. Arch. Surg., *40:*1176–1184 (June) 1940.
7. Rand, Carl W.: The Neurosurgical Patient. Springfield, Charles C Thomas, 1944, p. 442.
8. Roseman, Ephraim, and Taylor, Anne: Progress in the Treatment of Epilepsy. Am. J. Nursing, *52:*437–440 (April) 1952.
9. Walker, A. E., and Johnson, H. C.: Surgical Treatment of Epilepsy. Am. J. Surg., *55:*200–218 (Jan.) 1948.
10. Walker, A. E.: Treatment of Epilepsy by Cortical Excision. J. Pediatrics, *38:* 285–298 (March) 1951.

CHAPTER 39

Surgery of the Cranial Nerves

The cranial nerves are often affected in both intracranial injuries and brain tumors. Some of the nerves are more sensitive to pressure than others. For example, double vision (*diplopia*) caused by injury to one or more of the special motor nerves to the eye muscles, is often an indication of general increase in intracranial pressure, but corneal anesthesia is caused only by direct involvement of the trigeminal nerve or its nucleus in the brain stem. Unless the nerve has been permanently damaged, the successful removal of a tumor or the relief of pressure is followed by complete restoration of function. Of all the cranial nerves the tenth or vagus nerve is the only one carrying impulses essential for life.

If the vagus nerve is destroyed on one side only, there will be paralysis of the vocal cord on the same side, with consequent disturbance of phonation, and serious interference with the mechanism for swallowing. The latter difficulty may necessitate tube feeding. Destruction of both vagi is followed by respiratory difficulty (paralysis of both vocal cords) and inability to swallow without aspiration (loss of cough reflex and paralysis of glottis).

Tumors in the cerebellopontine angle often involve the tenth nerve as well as the fifth, seventh, and eighth, and the outcome depends upon the success of the surgeon in saving the tenth nerve. Paralysis of the facial muscles (which are innervated by the seventh cranial nerve) is another frequent complication associated with these tumors, as it is also with fracture of the skull and mastoid infection. When destruction of the intracranial portion of the facial nerve has occurred it is possible to secure partial return of function by anastomosing the extracranial portion of the facial nerve to the central portion of another nerve, usually the spinal accessory or the hypoglossal. When successful, this procedure restores tone to the paralyzed facial muscles, thus improving facial expression, and often a patient learns to control the newly innervated muscles quite well. There is, of course, paralysis of the trapezius muscle when the eleventh nerve is used for this purpose, but no serious deformity or disability results.

438

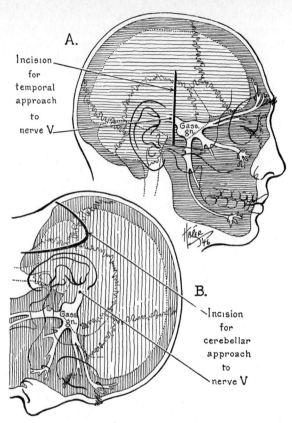

A.

Incision
for
temporal
approach
to
nerve V

Gass.
gn.

B.

Incision
for
cerebellar
approach
to
nerve V

Gass.
gn.

FIGURE 115. Surgical treatment of trigeminal neuralgia. *A*, Temporal approach to N. *V.; B*, cerebellar approach to N. *V.*

TRIGEMINAL NEURALGIA

The cause of this common and extremely painful affliction, also known as tic douloureux, is not known.

Symptoms. Trigeminal neuralgia is characterized by frequent attacks of almost unbearably severe pain occurring in the distribution of one or more of the branches of the fifth cranial nerve. The pain is sudden, shooting, or stabbing, and there is often a small area of face or tongue (*trigger zone*) the stimulation of which starts up an attack. Occasionally the pain is bilateral in distribution, indicating that both nerves are affected.

Treatment. The attacks may be abolished by any procedure which renders the nerve functionless. This may be accomplished in three ways: (1) by injection of alcohol into a part or the whole of the nerve; (2) by division of the branches of the nerve as they issue from the skull; and (3) by division of the nerve within the skull. In recent years a fourth method, namely, section of the pain fibers to the face within the medulla, has been devised. Tactile sensation would be spared by this procedure. However, the hazards of the operative procedure, along with the certain damage to contiguous structures, make the disadvantages far outweigh the advantages.

Of these methods, the third is followed by the fewest complications and recurrences. The muscles of mastication need not be paralyzed, and at times some sensation in the face and tongue of the affected side is preserved. One constant and enduring hazard after the operation is the anesthesia of the cornea which follows destruction of the nerve. The natural protective mechanism of the cornea is thus rendered defective, and corneal ulceration sometimes occurs, particularly when proper care is not taken to protect the eye at all times.

Nursing Care. The nurse should teach the patient to be responsible for the protection of his eye. A daily boric acid eye wash to cleanse the eye and the wearing of glasses fittted with a side shield to prevent foreign bodies from coming into contact with the eye help to prevent corneal irritation. The patient should be taught to look into every mirror he passes to detect any abnormality.

Herpes of the lips and face, originating from trauma, is another complication which is often very annoying. If this condition is persistent the nurse should help the patient to select a bland diet to prevent irritation.

Sometimes the patient may complain of losing particles of food between his teeth and cheek on the affected side. Until he is accustomed to the loss of sensation on the side of his face he should be warned to take care while eating to avoid biting his cheek. Good oral care should be emphasized by teaching the patient to cleanse his mouth after each meal.

GLOSSOPHARYNGEAL NEURALGIA

A rare form of tic involves the ninth nerve (*glossopharyngeal*) instead of the fifth nerve. In this form the distribution of the pain is limited to the portion of the pharynx supplied by the ninth nerve, but the pain is of the same type. Cure of this form is also effected by division of the appropriate nerve within the skull.

MÉNIÈRE'S DISEASE

Somewhat less frequent in occurrence than tic douloureux, Ménière's disease is an affection of the eighth cranial nerve.

Symptoms. Since this nerve is composed of two parts, the auditory branch which transmits the impulses of hearing from the ear, and the vestibular branch, which carries the impulses of equilibrium from the semicircular canals, two types of symptoms may be expected: (1) gradual loss of hearing (*deafness*) and noise in the ear (*tinnitus*); and (2) attacks of violent dizziness (*vertigo*) accompanied by nausea and vomiting. The attacks vary greatly in frequency, intensity, and duration. When severe they are incapacitating. The sensation is familiar to those susceptible to seasickness, or to those who remember the childhood experience of unwinding rapidly in a twisted rope swing. The vertigo is at times so severe as to cause the patient to feel as though he had been thrown to the ground. The deafness and tinnitus may be intensified during attacks. This disease also is occasionally bilateral.

Treatment. Cessation of the attacks of vertigo results from the division of the vestibular branch of the eighth nerve within the skull. Restoration of hearing does not follow operation, but whatever hearing the patient may have had may be preserved. The attacks of vertigo do not recur. During the immediate postoperative period, however, the patient may have intense dizziness, which gradually diminishes within a few hours or a few days, at most. Tinnitus is frequently abolished or improved. Other forms of treatment such as a salt-free diet or histamine injections may give temporary relief to some patients.

Nursing Care. The postoperative care should include close observation of the temperature, pulse and respirations. The patient sometimes has difficulty in voiding. Warming the bedpan, turning on the spigot so there is the sound of running water, and allowing the patient as much privacy as is possible help him to void voluntarily. If this is not successful the surgeon's permission may be sought to permit the patient to sit up in bed. This may be contraindicated, or the surgeon may prefer that the nurse give the patient an enema.

Since only a small amount of hair on the posterior part of the scalp has been shaved, in women the hair is often tangled and matted when the head dressing is removed. Dampening the hair with 70 per cent alcohol makes combing much easier.

Atttempting to walk at first often proves difficult because of the loss of balance on the operative side. When the patient stands or walks he feels that he is being pulled toward the side of operation. Teaching him to walk along the corridor with his hand against the wall prevents him from falling. He must be taught that he should learn to retain his balance by depending on his eyes. This patient needs frequent words of reassurance because at times he appears to have complete lack of confidence in himself.

SPASMODIC TORTICOLLIS

This curious condition, known also as wryneck, is very distressing. Spasmodic contraction of the muscles of the neck innervated by the spinal accessory nerves (*eleventh cranial nerve*) and the upper pairs of cervical spinal nerves produces grotesque deformity and disability. The cause of the condition is not understood. Surgical treatment is designed to paralyze the affected muscles by dividing the spinal accessory nerves and the upper cervical nerves. The resultant deformity and disability, however, may be considerable.

SUMMARY

The important functions of the twelve pairs of cranial nerves are especially apparent when the nerves are affected by injury or disease. Trigeminal neuralgia and Ménière's disease are common afflictions and can be cured by surgery.

VOCABULARY REVIEW

diplopia   *tinnitus*   *torticollis*
tic douloureux   *vertigo*

SUGGESTED READING

1. Christopher, Frederick: A Textbook of Surgery. 5th Ed. Philadelphia, W. B. Saunders Co., 1947, pp. 524–532.
2. Dandy, W. E.: Ménière's Disease, Its Diagnosis and Treatment. Arch. Surg., *16*:1127–1152, 1928.
3. Fedder, Helma: Trigeminal Neuralgia. Am. J. Nursing, *48*:370–371 (June) 1948.
4. Green, Robert E., and Douglass, Carleton C.: Intracranial Division of the Eighth Nerve for Ménière's Disease; A Follow-up Study of Patients Operated on by Dr. Walter E. Dandy. Ann. Otology, Rhinology and Laryngology, *60*:610–621 (Sept.) 1951.

5. Merritt, H. Houston: Trigeminal Neuralgia. Am. J. Nursing, *48:*368–370 (June) 1948.
6. Walker, A. E.: Relief of Facial Pain. M. Clin. N. America, *29:*73–97 (Jan.) 1945.

CHAPTER 40

Surgery of the Spinal Cord

Much that has been said about the brain (p. 411) applies equally to the spinal cord. It, too, is a soft structure composed of nerve cells and fiber tracts, invested by the same membranes, and enclosed in a nonexpanding sheath, the spinal canal. The cord is as susceptible to damage from compression as is the brain. The motor nerves and fibers are more easily damaged than are the sensory, but in time both are affected.

Fracture and dislocation of the spine are often complicated by injury to the spinal cord. The most important consideration is the realization that, since such damage to the cord as has already occurred is irreparable, no further damage must be permitted: therefore, the utmost care must be taken in transporting patients with spinal injuries and in carrying out therapeutic procedures.

Traumatic Paraplegia. Although severe injuries to the spine which damage the spinal cord and result in paralysis of the extremities have always occurred in civilian life, the rapid accumulation of large numbers of such patients during World War II served to focus attention on the problem. When the injury is in the cervical region, with paralysis of all four extremities and of all of the muscles of the chest and abdomen, the patient does not survive long. Injuries resulting in paralysis of the lower extremities only are compatible with life. The chief problems involved are the care of the lower urinary tract, the avoidance of decubitus ulcers, the maintenance of nutrition and the rehabilitation of the individual.[1]

DIAGNOSIS OF SPINAL CORD INJURIES

Localization. Pain is a common symptom since the spinal nerves are often affected and the distribution of the pain is often

[1] Brown, pages 766–790.

a localizing sign. The segmental distribution of the spinal nerves helps in the localization of cord lesions, since alteration of function may occur in those portions of the body which are served by spinal nerves situated at the site of the lesion or below it. For example, a tumor or an injury in the midthoracic region may cause loss of sensation in the legs and the loss of motor function of the legs, together with disturbance of bladder and rectal control, but there will be no impairment of the function of the arms.

Queckenstedt Sign. When a tumor has filled the available space in the spinal canal and the cord is compressed, obstruction to the flow of cerebrospinal fluid occurs. This spinal block can be observed by the absence of response to compression of the jugular vein, which normally causes a rise in spinal fluid pressure, as measured by spinal puncture (*Queckenstedt test*). The location of such a block can be visualized by roentgenograms taken after the injection of radiopaque oil into the spinal canal.

HERNIATED NUCLEUS PULPOSUS

Another complication of spinal injury, now frequently recognized, is rupture or dislocation of an intervertebral disk. Commonly causing low back and sciatic pain, this lesion may also simulate a spinal cord tumor. The proper treatment is removal of the disk.

Postoperative Nursing Care. After the operation the patient is placed in a bed which has had a fracture board placed beneath a regular mattress. The patient usually has severe pain in his back which may be relieved by opiates. Turning should be encouraged at least every hour; the nurse should assure the patient that he will not injure his back while turning. The dressings are examined frequently for bleeding. The ability of the patient to move both his legs with equal ease, and the presence of sensation in both legs should be carefully noted. The male patient often has difficulty in voiding. When all the measures that encourage voiding such as turning on the water in the room, and the giving of an enema or Prostigmin fail, the surgeon may permit the patient to stand up or to sit on the edge of the bed.

The surgeon usually orders that the patient wear a corset after he is discharged. The corsetière should measure the patient a day or two after operation so that the final fitting may be made the day he leaves the hospital. Conservative postoperative treatment consists in advising the patient not to return to work for three months and to refrain from lifting in the interim.

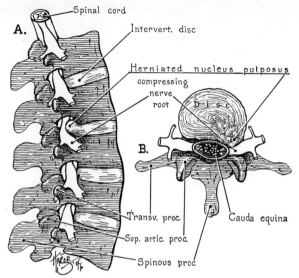

FIGURE 116. Herniated nucleus pulposus (ruptured intervertebral disk).

TUMORS OF THE SPINAL CORD

The same varieties of neoplastic and infectious tumors are found in the spinal cord as in the brain, and the general plan of treatment is the same. When such a tumor can be removed completely before serious damage to the cord has occurred, there will be return of function.

LAMINECTOMY

The spinal cord is exposed surgically by dividing the flat bony processes (*laminae*) of the vertebrae. The dura lies beneath the bone, and when it is opened the spinal cord and its pairs of spinal nerves are seen floating in spinal fluid. The motor and the sensory root of each spinal nerve are separate as they leave the spinal cord, uniting after they pierce the dura. This anatomic fact makes possible the division of sensory fibers (*chordotomy*) for the relief of intractable pain without producing paralysis of the affected part. In the closure of laminectomy wounds the bone is not replaced since the thick muscles of the back afford sufficient protection to the cord. As in surgery of the brain, there is no place here for rough handling of tissues, poor hemostasis, or lack of asepsis. In the postoperative period certain essential precautions must be observed.

Nursing Care

Great care must be taken to avoid injuring the spinal cord by movement of the temporarily weakened spine. Several nurses and/or attendants are needed to turn such a patient. Decubitus ulcers and urinary tract infection must be guarded against, since the sequelae of one or both of these commonly cause death following operation on or injury to the spinal cord.

The nurse needs to be especially watchful and careful when there has been a serious injury to the cord caused by an accident or by an infiltrating tumor. A sponge mattress and a cradle to elevate the bedclothes at the foot of the bed aid in preventing bedsores. Frequent bathing, massaging, and turning help to prevent decubitus ulcers. There should be a definite routine for carrying out the plan of nursing. At no time should the patient be allowed to remain in one position for more than a very few hours during the day or night. The bedclothes should be kept immaculate.

Voluntary urination is often inhibited. A hot enema sometimes increases the ability to void. When there is paralysis of the bladder, incontinence may be present with resultant irritation and maceration of the perineal skin. Permanent catheterization and tidal drainage of the bladder may be necessary, even though this often leads to urinary infection. Careful attention should be paid to distention and constipation. Incontinence of feces can be controlled in most cases by the administration of a daily enema given after breakfast.

Nursing Care Following Chordotomy. The terminal cancer patient who has unbearable pain from metastases from cancer is the most frequent candidate for chordotomy. Such a patient is usually undernourished, sleeps poorly, and is extremely uncomfortable even though large doses of sedatives and analgesics are given frequently.

The physical preparation is similar to that for either general or local anesthesia. The patient and/or a member of his family have been informed that the operation will be done to relieve pain, but in so doing the temperature sense will be lost.

When a unilateral chordotomy is performed, the patient will have analgesia on the side opposite beginning a few segments down from the operative lesion. A bilateral chordotomy produces complete analgesia and loss of temperature sense a little below the level of the operation. In addition, such a patient usually is incontinent for a few days after operation; incontinence is usually not permanent.

The release from pain which these patients gain is most gratifying, but they and those who care for them must know that thermal burning can take place without the patient's knowledge. Hot water bottles or other heating devices should not be permitted. The patient can feel, but the senses of pain and temperature which normally protect against injury have been lost.

SUMMARY

The most common lesion affecting the spinal cord and its nerves is the dislocation of an intervertebral disk. Serious injuries usually cause permanent paralysis necessitating long-term care and rehabilitation.

VOCABULARY REVIEW

paraplegia	*nucleus pulposus*	*chordotomy*
Queckenstedt	*laminectomy*	*analgesia*

SUGGESTED READING

1. Bruck, Helen: Nursing the Laminectomy Patient. Am. J. Nursing, *51*:158 (Mar.) 1951.
2. Cooper, Irving S., Craig, Winchell M., and Kernohan, James W.: Tumors of the Spinal Cord. Surg., Gynec. & Obst. *92*:183–190 (Feb.) 1951.
3. Hamby, Wallace: The Hospital Care of Neurosurgical Patients. 2nd Ed. Springfield, Charles C Thomas, 1948, pp. 113–135.
4. Mount, Lester A.: Injuries of the Spinal Cord. Am. J. Nursing, *45*:101–103 (Feb.) 1945.
5. Woodruff, Margaret B.: To Prevent Pressure Sores. Am. J. Nursing, *52*:606 (May) 1952.

CHAPTER 41

Nursing in Ophthalmology

Aristotle said that the eye is the chief organ through which objective reality is appreciated and that sight is the most comprehensive of all the senses. The importance of proper care of the eyes is obvious to all. In addition to disorders peculiar to the eyes, many ocular lesions are manifestations of such systemic diseases as diabetes, hypertension, nephritis, endocrine disturbances, syphilis, and brain tumors: indeed, the eye lesion is often the earliest cause of the patient's symptoms so that the ophthalmologist is the first doctor consulted. Because of the large number of general diseases that affect the eyes, ophthalmology is, perhaps, more closely related to general medicine than any other specialty.

Anatomy and Physiology of the Eye. The eye is a slightly oval globe situated within the orbit which, in turn, is a cone-shaped cavity formed by the bones of the skull. The orbit affords protection to the eye from external trauma. Because of the close

449

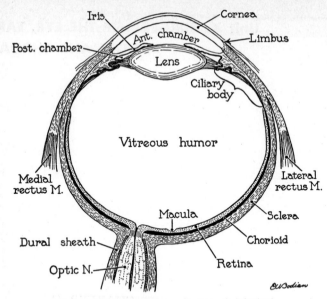

FIGURE 117. The eye (cross section of right eye).

anatomic relation of the orbit to the adjacent nasal sinuses, bacteria sometimes pass from infected sinuses through the bony barrier to involve the eye. Within this bony cavity the eyeball itself is held in a cushion of orbital fat which permits motion of the eye and also absorbs shock to the eye.

Muscles. Attached to each eye are six muscles, known as the extraocular muscles. For each eye there is one muscle above, one below, and one on each side; these are named superior, inferior, internal and external rectus muscles from their respective positions. Also there are superior and inferior oblique muscles which have a transverse course. These six muscles are innervated by the third, fourth, and sixth cranial nerves, and they all coordinate to accomplish the simultaneous movements of the two eyes.

Eyelids. The eyes are covered anteriorly by the lids, which are made up of skin, muscle (for opening and closing the lids), a stiff cartilaginous strip called the tarsus, and a thin inner covering of epithelium known as conjunctiva, which is a continuation of the conjunctiva which covers the globe and is known as the bulbar conjunctiva.

Glands. The lids contain two groups of secretory glands, the meibomian glands and the glands of Moll. These secrete lubricants for the front of the eyeball. At the outer margin of the orbit, just beneath its bony rim, lies the lacrimal gland which secretes the tears that bathe the front of the eye. The tears pass from the lacrimal gland downward toward the inner (*nasal*) portion of the cornea where they are drained off into the punctum, a small opening at the inner margin of each lid. Each punctum opens into a thin tube (*canaliculus*) which ends in the lacrimal sac. The lacrimal sac in turn lies in a bony fossa along the side of the nose. From this sac the tears finally pass through the nasal duct into the inferior meatus of the nose where they are absorbed by the mucous membranes.

Eyeball. The eyeball itself is a closed sphere about 1 inch in diameter. It is made up of three main coats or layers known as the sclera, choroid, and retina.

THE SCLERA. The sclera, or outer protective layer, is the thickest and is composed of fibrous tissue. It forms the posterior five sixths of the globe, the anterior one sixth being formed by the transparent cornea. The junction of clear cornea and opaque sclera is known as the limbus. The anterior portion of the sclera is covered by the bulbar conjunctiva, which is continuous with the conjunctiva covering the inner surface of the lids.

THE RETINA. The retina, or nerve layer, is the innermost coat of the globe. It is a thin tissue composed of the elements (*rods* and *cones*), which pick up an image, and the nerve fibers which conduct the image by way of the optic nerve to the brain. The retina covers the posterior two thirds of the globe, being attached posteriorly at the optic nerve and anteriorly at the ora serrata where it passes into the ciliary body. The retina has often been compared to the film in a camera because it is the portion of the eye that is sensitive to light. In the center of the posterior portion of the retina there is a 0.5 mm. area known as the macula lutea in which cones alone are found. It is with this area that we are able to see small objects. In the remainder of the retina the rods predominate and only large objects can be distinguished. Vision in the dark, however, is best when using the peripheral area of the retina.

THE CHOROID. The choroid, or nutrient layer, lies between the retina and the sclera. It consists of many blood vessels in a supporting structure of connective tissue. These vessels bring nourishment to the retina, the vitreous humor, and indirectly to the lens. The iris, ciliary body, and choroid are spoken of collectively as the uveal tract, and are so intimately associated that when one portion becomes diseased the others are usually affected also.

CILIARY BODY. Anteriorly the choroid passes into the ciliary body, an elevated body from which the lens is suspended by many thin fibers called zonular fibers. The ciliary body has two functions, namely, the formation of the aqueous humor, and the changing of the lens from thin to thick to enable the person to see equally clearly for far and near objects (power of accommodation).

IRIS. Continuous with the ciliary body, and hanging behind the cornea like a curtain, is the iris. This is a pigmented membrane, circular in form, which gives to the eye its characteristic color (e.g., brown or blue).

PUPIL. The iris is perforated in the center by an opening of variable size known as the pupil. Dilatation and contraction of the iris govern the size of the pupil, which in turn controls the amount of light entering the eye.

THE MEDIA. The clear translucent portions of the eye, that is, cornea, aqueous, lens, and vitreous, are spoken of collectively as the media of the eye.

The lens, a clear biconvex body, is suspended between the aqueous and vitreous chambers. Just in front of the lens lies the iris.

The smaller aqueous chamber is the space between the lens and the posterior surface of the cornea. It is filled with aqueous humor, a clear watery fluid which is secreted constantly by the ciliary body. This passes through the pupillary space, brings nourishment to the lens and cornea, and is drained off by the canal of Schlemm in the angle formed by the root of the iris and the periphery of the cornea.

The vitreous chamber lies between the lens and the retina and is filled by a gelatinous substance called the vitreous humor which is largely responsible for maintaining the shape of the eyeball.

Image Formation. The optic nerve passes from the posterior pole of the eye through an opening in the orbit into the cranial cavity where it meets the nerve from the other eye and joins the brain. Here the nerves partially cross and continue backward on each side along the temporal and parietal lobes as the optic tracts and radiations, to end finally in the occipital or posterior lobes of the brain. Light rays from an object pass through the cornea, aqueous humor, lens, and vitreous, and are bent (refracted) by these structures so that the rays strike the retina. The stimulus of the light is picked up by the rods and cones, and is carried along the optic pathways of the brain to the occipital lobes, where finally the seen image is registered upon the conscious mind of the individual (Fig. 110, p. 425).

METHODS OF EXAMINING THE EYE

Much of the eye can be examined directly; even the interior of the eye, because of the transparency of the cornea, lens, and humors, can be visually examined. In addition, careful tests can be made of the functional ability of the eye. The muscles which control the movements of the eye in its orbit (extraocular movements) are tested by having the patient observe a moving object, usually the examiner's finger. Pupillary reactions are tested by means of strong light, and by making the patient shift his gaze from nearby to distant objects (*accommodation*).

Instruments. When inspecting the lids, conjunctiva, and cornea the ophthalmologist may wear a pair of magnifying spectacles (a *loupe*) or use a special binocular microscope. By means of a fine beam of light projected through the transparent media of the eye from a *slit lamp* it is possible to detect opacities in the different media. The retina itself is directly observed by means of the *ophthalmoscope;* through the peep-hole in this instrument the examiner can see the illuminated retina and its blood vessels. The *perimeter* is used to outline tthe extent of the visual fields, and the *tonometer* is used to measure the tension of the globe.

REFRACTION

By refraction is meant the determination of the refractive error in the eyes of the patient. Refractive error is a term which is used to signify a failure on the part of the various light-transmitting portions of the eye to bring the light rays into a correct focus on the retina. It is the commonest cause of defective vision (poor eyesight). The amount and nature of the existing refractive error are measured both directly and by means of trial lenses. The ophthalmologist can then prescribe for the patient the spectacle lenses needed to bring all the light rays to a proper focus on the retina. When this is done, normal vision is the result. The fundamental refractive errors are myopia, hyperopia, and astigmatism. All of these conditions cause blurring of the image. They may be found alone or in any combination.

Myopia. Myopia (near-sightedness) is caused by an overlong anteroposterior diameter of the eyeball, which causes the light rays to focus in front of the retina.

Hyperopia. This condition (far-sightedness) occurs when the eyeball is too short, so that the rays focus behind the retina.

Presbyopia. Presbyopia is a refractive condition, occurring between the ages of 40 and 43, wherein one is unable to see near objects clearly. As we grow older, the fibers of the lens harden and the muscles that make the lens fat and thin weaken, thereby bringing about a lessening of the power of accommodation. This causes near objects to be blurred and a magnifying lens is then necessary to enable the person to read. At first, a weak lens suffices but this has to be strengthened about every two years as the person grows older. If one already uses a glass for distance vision, bifocals will be necessary when he becomes presbyopic.

Astigmatism. Astigmatism results from asymmetry of the corneal curvature, so that rays in the perpendicular plane do not focus at the same point as rays in the horizontal plane.

Cycloplegics. In all patients under the age of 40 years refraction should be done when the eye is under the influence of a *cycloplegic* (a drug which paralyzes the muscles of accommodation). In children up to the age of 12 atropine is used; in patients between 12 and 40 homatropine is the cycloplegic employed. After the age of 40 no cycloplegic is necessary because the power of accommodation has become relatively weak.

OFFICE NURSING
(See also p. 469)

When employed as office nurse for an ophthalmologist, the nurse is expected to instil drops, give irrigations, sterilize and care for instruments, drops and supplies, and assist with the removal of foreign bodies, other minor operations, and dressings. The eye is an exquisitely sensitive organ; because of this it is necessary to limit the strength of local applications and to be extremely careful in the manner of their application.

Atropine Poisoning. In some patients atropine causes toxic symptoms, including flushing of the face, dryness of the throat, skin rash, vomiting, rapid pulse, excitability, and occasionally delirium. A less serious, occasional result of the prolonged use of atropine is a local reddening of the skin of the eyelids. This disappears when use of the drug is discontinued. Individuals who are either very young or blonde or both, seem more susceptible than others. If any of these symptoms appear the doctor should

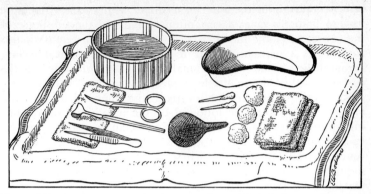

FIGURE 118. Dressing tray. All items are sterile, and include forceps, lid retractor, iris scissors (for removing sutures), basin containing irrigation solution, irrigating syringe, curved basin, toothpick swabs, cotton and gauze.

be notified at once. For patients known to have or suspected of having sensitivity to atropine, scopolamine hydrobromide is used rather than atropine.

INJURIES AND THEIR COMPLICATIONS
Foreign Bodies

The commonest source of injury to the eyes is due to their constant exposure, and is most frequently encountered in a windy and dusty environment. We have all been through this unpleasant experience, some more frequently than others because the reflex that closes the lids varies greatly in speed; people with a slow reflex suffer foreign bodies more often. Many foreign bodies are removed with the corner of a gauze square or a clean handkerchief, but this practice should be discouraged because of the danger of introducing infection into the eye. All cases in which the foreign body is stuck firmly require the aid of a doctor.

Treatment. The eye is first anesthetized with a drop or two of Pontocaine or other local anesthetic, and the patient is comfortably seated with his head in a good light. An effort is first made to remove the foreign body with the end of a sterile toothpick swab; and if this fails a sterile instrument called a spud must be used to pick the body off the cornea. The spud has a thin narrow blade which can be inserted beneath the foreign body to loosen it from the underlying cornea. Since the cornea is only 0.5 mm. thick in some areas, great care is necessary to prevent penetration of the anterior chamber. In the case of metallic foreign bodies a ring of rust often remains in the substance of the cornea after the metal particle itself has been removed; this rust causes a permanent scar if neglected. Its removal is best accomplished by the use of a small dental burr which grinds the rust away while doing the least possible damage to the cornea.

Removal of foreign bodies requiring more than minimal manipulation should be followed by the instillation of a lubricant into the eye and the application of an eyepad to the eye. In addition, in severe cases atropine should be instilled to prevent the traumatic iritis which so often results. These patients should be observed on the day following treatment to be sure that no infection is beginning.

Foreign bodies moving at high velocity occasionally penetrate the eyeball. If the damage to the globe is considerable, enucleation (removal of the eyeball) is usually necessary. Small fragments of steel or other metals, however, sometimes are driven into the eyeball without causing more than a tiny puncture wound. Such foreign bodies must be removed; this is done by first localizing the foreign body by x-ray and then using a strong electromagnet to draw the fragment out of the globe.

Hematoma of the Orbit

The ordinary "black eye" is of common occurrence. The treatment of this condition consists in the application of cold compresses for the first twenty-four hours to reduce the bleeding into the tissues. It is, of course, this bleeding that accounts for the discoloration and swelling about the eye. After twenty-four hours hot compresses are applied to hasten the absorption of the blood. The classic remedy of applying a beefsteak to a black eye is in reality nothing more nor less than a form of compressing. Another old-fashioned remedy, however, applying leeches to a black eye, is harmful because this increases the bleeding instead of checking it.

Lacerations of the Lids and Eye

These are not so frequent as might be expected considering the large number of people who wear glasses. The rapid lid-closing reflex saves many an eye when glasses are broken. Lid lacerations should be repaired by an ophthalmologist, if one is available, because these lacerations require an entirely different technic than do lacerations in other areas in order to prevent an ugly and damaging V-shaped notching of their healed margin.

Lacerations of the globe itself, though infrequent, are most serious because of the likelihood that they will be followed by reduction of the vision. Patients suffering this condition should be seen by an ophthalmologist as soon as possible, as early operative attention is essential. Wounds of the cornea may be closed by a corneal suture which pulls the lips of the wound together directly, or they may be held together by a conjunctival flap which has been undermined from above or below and drawn over the cornea to cover the wound completely. After the cornea has healed the conjunctival flap is released and it returns to its former normal position. In either case any protruding portion of the inner structures of the eye, such as the iris, lens, vitreous, or uveal tract, must be excised before the wound is closed. Such tissue should never be replaced in the eye because of the danger of introducing infection with it. Lacerations of the sclera and conjunctiva are closed edge to edge. In the case of scleral perforations, cautery punctures are made around the involved areas in an effort to prevent the underlying retina from becoming detached.

Sympathetic Ophthalmia

All lacerations of the globe involving the uveal tract are potential sources of further danger. One fourth of one per cent of all such injuries are followed by sympathetic ophthalmia, an extremely serious complication. In this condition the uninjured eye develops a destructive inflammatory reaction which, prior to the introduction of cortisone, always resulted in great reduction of the vision of both eyes. Why or how this occurs is not understood. It has not been observed earlier than twelve days following the injury to the first eye, and never developed after the early removal of an injured eye. Because of the grave nature of this condition, the possibility of its development in all cases of injury to the uveal tract must be kept in mind, and treatment with cortisone begun at the earliest suspicion. The success of this treatment saves many eyes which in previous years would have been removed.

Enucleation. Where sympathetic ophthalmia is suspected or where a laceration has been so great as to have allowed the escape of the contents of the globe, or in cases of malignant intraocular tumor, the eye must be removed. This operation is called enucleation. In it the conjunctiva is incised completely around the limbus and is separated by blunt dissection from the underlying structures. Next, the four rectus muscles are identified and divided from their attachments to the globe; sutures are placed in their cut ends. The globe is then separated from Tenon's capsule, which is the muscle cone that surrounds the posterior portion, back to the posterior pole where the optic nerve leaves the globe. The optic nerve is then divided a few millimeters from the globe so as to be sure not to enter and collapse the globe, and the eyeball is lifted out of the orbit. Bleeding is controlled with warm sponges. A plastic ball, a little smaller than the globe, is placed in Tenon's capsule, the capsule and the rectus muscles are closed over this implant, and finally the conjunctiva is closed. On healing this leaves a useful stump on which can be worn a concave prosthesis, colored to match the other eye. In successful cases movement of this artificial eye is so good that it is difficult to distinguish it from the normal eye.

Evisceration. When there is infection within the eyeball, this procedure is used in place of enucleation. The cornea and a thin rim of adjacent sclera are removed; through this opening the contents of the eyeball are taken out, leaving only the sclera.

Retinal Detachment

The retina is attached to the underlying structures of the eye only at the anterior and posterior borders. Over the remainder of its surface it is held in contact with the choroid by pressure of the semisolid mass of vitreous humor that fills the vitreous chamber. Blows to the eye and degenerative processes produce tears in the retina through which the humor enters; this causes elevation or separation of the thin retina from the choroid. Such an elevation is known as a retinal detachment. The visual field is lost over the area corresponding to the detachment and when the macular area is involved the visual acuity is greatly reduced. In an occasional case the retina will flatten out and become reattached if the patient is made to lie on his back in bed. Such cures, however, are extremely rare, and in almost all cases surgery is necessary.

In operations for retinal detachment the first object is to locate the tear in the retina. This is done by means of the ophthalmoscope, and the position of the tear is outlined on the outer surface of the eye. After the back of the eye has been exposed, electrocautery punctures are made through the sclera in such a way as to surround the tear, and the subretinal fluid is permitted to escape either through the puncture holes or, if necessary, through a larger hole made with a knife. When the fluid has escaped the retina can flatten out into its normal position again, and the sterile inflammation produced by the punctures seals off the tear and holds the retina in contact with the choroid.

Nursing Care. After operation the patient must remain flat on his back for ten days to allow healing to take place. During most of this time he must have both eyes bandaged to prevent their movement, for such movement might prevent or delay healing. After this he must wear pin-hole glasses; these discourage excessive movement of the eyes by admitting light only through small central openings, thus permitting the wearer to look straight ahead only. The patient is allowed up and out of bed very gradually and his activity must be curtailed for four to six months after a successful operation. From the above outline of the postoperative treatment it is obvious that this is an unpleasant period for the patient. For this reason the nurse can be extremely helpful by making the patient as comfortable as possible, and by offering constant encouragement. Some surgeons are now permitting early ambulation, lavatory privileges, and sitting up in bed. If, as claimed, the end-results in the treatment of detachment are equally good, this regimen is preferable.

DISEASES

Styes

A stye is an infection of the small lubricating glands in the margins of the lids. It appears as a red elevation on the lid margin and is painful.

Treatment. Yellow oxide of mercury ointment was the time-honored treatment for styes. This gave nothing more than slight comfort and, since the advent of chemotherapy, has been discarded. The most helpful form of treatment is the application of hot compresses. The addition of chemotherapeutic drugs locally hastens a successful outcome. In most instances, the inflammation subsides, but sometimes suppuration occurs, just as in a furuncle, at which time the stye should be incised and drained.

Chalazia

A chalazion is a cyst of the meibomian glands of the tarsal plate of the lids. It presents a small lump in the lid which is hard and painless. If infected the redness and pain characteristic of infection everywhere are present here also.

Treatment. The infected case is treated by hot compresses, followed by incision and drainage at the proper time. A small percentage of noninfected chalazia become reabsorbed after massage. In most cases this fails and they must be removed surgically.

Conjunctivitis

This condition can be divided into three large groups according to causative agents: (1) traumatic (mechanical, thermal, or chemical), (2) infective, and (3) allergic. The symptoms differ somewhat in the three types but, in general, are as follows: redness of the conjunctiva; discomfort varying from a slight feeling of grit in the eyes in mild cases to actual pain in severe cases; lacrimation and photophobia (intolerance to light); marked itching and burning of the eyes in the allergic type; and a purulent discharge in the infective type. Of course, all of these symptoms vary with the severity of the case.

Treatment. The history usually serves to separate those cases in the traumatic group. These are treated by the removal of the causative agent followed by irrigations and mild antiseptic drops until the conjunctiva heals. In the infectious group, the specific organism can be isolated and identified by culture, and the chemotherapeutic or antibiotic agent known to be most effective against this organism is then used. However, since the advent of the wide spectrum chemotherapeutic and antibiotic drugs, the usual method of handling this group is to use the drug of widest spectrum, resorting to culture only in the few cases where this method fails. A solution of zinc sulfate, boric acid, and adrenalin is very effective against the milder forms and every ophthalmologist uses his own variation of this extensively. Antibiotics have greatly facilitated the treatment of the infectious types of conjunctivitis, but occasionally, especially when used indiscriminately, they cause allergies. The third group, allergic forms of conjunctivitis, presents a rather characteristic appearance, being pale and smooth with much itching and no discharge. Antihistaminic or cortisone drops are sometimes helpful, but may prove disappointing. Of course, if the allergen can be determined and removed, recovery follows quickly.

Ophthalmia Neonatorum

Until the instillation of silver nitrate into the eyes of all newborn infants became mandatory, gonorrheal conjunctivitis was the greatest single cause of blindness; Credé's procedure greatly reduced the incidence of blindness from this source. Once the disease had developed, its treatment was a formidable ophthalmologic problem, and many eyes were lost until the introduction of the sulfonamides and penicillin.

In gonorrheal conjunctivitis the eye presents a severely inflamed appearance, with much swelling and profuse discharge. The eye rapidly closes because of the edema of the lids; later the ulcerated cornea perforates and the eye is lost. Since the advent of chemotherapy, however, treatment has become successful. The gonococci disappear within two to four days and the eyes are clear in a week. None of the damaging sequelae that nearly always accompanied longstanding infection is seen now. In treating such patients the nurse must be extremely careful to maintain the strictest isolation technic not only for the safety of others but in her own interest as well.

Trachoma

This disease, fortunately, is not very common in the United States, but it is widespread in China, India, and Egypt, causing blindness in a tragically large proportion of the population. The mode of its transmission is not known, though it has recently been shown to be caused by a virus. It begins as a mild injection of the conjunctiva, followed by the formation of follicles and the ingrowth of fine blood vessels into the superior portion of the cornea. This group of vessels is called a pannus, and is characteristic of trachoma. In the later stages of the disease the tarsus of the lids becomes scarred, and as this scarring progresses the lids are inverted (*entropion*) and the lashes are made to rub on the cornea. Finally the cornea becomes hazy and the vision is greatly reduced.

This disease is extremely chronic and the older forms of treatment served only to check its progress. Chemotherapeutic and antibiotic agents, however, have been discovered to be dramatically effective in the treatment of trachoma; indeed, it seems probable that the disease may some day be entirely eradicated.

Corneal Ulcers

Any abrasion of the corneal epithelium is a corneal ulcer. Small abrasions may be outlined with the use of fluorescein: if they are uncomplicated they will heal in a few hours without leaving a scar. The only treatment necessary is the instillation of a lubricant such as castor oil to promote healing and to relieve the pain caused by the rubbing of the lids over the denuded corneal surface.

Larger ulcers involve the deeper layers of the cornea and upon healing leave a scar. The ultimate damage to the visual acuity depends on the position of the scar on the front of the eye, for if it is centrally placed it will be in the line of vision, whereas a peripherally placed scar does not reduce the vision significantly. Corneal ulcers are traumatic or infectious in nature; in some cases a traumatic ulcer becomes infected.

Treatment. In the treatment of all but the mildest corneal ulcers the iris should be put at rest by the daily instillation of atropine. Hot compresses are helpful in all cases and irrigations are used when there is a purulent discharge. There are some rare forms of ulceration of the cornea that occasionally resist all forms of treatment; the eye may be lost following the perforation of such an ulcer with consequent development of *enophthalmitis* (inflammation of the interior of the eye).

Traumatic Ulcers. Traumatic ulcers are treated by the application of lubricants and antibacterial ointments and heal rather quickly when no complication occurs.

Infectious Ulcers. Ulcers caused by infection take longer to heal but respond well to the application of the chemotherapeutic and antibiotic drugs. In all cases of corneal ulcer, the eye should be covered with an eye pad until the cornea has healed.

Keratitis

Inflammation of the cornea is called keratitis. The chief symptoms of this condition are severe pain in the eye, redness, and watering of the eye (excessive lacrimation). Keratitis may be a complication of syphilis, tuberculosis, or herpes; in such instances, when the cause can be recognized, specific treatment is directed at the causative infection. Often, however, no cause can be found for keratitis.

Nonspecific general therapeutic measures are employed in the treatment of patients who have a keratitis of unexplained origin. These measures include the use of atropine, hot compresses, and local application of sulfonamides and antibiotics. Cortisone also is helpful in some instances.

Uveitis

The inflammation of any portion of the uveal tract is called uveitis. The iris, ciliary body, and choroid constitute the uveal tract. Inflammation of the individual portions of the tract occurs (iritis, cyclitis, and choroiditis), but in some cases the inflammation involves more than one portion. The symptoms of uveitis include redness of the globe which is most noticeable adjacent to the limbus, pain in the eye, photophobia, and a gradual decrease in the vision. Uveitis may be a manifestation of several general diseases. It occurs along with other signs of the disease, or it may be the first manifestation to appear and in these latter cases it is important that the specific nature of the underlying disease be recognized so that it can be cared for properly. Syphilis and tuberculosis are the two diseases that most frequently cause lesions in the uveal tract. In these the treatment is to be directed at the systemic condition. In addition, hot compresses and atropine drops several times a day are employed locally, as in the case of all types of uveitis.

Foci of infection are another cause of uveitis. Where these exist and can be eradicated, the eye will clear rapidly. Here again the hot compresses and atropine to the eye itself are indicated.

Finally there is a third large group of cases of uveitis in which no definite cause can be found. These are divided into the granulomatous and nongranulomatous types. In the granulomatous variety cortisone is helpful; in some instances the local application of drops or ointment suffices, but in others oral or parenteral therapy is necessary. Cortisone has little apparent effect in the nongranulomatous uveitis. In these cases the usual local therapy is supplemented by oral administration of the sulfonamides or antibiotics and by foreign protein fever therapy. Salicylates in rather large doses are advised by some ophthalmologists.

Foreign Protein Therapy. This is a form of nonspecific treatment frequently used in inflammatory conditions of the eye. It consists in the production of an elevation of the temperature of the patient by means of the injection of a protein substance. Typhoid-paratyphoid or diphtheria vaccines given intravenously, or sterile milk injected intramuscularly, are the proteins ordinarily used. A course of treatment is begun with small doses, increasing in amount every other day; the size of the dose and the number of injections are governed by the severity and the tenacity of the infection. The patient's temperature should be taken every hour following each injection until it has returned to normal. Codeine may be given during the period of temperature elevation to relieve the discomfort that accompanies the fever, but aspirin and other antipyretics are contraindicated since the production of fever is the object of this form of therapy. Fever of a higher degree can be induced by means of the heated chamber, and this is occasionally employed in the treatment of some eye diseases.

Retinitis

Inflammation of the retina, also, is caused by many systemic diseases, and the nature of the underlying disease can often be diagnosed from characteristic changes seen in the retina. Diabetes, arteriosclerosis, nephritis, syphilis, tuberculosis, and many other systemic diseases produce retinal lesions. As in the case of uveitis, when the presence of a specific disease can be determined as the cause of the retinitis, the treatment is directed toward the disease. The symptoms of retinitis may be so slight as to escape the notice of the patient unless the macular region of the retina is involved, in which case the vision is seriously reduced. There is no pain, redness, or watering of the eye to call the patient's attention to the presence of the lesion. On ophthalmoscopic examination the fundus shows exudates, hemorrhages, and edema of the retina. Changes in the vision and in the visual fields are present in many cases, and it is usually these that cause the patient to seek help.

Papilledema and Optic Atrophy

Inflammation of, or pressure on the optic nerve produces edema of the head of the nerve where it enters the eyeball (*optic disk*). The swollen nerve head actually protrudes into the eye; this is called papilledema or choked disk. It occurs in diseases which involve the central nervous system, and is also produced by increased intracranial pressure (see Chap. 37, page 416). Following prolonged papilledema the nerve fibers die, and the dead-white, flat disk of optic atrophy becomes apparent. In papilledema and in optic atrophy the visual acuity becomes progressively reduced and finally complete blindness may result.

Glaucoma

In this disease the pressure within the eyeball becomes too high. Normally the aqueous humor is formed and absorbed at a constant rate. In glaucoma the fluid is secreted more rapidly than it is absorbed, so that the volume of the globe is increased and the intraocular tension is elevated. When this elevation is gradual the symptoms are slight and may not be noticed by the patient until extensive and irreparable damage has been done. When the tension rises rapidly, however, symptoms are severe and cause the patient to seek immediate attention because of the great pain and the loss of vision. An increase in tension causes pressure upon the optic nerve, damaging the nerve fibers and reducing the visual acuity. Such elevation of the tension must be relieved rapidly if permanent damage to the eye is to be avoided. In some cases of glaucoma this can be accomplished by the use of miotics and by the enforcement of rest in bed. The miotics contract the pupil and open the drainage angle of the anterior chamber, thus allowing the normal rate of drainage of the aqueous humor to be resumed. When medical treatment fails to control the tension, more radical surgical treatment must be used.

OPERATIONS FOR THE RELIEF OF GLAUCOMA

Many types of operation have been devised for the treatment of glaucoma; all have as their common aim the establishment of an artificial passage for the release of excess aqueous humor from the globe and in this manner a reduction of the tension.

Iridencleisis, iridotasis, and corneal trephine are the most widely used operations in the treatment of chronic glaucoma. Basal iridectomy is the operation of choice in the acute type, cyclodialysis in the glaucoma (aphakic) type which follows cataract extraction, and goniotomy in the congenital variety.

Iridencleisis; Iridotasis. In these two operations a conjunctival flap is made around the superior portion of the cornea; the globe is entered with a keratome, the iris pulled out of the anterior chamber at this point and deposited on the adjacent sclera; the conjunctival flap is closed with several sutures. Thus a tract is created along the extruded portion of the iris by which the fluid can escape from the eyeball to be absorbed under the conjunctival flap. The difference in the two operations is only in the handling of the iris.

Corneoscleral Trephining. In the trephine operation a conjunctival flap is dissected and the underlying cornea is split into two thicknesses. A small opening into the anterior chamber through the deeper half of the cornea is made with the trephine at the limbus. The superficial layer of cornea and conjunctival flap are then replaced and sutured, and on healing there remains a small opening through which fluid can escape to be absorbed under the flap of conjunctiva as in the other operations.

Basal Iridectomy. In this operation, the anterior chamber is entered and a large portion of the iris is excised.

Cyclodialysis. Quite different in technical detail from the preceding operation, this method provides also a means for fluid from the anterior chamber to escape, but in this instance into a space prepared between the choroid and sclera.

Goniotomy. In congenital glaucoma, there is an abnormality in the angle of the anterior chamber which closes it. This procedure is designed to open the angle mechanically.

After-care. All patients with glaucoma should be under the care of an ophthalmologist for the remainder of their lives as no type of operation is permanently successful in all cases, and a recurrence may develop at any time. Often several operations are necessary to bring the tension under control, and sometimes blindness cannot be prevented.

Operations for glaucoma usually fail to produce good results in Negroes. This is thought to be due to the racial tendency toward excessive scar formation, thus interfering with the continuous function of newly made drainage channels.

Cataract

A cataract is an opacity of the lens. Cataracts may be congenital, the result of trauma, or secondary in nature, such as those which occur in diabetes and several other diseases. The commonest variety is the senile cataract. The cause of the senile type is not known, though most experimental evidence on the subject points to some interference in the metabolism of the lens as the underlying factor in its formation. Senile cataract usually begins in the fifth or sixth decade of life, develops slowly over a period of years, and nearly always involves first one eye and then the other. The only symptom of a cataract is the gradual decrease in the visual acuity of the involved eye. This is frequently described by the patient as a veil drawn over the eye. As the opacity of the lens becomes denser, the vision of the eye grows progressively worse. This process is called maturation of the cataract, and when full maturity has been reached the vision is limited to the perception of light alone. On examination a cataract appears as a white object filling the pupillary space and preventing the visualization of any of the details of the eye behind the lens.

OPERATIONS FOR CATARACT

There is no medical treatment to cure cataracts or to prevent their progression. The only effective treatment is surgical, consisting in the removal of the opaque lens.

Discission. For congenital cataracts, however, and for some traumatic ones, an operation is performed in which the capsule of the lens is opened with a thin needle knife and the lens fibers are pierced (*discission*). This procedure allows the aqueous humor to come into contact with the lens substance, which is then absorbed by the aqueous. This type of operation is successful only in young patients. For all other types of cataracts the eyeball must be opened and the opaque lens extracted. This can be done by two methods, the extracapsular or the intracapsular extraction, both of which are widely used.

Extracapsular Operation. In the extracapsular operation the globe is opened by an incision along the limbus over the upper half of the eye. The cornea is then lifted up like the hood of an automobile; the iris is pulled out and a portion excised, the capsule of the lens is incised, and as much of the lens substance as possible is expressed from the eye. The globe is closed either by sutures through cornea and sclera, or by the less effective method of sutures in the conjunctival flap. On healing, the posterior capsule of the lens, which has been left in the eye, may become opaque and act as a thin curtain before the vision. Discission is then necessary to obtain clear vision.

Intracapsular Operation. The newer method, intracapsular extraction, is steadily growing in popularity among ophthalmic surgeons. In this operation the opening and closing of the eye are performed in the same manner as for the extracapsular method, but here the lens is grasped with smooth forceps and extracted within its capsule. The intracapsular technic is a bit more difficult to master than that of the extracapsular operation, but this operation has two important advantages. First, the cataract can be removed at an earlier stage of maturity, thus shortening the unhappy period while the patient waits in a state of reduced vision for the lens to become completely mature, which is a requirement for the extracapsular operation; second, no discission is necessary after the intracapsular method because in it the posterior capsule of the lens has been removed with the rest of the lens.

Trials are being made, at present, of a method in which a substitute lens of plastic material is placed in the eye when the cataract is removed. If successful, this method will result in greatly improved vision after operation.

Postoperative Care. The postoperative care is the same for the extracapsular and intracapsular operations. Until recently both eyes were bandaged at operation and the patient required to be quite flat and still for several days—a most trying time for the patient. Now many surgeons follow a much less rigid and more comfortable postoperative routine. The unoperated eye is left uncovered from the start. A pillow is placed beneath the head, and in a few hours the back of the bed is elevated. In two or three days the patient is started up in a chair. The eye is first dressed one and a half or two days following operation and each day following this. If everything has gone well the patient is discharged on the seventh or eighth postoperative day, with instructions to return to the surgeon's office for observation at regular intervals. After operation, the eye is moderately inflamed, but this redness gradually clears as healing progresses and the eye is usually white again at the end of a month. Three to four months after operation the eye is usually ready for refraction and for the prescription of a permanent pair of glasses. However, temporary glasses can be prescribed when the patient leaves the hospital, as long as they understand that the healing process continues for three or four months, and the refraction may change until this is complete. A strong spectacle lens is required to take the place of the surgically removed lens of the patient. If the eye is normal in all other respects, normal vision will be regained with properly fitted glasses.

Strabismus

In this condition there is inability to direct the two eyes at the same object because of a lack of coordination of the extraocular muscles. The eyes may diverge, converge, or deviate in a vertical direction, and the condition can be congenital or paralytic in nature. When it occurs early in life the patient has no complaint other than the distressing appearance of crossed eyes. In young patients it is important to correct the strabismus at an early stage so as to ensure the proper development of the macular area and, therefore, vision in the deviating eye. When strabismus occurs after the development of the macular area, double vision immediately results.

Some cases of strabismus respond to muscle exercises or to the wearing of glasses, but most patients require surgical treatment. The operations for the correction of strabismus consist in the moving of the faulty muscle or muscles forward or backward from their old attachments to the globe. Unfortunately there is no precise means of estimating how much to move the attachment of a muscle in order to correct a given amount of deviation of the eyes, so that several operations may be necessary to cure the squint. Muscle training and exercise, known as orthoptics, combined with surgery are extremely helpful in the treatment of strabismus.

Postoperatively the patients are permitted much more freedom and comfort than after most eye operations. The eyes must be bandaged for a time, but the head can be moved about and the patient is not confined to bed.

Neoplasms of the Eye

The ophthalmic surgeon is called upon to treat tumors arising both in the eye and in the orbit. Fortunately such neoplasms are not very common. Intraocular tumors arise from the retina, choroid, or iris, or may be metastatic growths from malignant neoplasms located elsewhere in the body. Occasionally, it is possible to remove a small tumor of the iris and save the eye; most intraocular tumors require enucleation. Extraocular tumors may arise from any of the orbital tissues, and may cause exophthalmos. If benign, these can usually be removed without too much disturbance of the function of the eye. When malignant, exenteration of the orbital contents is carried out. Roentgen ray and radium therapy must be used with extreme caution, as the lens is particularly susceptible to radiation; a cataract may result from insufficient protection of the lens.

NURSING CARE IN OPHTHALMOLOGY
Light

In most diseases of the eye strong light causes discomfort to the patient (*photophobia*) and in some instances it may cause great pain. The natural protective reflex, squinting, can result in a squeezing of the lids that may seriously harm the diseased eye. It is obvious, therefore, that the nurse must know of this danger and must take the necessary precautions to protect her patient from excessive light. The patient should always be shielded from strong sunlight as well as from strong artificial light. On the other hand it is important not to keep the room in the depressing gloom of too much darkness. A happy medium can be maintained. Eyes that are being unbandaged for the first time after operation are particularly sensitive to light, and it is at this time that the compression produced by squinting can do the most damage. It is wise, therefore, to have the room moderately dark during the changing of dressings unless the doctor specifies otherwise.

Drops

The nurse may be called upon many times a day to instill drops into the eye. The eye is a sensitive organ and use of the wrong drugs may cause damage. Also, some drugs, regularly used in the treatment of specific eye conditions, are contraindicated in other conditions, and will do irreparable damage if used by mistake. Therefore the importance of being certain that one has the prescribed solution of the proper drug cannot be too strongly emphasized.

Technic of Administration. The patient should be in a comfortable position. When she is dealing with a bed patient the nurse may stand at either side of the bed and face the patient's head. The dropper is held in the right hand while the forefinger of the left hand depresses the lower lid as the patient is directed to look upward. A drop is then allowed to fall at the inner aspect of the eye, care being taken not to touch any part of the eye with the dropper. The drop should not be instilled at too great a distance from the eye in order to prevent the shock to the patient that would result from drops hitting the eye forcefully. If the patient is ambulatory, he is seated comfortably in a chair with the head tilted slightly backward on a headrest. The nurse stands in front and a little to one side, using her hands in the manner described for delivering the drop to bed patients. It is quite important when applying pressure to open a lid that none of the pressure reaches the eyeball itself. In children who refuse to open their lids the drop may be deposited at the inner junction of the closed lids with the head bent backward; when they do open their lids the solution will run into the eye.

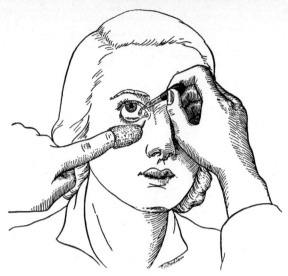

FIGURE 119. Method of instilling drops into eye. The left index finger is wrapped in a sterile gauze sponge.

Care of Solutions and Instruments. Signs of deterioration of solutions such as sedimentation or change in color should be looked for by the nurse. If any doubt exists as to the freshness of a solution it should be discarded and a fresh preparation used. It would be ideal to have a separate bottle and dropper for each instillation, but obviously this is impossible because it entails too great waste of time and material. When possible a fresh dropper should be used for each instillation, but since even this is not always practicable the greatest care must be exercised to prevent contamination of the dropper; if it has been contaminated it must not be returned to the bottle under any circumstances. The glass pipet with rubber bulb on one end is the usual instrument for instilling drops. The glass portion of this instrument is easily sterilized, whereas the rubber portion undergoes deterioration, so care must be used to draw the solution up into the glass part only. A dropper must never be used for a second solution unless it has been resterilized.

When the nurse is giving drops she must take care not to get any of the solution on her own hands, for from there into her eyes is an easy journey. Everyone who has worked in ophthal-

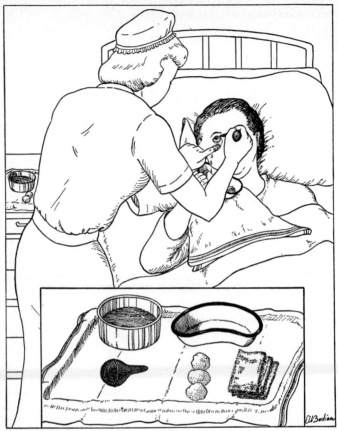

FIGURE 120. Technic for irrigating eye. Insert shows irrigation tray containing basin of solution, curved basin, rubber irrigating syringe, cotton and gauze. Note that left index finger of nurse is covered by sterile gauze.

mology for any length of time has had the experience of blurred vision and dilated pupils as the result of carelessness in administering atropine.

Irrigations

These are indicated in inflammatory conditions of the conjunctiva, as part of the preoperative clean-up and postoperative care, and following the instillation of fluorescein when staining the cornea. The apparatus used in this treatment consists of a simple rubber syringe (a rubber ear syringe is most convenient), or a glass undine; when these are not available an ordinary eye-dropper may be used to deliver the solution into the eye. Cotton or a curved basin is used to catch the solution as it runs from the eye. Boric acid is the most commonly used solution for irrigations of the eye. The solution should be warmed, and it should be tested by letting a few drops fall on the wrist to make sure that it is not too hot.

Technic. The patient should be either flat in bed, or in a treatment chair with the head supported on a headrest. The curved basin or cotton to catch the solution as it leaves the eye is held at the side of the face by the patient or by an assistant. The nurse giving the irrigation stands in front of the patient in order to have full view of what she is doing. The lid margins should be cleansed of foreign matter such as dust, secretion, or crusts by gentle wiping with cotton. The lids of the eye are held open by the fingers of one hand while the syringe is held in the other hand. The stream of fluid is gently directed onto the eyeball from the nasal portion toward the outer angle, care being taken that none runs over the bridge of the nose into the other eye. The irrigation should be continued until the conjunctival sac is completely free of secretion and foreign matter. As in the case of the eyedropper, the syringe should not be allowed to touch the eye. At the completion of this treatment the skin of the lids and adjacent areas should be dried with cotton.

Hot Compresses

Moist heat is used to relieve pain and to increase the circulation in inflammatory conditions. Superficial and deep inflammation of the globe, as well as of the lids and orbit, responds well to the application of heat. This is best applied by gauze or cotton compresses large enough to cover the whole orbital area. The patient should be lying in bed, and the pillow and the patient's chest should be covered with a towel to prevent wetting. The skin of the lids should be wiped clean as in irrigations, and a little petrolatum applied to this area to prevent the maceration of the skin that otherwise follows frequent compressing. The gauze or cotton pads are soaked in a basin of boric acid solution heated on a hot plate at the bedside. The solution is kept between 115 and 120° F.; care must be taken that it does not become hot enough to burn the patient. The pads are grasped at

TABLE 3. Drugs Commonly Used in Ophthalmology

NAME	STRENGTH OF SOLUTION	MODE OF USE	EFFECT	REMARKS
ANTISEPTIC SOLUTIONS				
Gantrisin	4%	Instill 2 drops	Antiseptic	Used in external infections of eyes
Sodium sulfacetamide (Sulamyd)	30%	Instill 2 drops	Antiseptic	Used in external infections of eyes
Aureomycin		Instill 2 drops	Antiseptic	Used in external infections of eyes
Terramycin	0.5%	Instill 2 drops	Antiseptic	Used in external infections of eyes
OINTMENTS				
Yellow oxide of mercury	1.2%	Apply to lids	Mildly antiseptic	Used in styes and blepharitis (least effective)
Epinephrine bitartrate	2%	Apply to eye	Dilates	Used where strong mydriatic is required
Gantrisin	4%	Apply to eye	Antiseptic	Used in external infections of eye
Sodium sulfacetamide (Sulamyd)	10%	Apply to eye	Antiseptic	Used in external infections of eye
Sulfathiazole	5%			
Myciquent	½%	Apply to eye	Antiseptic	Used in external infections of eye
Bacitracin	500 units per gram	Apply to eye	Antiseptic	Used in external infections of eye
Cortisone	1.5%	Apply to eye	Blocks allergic reactions	Used in iritis and uveitis to block inflammatory reactions while underlying cause is searched for and treated

ANESTHETICS

Drug	Strength	Dose	Action	Remarks
Cocaine hydrochloride	5%	Instill 1-3 drops	Anesthetizes cornea; dilates pupil	May damage cornea or cause glaucoma
Pontocaine hydrochloride	½%	Instill 1-3 drops	Produces anesthesia	No harmful side effects
Holocaine hydrochloride	1%	Instill 1-3 drops	Produces anesthesia	No harmful side effects
Butyn sulfate	2%	Instill 1-3 drops	Produces anesthesia	No harmful side effects
Procaine	1-2%	Injection	Produces anesthesia	Used for surgery of lids and orbit

MYDRIATICS AND CYCLOPLEGICS

Drug	Strength	Dose	Action	Remarks
Atropine sulfate	½-3%	Instill 1-2 drops	Dilates pupils; paralyzes muscles of accommodation	The most widely used drug in ophthalmology
Homatropine hydrobromide	2-5%	Instill 1-2 drops	Dilates pupil	Used for eye examinations
Euphthalmine hydrochloride	5%	Instill 1-2 drops	Dilates pupil	Short in duration—useful in older patients

MIOTICS

Drug	Strength	Dose	Action	Remarks
Pilocarpine hydrochloride	1-2%	Instill 1-2 drops	Contracts pupil	Used in glaucoma
Eserine salicylate	¼-1%	Instill 1-2 drops	Contracts pupil	Used in glaucoma

OTHER DRUGS

Drug	Strength	Dose	Action	Remarks
Epinephrine	1-1000	Instill 1-2 drops	Dilates pupil; contracts blood vessels	To control hemorrhage
Dionin	1-5%	Instill 1-2 drops	Relieves pain	Smarts immediately on instillation
Fluorescein	2%	Instill 1 drop	Stains corneal abrasion	Remove excess by irrigation
Antistine	½%	Instill 1-2 drops	Antihistamine	Used in allergic conjunctivitis
Cortisone	0.5% and 2.5%	Instill 1-2 drops	Blocks allergic reaction	Used in inflammations while underlying cause is searched for and removed

each end, twisted to squeeze out the excess fluid, and then smoothed out gently on the closed lids. When the compress cools it is replaced by a hot one every one or two minutes to ensure that constant heat reaches the eye for a period of fifteen or twenty minutes at each treatment. The frequency of the treatments is governed by the severity of the condition being treated. The lids are dried and the petrolatum is removed at the end of each treatment. The compress pads and basin are sterilized between treatments and put away for the next treatment of the same patient.

Cold Compresses

These are helpful in controlling bleeding into the anterior chamber or in edema of the lids (*chemosis*). They are also recommended in the early stages of conjunctivitis to decrease discomfort and secretion, but should not be used in late or deep-seated infections. Cold compresses are given in the same manner as that described for hot compresses, except that ice is used in the solution in place of heat.

Ointments

Drugs used in the form of ointments are best applied by means of sterile glass rods to the inner margin of the lower lid of the eye. The patient is instructed to hold the lids closed for five minutes to allow the ointment to spread and be absorbed.

Powders

The application of powder to the eye is made simply by dusting the powder from a sterile tongue depressor or spatula onto the eye. A drop of Pontocaine beforehand makes the application more comfortable, as the powder acts as a foreign body before it has been dissolved by the tears.

Preparation for Operation

Before operation the patient should have a general physical examination and such special examinations as are indicated. For most eye operations the eyelashes are cut short and an irrigation is given at bedtime on the night preceding operation. A mild sedative is given to ensure the patient a good night's rest. Most patients are naturally apprehensive at this time and the nurse can do a good deal to allay nervousness. In preparation for major operations a soap solution enema is given in the evening before operation and breakfast is omitted. Tea and toast are given at breakfast time if local anesthesia is to be used. For afternoon operations breakfast is given and lunch omitted or replaced by tea and toast.

Postoperative Care

After operation the patient must be made as comfortable as possible. It is important after most operations that the patient keep his head quite still and that he refrain from any strain such as coughing, vomiting, and the like. The nurse must make it plain that she is there to meet the patient's every need and that he must be completely inactive, allowing everything to be done for him no matter how trivial it may seem. Backache is one of the commonest postoperative complaints, as these patients must lie in one position for a long period. This can be greatly relieved by frequent gentle backrubs.

The patient has both eyes covered and therefore feels shut off from his surroundings. Here again the nurse can help by offering frequent reassurance. Occasional patients, particularly those of advanced years, become confused (disoriented) after some time in the utter darkness; nothing less than permitting the opening of the unoperated eye to allow them to reestablish contact with their surroundings will clear this state of confusion. The decision to remove the bandage should be made only by the doctor; he must be notified whenever a patient becomes disoriented. Any severe pain in the eye following operation is also an indication for notifying the doctor.

When the patient is sleeping it is the job of the nurse to prevent undue movement of the head or touching of the eyes with the hands. In small children enforced restriction by means of a jacket, sheet, or other restraint is necessary to keep the hands away from the eyes. In most cases children's hands can be kept at a safe distance from their eyes by a cuff stiffened with tongue depressors which is fastened around their arms so as to prevent bending at the elbow.

SUMMARY

Ophthalmologic surgery is undertaken to correct squint, to save vision by replacing a detached retina, by removing a cataract, or by relieving the pressure in glaucoma. Injury, infection, and neoplastic disease may lead to loss of vision and to loss of the eye itself. Apprehension and even psychotic confusion are of common occurrence, but good nursing prevents or minimizes them.

VOCABULARY REVIEW

conjunctiva	hyperopia	glaucoma
media	astigmatism	cataract
uveal tract	stye	strabismus
ophthalmoscope	chalazion	cycloplegic
myopia	keratitis	discission

SUGGESTED READING

1. Blake, Eugene M.: Glaucoma. Am. J. Nursing, 52:451–452 (April) 1952.
2. Chace, Robert R.: Treatment of Cataract. Am. J. Nursing, 48:150–152 (March) 1948.
3. Lord, Helen May: Nursing Care in Corneal Ulcer. Am. J. Nursing, 49:378–380 (June) 1949.
4. Rones, Benjamin: The Eyes and Vitamins. Am. J. Nursing, 52:728–729 (July) 1952.
5. Ruedemann, Albert D.: Headaches Caused by Eye Defects. Am. J. Nursing. 52:1093–1094 (September) 1952.
6. Shaw, Cora L.: Nursing Care of Patients with Cataract. Am. J. Nursing, 48:153–155 (March) 1948.
7. Sinescal, Arthur A.: Trachoma. Am. J. Nursing, 52:1508–1510 (December) 1952.
8. Weaver, Helen E.: The Nurse and Sight Conservation. Am. J. Nursing, 51:553–555 (September) 1951.
9. Weaver, Helen E.: Glaucoma: A Problem for the Public Health Nurse. Pub. Health Nursing, 41:93–94 (February) 1949.
10. Weiss, M. Olga: The Psychological Aspects of Nursing Care for Eye Patients. Am. J. Nursing, 50:218–220 (April) 1950.

CHAPTER 42

Nursing in Otolaryngology

INTRODUCTION

The organs of the upper part of the respiratory tract include the ear, the nose, the paranasal sinuses, the pharnyx, and the larynx. In addition to housing the end-organs of the special senses of hearing, equilibrium, and smell, the upper respiratory tract serves as the entrance to the lungs, and contains the apparatus

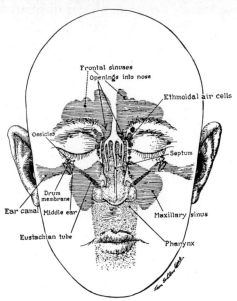

Frontal sinuses
Openings into nose
Ethmoidal air cells
Ossicles
Septum
Drum membrane
Ear canal Middle ear
Maxillary sinus
Eustachian tube
Pharynx

FIGURE 121. Diagram to show the locations and intercommunications of the nose, the paranasal sinuses, the ears, the pharynx, and the mouth.

for producing sound (*phonation*). The inner surfaces of the components of the tract are lined by a continuous sheet of epithelial cells, which are in some places similar to the squamous cells of the skin, and in other places are mucus-secreting cells. This sheet of cells (*membrane*) is constantly exposed to the air we breathe, and to all the noxious substances that are found in air, including dust, pollen, bacteria, viruses, and the like. It is not surprising that infections and other diseases of the upper respiratory tract are common. Special instruments, technics, and knowledge are necessary for the proper examination of the tract, and for the diagnosis and the care of its diseases. Largely for these reasons otolaryngology was one of the earliest surgical specialties to be developed.

The various parts of the upper respiratory tract are usually spoken of as though they were entities in themselves, and it is true that most of these parts have special characteristics and individual functions; it is important, however, to realize that all are in communication with one another, so that infections spread easily. It is also true that the damage caused by disease in one

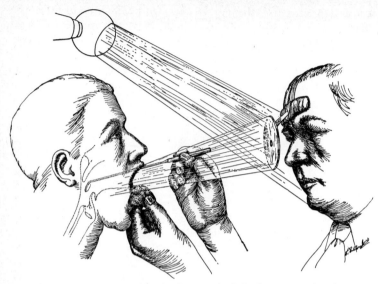

FIGURE 122. The use of the head mirror and of the laryngoscopic mirror enables the examiner to see the vocal cords.

component of the tract may cause changes in function in other components.

METHODS OF EXAMINING THE UPPER RESPIRATORY TRACT

The otolaryngologist must learn to peer through tiny apertures, into dark cavities, and around corners. One of the most useful devices in his armamentarium is the head mirror. This is a curved mirror with a peep-hole through its center; it is worn on the forehead of the examiner so that he may look with one eye through the peep-hole; at the same time the mirror reflects a focused beam of light at the patient from a source of light placed to one side of the patient's head. Using the head mirror, the examiner looks into the nostrils, which he spreads with a nasal speculum, and into the pharynx while he holds the back of the tongue down with a tongue depressor. By means of a small mirror held at a 45 degree angle in the pharynx over the epiglottis, it is possible to see down into the larynx and to observe the action of the vocal cords. Modern ingenuity has supplemented these simple tools with electrically illuminated tubes, some of which are equipped with magnifying lenses; the otoscope is used to visualize the ear drum (*tympanic membrane*); the pharyngoscope enables the examiner to see the posterior nasopharynx, including the orifices of the eustachian tubes; the laryngoscope, a short form of bronchoscope, can be passed directly into the larynx.

Transillumination. Information as to the condition of the paranasal sinuses, specifically the maxillary and frontal sinuses, may be gained by transillumination. In this examination a light is placed in the mouth of the patient, the lips are closed, and the room is darkened. Normal sinuses, because they contain air, transmit the light well, whereas diseased sinuses remain dark. Properly taken roentgenograms furnish the same information more reliably, and show the condition of the ethmoid and sphenoid sinuses, as well as of the mastoid cells.

Tests of Hearing and Equilibrium. It is also the function of the otolaryngologist to examine the patient's hearing and sense of equilibrium.

Audiometric Tests. Much can be learned by the use of a tuning fork, but more accurate determination of the exact amount of hearing in each ear can be made by the use of the audiometer, an electronic device which can produce pure tones of any desired pitch or intensity. During the examination the hearing of the ear not undergoing the test is masked by directing into it a buzzing sound, so as to prevent the crossing over to it of sound from the other side through conduction by the bones of the skull.

Caloric and Spinning Tests. The function of the vestibular apparatus (that is, to maintain equilibrium) is tested by the caloric test and by spinning the patient in a tilting chair. In the caloric test ice water is dropped on the ear drum, a violent stimulus which, in a normal subject, immediately produces vertigo. Anyone who has, as a child, spun in an untwisting rope swing can appreciate the tilting chair test. In this manner the fluid in the semicircular canals is set into motion and the response of the patient is observed.

THE NOSE AND THE PARANASAL SINUSES

Anatomy and Physiology. The external nose consists of bone and cartilage covered with muscles and skin. Internally the nasal septum, composed of cartilage and bone, divides the nose into two cavities. On the lateral wall of each nasal cavity are three elongated, shell-like bones covered with thick, vascular mucous membrane, called the turbinates. The space between the inferior turbinate and middle turbinate is known as the middle meatus. It is into this region that the nasolacrimal duct opens. The superior meatus is just above the middle turbinate. The middle and superior meatuses are of clinical importance because it is into these two spaces that the nasal sinuses drain.

The paranasal sinuses are eight in number—on each side, there are the frontal, maxillary, sphenoid, and ethmoid. They are normally filled with air and lined with thin mucous membrane. As in the nose, the outer layer of this membrane is covered with ciliated epithelium. All the sinuses communicate with the nose through their various openings or ostia. The frontal sinuses lie in the frontal bone, one above each eye. They vary greatly in size or may be absent. Each frontal sinus drains into the middle meatus on the same side. The maxillary sinuses lie in the superior maxillary bone in each cheek and they also open into the middle meatus. The ethmoid sinuses are a group of tiny cavities which lie on each side of the nose between the middle and superior turbinates and the orbit. They communicate with both the middle and superior meatuses. The sphenoid sinus is also paired, each one lying in the sphenoidal bone and separated from its fellow by a bony partition. This sinus drains into the superior meatus.

The functions of the nose are respiratory, olfactory, and phonatory; of these the respiratory function is by far the most important. The nose warms, moistens, and filters the inspired air before it enters the lungs. As air is drawn through the nose, its temperature is raised or lowered as required to approximate body temperature. The nasal mucous membrane is covered with a thin layer of mucus; some of this moisture is taken up by the inspired air. Possibly an even more important function of the mucous layer is to catch small dust particles, bacteria, and the like, on its surface. The layer of mucus is not stationary, but is kept in constant motion by the action of the cilia. This whip-like action of the cilia causes the mucus to move toward the throat. Thus, entrapped particles are carried to the throat and swallowed, rather than drawn into the lungs. The ends of the olfactory nerve are located in the upper one third of the nose. It is by means of this nerve that we appreciate flavors. The nose and sinuses together with the throat and chest act as resonant chambers and give quality (timbre) to the voice.

Disturbances of the Nose

FURUNCLE

The vestibule of the nose is lined with skin and with short hairs called vibrissae. Not uncommonly one or more of these hair follicles become infected, giving rise to a furuncle. These furuncles should never be squeezed or picked as this procedure may cause the infection to spread along the veins of the nose to the venous sinuses of the brain.

Treatment. It is, however, safe to apply 2 per cent yellow oxide of mercury ointment to the inflamed area. The more severe infections should be treated with hot compresses. Such procedures will usually cause the furuncle to become localized and eventually to rupture spontaneously. Penicillin is administered in serious cases.

EPISTAXIS

Nasal hemorrhage is a common ailment. It may result from injury to the nose, operation, ulceration, hemophilia, nose-picking in children, or hypertension. Considerable blood may be lost. Fortunately, the commonest site of the bleeding is the anterior portion of the septum where there is a rich anastomosis of blood vessels.

Treatment. Often the bleeding can be controlled by simply pressing the nostrils between the fingers for a few minutes, or introducing into the nostril a small pledget of cotton saturated with adrenalin. The patient should be placed in the semirecumbent position. If the bleeding is severe and the patient is restless, he should be given morphine.

Electrocautery. Bleeding is apt to recur unless the area is cauterized. Under direct vision, a small cotton pledget moistened with a few drops of 10 per cent cocaine solution containing adrenalin is placed over the bleeding point. In the majority of cases this stops the hemorrhage and also anesthetizes the area, which is then touched with a silver nitrate stick or coagulated with electrocautery.

Profuse Hemorrhage. Occasionally the hemorrhage is too profuse to be controlled by these methods, or it may be from higher in the nose. In this event the nose must be packed with ½ inch gauze which has been well saturated with petrolatum. This packing should not remain in the nose for longer than twenty-four hours; if left for a longer period of time, it becomes foul and may give rise to an infection of the sinuses.

FOREIGN BODIES

Children are prone to introduce small foreign bodies, such as beads, peas, beans, and so on, into the nose. Beans and peas may even sprout, but any foreign body will cause swelling of the mucous membrane of the side where it is located, with resultant nasal obstruction. There is also a discharge (often purulent) from the nostril.

Removal. Removal can usually be accomplished after the application of 10 per cent cocaine solution with adrenalin on a cotton pledget. Occasionally a general anesthetic has to be administered.

FRACTURES

Fractures of the nose commonly involve the nasal bones and the septum; occasionally the septum alone is fractured. These structures may be displaced laterally or anteroposteriorly, or there may be a combination of the two. After injury there is usually a brisk nosebleed, which subsides spontaneously within a short time. Swelling of the soft tissues soon follows. Often the external deformity may be noted on simple inspection, or actual crepitus may be felt. On examination of the interior of the nose, the septum is seen to be deflected to one side or the other. An x-ray film will show a crack in the nasal bones and any displacement of the fragments.

Treatment. If there is no displacement of the bone and if the deflection of the septum is minimal, no treatment is required. If, however, the nasal bones are depressed or the septum is seriously displaced, these structures should be replaced in their normal position. This is done by manipulation under anesthesia. Packing is not required after the fracture has been reduced as the bones and the septum tend to stay in position once the proper alignment has been made.

DEVIATION OF THE NASAL SEPTUM

Deviation of the nasal septum is either traumatic or developmental in origin. An untreated fracture of the nose may result in a permanent deflection of the septum. In other instances, because of some unknown factor in the growth of the nose, the septum becomes thickened or is displaced into one nostril. Sufficient septal deflection causes respiratory obstruction. Often the patient has repeated colds and complains that a cold persists for several weeks; a patient with a severe septal deflection will give a history of repeated attacks of acute sinusitis on the affected side, due to blocking of normal drainage from the sinuses.

Submucous Resection. Operative treatment is indicated if the deflection is obstructing ventilation or drainage. The operation to correct a deviated septum is called submucous resection; it is performed under local anesthesia. The patient is allowed to have breakfast. He is given 0.2 gm. of phenobarbital half an hour before the scheduled time for operation for the purpose of counteracting any toxic effects of cocaine. The patient may be seated in an ordinary office chair or, if the operator prefers to stand, the patient may be placed on an operating table, one end of which is elevated to serve as a back rest. The septum is anesthetized by the application of cotton tampons moistened with 20 per cent cocaine solution containing adrenalin. These tampons should have the excess cocaine solution squeezed from them before insertion in the nose, thus preventing a large amount of the cocaine from being swallowed and lessening the possibility of overdosage. The cartilage and bone of the nasal septum are removed from beneath the mucous membrane. When this is done completely the remaining septum (largely mucous membrane) should be in the midline. A petrolatum gauze pack is inserted into each nostril to hold the flaps of mucous membrane together and to control bleeding. These packs should be removed early the next day.

Nursing Care. The patient should remain in bed until after the packs are removed. For the first three or four hours he is placed in semi-Fowler's position and ice compresses are applied to the nose. There is remarkably little postoperative pain and what little discomfort there is may be readily controlled with codeine and aspirin. The patient may be placed on whatever diet is desired. These patients should be watched carefully for any evidence of excessive bleeding.

Diseases of the Paranasal Sinuses

SINUSITIS

Infection of the lining membrane of the sinuses may be acute or chronic. Any sinuses may be involved, but the ethmoid and the maxillary are the ones most commonly affected. The common cold is the usual forerunner of acute sinusitis; chronic sinusitis results from the neglect of acute sinusitis. A deviated nasal septum or swelling of the mucous membrane due to allergy (allergic rhinitis) may interfere with the drainage of an acutely infected sinus to such a degree that a chronic infection results. Infection of the roots of the upper bicuspid and molar teeth at times causes chronic infection of the maxillary sinuses as the roots of these teeth lie close to the floor of the sinus.

An infected sinus may be a focus of infection in such diseases as bronchitis, bronchial asthma, bronchiectasis, nephritis, arthritis, and certain diseases of the eye.

INFECTION OF THE ETHMOID SINUS

Acute Ethmoiditis. In nearly every severe head cold there is an accompanying ethmoiditis. The patient complains of a stuffy sensation in the nose and there is profuse mucopurulent nasal discharge. Often there is headache between the eyes and pain on movement of the eyes. There is edema of the nasal mucous membrane and purulent discharge above and below the middle turbinate.

Treatment. Reestablishment of drainage may be accomplished by the local application of agents such as cocaine, ephedrine, neosynephrine, Privine, and Paredrine which cause shrinking of the congested mucous membrane.

Chronic Ethmoid Sinusitis. Here the symptoms are those of persistent nasal obstruction on the involved side and nasal discharge. Headache is frequently not present, but the patient may complain of an impaired sense of smell. On examination a discharge is seen above or below the middle turbinate, depending on whether the posterior or anterior ethmoid sinuses are involved. Frequently polyps are seen in these regions. A polyp is an edematous overgrowth of the chronically infected mucous membrane. In appearance it closely resembles a peeled grape. Polyps vary greatly in size and number, and may grow to fill the entire nostril. Nasal allergy and neoplasm of the sinuses cause polyps as well as infection.

Treatment. Occasionally a mild chronic ethmoid infection responds to conservative treatment, but the majority of the cases require operation. The preparation of the patient is the same as for submucous resection (p. 485). The operation is performed under local anesthesia. The middle turbinate is removed and the ethmoid cells thus exposed are removed by biting them away with an ethmoid rongeur. If the patient has a deviated nasal septum this should be straightened. The nose is packed with petrolatum gauze. The after-care of the patient is similar to that given after submucous resection.

INFECTION OF THE SPHENOID SINUS

This condition often accompanies an infection of the corresponding posterior ethmoid sinus, and may be either acute or chronic. Often the only symptoms of either type of infection are nasal obstruction and discharge from the nose. Because of the position of the sinus the discharge is frequently postnasal (accumulating in the throat). If headache is present there is nothing typical in its location; headache in the occipital region, however, is suggestive of a sphenoidal infection. There is discharge above the posterior end of the middle turbinate. An x-ray examination may show clouding of the sinus.

Treatment of Acute Form. The milder acute infections usually respond to daily shrinking of the nasal mucous membrane in the region of the sphenoid orifice, but the more severe acute infections sometimes require irrigation of the sphenoid through the natural ostium.

Operation for Chronic Form. If a chronic sphenoid infection is present, the posterior end of the middle turbinate is removed under local anesthesia and the sinus orifice is enlarged with sphenoid rongeurs. The interior of the sinus should never be curetted because of possible injury to the optic nerve or carotid artery. Many operators routinely enlarge the sphenoid orifice at the time of the performance of an operation on the ethmoid sinuses. The postoperative care consists primarily of irrigations of the sinus through the enlarged ostium.

INFECTION OF THE MAXILLARY SINUS

Acute Form. The patient who has acute maxillary sinusitis complains of nasal obstruction and discharge; in addition, headache above the eyes (*frontal headache*) is commonly present. Often the patient complains of pain in the face and in the upper teeth on the involved side, or simply of a fulness in this region. There is discharge under the middle turbinate, and the sinus does not transilluminate clearly. Roentgenograms are much more accurate than transillumination in diagnosing maxillary sinusitis, and may show diffuse clouding or a level of fluid (that is, pus) in the sinus.

Treatment. At first the treatment consists in efforts to reduce

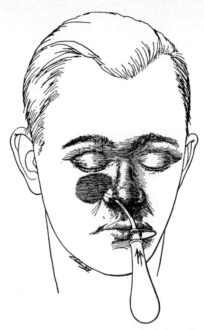

FIGURE 123. Establishing drainage of an acutely inflamed maxillary sinus by introducing a trocar into the sinus.

the swelling of the nasal mucous membrane in order to promote drainage. Codeine with aspirin is given every four hours if there is much discomfort. If definite improvement is not shown in forty-eight hours, the sinus should be punctured and the pus washed out. To do this a cotton-tipped nasal applicator moistened with a few drops each of 20 per cent cocaine solution and 1 in 1000 adrenalin is introduced beneath the anterior end of the inferior turbinate and is allowed to remain about twenty minutes. Then a curved trocar is put through the thin bone under the inferior turbinate. The patient leans forward and holds a basin under his chin. Warm sterile normal saline is gently forced through the trocar and comes out through the natural ostium, carrying pus with it. If desired, a culture is taken. These irrigations should be carried out every day or every other day until the washings return clear.

Chronic Form. Chronic maxillary sinusitis is characterized by long standing nasal discharge and obstruction. There may be frontal headache, but, unless there is an acute infection, pain in the face and upper teeth is not present. The lining membrane becomes thickened and may contain microscopic abscesses. Discharge or polyps, or both, are present in the middle meatus. The sinus is dark on transillumination and cloudy on x-ray examination.

Treatment. Occasionally three or four punctures and irrigations of the sinus will clear up the infection if polyps are not present, but the greater number of patients will require a radical antrum (Caldwell-Luc) operation.

TECHNIC OF CALDWELL-LUC OPERATION. This operation is best performed under general anesthesia. The preoperative preparation is the same as that for any patient undergoing general anesthesia. The head of the operating table should be lowered slightly to prevent aspiration of blood and mucus. A postnasal pack is inserted to prevent blood from draining into the pharynx. An incision about 1½ inches long is made in the mouth along the upper gum above the canine teeth; the periosteum is elevated with a periosteal elevator and the bone exposed. With a perforator an opening is made into the maxillary sinus and the opening is enlarged with bone forceps. The lining mucous membrane is completely removed from the sinus with forceps. An opening is then made into the sinus beneath the inferior turbinate. A small petrolatum gauze pack is placed in the antrum and one end brought out through the opening under the inferior turbinate. The incision over the canine fossa is sutured.

Nursing Care. The patient is placed in bed face down with a pillow under his chest until the swallowing reflex returns. He may then be placed in semi-Fowler's position. Ice compresses are applied to the face for five or six hours to help prevent swelling. Morphine may be administered every four hours if necessary to control pain. The patient is given a liquid diet for two or three days, and is watched carefully for signs of excessive bleeding. The pack is removed the day after operation. Postoperative care consists of irrigations through the opening into the sinus under the inferior turbinate until the washings return clear.

INFECTION OF THE FRONTAL SINUS

Acute Form. The cause of acute frontal sinusitis is identical with that of acute ethmoid or maxillary sinusitis. Frontal headache and pain above the eye are nearly always present. The patient usually awakens in the morning with no discomfort, but after he has been up for several hours the headache and pain appear and are extremely severe. Examination reveals the same findings as in acute ethmoiditis. In addition the anterior wall of the frontal sinus is tender on light percussion, a finding characteristic of the disease. The involved sinus does not transilluminate clearly and x-ray examination shows cloudiness or a fluid level in the sinus.

Treatment. Treatment consists in shrinking the nasal membrane in the region of the nasofrontal duct, under the anterior end of the middle turbinate. The application of moist or dry heat to the involved sinus is of benefit. Codeine and aspirin should be given for relief of pain. If after several days of this treatment improvement does not take place, the sinus should be irrigated. This is accomplished by introducing a curved frontal sinus cannula into the sinus through the nasofrontal duct after cocainization of this area. The sinus is gently irrigated with warm sterile normal salt solution, a small rubber bulb being attached to the cannula. Sometimes the anterior third of the middle turbinate must be removed before this procedure can be carried out.

TREPHINING. In obstinate cases the author prefers trephine of the sinus to irrigation. This is accomplished under general anesthesia. The eyebrow is shaved off on the involved side. A pack is placed in the nasopharynx to prevent aspiration of pus. Cotton pads moistened with warm normal salt solution are placed over the eyes. An incision about 1 inch long is made through the inner third of the eyebrow. With a perforator a small opening is made through the anterior bony wall of the sinus. At this point in the operation the mucous membrane of the sinus often bulges into the wound, and is incised; the pus is gently removed with suction. A short length of soft rubber tubing is placed through the opening into the sinus and anchored to the skin edges with a suture. The wound is left wide open and dressings are applied. The relief of pain and headache is most dramatic. On the second day after operation the drain is removed and the sinus irrigated through the wound with warm sterile salt solution. These irrigations are carried out daily until there is no pus in the washings. The wound is then allowed to heal.

Chronic Form. Chronic frontal sinusitis may give rise to osteomyelitis of the frontal bone, brain abscess, extradural abscess, or meningitis. Because of the danger of these complications it is the most serious of the chronic sinus infections. The symptoms are frontal headache and a purulent nasal discharge. Rarely is there tenderness over the involved sinus unless there is a superimposed acute infection. As in acute frontal sinusitis, a discharge is visible under the anterior end of the middle turbinate, and nasal polyps may be seen in this area. There is frequently an associated chronic infection of the ethmoids. The infected sinus tranilluminates poorly and an x-ray film shows clouding.

Treatment. Any treatment other than operative is of no avail. If the ethmoid sinuses are infected they, too, should be operated upon.

TECHNIQUE OF OPERATION. The radical operation for chronic frontal sinusitis is performed with the patient under general anesthesia. The preoperative preparations are identical with those for trephining (p. 490). An incision is made through the eyebrow for almost its entire length. The bone of the entire anterior wall and part of the floor of the sinus are removed with rongeurs. The entire mucous membrane lining of the sinus is removed with a curette. The resulting bony cavity is carefully inspected for any areas of infection (*osteomyelitis*); if any are found, all diseased bone is removed. The nasofrontal duct is then enlarged with a rasp. A piece of soft rubber tubing is placed in the sinus at the inner angle of the wound and sutured to the skin edges. The flaps of periosteum, muscle, and subcutaneous tissue are closed with catgut; the skin edges are closed with fine silkworm gut. The drain is removed on the second day after operation. Postoperative care consists of irrigations of the sinus through the enlarged nasofrontal duct.

CHEMOTHERAPY AND ANTIBIOTICS IN SINUSITIS

The systemic effects upon the patient with sinusitis are variable: some patients are systematically ill, with fever, anorexia, and malaise, whereas others complain only of the local symptoms.

In recent years the treatment of acute sinusitis, and to a less extent chronic sinusitis, has been revolutionized by the introduction of the various antibiotics. In the acute cases, the subjective symptoms are usually reduced both in severity and duration. It is also most significant that the frequency of complications has been tremendously reduced. In some cases of chronic sinusitis, the administration of antibiotics has resulted in improvement to such a degree that operation has been found unnecessary. In an even greater number of cases antibiotics given preoperatively and postoperatively have greatly reduced the period of convalescence, and the incidence of complications due to a spreading of the infection.

Instead of trying one antibiotic after another in a hit or miss manner, one should get a culture of the discharge as it comes from the sinus. After the offending organism or organisms are isolated, it is a relatively simple laboratory procedure to determine the sensitivity of the organisms to the various antibiotics. Naturally, the antibiotic chosen is the one to which the organisms are most sensitive.

NEOPLASTIC DISEASE OF THE NOSE AND SINUSES

Many varieties of neoplasms occur in the nose and accessory sinuses, but the commonest tumor is carcinoma. Here, as elsewhere, the onset is insidious and painless; the first complaints of the patient are either the result of infection which follows obstruction caused by the neoplasm, or are due to metastases in the lymph nodes of the neck, in the mediastinum, or in the bones of the skull. By the time symptoms direct attention to the tumor it has usually spread beyond the local limits of its origin, so that surgical treatment is futile; in some types of carcinoma good results follow radiation therapy, but in general the prognosis is unfavorable.

THE PHARYNX AND THE LARYNX

Anatomy and Physiology. The pharynx is that part of the upper respiratory tract which is continuous with the posterior portions of the nose and mouth. The inferior portion of the pharynx is continuous with the larynx and esophagus; the pharynx is thus common to both the respiratory and the alimentary tracts. The lining membrane of the pharynx is epithelial, and in the upper portion (nasopharynx) the surface cells are ciliated. Beneath the epithelial surface are many mucous glands and much lymphoid tissue. There is usually a mass of lymphoid tissue located along the roof and posterior wall of the pharynx on each side; these masses constitute the adenoids. There are also several sets of muscles in the pharyngeal wall which are necessary for swallowing and aid in phonation. On the upper lateral wall of the pharynx on each side is found the orifice of the eustachian tube, a duct which leads directly into the cavity of the middle ear. In the lower pharynx, lateral and posterior to the base of the tongue, are large, oval masses of lymphoid tissue; these are the tonsils.

The larynx is a semirigid tube joining the lower pharynx and the upper trachea. It is lined with the characteristic mucous membrane of the respiratory tract and owes its rigidity to the support given by the hyoid bone, and the arytenoid, cricoid, and thyroid cartilages. The upper end of the larynx (*glottis*) is immediately behind the tongue, and is guarded by a trapdoor-like structure, the epiglottis, which covers the opening during swallowing, thus preventing the entrance of food, fluid, or other foreign material into the larynx. Within the larynx are the vocal cords, two folds of fibrous tissue covered with squamous epithelium, which project into the lumen. The position of the cords, the vibration of which produces the sound of the voice, is determined by the action of the intrinsic muscles of the larynx. These muscles, and also those which control the position and movements of the epiglottis, are activated by the tenth cranial nerves.

Adenoids

The commonest disorder of the nasopharynx is chronic infection and hypertrophy of the adenoid (lymphatic) tissue. Following the repeated colds of infancy and childhood, the adenoids may become large enough to obstruct the opening between the posterior nose and the nasopharynx, resulting in habitual mouth breathing. Hypertrophy of the adenoid tissue, furthermore, may cause blocking of the orifices of the eustachian tubes, the chief cause of middle ear infection (*otitis media*) and deafness in children; it is also the important factor in aerotitis, a common complaint among aviators. Diagnosis of infected, hypertrophied adenoids is readily made upon inspection of the nasopharynx by means of the nasopharyngoscope.

Treatment. Treatment consists in the surgical removal of the adenoid tissue, or in its destruction by radiation. The surgical procedure (*adenoidectomy*) is usually combined with removal of the tonsils (*tonsillectomy*) and is described with that operation. It is impossible to remove all the lymphoid tissue surgically, however, and any remnants may hypertrophy to cause recurrence of the condition. The results of irradiation are more satisfactory; for this purpose the brief application of radium or its gaseous emanation (radon) is used. The radium applicator is introduced gently through the inferior meatus of each nostril of the recumbent patient. The exposure is brief and must be carefully timed to secure adequate radiation without causing a burn from overexposure.

Tonsillitis

Acute Form. The symptoms of acute tonsillitis are sore throat, pain and difficulty in swallowing, and malaise. Fever is usually present. The commonest cause of the infection is the streptococcus, but the possibility of diphtheria and of Vincent's angina must be considered. Scarlet fever also begins with a sore throat, and it is a good general rule that patients with acute tonsillitis be isolated promptly. The tonsils are swollen and red, and often there are patches of white or yellowish exudate on the surface. The lymph nodes of the neck are enlarged and tender. Smears and cultures of the tonsillar exudate must be made in order to identify the causative bacteria.

Treatment. Treatment consists in local measures combined with systemic therapy to combat the infection. The sulfonamides and penicillin are effective. Rest in bed, liquid or soft diet, adequate fluids, and codeine and aspirin are prescribed. Mild cases respond to this treatment; severe cases should be treated with sulfadiazine or penicillin (or both), the former by mouth and the latter intramuscularly.

TONSILLECTOMY

Indications. There are several reasons for removing the tonsils. Repeated attacks of acute tonsillitis lead to the persistent presence of pathogenic bacteria, causing low-grade chronic tonsillitis; this condition seems to cause further acute flare-ups, and also acts as a focus of infection which may have harmful effects in other parts of the body. In addition to chronic tonsillitis, other indications for tonsillectomy are the presence of persistently enlarged cervical lymph nodes, repeated attacks of otitis media, and the occurrence of such systemic diseases as infectious arthritis, rheumatic fever, or chronic nephritis.

Technic. Tonsillectomy and adenoidectomy are usually combined into one procedure; T. and A., as it is familiarly called, is possibly the most frequently performed operation. Tonsillectomy is readily carried out under either local or general anesthesia, but the combined T. and A. requires a general anesthesia. At least six weeks should elapse between the most recent acute infection of the upper respiratory tract and the operation. During the

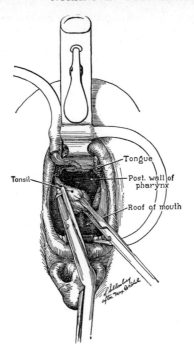

FIGURE 124. Tonsillectomy.

operation the operating table should be inclined about 15 degrees, with the patient's head lower than his feet, so as to reduce to a minimum the possible aspiration of blood or tonsillar debris. Adenoid tissue is scraped from the nasopharynx by means of a curette, and bleeding is checked by packing with gauze. Each tonsil is then grasped and dissected free with scapel and scissors. Catgut sutures are used to control bleeding from the tonsillar fossae. Constant suction is employed to keep the throat dry, thus preventing aspiration.

Nursing Care. The postoperative care is like that given patients after any general anesthesia (p. 81). On return from the operating room the patient is placed face downward, with a pillow under his chest until the swallowing reflex returns. While he is in this position there is no danger of aspiration because the secretions will drain out of the mouth. An emesis basin and a generous supply of gauze or paper tissue is provided for the expectoration of blood, mucus, and saliva. An ice collar is applied immediately. As soon as the patient is conscious he is placed in Fowler's position.

Bleeding is the chief complication; when the blood is expectorated it is bright red, but when it is swallowed and then vomited the mixing with the gastric juice produces a reddish brown color. If the patient is not fully awake or is dozing when the bleeding starts he may be observed to swallow frequently. A steady increase in pulse rate or the frequent expectoration of bright red blood should be reported to the surgeon.

Water and cracked ice are given as soon as nausea ceases. Codeine is usually given the first day. On the second day, gargles of normal salt solution or aspirin in suspension are helpful to relieve discomfort. If aspirin in chewing gum is given about one half hour before mealtime, a semi-liquid diet can be taken with little discomfort. Orange, grapefruit, and lemon juice are excluded from the diet. Fluids should be forced to three liters daily and must be offered regularly and the patient encouraged to drink.

Adults are usually discharged from the hospital on the third or fourth day after operation, but children commonly leave the hospital on the second day. The adult is instructed to be a convalescent for at least one week, and should gargle twice or three times daily, drink three liters of fluids daily, and refrain from strenuous exercise.

Peritonsillar Abscess

This condition, also called quinsy, is a complication of the spread of infection from the tonsil into the adjoining pharyngeal wall with abscess formation. The symptoms are the same as those of a severe tonsillitis, usually with localization to the affected side. Swelling of the pharynx is readily seen, and fluctuation can be felt.

Treatment. The treatment is incision and drainage, release of the pus causing almost instantaneous relief of pain. Great care must be used to prevent aspiration of any of the pus or blood.

Laryngitis

Inflammation of the larynx is a common complication of infections of the upper respiratory tract. The consequent edema and thickening of the mucous membrane and vocal cords result in hoarseness and cough; there may be actual loss of voice and, in severe cases, respiratory obstruction which is due in part to spasm

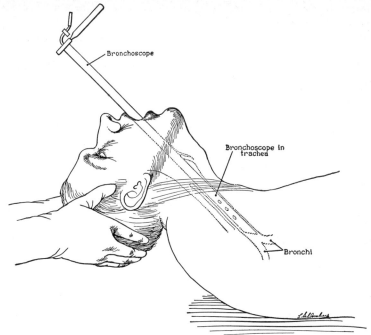

Bronchoscope

Bronchoscope in trachea

Bronchi

FIGURE 125. Bronchoscopy.

of the laryngeal muscles. One form of laryngitis occurring in infancy and childhood is called croup. Diphtheria produces the most serious variety of laryngitis, as the inflammatory exudate (*diphtheritic membrane*) may produce mechanical obstruction to the passage of air. In such a case, in addition to treating the infection, a breathing tube is inserted from the mouth into the trachea to prevent asphyxiation; this is called intubation. The tube is retained until the obstruction subsides. Less severe forms of laryngitis respond well to inhalation of steam generated by a croup kettle.

A chronic type of laryngitis occurs after repeated upper respiratory tract infections, or after prolonged abuse of the voice; actual thickening of the vocal cords results, but the symptoms disappear upon removal of the cause and a proper period of rest.

Neoplasms of the Pharynx and Larynx

Both benign and malignant tumors arise in the nasopharynx, more often in adults than in children; malignant tumors are the more frequent. The same symptoms are produced by these as are produced by hypertrophy of the adenoids (p. 493); in the later stages nosebleed is common. Impairment of hearing usually follows, and metastasis to the cervical lymph nodes is the rule. Cure seldom follows surgery, but irradiation is more successful. Tonsillar tumors also are usually malignant and are treated more successfully by radiation than by surgery. Biopsy, however, should be routinely performed in order to establish the correct diagnosis.

The prognosis is more favorable in laryngeal tumors. Benign epithelial papilloma, a tassel-like or cauliflower-like growth, is a common lesion; it causes persistent hoarseness, and is permanently cured by surgical removal, performed through a laryngoscope.

Cancer of the larynx is also a common disease; since it gives rise to the early symptom of hoarseness, it is often curable. The larynx is removed (*laryngectomy*), necessitating a permanent tracheotomy. The voice is lost, but an artificial larynx is available, by means of which the patient can make himself heard and understood.

TRACHEOTOMY

The purpose of this operation is to produce an opening through the neck into the trachea for the purpose of respiration. Permanent tracheotomies are necessary after laryngectomy and in patients having constriction of the upper larynx resulting from disease or injury. Tracheotomy is often an emergency procedure as well, in order to prevent asphyxiation when sudden obstruction of the larynx occurs, as in severe infections of the upper neck (e.g., Ludwig's angina), angioneurotic edema, or hemorrhage. Since death from asphyxia occurs in a few minutes, a sterile tracheotomy set must be available in every hospital ward in which there are patients who have diphtheria, other laryngeal disease, serious infection of the neck, or recent operations about the neck.

Technic. The operation may be performed swiftly and easily. Procaine infiltration of the skin is the only anesthesia necessary, and even that is not needed for a patient who is in extremis. A short vertical incision is made in the skin of the lower neck directly over the trachea. The deep fascia is incised and the neck muscles are retracted to either side, exposing the trachea. If care is taken to stay below the isthmus of the thyroid gland, practically no bleeding is encountered. The trachea itself is then

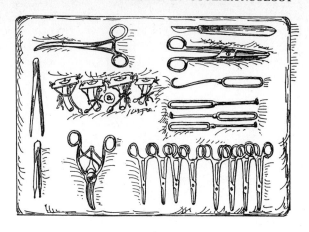

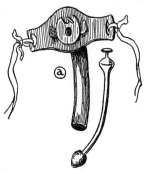

FIGURE 126. Tracheotomy set. This tray of instruments is dry-sterilized and kept on the ward for emergency use. Each tracheotomy tube (a) consists of three parts made to fit each other: outer or guard tube, inner tube, and obturator.

incised and three cartilaginous rings are divided. Air rushes in and out as soon as the trachea is opened, and the patient's relief is immediate. A tracheotomy tube of the proper size is then inserted and strapped to the neck. Fortunately the tracheal mucosa at this level is quite insensitive, so that the tube is well tolerated. The wound about the tube is loosely packed with gauze, and no attempt is made to close it as there is always bacterial contamination from the open trachea.

Wounds of the trachea, either operative or traumatic, have a tendency to heal rapidly; it is necessary, therefore, to keep a tube

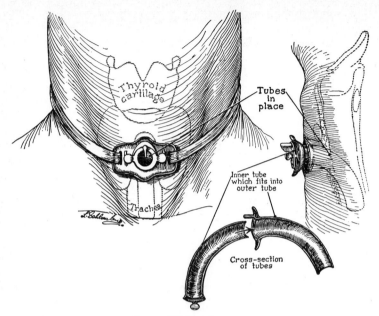

FIGURE 127. Tracheotomy.

in the trachea constantly if the surgeon wants the tracheotomy to be permanent. When, on the other hand, the tracheotomy is no longer needed, the tube is removed; complete healing occurs in two to three weeks.

Tracheotomy tubes are made of noncorrosive metal, and in various sizes. The outer or guard tube should fit the trachea snugly. The inner tube fits exactly into the guard tube, and may be removed at will by the nurse or the patient for cleaning and removing obstructing clots of mucus. The guard tube should be changed or adjusted only by the surgeon, however, since it is often difficult to replace.

Nursing Care. A patient with a newly inserted tracheotomy tube is most conveniently cared for in a private room. The constant attention of a nurse is required for at least a few days, often much longer, depending upon the case. The patient is voiceless, and so cannot call for help or, if a baby, cry aloud.

Fluids are given soon after operation; diet as tolerated may be administered the following day. Antibiotic agents, usually penicillin and streptomycin, are given routinely for the first few days.

The room should be humidified in cool weather, but the temperature should be kept at 70° F. Opiates and atropine must not be given and the surgeon often writes an order to this effect. Opiates would decrease the cough reflex and atropine would dry up the secretions; both are contraindicated.

Equipment. The complete care of the patient is accomplished in the safest and easiest manner when the room is equipped with all the necessary facilities. Articles for this purpose include a suction apparatus to which is attached a rubber catheter that fits the tracheotomy tube, a bottle filled with sterile salt solution in which the catheter is rinsed, a jar of sterile sponges, a sterile forceps in 1 per cent lysol, a sterile covered basin containing one obturator which fits in the tracheotomy tube, one complete tracheotomy tube which is the same size as the one in the trachea, an electric hot plate, a 2-quart covered basin half filled with water, pipe cleaners, wire applicators, absorbent cotton, a small bowl of hydrogen peroxide, silver polish, pencil and paper, paper or gauze wipes, and a paper bag pinned to the bed within easy each. When the room is fully set up the nurse feels secure and independent because not only can she take care of the patient more efficiently with all the facilities at hand, but also because she does not require aid from others.

Insuring Patency. The nurse must understand that the tracheotomy is not the ultimate object but is only a means to pipe air into the lungs. Her primary responsibility is to ensure free passage of air through the tube by keeping the tube patent. There is usually considerable discharge of secretion which, when not coughed out, must be removed by suction; a clogged tube causes asphyxiation in a few minutes. The coughing and rattling sound produced by the mixture of mucus and air are an indication for suction. The patient should be taught not to cough forcibly to expel the mucus but to indicate to the nurse when suction is necessary for removal of excess mucus. It is difficult even for an adult to cooperate in this way; in the case of a child it is impossible. Forceful coughing may cause hemorrhage. When the secretions are forced out they should be wiped away quickly and gently before they are inspired through the tube.

Breathing is less difficult when a thin layer of moistened gauze saturated in 2 per cent sterile boric acid solution is placed over the opening of the tube so that the air is humidified and filtered. The excess solution is expressed so that there is no dripping. After the sponge is unfolded it is placed over the mouth of the tube and is held in place by tucking it under the tape about the patient's neck.

The apprehension of the patient which is frequently encountered is often attributable to his frightening experience of partial or complete laryngeal obstruction before operation. The nurse should be reassuring and calm. She should give him detailed explanations concerning his care so that if he is an adult he is unconsciously learning how to care for himself. When constant attention is no longer necessary the patient should have a bell placed within reach so that he can summon a nurse quickly.

Care of the Tube. The surgeon usually orders that the inner tube be cleaned every hour for the first few days and as often as the nurse feels that it is necessary after that period. The removal of the inner tube is not difficult but it should be done gently and smoothly. A slight jerk of the tube may start violent coughing. While the guard tube is held firmly with the left thumb and forefinger, the inner tube is withdrawn with the right hand. The tube is cleaned by placing it in a bowl of hydrogen peroxide to harden the mucus so that it is more easily removed. When the tube is small in size a pipe cleaner is repeatedly inserted and drawn through the tube until the tube appears entirely clean when it is inspected in a good light. Absorbent cotton on a wire applicator is more satisfactory for cleaning larger tubes. Tarnishing occurs quickly; the use of silver polish will keep the tube shining. While the tube is being cleaned dents and irregularities are prevented by handling it without force. An improperly fitting inner tube is dangerous and also wasteful because it requires the discarding of all three parts. The tubes are handmade and are interchangeable only when more than one was originally made for the guard tube. The inner tube is boiled for one minute in the basin on the hot plate. It is reinserted with the same precautions with which it was removed.

Decannulation. The insertion of a tracheotomy tube is often a temporary measure. In such cases, before removal of the tube, the patient must be made to breathe normally by a gradual obstruction of the tube. Part of a cork is placed in the mouth of the tube, and if there are no signs of respiratory distress or obstruction the size of the cork is increased until the tube is completely obstructed. When the patient is comfortable and shows no ill effects, the tube is removed and the opening is permitted to heal. This process usually takes several days and is known as decannulation.

Learning to Talk. Patients with a tracheotomy should not be permitted to whisper but should be encouraged to converse in writing; they are able to talk if a cork is inserted in the tube or when the tube is removed and the trachea is closed. Patients with total laryngectomy will not be able to talk in the natural manner and must wear a tube permanently. They can learn to talk by two methods; the most useful is by means of an esophageal voice. This method is acquired by the mastery of the ability to swallow air, to force it back from the stomach and to form words out of the belch when it returns. The voice sounds like that of a patient who has a severe case of laryngitis but it is quite understandable, and is indeed a source of great enjoyment and satisfaction to the patient. This process of learning requires much patience, persistence and initiative. It is accomplished most easily under the direction of an instructor.

Care of Tube by Patient. When a patient is to be discharged with a tracheotomy tube it is essential that he be able to care for himself without hesitancy or apprehension. If a child, the person responsible for him is taught by demonstration of the changing and cleaning of the tube. When possible, instruction is begun several days before discharge so that practice under the supervision of a nurse may be carried out to make certain that the care is completely understood.

THE EAR

The external ear is composed of skin and cartilage, and the external opening (*external auditory meatus*) leads to the ear drum (*tympanic membrane*), a tightly stretched diaphragm which receives sound waves and accurately transmits their vibrations. The ear drum forms the external wall of a small cavity called the middle ear. Within the middle ear are the three ossicles (*malleus, incus,* and *stapes*), a chain of tiny articulated bones joining the ear drum and the internal ear, and serving to transmit the vibrations of sound to the internal ear.

Leading off from the cavity of the middle ear is the eustachian tube, which opens into the nasopharynx; this tube has for its function the equalization of air pressure between the middle ear and the atmosphere. The middle ear, internal ear, and mastoid cells are all within the temporal bone of the skull. The mastoid cells are similar to the accessory nasal sinuses, but communicate through a minute opening with the cavity of the middle ear. The internal ear is composed of the spiral cochlea, which contains the auditory nerve endings which are stimulated by the sound vibrations, and the three semicircular canals, each perpendicular to the others, which are the end organs of the special sense of equilibrium.

Surgery of the External Ear

Congenital Deformities. These are relatively common. The ear may be partly or almost completely absent, or it may be large and prominent. Such deformities often cause the afflicted child to be an object of ridicule and may give rise to serious personality disturbance; fortunately a skilful plastic surgeon can do much to repair the disfigurement.

Trauma. Because of its exposed position, accidental injury is fairly frequent, but the ear has an excellent blood supply and even the severest lacerations heal admirably if properly treated.

Inspissated Cerumen. Another exceedingly common affection is the accumulation of wax (*cerumen*) in the external auditory meatus, which causes impairment of hearing and sometimes pain; this is removed gently under direct vision, although it is necessary at times to soften the wax by the application of a drop or two of oil.

Foreign Bodies. Children and psychotic patients insert foreign bodies into the external meatus, with resultant pain and inflammation; as a rule these objects are easily removed.

Inflammation. A condition troublesome to cure is chronic inflammation (*external otitis*) of the meatus caused by fungus infection. This is common, particularly in those who engage in aquatics; the symptoms are itching, discharge, and pain. The local application of various chemical disinfectants is helpful in some cases, but no specific therapy has been devised. The use of boric acid powder containing 1 per cent iodine has proved useful in treating this condition.

Carcinoma. Cancer of the external ear is also a common lesion. It is treated by a combination of radical excision and radiation therapy, which is sufficient if the deeper tissues are not invaded at the time treatment is undertaken.

Diseases of the Middle Ear

ACUTE OTITIS MEDIA

Acute purulent inflammation of the middle ear cavity is common, especially in children. The pathogenic bacteria gain entrance through the eustachian tube, so that the disease is a complication of acute infection of the upper respiratory tract, particularly if there is infected adenoid tissue about the pharyngeal orifice of the eustachian tube. Coughing, sneezing, or anything which causes sudden elevation of the intrapharyngeal air pressure tends to force air and bacteria into the middle ear. Aerotitis, an occupational disease among aviators, is a middle ear infection produced in this manner. The symptoms are severe earache and impairment of hearing. Fever and leukocytosis occur. On examination the ear drum on the affected side is seen to be inflamed and bulging.

Treatment. As in any purulent infection, the proper local treatment is to establish drainage early in order to prevent complications; this is done by making a tiny incision through the ear drum (*myringotomy*). General anesthesia is necessary. Relief of pain is almost immediate, and in the uncomplicated case healing of the drum without impairment of hearing takes place after a few days of drainage.

Less severe attacks of acute otitis media are successfully treated by sulfonamide or penicillin therapy, as the usual bacterial invaders are streptococci, staphylococci, or pneumococci, against which these agents are most effective. In patients in whom the drum is red but not bulging, the need for myringotomy may be averted if chemotherapy is started at once. The prevention of otitis media, however, is the best safeguard against loss of hearing or more serious complications; this has already been discussed under the subject of infected nasopharyngeal adenoid tissue (p. 493).

Complications. The complications of repeated attacks of otitis media or of improperly treated or neglected otitis media are serious. These include scarring of the drum, chronic perforation of the drum, osteomyelitis of the ossicles, mastoiditis, and permanent impairment of hearing; occasionally brain abscess or meningitis follow, and death is not unknown. These complications may occur even in a promptly treated case if the infection is overwhelming, and in such cases chemotherapy (sulfonamides and penicillin) is often life-saving.

MASTOIDITIS

Infection of the mastoid cells of the temporal bone is a serious complication of otitis media. It is indeed fortunate that this infection responds well to therapy with sulfonamides or penicillin or both; before the days of chemotherapy mastoiditis was a prolonged illness, usually requiring surgery.

Mastoiditis is suspected if purulent discharge persists after acute otitis media, or if there are pain, tenderness, and redness over the mastoid process of the temporal bone. Fever and leukocytosis are variable. Roentgenograms may show clouding of the mastoid cells.

Treatment. Rest in bed, antibiotic therapy, adequate diet and fluids, and narcotics for the relief of pain, are begun at once. The majority of patients show improvement within twenty-four to forty-eight hours, and the symptoms and signs subside in a few days.

Mastoidectomy. If the discharge from the ear persists for from three to four weeks, any infection in the sinuses or nasopharynx should be searched for and eliminated. If the discharge from the ear persists another two or three weeks, a simple mastoidectomy should be done or chronic mastoiditis with permanent damage to hearing may result. Fortunately, due entirely to the sulfonamides and the antibiotics, a simple mastoidectomy is a very rare operation, whereas fifteen years ago it was an exceedingly common one.

The simple mastoidectomy is performed on those patients in whom the infection is limited primarily to the mastoid cells. The operation is performed under general anesthesia. A curved incision is made behind the ear, and the bone of the mastoid process is exposed. All infected mastoid cells are removed with rongeurs and curette, taking care not to injure the facial nerve which controls the movements of the facial muscles. This nerve passes through the temporal bone and may be in extremely close contact with the infected mastoid cells. Two other important structures which must be looked for and avoided are the lateral venous sinus of the brain and the dura mater. The wound usually heals in a matter of weeks, the ear ceases to discharge pus, and the hearing returns to normal.

An ear that continues to discharge pus for a long time (a matter of months or years) does so because there is a chronic infection in both the mastoid cells and the middle ear. These infections rarely respond to antibiotics or sulfonamides. To eradicate this infection a radical mastoidectomy is required. This operation is similar to the simple mastoidectomy, but in addition to removing the mastoid cells the drum is removed, and also all middle ear structures with the exception of the stapes. After this operation, the hearing does not return to normal. In fact, it may be even further reduced.

It is important to remember that if acute otitis media is adequately treated, there will be fewer and fewer cases requiring a radical mastoidectomy.

NURSING CARE. Before operation, the head is shaved on the affected side for a distance of about 3 inches around the ear. The preoperative preparation is like that given any patient who is to have general anesthesia. After operation routine care is given the patient; but when there is a sudden or gradual rise in temperature the nurse should be aware of its significance. Many times it is indicative of the dangerous complications which can follow mastoid infections and it should be reported to the surgeon immediately.

Deafness

Loss of hearing is a common complaint, even among children; it constitutes a serious handicap. The problem is being handled in three ways. Efforts are being made to prevent deafness by reducing the incidence of ear infections; along this line it has been found that the routine examination of school children followed by radiation of the nasopharynx of those who need it reduces to a large extent the incidence of defective hearing. In the second place, the attempt is made by the use of electronic amplifying devices to render seriously impaired hearing serviceable, and to further decrease the deaf patient's handicap by teaching him lip-reading. Lastly, continuing efforts are being made to learn more about the causes of deafness and to perfect procedures which will restore hearing that has been lost.

Defective hearing is of two types: conductive deafness, in which the loss of hearing is due to impaired conductive powers of the drum, ossicles or wall of the middle ear as a result of injury or disease; and nerve deafness, in which the impairment is due to injury or disease of the cochlea or the auditory nerve. Patients who have only a moderate hearing loss of either the conductive or nerve type are greatly benefited by the use of a properly fitted hearing aid.

One common type of conductive deafness is otosclerosis. It usually affects young people in their twenties. There is often a strong family history of otosclerosis, as a woman with the disease may transmit it to her children. In otosclerosis new bone forms around the stapes and thus prevents movement of this ossicle. Fortunately, a well-fitted hearing aid enables these patients to hear amazingly well. In recent years an operation has been devised, the fenestration operation, popularly called "window operation," which holds out great hope for these patients. In this operation a tiny opening is made in one of the semicircular canals. This procedure apparently allows the sound waves to by-pass the drums and ossicles and enter the inner ear directly.

SUMMARY

The majority of patients who have diseases of the ear, nose or throat do not require hospitalization. Serious infections, if neglected, can lead to deafness and even death; fortunately, most serious infections are now readily controllable by antibiotic therapy. Patients who have a tracheotomy need constant, expert nursing until they have been trained to care for themselves.

VOCABULARY REVIEW

laryngoscope	*otitis media*	*tracheotomy*
pharyngoscope	*aerotitis*	*decannulation*
adenoids	*epistaxis*	*mastoiditis*
audiometer	*tonsillectomy*	*fenestration*

SUGGESTED READING

1. Conley, John J.: Tracheotomy. Am. J. Nursing, *52:*1078–1081 (Sept.) 1952.
2. Bellam, Gwendoline: Tonsillectomy Without Fear. Am. J. Nursing, *51:* 244–245 (April) 1951.
3. Gardner, Warren H.: Rehabilitation After Laryngectomy. Pub. Health Nursing, *43:*612–615 (Nov.) 1951.
4. Greene, James S.: Speech Rehabilitation Following Laryngectomy. Am. J. Nursing, *49:*153–154 (Mar.) 1949.
5. Hall, James T., and Sadler, Julia Bland: Nursing Care in Tonsillectomy and Adenoidectomy. Am. J. Nursing, *47:*537–539 (Aug.) 1947.
6. Hardy, William G.: Teamwork in the Prevention of Hearing Impairment in Children. Pub. Health Nursing, *43:*278–279 (May) 1951.
7. Holmquist, Emily W.: Nursing the Adult Tracheotomized Patient. Am. J. Nursing, *47:*310–314 (May) 1947.
8. Jackson, Chevalier, and Jackson, Chevalier L.: Diseases of the Nose, Throat and Ear. Philadelphia, W. B. Saunders Co., 1945, pp. 269–278.
9. Is Your Patient Deaf? Am. J. Nursing, *52:*578 (May) 1952.
10. Lewis, Donald K.: Deafness. Am. J. Nursing, *52:*575–578 (May) 1952.
11. Martin, Hayes, and Ehrlich, Harry E.: Nursing Care Following Laryngectomy. Am. J. Nursing, *49:*149–152 (Mar.) 1949.
12. Proctor, Donald F.: Preventing Deafness in Children. Am. J. Nursing, *49:* 45–47 (Jan.) 1949.

CHAPTER 43

Deformities of the
Bones, Joints and Muscles

INTRODUCTION

The skeleton forms the framework of the body, and its constituent bones are individually rigid. The body, nevertheless, possesses great flexibility and a variety of movements, achieving that result from the many joints within the framework and from the powerful action of the skeletal muscles. Abnormality of growth, injury, or disease can so alter any of these structures that proper function is partly or entirely lost.

About two hundred years ago a French physician conceived the idea that some of the musculoskeletal deformities of the adult might be the consequence of improper posture during childhood, and, if so, they were preventable. He began, therefore, to advocate the importance of correct posture in children, and for this new concept he coined the term "orthopedics," meaning literally

509

"the straight child." From this beginning the specialty of orthopedic surgery has come to include all aspects of the surgical care of the musculoskeletal system.

Growth and Repair of Bone. In the fetus the skeleton is at first composed of cartilage. The large cells of this tissue produce a light-weight, firm, clear substance called hyaline cartilage. It is tough, but without the rigidity of bone. As the infant grows this cartilage is replaced by bonelike (*osteoid*) tissue, which has the characteristic architecture of bone but is not yet hard. The bone-forming (*osteogenic*) cells arise from the sheath of the bone (*periosteum*) and, like cartilage cells, are originally derived from primitive connective tissue cells. Later, bone making (*ossification*) takes place in the bone ends (*epiphyses*) and in the shaft (*diaphysis*), calcium salts being deposited in the osteoid tissue. This calcification is responsible for the natural hardness of bone.

In all the long bones, however, there is a zone between the shaft and the bone end in which cartilage cells persist and continue to grow. It is the activity of this zone, known as the epiphyseal line, which accounts for the elongation of the bones during the growth of the child. In the adolescent, between the ages of 17 and 20, this cartilage is finally replaced by bone; the epiphyses are thus united with the shaft, and the person grows no taller.

Repair of damage caused by injury or disease is accomplished by a process very similar to the original formation of bone. The blood clot which occurs as a result of a fracture is organized into granulation tissue, and this is then transformed into osteoid tissue, which finally becomes calcified bone. The same process occurs when granulation or scar tissue forms in the course of healing in bone infection. As a rule, the repair of bone is carried out so efficiently that the natural architecture is almost completely restored, and later little trace of the injury remains.

Influence of Diet. For the proper formation of bone an adequate diet is essential. A deficiency of vitamin C causes scurvy, which, in babies, results in deformed bones because of interference with growth at the epiphyseal line. More common, however, is rickets. In this disease, caused by deficiency of vitamin D, the bones are not properly calcified, permitting deformity of the abnormally soft bones which bend under the weight of the body or from the pull of the muscles. Sufficient calcium and phosphorus salts must be contained in the diet, or calcification cannot be completed. Softening of the skeletal bones may occur in

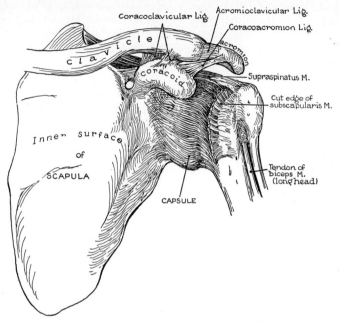

FIGURE 128. Shoulder joint.

women during pregnancy or lactation unless the mother's diet contains calcium in excess of the usual need, for calcium goes into the fetal bones, or into the breast milk, even when the mother is suffering from deprivation.

Influence of Glandular Secretions. The influence of the hormone secreted by the parathyroid glands in controlling calcium and phosphorus metabolism is now well known, and bony changes occur as a result of disorders of these glands (see Chap. 34). Oversecretion (hyperparathyroidism) permits loss of calcium from the body, with consequent softening of the bones.

Mechanics of the Joint. The least movement of the body requires the use of one or more joints, and these marvelous structures serve so efficiently and so faithfully that the ordinary person scarcely heeds their existence until he is confronted by painful or impaired function. In general, the joints and their accessory structures are designed to furnish motion without friction; they must also be strong enough to withstand stress and strain.

Each bone of the skeleton is articulated, that is to say, it is connected with another bone or several other bones by means of a joint or joints. The several kinds of joints are classified according to the sort of motion permitted. Thus, without entering into a highly technical consideration of the subject, one finds these chief varieties: hinge joints, permitting motion in one plane; gliding and rotary joints, permitting motion in two planes; and ball-and-socket joints, permitting motion in all three planes. The knee joint and the joints of the fingers are examples of the hinge; the wrist and ankle are gliding joints; the shoulder and hip are ball-and-socket joints.

The end of every bone entering into an articulation is covered with fibrocartilage, a tough substance which protects the bone end from injury and wear. The entire inner surface of each joint is lined with a smooth self-lubricating membrane, the synovium. Composed of connective tissue cells, this lining membrane secretes a glairy fluid, the synovial fluid, which serves to lubricate the joint surfaces, a very small amount being sufficient for this purpose.

The entire joint is contained within an envelope of tough fibrous tissue, the capsule. The integrity of the joint is further maintained by the supporting ligaments. These are, in reality, strategically placed thickenings of the articular capsule, which provide stability to the joint and act to prevent movement of the articulating bones beyond the natural limits of the joint. As a rule, the ligaments are situated where the muscles about the joint are weakest.

Small accessory sacs of synovial fluid are located outside of the joints to prevent undue friction from the rubbing motion of such muscles and tendons as overlie the joints. These structures are called bursas. Although the location of the larger ones is constant, there is a considerable variation in the size and number of the bursas to be found about any given joint.

Impaired Function. As the result of injury or disease, various kinds of damage to the different joint structures occur. The articular cartilages, in particular, fail to heal when damaged, so that impairment of joint function follows. The synovial membrane, however, is capable of complete regeneration; but occasionally, when opposite surfaces are injured or diseased, the repair may result in the adhesion of the opposing surfaces. If only a few adhesions form, the joint function is not severely impaired; but numerous dense adhesions may result in severe loss of motion (*fibrous ankylosis*). Under favorable circumstances, joint capsule and ligaments heal readily with complete return of function; but following loss of substance due to repeated injury or to disease these structures may become weak or useless.

When a joint has been badly damaged, healing is sometimes accompanied by excessive scarring, followed by calcification. The final result is complete immobilization of the joint (*bony ankylosis*). Occasionally, on the other hand, as the result of injuries that destroy the supporting ligaments and otherwise weaken the joint capsule, an unstable joint is produced.

Anatomy and Physiology of Skeletal Muscle. In contrast to the smooth involuntary muscle found in the gastrointestinal tract and elsewhere in the body, the fibers of skeletal (*voluntary*) muscles appear striped (*striated*) when seen under the microscope. These muscles, which are able to produce bodily motion by virtue of their ability to contract, usually arise from one bony surface (*origin*) and are attached (*insertion*) to some point on the surface of another bone by means of a fibrous band (*tendon*). Thus, the muscles act upon the bones like a force applied to a lever, the fulcrum being the joint.

Voluntary muscle is controlled by the central nervous system; if this nervous telegraph system is interrupted at any point between brain and muscle the person can no longer exert his will over the contraction of the muscle, and its function is lost. Each muscle of the body has a well-defined function, and all of the muscles are so arranged that each has an adversary, an opposing muscle. As no muscle is ever completely relaxed unless paralyzed, the coordinating action of the central nervous system is of the utmost importance since motion is accomplished only by simultaneous contraction of one group of muscles and relaxation of the antagonistic muscles. Flexion of the index finger (the beckoning gesture), for example, requires not only contraction of the flexor muscles but also simultaneous and equal relaxation of the extensor muscles. In extending the finger this process is reversed.

Effects of Injury. Striated muscle fibers are highly specialized structures; if injured, they die and are replaced by scar tissue. The loss of muscle tissue is permanent, and although hypertrophy of the remaining fibers may compensate for a small loss, an extensive loss of tissue results in reduced power. Interestingly enough, muscle fibers atrophy when not used for a long time. Extremities immobilized because of injury or disease should be treated to prevent the atrophy of disuse, lest permanent loss of power result. The local use of heat, passive movement, massage, and electrical stimulation aid in preventing atrophy.

CONGENITAL AND ACQUIRED DEFORMITIES

Deformities are common; some are congenital, being already present at birth, and others make their appearance later in life. There is also a variety of causes for these deformities. Some are hereditary, the defect descending from generation to generation; some are the result of nutritional deficiency; and others follow improper postural habits or mistreatment of the body, as from poorly fitting shoes. Additional deformities occur when, through disease of the central nervous system, there exists an imbalance of muscle tone. That deformities result from injuries or from the ravages of neoplastic or infectious disease is well known; these will be considered later.

Chondrodystrophia Fetalis. This is a hereditary deformity the chief feature of which is the improper development of the fetal cartilages. This inherited characteristic is responsible for the occurrence of many of the dwarfs seen on the stage and in the circus.

Curvature of the Spine

From a functional standpoint it is inadequate to think of the spine as a collection of two dozen or so assorted vertebrae. On the contrary, the spine is a complicated organ composed of numerous ligaments, muscles, and vertebrae, each purposefully designed and placed. The spinal cord is housed within the spine, and the paired spinal nerves issue from it. The head is supported by the spine, which also serves as the point of attachment for the many muscles of the shoulder girdle, the pelvis, and the trunk. Furthermore, the spine is amazingly flexible, permitting a wide range of motion in every direction. The anatomic construction of the spine is such that, in addition to its other functions, it acts as a shock absorber so that the numerous jolts received in walking or other activity are equally distributed.

In a normal person standing upright the spine is straight in the lateral plane, but in the anteroposterior plane it has several gentle curves. There is a slight convexity anteriorly in the cervical and lumbar regions, whereas the convexity is posterior in the thoracic and sacral regions. There are four possible deviations from the normal, including lateral curvature (*scoliosis*), **exag-**

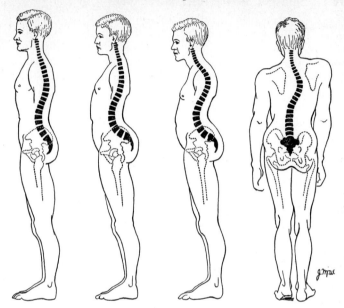

FIGURE 129. Curvature of spine. Left to right: normal; lordosis (swayback); kyphosis (hunchback); scoliosis (lateral curvature).

gerated anterior convexity or sway-back (*lordosis*), exaggerated posterior convexity or humpback (*kyphosis*), and rotation on the long axis. As a rule, two or more of these abnormal curvatures are combined, one or more secondary curvatures compensating for the primary deformity.

Causes. In the light of present knowledge it seems likely that nearly every deformity of the spine has a true pathologic basis, and that few curvatures are the result of poor habits of posture. Parents who note poor posture in their children should consult an orthopedic surgeon; little improvement results from admonishing the child to "stand straight!" Common causes of spinal curvature are rickets, inequality in the length of the legs, flat feet, congenital malformation of vertebrae, high heels, abnormalities of growth including unequal rate of growth of bones and muscles, neurologic disorders such as poliomyelitis, poor eyesight, infections and tumors of the spine, and injuries.

Treatment. The treatment naturally depends upon the cause and type of the curvature. If the lesion is a longstanding one, with structural deformity, little can be done; but if treatment is started at the beginning of the deformity, much can be accomplished in the way of prevention and restoration. Of first importance is the treatment of the disease which is affecting the spine, so that further deformity will be prevented. Next is the use of mechanical measures to compensate for abnormalities, as the use of a thick-soled shoe to lengthen a short leg, thus leveling the bony pelvis. When the curvature is due to muscle weakness a brace may be provided to do the work of the paralyzed muscles, thus serving as antagonist to the remaining muscles which, if unopposed, would pull the spine out of line. Muscles not hopelessly damaged may be strengthened by special exercises designed to overcome local muscle weakness.

BACKACHE

This commonest of complaints is attributable to man's way of living, his upright posture and method of locomotion, and the many ways in which he uses his back. Injury and disease, too, cause backache, the severity of which may seem out of all proportion to the nature of the injury or disease. It is also important to remember that pain felt in the back may be referred from elsewhere; thus pain from a stomach ulcer or a gallstone is occasionally felt only in the back, and must be differentiated from true backache.

When the spine is permitted or forced for long periods to assume curves which are more extreme than normal, the spinal muscles become fatigued and painful spasm occurs. This type of backache commonly follows long hours of sitting in an improper attitude or sleeping upon a bed which does not support the body correctly. Upon resumption of normal posture the muscles soon become rested, and the pain disappears. Prevention of further backache depends upon the avoidance of cramped or slouching positions, and upon the use of a mattress and a bed spring which are firm enough to support the body without sagging. An additional measure for the prevention of further trouble is postural training, composed of exercises carefully designed to strengthen those muscles which aid in supporting the back, notably the abdominal muscles.

The use of high heels by those not accustomed to them or the wearing of flat heels by those habituated to high ones often causes severe backache because the tipping of the pelvis requires a compensatory bending of the spine. The natural lumbar lordosis may be badly exaggerated by the forward pull of the heavy abdomen of an obese person or during pregnancy, and again backache is the result.

Those of us who never forsake the city become used to walking on hard sidewalks and streets and do not realize how well the spine absorbs the jolt caused by each step; but that this pounding often causes backache is thoroughly appreciated by the country-man who visits the city. Often, too, people are careless about rundown heels and walk about on the exposed nails, which do not absorb the shock as do rubber or leather heels.

When the spine is deformed by disease, backache often accompanies the constant muscular effort to overcome the abnormal curvature. A brace, properly adjusted to aid the muscles, is the most effective means of relieving the pain. Occasionally, backache is the result of abnormal mobility of the spine, which causes over-activity of the muscles and ligaments. A brace may not be sufficient, and at times operation is indicated. Mechanical defects must first be corrected, if possible, before fusion is considered. Fixation of the spine is accomplished by a fusion or bone-grafting procedure to bring about ankylosis of the intervertebral joints.

Deformities of the Legs and Feet

Congenital and acquired deformities of the lower extremities are far more common than those of the upper. With respect to the congenital deformities, no adequate explanation of this disparity has been offered, but the production of acquired deformities of legs and feet is no doubt encouraged by the strain of weight bearing and by the unconcern of many people in their selection of style and fit of shoes.

DISLOCATION OF THE HIP

In common with some other congenital deformities, dislocation of the hip is not apparent at birth. In most instances the dislocation is due to an abnormal forward rotation (*anteversion*) of the neck of the femur, so that there is both failure of the femoral head to press into the hip socket (*acetabulum*) and stretching of the joint capsule. Occasionally the dislocation is due to abnormal shallowness of the acetabulum. In either case, the head of the femur is not firmly fixed in its socket, and when the infant begins to stand the head of the femur gradually slides upward and backward. It is interesting that congenital dislocation of the hip is more common in female infants, and that it is rare in Negroes. In about half the cases the deformity is bilateral. Congenital dislocation of other joints is rare.

This deformity may affect one or both legs, and attention is called to it by a rapidly progressive limp or waddle as the baby learns to walk. Occasionally a diagnosis of this condition, particularly if it is unilateral, can be made before weight bearing begins. A sharp-eyed nurse may note a difference in the crease of the buttock (gluteal fold) with widening of the perineum.

Treatment. The condition should be treated as soon as recognized; and, in babies of 2 years or under, cure usually results from manipulation followed by fixation in a plaster cast for six to eighteen months. Lorenz, a Viennese surgeon, introduced this method, which was widely publicized under the title of "bloodless surgery." Open reduction is sometimes necessary, however, particularly if the joint capsule is badly deformed or if the acetabulum fails to grow properly. The most successful procedure is the "shelf" operation, in which the acetabulum is deepened.

CLUBFOOT

Those well versed in romantic literature think of clubfoot (*talipes equinovarus*) as a common congenital deformity, and so it is; yet scarcely a person thus deformed is seen on the streets, a tribute to the success of the modern treatment of that condition. To visualize the deformity, one may picture a person walking with foot turned inward in an extreme manner so that his weight is actually borne on the outer surface of his ankle. A normal foot can assume the position of a clubfoot, but the clubfoot is fixed in that position. It is thought that imbalance of muscular pull is responsible for the production of this deformity, although malposition in utero has also been suggested. There are other varieties of clubfoot in addition to the equinovarus, but the latter is the commonest; 85 per cent of all cases are of that type.

Treatment. Treatment is begun in the first weeks of life; if it is not, structural changes in the bones develop, lessening the chance of cure. The deformed foot and ankle are manipulated into correct position in gradual stages, the gain being maintained each time by the use of a plaster cast. Finally, as walking begins, a light brace is used until the muscle balance is sufficiently restored to prevent recurrence.

When treatment of a clubfoot has been postponed or neglected until bony changes have already occurred, a wedge osteotomy

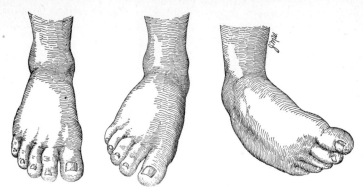

FIGURE 130. Left to right: normal; flatfoot (pes planus); clubfoot (talipes equinovarus).

can be performed. This operation straightens the foot, but such a foot is usually weak and functions poorly.

FLATFOOT

Flat foot (*pes planus*) is an extremely common disability; interestingly enough, however, many people have flat feet which do not cause symptoms. In other words, it is not the flatness of the foot which causes trouble; it is a question of its relation to the function of the whole weight-bearing mechanism. Thus, one person may have a perfectly functioning leg and foot with flat arches, whereas another may have poor function with high arches. In the latter case it is a disturbance of the arches which is likely to produce symptoms.

There are two arches in the foot, the long arch (from heel to toes) and the transverse (*metatarsal*) arch. The weight of the body, transmitted through the tibia, should be equally distributed to the heel and to the ball of the foot.

If the foot is turned outward (*pronated*), it is seen that the line of weight bearing passes medially to the midpoint of the arch, throwing great strain on the medial ligaments and calf muscles which support the long arch. If these structures are unequal to the task, the unsupported arch gives way, and a flatfoot is acquired with resultant pain and deformity. This is but one of the many types of acquired flatfoot.

Treatment. A lift along the inner edge of the heel and sole of the shoe will shift the line of weight bearing laterally. This measure, combined with exercises to strengthen the muscles support-

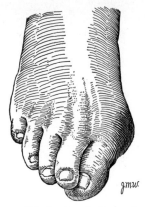

FIGURE 131. Bunion (hallux valgus).

ing the arch, and training to make the patient turn his foot straight ahead as he walks, will as a rule relieve the symptoms. As in other orthopedic conditions, unless treatment is undertaken early, structural changes take place that prevent a good functional result. The use of a plate to support the arch is occasionally necessary, but will not relieve the symptoms unless the underlying causes are treated as well.

Metatarsal Pain. High heels, by throwing an undue amount of weight upon the ball of the foot, may produce a flattening of the metatarsal arch. Here, again, relief of symptoms depends upon the restoration of normal weight bearing, and a support beneath the metatarsal arch will not relieve the pain if the patient continues to wear high heels.

BUNION

Hallux valgus, the deviation of the great toe toward the second toe, is a deformity produced by ill-fitting shoes and is generally associated with anterior arch weakness. Less severe bunions are cured by the wearing of wide shoes.

Deformities Caused by Dietary Deficiencies

The deformities which occur in association with scurvy and rickets have been mentioned (p. 510).

Osteochondrosis. This term has been suggested for another type of deformity which may be the result of a deficiency, but which is at present of unknown etiology. The various growth centers (*epiphyses*) are affected, and fragmentation of hyaline articular cartilage takes place with temporary pain and loss of function. When occurring in the hip it is known as Legg-Perthes disease; when in the bony prominence below the knee, as Osgood-Schlatter disease. The spine and the upper extremity may also be affected.

Treatment by the use of splints is designed to prevent further deformity. Rest, adequate diet, and physiotherapy are also advisable.

Deformities Caused by Disease of the Nervous System

POLIOMYELITIS

Poliomyelitis (*infantile paralysis*) is an acute contagious disease affecting the spinal cord. It is caused by a filtrable virus. There is no infection of the musculoskeletal system; but as a result of injury to the motor nerve cells of the spinal cord, various skeletal muscles may be seriously weakened or paralyzed, a state which may be temporary or permanent.

Treatment. In all cases of poliomyelitis in which any muscular weakness is apparent, orthopedic treatment is begun just as soon as the acute febrile illness has subsided. The purpose is threefold. Weakened or paralyzed muscles must be supported at once with splints, or else the antagonistic muscles, if stronger, will produce deformity; secondly, weakened and paralyzed muscles must be stimulated by physiotherapy and graduated exercises, so that a maximal amount of function may be regained; and finally, where there is permanent loss of muscle power, substitution must be made either by the use of braces or by corrective operations which lengthen contracted tendons or add stability to joints rendered weak by paralyzed muscles.

If the muscles of respiration and the diaphragm are weakened, the disease may prove fatal. It is in these cases that the "iron lung" (*respirator*) has occasionally been life-saving. Of particular benefit to the patient convalescing from poliomyelitis is the water bath or swimming pool, for the weakened muscles can often move an extremity as it floats in water, relatively uninfluenced by the pull of gravity.

Kenny Method. The Kenny method, named for the Australian nurse who popularized it, has as its basic concepts the maintenance of normal position and the reeducation of muscles. According to Miss Kenny, the pain in poliomyelitis is due to the severe contraction (spasm) of the affected muscles. During the acute stage of the illness the patient is kept on a thin mattress upon a wooden flooring (fracture board) instead of springs; a second board is set at right angles at the foot of the bed, and the patient's feet are placed against this to prevent footdrop; no further splinting is done. The patient is made as comfortable as possible by the use of pads, pillows, or blankets as supports for the affected parts. These are gradually removed as the pain subsides. During the acute muscle spasm, hot wet packs are applied to the muscles involved. These are continued until the spasm is relieved. While the patient is critically ill, the packs are given only to the chest and neck to avoid tiring the patient; during this time the patient is handled as little as possible; alcohol rubs are omitted because they are said to increase spasm. Later, active and passive exercises are used. The carrying out of the Kenny treatment is entirely a nursing procedure.

SPASTIC PARALYSIS

A very different type of lesion of the nervous system produces an equally tragic deformity of the musculoskeletal apparatus. In Little's disease (spastic paralysis of children) severe spasticity of the muscles of two or all of the extremities is due to a cerebral lesion. This disease has been ascribed to congenital brain defects, and also to intracranial injury from prolonged or violent childbirth. The extreme spasticity of the muscles prevents normal movement. Sudden stimuli may provoke immediate extension of arms and legs as a response. If walking is possible, it is with a mincing, tiptoe gait. Frequently the brain abnormality is such that there is little or no mental development, although many sufferers have normal intelligence. Coordination is sadly lacking.

No form of treatment has resulted in a cure, although careful muscle training, at times combined with operations on the motor nerves, may restore a useful degree of voluntary control over the spastic muscles. These patients are most effectively handled in the "hospital schools."

THE HOSPITAL SCHOOL

The care of severe musculoskeletal deformities, and often of infections and injuries as well, is usually a long-term problem. If the patient is a child, there is apt to be much loss of school and of the normal play and social activities which are so important to the normal growth and development of the individual. If the patient is an adult, the problem is likely to be one of adjustment to the deformity, and of retraining the individual. The social and economic significance is obvious. Because of the special problems involved in the way of program, staffing, and equipment, it has been found best to develop specialized institutions designed to provide a combined program of medical care, education and rehabilitation.

SUMMARY

The smooth action of the muscles upon the jointed framework of the human body makes possible the variety of movement of which man is capable. Congenital and acquired deformities can prevent a child from taking a normal part in living and can take away from an adult his livelihood and place in society. The correction of musculoskeletal deformity is often a long-term problem, best handled in special institutions in which medical care, educational and rehabilitory facilities are combined.

VOCABULARY REVIEW

orthopedic	*bursa*	*clubfoot*
ligament	*ankylosis*	*bunion*
synovial	*kyphosis*	*poliomyelitis*
	scoliosis	

SUGGESTED READING

1. Allen, Lucy E.: Congenital Dislocation of the Hip. Am. J. Nursing, *47:* 722–726 (Nov.) 1947.
2. Billig, Harvey E., Jr.: The Specialist Looks at Everyday Medical Care in Industry: Orthopedics. J.A.M.A., *146:*1179–1183 (July 28) 1951.
3. Ferderber, Murray B.: Rehabilitation Program for the Aged in Two County Institutions. Pub. Health Nursing, *44:*664–667 (Dec.) 1952.
4. Grice, David S.: Talipes Equinovarus Diagnosis and Treatment. Am. J. Nursing, *51:*707–709 (Dec.) 1951.
5. Howorth, M. Beckett: Your Feet and Your Shoes. Am. J. Nursing, *52:* 1368–1372 (Dec.) 1952.
6. Knocke, Lazelle S.: Some Common Types of Braces. Am. J. Nursing, *52:*868–869 (July) 1952.
7. Ladd, Margaret P.: The Bent Pin: Posture, Industry, Nurse. Pub. Health Nursing, *39:*609–612 (Dec.) 1947.
8. Lewin, Philip: Orthopedic Surgery for Nurses. Philadelphia, W. B. Saunders Co., 1947, pp. 138–148.
9. Leavitt, Darrell et al.: Scoliosis. Am. J. Nursing, *50:*198–202 (April) 1950.
10. Macdonald, Mary: Talipes Equinovarus, Nursing Care in the Community. Am. J. Nursing, *51:*711–712 (Dec.) 1951.
11. Stimson, Barbara: Backache, Am. J. Nursing, *51:*672–674 (Nov.) 1951.
12. Williams, Barbara J.: Talipes Equinovarus, Nursing Care in the Hospital. Am. J. Nursing, *51:*710–711 (Dec.) 1951.

CHAPTER 44

Musculoskeletal Injuries

Injuries to the musculoskeletal system are in fact wounds of the muscles, tendons, joints, with or without attendant injuries to the bones. As with all wounds, these are open or closed, and they may be produced in a variety of ways. Muscles, tendons, and the ligamentous portions of joints may be severed in a deep lacerated wound, or they may be avulsed by an object striking with the force due to high velocity. Although bone is often exposed by a deep laceration, it is not easily divided; it is frequently shattered, however, if struck with great force. War wounds and those resulting from industrial, railroad, or automobile accidents are commonly open, whereas the injuries received in civil life as a result of accidents occurring in the home or in athletics are usually closed.

The treatment of open wounds has been discussed in Chapter 2 (p. 13). Wherever possible, divided tendons, nerves, muscles, and joint structures are approximated by sutures, but often this ideal treatment is not possible. In these deep wounds infection by spore-bearing bacteria (e.g., tetanus, gas gangrene) is always a possibility, and adequate preventive measures must be taken, including cleansing of the wound, débridement, and the use of antitoxin and antibiotics. Experience gained during World War II has shown that it is exceedingly dangerous to attempt immediate closure of fresh battle wounds of the extremities because of the likelihood of anaerobic infection. Following débridement these wounds are left wide open, and are lightly packed with sterile gauze. Secondary closure may be carried out several days later.

Healing is facilitated and the patient's comfort increased, especially when transportation is necessary, by the use of adequate splints. Prolonged immobilization of muscles, tendons, and joints, on the other hand, leads to disastrous stiffening with loss of function. In patients who have had suture of divided tendons, motion must be begun as soon as the healing is sufficiently strong to permit of it. Movements must be restricted at first, then gradually increased up to full performance.

In civil life closed wounds of the musculoskeletal system are more common than open wounds. These injuries include tearing of the muscles, tendons, or joint structures, dislocation of the joints, and fracture of the bones; two or more are usually combined. Hemorrhage always occurs and pain, tenderness, swelling, and disability are regularly present. Such wounds are produced by blows, by falls, by lever action, and by any violence that forces a muscle, a joint, or a bone beyond its normal limits. In this last category are included those injuries which are the result of sudden forceful muscular contraction, for example, the "pulled tendon" of the sprinter and the fractured humerus of the baseball pitcher.

INJURIES TO JOINTS

Any trauma to a joint which is severe enough to damage the synovial membrane causes an effusion of serous fluid. The familiar "water on the knee" is an example of such an effusion into a joint (*hydrops*), and commonly follows a severe injury to the knee.

When a joint is subjected to violent movement beyond its normal limits the result is (1) tearing of the supporting ligaments, muscles, and tendons (sprain); (2) tearing of ligaments and avulsion of bony insertions (fracture-sprain); (3) tearing of the joint capsule with dislocation; or (4) dislocation with fracture. The clinical symptoms and signs of these related injuries differ chiefly in degree, and often it is only by x-ray evidence that a correct diagnosis can be made. Immediate pain and swelling occur in all, and the deformity and disability (loss of function) are sometimes pronounced.

The joints most frequently injured are the ankle, wrist, knee, elbow, shoulder, and hip, and the type of injury is usually characteristic. Thus simple sprains (i.e., without fracture) of the ankle are of common occurrence, but sprains of the wrist are complicated by fracture of the scaphoid or the distal end of the radius. Injuries to the knee usually result from lateral or twisting strains, with damage to the semilunar cartilage and crucial ligaments, structures not found in the other joints. The characteristic injury to the elbow is a fracture dislocation; the hip and shoulder are commonly dislocated without fracture.

Treatment. Treatment depends upon the nature of the injury, and to be successful, therefore, must be based upon correct diagnosis. Simple sprains are treated by rest and immobilization, which permit the torn structures to heal. Elevation of the part

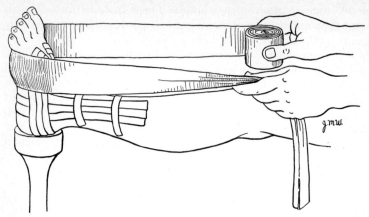

FIGURE 132. Method of applying adhesive tape to support a sprained ankle. Note that patient holds bandage beneath sole of foot to maintain desired position during application of adhesive. Care in taken that no adhesive strap completely encircles the extremity, in order that there will be no constricting band when swelling occurs.

and hot applications will reduce the swelling and relieve the pain. Immobilization can be adequately maintained by the use of properly applied adhesive strapping which fixes the part in the position best suited for healing. Thus an ankle which is sprained by inversion of the foot should be strapped with the foot in eversion. Weight bearing is avoided for the first forty-eight to seventy-two hours, after which it may be gradually resumed. Massage and hot applications accelerate healing, and full use is permitted in seven to ten days.

Fracture-sprains must be treated as are other fractures, with adequate reduction and fixation; fracture-dislocations are treated in the same way, although these often require special methods of treatment.

Simple dislocations are treated by reduction of the dislocation, followed by immobilization of the joint to permit healing of the damaged capsule and ligaments. Most dislocations are easily reduced if the patient is anesthetized sufficiently to secure relaxation of the muscles. Traction on the extremity in a direction exactly opposite to that of the force which caused the injury usually brings the displaced bone end into position. In reducing dislocations there is need for expert manipulation without undue force, for ill chosen, violent maneuvers may succeed only in frac-

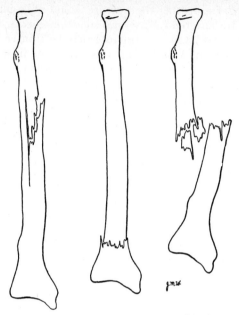

FIGURE 133. Types of fracture. Left to right: greenstick, impacted, and comminuted.

turing the displaced bone or in further traumatizing the joint capsule and other related structures. The use of a sling, or of a Velpeau bandage which fastens the arm against the thorax, is sufficient for the immobilization of shoulder and elbow dislocations. In dislocations of the hip, however, weight bearing must not be permitted until torn capsular structures have had time to mend. Rest in bed usually provides adequate immobilization.

Following repeated dislocations the joint capsule and ligaments sometimes become so weak or relaxed that dislocation occurs after minimal trauma or even during normal activity. Operative treatment is usually necessary for the cure of this habitual dislocation, some type of plastic procedure being required to reestablish joint stability.

FRACTURES

If the skin over the broken bone is intact the fracture is considered simple; in compound fractures there is an open wound. An incomplete fracture is called a greenstick fracture. If the fragments are driven together the fracture is said to be impacted, but if the bone is shattered into several small fragments, the fracture is comminuted. The line of fracture may be transverse, oblique, spiral, or T-shaped. A pathologic fracture is one in which a bone is broken by a force far less than that required to fracture it normally; this type occurs only in bones weakened by preexisting disease, such as syphilis, derangements of calcium metabolism, or neoplasm.

The diagnosis of a fracture can nearly always be made upon the history of the injury and the appearance of the part, but should be confirmed by x-ray examination. Properly taken roentgenograms furnish additional information as to the nature and position of the fragments, and may even disclose an unsuspected fracture. Accurate details of the manner in which the injury was received are of value, since many types of injury are produced in characteristic ways. Pain, swelling, deformity, and disability occur constantly and are diagnostic. The alterations of normal landmarks and the limitation of motion are sufficient for a presumptive diagnosis of fracture without an attempt to elicit the barbarously painful sign of crepitus (grating of one bone end upon the other).

Treatment of Fractures

It must be remembered that severe trauma to the adjacent soft parts always accompanies the breaking of a bone, and that there will be hemorrhage and often shock. Whether the shock is solely the result of loss of blood or fluid into the tissues, or is in part due to the severity of the painful stimuli, is a moot point; in any case the condition requires prompt treatment. The emergency treatment of a fracture or suspected fracture, therefore, is to apply a splint which will temporarily immobilize the broken bone. This treatment serves to reduce the element of shock, to prevent conversion of a simple fracture into a compound one, and to make transportation of the patient more feasible. Application of the often repeated aphorism, "Splint 'em where they lie," has saved many lives.

Reduction and Fixation. In reducing (setting) fractures the general principle is to bring the more easily controlled fragment into line with the less controllable fragment. When the fracture is reduced—that is to say, when the fragments are correctly aligned—the broken bone is immobilized by some means, usually a plaster cast, until bony union occurs. The final step in treat-

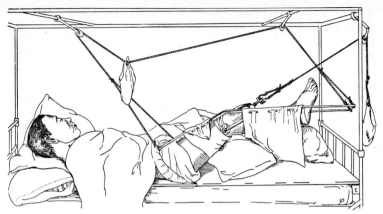

FIGURE 134. Skeletal traction. Fracture of femur is being reduced by traction applied through lower end of femur by means of a Kirschner wire. Countertraction and support of the Thomas splint are accomplished simultaneously by the overhead pulleys and weight.

ment is the restoration of function by graded exercise and physiotherapy as soon as the union is sufficiently strong.

The majority of simple fractures can be reduced satisfactorily by manipulation of the fragments while the patient is under the influence of an anesthetic agent; the fragments are immobilized in a plaster cast which is applied at once. There are many fractures, however, which for a variety of reasons cannot be treated so simply. In the first place, the bone may be broken obliquely, so that the ends slip upon each other; or there may be many small fragments which do not fit together solidly. Another factor is the pulling action of the strong muscles, which may cause slipping and overriding of the bone ends. In addition to simple manipulation there are at least four methods of securing reduction and fixation. These are skin traction, skeletal traction, external fixation, and open reduction with or without internal fixation. It must be emphasized that no single method produces satisfactory results in every type of fracture; the experienced surgeon secures good results by selecting the best method for each fracture.

Traction. In reduction by skin or skeletal traction the distal fragment is slowly pulled into line with the proximal fragment by means of a weight. Anesthesia is unnecessary, but narcotics to relieve pain are required during the hours or even days necessary to accomplish reduction by this means. In skin traction the pull of the weight is transmitted to the extremity by means of adhesive tape attached to the skin distal to the fracture. This method is simple and effective, but it has disadvantages. The adhesive tape frequently slips or tears, and it will not withstand a strong pull, so that occasionally it will not bear a weight suficient to overcome the powerful pull of the muscles. In skeletal traction a steel wire (Kirschner wire) or a pin (Steinmann pin) is driven through the distal end of the broken bone; this may be done easily under local anesthesia. The weight is then attached by means of ropes and pulleys, and a much more direct and forceful pull can be obtained. In either method the extremity is maintained in the optimal position by means of a splint which fits snugly against the pelvis or shoulder girdle, affording countertraction. In using traction methods it must be remembered that there is little effect without countertraction; an unopposed weight will only pull the patient down or across the bed as the case may be. Countertraction may be obtained by the use of weights opposed to those pulling on the distal fragment, or by tilting the bed and using the pull of gravity upon the patient as the counterweight. When reduction has been obtained by traction and sufficient union has occurred to prevent slipping of the fragments, a plaster cast may be applied and the traction discontinued.

External Fixation. For external fixation, mechanical devices such as the Roger Anderson or Stader anatomic splints are available. By means of two or more wires or pins inserted into the bones, the fragments are aligned and fixed. These splints are especially useful in badly comminuted fractures of the long bones (such as an injury from an automobile bumper).

Internal Fixation. Internal fixation may be secured in various ways. By an open operation the fragments are exposed, aligned under direct vision, and fixed by means of wire, vitallium plates, or screws. This direct method of reducing fractures is used when simpler means are inadequate. Another method is the use of a nail driven through the skin into the fragments. This is especially useful in treating fractures of the head of the femur, as it obviates the use of the cumbersome hip spica cast, shortens the length of time to be spent in bed, and permits early use of the leg. The fragments are aligned under the fluoroscope; with local anesthesia and aseptic precautions a metal (vitallium) nail is driven through the neck of the femur into the head, fixing them to-

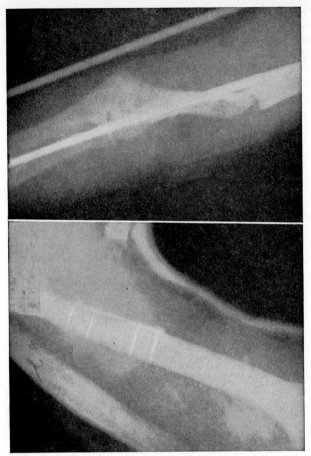

FIGURE 135. X-rays of fracture of right humerus. *Upper,* Before reduction; *lower,* fracture reduced and fragments held in place by means of vitallium plate and four screws.

gether. In some fractures of large long bones, such as the femur, an intramedullary pin is used; in this method a metal bar is placed in the marrow cavity on either side of the fracture.

Treatment of Compound Fractures

The open wound which is always a part of a compound fracture may permit contamination of the broken bone by fragments of clothing, particles of street dirt, or other foreign material. In addition to these sources of infection, bacteria lying on the skin may reach the depths of the wound. It must be remembered that the spores of B. welchii are often recoverable from the skin of the perineum and upper thighs. A second factor, of equal importance, is the crushing and devitalization of muscle incident to the fracture of the large bones. This traumatized tissue serves as an ideal culture medium for the growth of bacteria, particularly the anaerobes. It is obvious, furthermore, that this type of injury is also likely to produce shock.

In former times it was considered proper to convert a compound fracture into a simple one by closing the wound and treating the fracture in the same way a comparable simple one would be treated. World War I added the invaluable step of débridement, the removal of all devitalized tissues. And now, as an outgrowth of World War II, a different technic has been evolved. In this method débridement and reduction are followed by simple packing of the open wound with sterile gauze and application of a plaster cast. When feasible, a secondary or delayed closure of the wound is carried out. The final result is excellent, and the mortality very low. It is probable, however, that the first described method is often more satisfactory for the treatment of compound fractures sustained in civil life, where earlier treatment is the rule.

Penicillin is used, and should be administered in large doses from the outset of treatment, as its greatest value in this field lies in the prophylaxis of infection. Tetanus antitoxin must be given as well. The condition of the extremity and that of the patient must be watched so that the onset of a gas bacillus infection may be detected early. Penicillin and wide surgical exposure of the infected area will at times suffice to cure an early gas infection, but in the later stages a radical amputation may be necessary.

Complications of Fractures

Ischemic Palsy. Hemorrhage and swelling accompany every fracture, and in a closed space may compress the blood vessels, thus shutting off the circulation of the blood. The anatomic arrangement in certain locations, particularly in the region of the elbow, forearm, and leg, favors this constriction. The resultant lack of blood (*ischemia*) produces death of the tissue; thus there may be actual loss of skin or muscle. This serious complication, known as ischemic palsy, is preventable. Care must be taken that casts or circular bandages are not too tight:

for this reason the fingertips or toes are always left exposed so that the condition of the circulation may be constantly observed. If cyanosis, undue pain, or swelling develops, the cast or bandage must be loosened at once, or permanent damage will result.

Deformity. Improper reduction of a fracture often leaves permanent deformity and disability, particularly if a joint has been injured. Nature accomplishes wonders, however, and if the patient is intelligent and cooperative, much can be done toward the restoration of function. It is well to remember that early motion is imperative in fractures about the wrist, elbow, and shoulder, where mobility is important; prolonged immobilization, on the other hand, is required when weight bearing is the important consideration, as in fracture of the lower spine, leg, and foot.

Embolism. The marrow cavity of a long bone contains many blood vessels and much fat. It is easy, therefore, in the course of a fracture for droplets of fat to enter the veins, and fat embolism does occur as a complication of severe or multiple fractures. Paralysis and mental confusion are observed, and there may be pulmonary and renal complications. Death may result from massive embolism, but this is uncommon.

Nonunion. Nonunion is an occasional complication of fractures, and is difficult to treat successfully. A number of causes may be listed, including insufficient fixation, which permits too much motion at the fracture line; interposition of muscle between the bone ends; infection of the bones; syphilis; neoplastic disease; old age; and dietary deficiency. Each of these causes necessitates specific treatment, but occasionally there is no apparent cause and no treatment is successful. In such a case the line of fracture is not bridged by bony healing; instead, there is a fibrous union, with loss of stability and, at times, formation of a false joint.

SPINAL INJURIES

The common types of spinal injury include compression fracture of the vertebral bodies, dislocation, fracture of the spinous or articular processes, and rupture of the intervertebral disks. Of first importance in the consideration of spinal injuries is the possible presence of injury to the spinal cord, a grave complication (see Chap. 40). In the absence of damage to the spinal cord, spinal injuries may be successfully treated by reduction when possible, followed by the application of a plaster jacket or

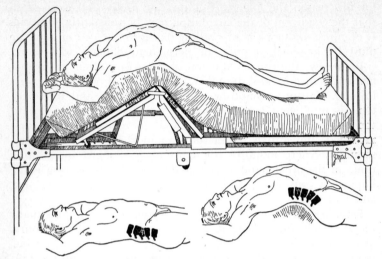

FIGURE 136. Reduction of compression fracture of lumbar vertebra by hyper-extension. The Gatch frame is reversed, and the spring is re-enforced with a hinged fracture board. Lower figures show effect of hyperextension upon the compressed vertebra.

metal brace which immobilizes the spine until healing has occurred.

Dislocations and fracture-dislocations usually occur in the cervical spine, and follow falls upon the head, as in diving into shallow water. In these there is a high incidence of serious damage to the cord, usually with fatal outcome. Compression fractures are common in the lower thoracic or lumbar region as a result of a fall in the sitting postion. In these fractures cord injury is less common, and cure follows proper reduction and immobilization. Avulsion fractures of the spinous or transverse processes are usually due to sudden twisting injuries and to violent muscular pull. Painful but not serious injuries, these fractures respond well to proper fixation. The diagnosis and treatment of dislocated or ruptured intervertebral disks are described in Chapter 40.

Muscular and ligamentous sprains of the back are common, usually resulting from weight lifting with the back bent at a disadvantageous angle, or from a twisting, reaching motion as, for example, in placing a heavy object on a high shelf. The more serious of these sprains injure the lumbosacral articulations, and are extremely painful and disabling. In mild injuries, adhesive strapping, rest, and heat are sufficient to obtain a cure; but in severe lumbosacral injuries a brace, or occasionally spinal fusion, a surgical procedure designed to immobilize the joint by a splint of grafted bone, may be required.

NURSING CARE IN MUSCULOSKELETAL INJURIES

The nursing care of orthopedic patients presents many problems not encountered in caring for other types of surgical patients. Such patients are of all ages; the individual, aside from the present injury, may be either physically fit or suffering from a chronic illness such as tuberculosis. The orthopedic patient is often hospitalized for long periods of time—months or even years —during which he may be able to do little for himself. It is not enough to see that such a patient's bed is changed, his tray brought, and his elimination regular. Means must be found to occupy his mind, so that it is not warped by the long confinement to bed; in addition, care must be taken to keep the body of the patient as fit as though he were active, so that muscles do not lose their power, nor joints stiffen through disuse.

There are numerous technical matters pertaining to orthopedic care that must be mastered. These include familiarity with the preparation and use of plaster casts and orthopedic appliances and apparatus, the care of the patient after they have been applied, and a knowledge of physiotherapy and occupational therapy. As a guiding principle, it is to be remembered that proper care will preserve the function of the musculoskeletal structures but the restoration of lost function is difficult or impossible.

Care of Patients in Traction Apparatus

The apparatus rigged up for the purpose of applying traction often appears complicated but is usually simple in principle. It is the duty of the nurse to understand fully what result the surgeon seeks and how this is to be accomplished. The cooperation of the patient is invaluable and may be encouraged by a simple explanation of what is being done. It is often necessary for the nurse to readjust the apparatus because dressings may slip, the splint may be disarranged, ropes may jam in the pulleys, and so on. In making the adjustments, however, the nurse must take care that there is no disturbance of the fundamental principles, that is, there must be no change in the amount of weight used or in the direction of the pull. These considerations are particularly important when moving the patient, as in changing his position or in taking him to the x-ray department.

Care of Immobilized Patients. Patients in head traction in the treatment of cervical spine injuries are a problem because of the necessity for immobilization. Traction is applied to the head by means of a padded halter passing beneath the occiput and chin, or by a wire or tongs inserted directly into the skull. Counter-traction is furnished by elevating the head of the bed on blocks so that gravity pulls the patient toward the foot of the bed. The countertraction permits turning the patient. Turning the patient with head and body in a straight line is necessary. The frequency for giving back care depends on such factors as the condition of the skin, incontinence and emaciation.

A full, adequate diet is essential to the proper repair of bone. Eating too fast often produces discomfort, if not actual nausea, therefore it is wise to offer the food in small amounts. The patient should be told what food is being served to him. Because of the mechanical difficulties involved in immobilization, the patient is forced to depend largely upon the nurse for his fluid intake. However, by the use of a drinking tube or similar device, adequate fluids may be given. A clean mouth is not only more comfortable but is also an aid in preventing infection. Regular brushing of the teeth and frequent use of mouthwashes are important.

Care of Patients in Casts

Technic of Applying Plaster Casts. Plaster of paris bandages are made by rubbing powdered plaster (calcium sulfate) into the meshes of rolls of crinoline cut into the desired width (2 to 8 inches). Just before actual use the roll is placed on end in a bucket of warm water. Air bubbles will rise. The roll is thoroughly wet when no more bubbles appear. Excess water is removed by grasping the roll at either end and pulling gently; but twisting is avoided as it causes too much plaster to be lost. Plaster casts may be padded or unpadded, depending upon the nature of the case and the surgeon's preference; padding is more commonly used and consists of glazed cotton and heavy felt. Sometimes stockinette is applied to the skin first. In unpadded casts the plaster is applied directly to the skin. The bandage is applied turn upon turn, even, moderate pressure being used. The greatest care must be taken to avoid wrinkles or dimples in the cast as such irregularities are apt to cause pressure sores.

Plaster Room. In applying fresh plaster it is impossible to avoid spilling small amounts on the floor and elsewhere; therefore it is desirable to have a special room for this purpose. A sink with a specially constructed drain and trap is also advisable, as plaster washed from the hands or remaining in the buckets used for moistening the bandages will quickly plug the ordinary drainpipe. Supplies needed for the plaster room are the following:

Acetic acid, 5%
Alcohol, 70%
Ammoniated mercury ointment, 5% (sterile)
Benzine
Boric ointment (sterile)
Compound tincture benzoin
Ether
Procaine, ½%
Stearate of zinc powder
Talcum powder
Petrolatum (sterile)
Zinc oxide ointment (sterile)

Alcohol lamp
Culture tubes (sterile)
Syringe and needles for procaine
Syringe (Chetwood)

Adhesive tape, 3,2,1, and ½ inch
Cotton pads
Crinoline, starched, 6 and 3 inch
Elastic bandages
Felt padding
Gauze bandages (unsterile), 6,4,3, and 2 inch
Gauze rolls, wide and narrow (sterile)

Glazed cotton bandages, 6,4,3, and 2 inch
Muslin bandages (unsterile) 6,4,3, and 2 inch
Plaster bandages 6,4,3, and 2 inch
Slings (muslin)
Sponge rubber
Stockinette, 10,8,6,4,3, and 2 inch
Surgical dressing cart (equipped as for surgical ward)
Webbing straps and buckles

Tape measure
Bandage scissors (large)
Plaster shears
Plaster knives
Cast spreader
Bending irons
Orthopedic table with attachments
Hammer
Hatchet
Mallet
Saw
Sandbags
Splints: airplane, basswood, coaptation, and Thomas
Throat sticks

Care During Setting of the Cast. As the moisture evaporates, the cast hardens (sets). The initial setting, however, does not make the cast firm. Great care must be taken in the handling of a wet cast. When any lifting is necessary the cast should be supported with the entire hand. Lifting with the finger tips causes indentations which may cause pressure areas. Two factors that are important in drying a cast are: good circulation of air around the cast and even drying by turning the patient frequently. In a warm climate, where there is no danger of chilling the patient, an electric fan may be used to speed the drying. It is important that the drying plaster cast be firmly supported until it has set. In the case of large body casts this may require many hours. Failure to observe this simple precaution of proper support results in the cracking of the cast, which necessitates the application of a new one.

The cast is usually supported with pillows. Extremities in casts should be elevated and supported. A straight leg cast may be supported by placing three pillows on an inclined plane from the heel to the hip; one pillow is placed lengthwise under the upper leg, and the other two are placed under the lower leg. This provides for even support. Whenever there is a concavity in the cast it should be supported. A small pillow placed crosswise at the level of the lumbar curve will give support when a body cast has been applied.

During the drying process the patient's extremities are watched carefully for signs of constriction of circulation: cyanosis, swelling, and pain. The patient frequently complains of tightness of the cast and pain. These complaints must be relayed to the doctor. Special effort must be made for the patient to describe what the pain feels like, for if he says it is "burning" there is urgent need to notify the surgeon immediately. Such pain does not usually last long, but it signifies terrific pressure which will result in necrosis with loss of sensation if the pressure is not relieved. These signs and symptoms must be reported immediately in order that the surgeon may, by cutting the cast, release the constriction and prevent the development of ischemic palsy. Plaster on the exposed toes and fingers should be washed off with a damp cloth. The edges of the cast should be bound with adhesive tape to prevent crumbling and to strengthen the edges.

Turning the Patient. The bed is prepared for the patient by putting a fracture board underneath the mattress. It is hardly necessary to say that a patient in a large body cast is practically helpless. In many instances assistance in feeding is needed. Complete turning must not be omitted in any case even though the patient is able to stay on his face for only a short time. For turning patients in large body casts at least two nurses or attendants are needed. One stands on each side of the bed. The patient is moved to one edge (toward side of injured extremity) and is instructed to hold his arms tightly to his sides. The closer nurse elevates her side of the patient by lifting with one hand beneath the patient's chest and the other beneath his thigh; the second

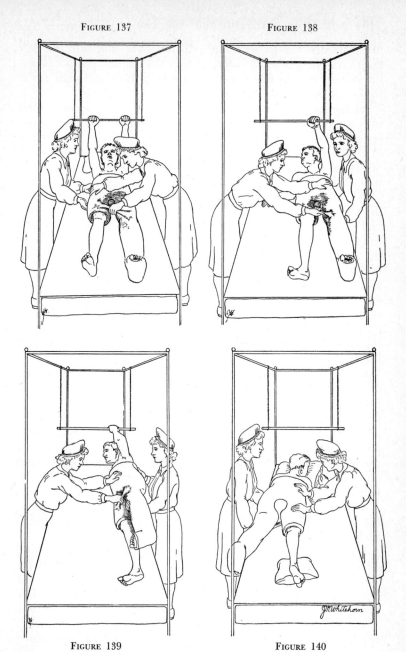

FIGURE 137   FIGURE 138

FIGURE 139   FIGURE 140

FIGURES 137–140. Method of turning patient in cast.

nurse steadies the patient and helps to lower him into the new position as he gradually is turned over toward her. Small changes in position may be effected by the use of pillows and pads at the back and between body surfaces.

Prevention of Pressure Sores. The prevention of pressure sores calls for the use of every method and device known, and for ingenuity in creating new ones. Regular care, including inspection of all pressure areas, rubbing, keeping the skin dry, and the relief of pressure as far as possible, are the simplest modes of prevention. Rough edges of casts may be taped with adhesive or covered with cotton pads. The most commonly used materials for protecting the perineal region from excretions are waterproof plastics, and oiled silk or oiled muslin. The material is cut in 4 or 5 inch strips which are tucked under the cast. They are held in place on the outside of the cast by adhesive or mending tape. Oiled paper may also be used for this purpose, but it has very little durability and must be changed frequently. An extremity may need to be elevated to relieve pressure at the edge of the cast. Bed cradles or similar devices are used to relieve the pressure of the bedcovers on the toes. Pressure on the heels is relieved by the use of a cotton "doughnut" or by a pillow placed underneath the leg so that the heel will extend over the edge.

Orthopedic Bed. Modern orthopedic beds allow for the introduction of the bedpan below the level at which the patient lies; this not only is easier and more comfortable but also aids in the prevention of pressure sores. The bedpan should be carefully adjusted so that the flesh of the buttocks rests on the edge of the pan. When the edge of the cast rests on the pan, urine will follow the buttocks up under the cast. Elevating the head of the patient on not less than one pillow while he is using the bedpan also helps to prevent him from moistening the back under the cast. A soft pillow or several cotton pads placed between the edge of the pan and the cast will make the patient more comfortable, if such a bed is unobtainable.

BALKAN AND BRADFORD FRAMES. There are other mechanical devices which aid in the maintenance of position and simplify the care of these patients. The Balkan frame may be built into the bed, or the portable wooden frame may be attached to any hospital bed. It provides support for the apparatus used in traction. A trapeze or other overhead support placed within the patient's reach provides help to the patient in turning and an opportunity for limited exercise. The Bradford frame is a rectangle of iron piping over which canvas is laced tightly. The canvas is put on the frame in two sections, with space enough at the buttocks so that the bedpan may be used without disturbing the patient's position. A valuable feature of the Bradford frame is that it may be bent at any point into the angle the surgeon desires, for the purpose of providing hyperextension. The features of both the Bradford and the Balkan frame are built into the modern fracture bed.

Removing the Cast. When the cast is to be removed, a plaster cutter, plaster knife, and scissors are needed. The cast is dampened along the line of anticipated incision and cut. The removal of the cast is a long awaited event, and to prevent undue worry and depression on the part of the patient he should be warned that all the joints which were in the cast will feel transitory stiffness and soreness. After the cast is removed, gentle washing of the part with warm water, mild soap and a soft cloth followed by the application of a little oil is indicated.

Care of the Convalescent Patient

Crutches. Crutches should be 1 inch shorter than the distance between the axilla and the heel, and should be fitted with rubber tips to prevent slipping. The patient should wear a shoe on the normal foot to offer better support and to allow the injured extremity to swing clear of the floor. The patient is instructed to bear his weight on his hands instead of in the armpit as the pressure due to bearing weight upon a crutch in the axilla is apt to damage the nerves and cause paralysis of the arm (*crutch palsy*). He is taught to bend forward from the hips. Since it is often necessary that crutches be used for many months, good posture must be learned. Unless the patient is warned he may concentrate his weight on the ball of the foot, flex the hip, and rotate the knee outwardly. He should be permitted to walk only a few steps the first day. The nurse should be at his side to prevent falls until he feels secure and has acquired ease and rhythm in his walk. The tendency to walk with chin on chest and eyes directed to the floor becomes a habit because of insecurity. Attention should be called to this detail when the patient learns to walk.

The patient moves both crutches forward together with the injured extremity, bearing the weight on the good leg. Then his weight is shifted to the crutches, and the good leg is brought forward. Short steps, caution, and the development of a smooth rhythm are then in order. The arm rest may be made more comfortable by being padded with sponge rubber or with cotton pads, but the patient must be cautioned against bearing his weight on the axilla.

Walker. For patients who have not been on their feet for a long time or for those who are timid about using crutches, a device called a walker is useful in the period of learning again how to walk. The walker is a circular metal frame mounted upon small wheels or casters; the patient stands inside the frame, supporting his weight by his hands. The walker may also be fitted with a seat or straps to aid in weight bearing.

Braces. In convalescence from bone disease or injury and in the correction of deformity, braces are frequently used. These are made of strong, light-weight materials such as aluminum, leather, or steel. They are used chiefly for the leg (walking calipers), the spine (Taylor spine brace), the arm or elbow, and for the neck. Removal of the brace is ordered by the doctor. Because the effectiveness of a brace depends upon a snug fit, it is a part of nursing care to see that the brace is correctly placed and adequately fastened.

Physiotherapy

The use of modern physiotherapeutic methods, including massage, passive motion, exercises, water baths (hydrotherapy), baking, diathermy, and sunlight (heliotherapy), constitutes one of the most important steps in the rehabilitation of patients who have had injury or disease of the musculoskeletal system. Nearly every hospital has trained technicians to carry on this work, but often it is the responsibility of the nurse to see that the patient follows instructions and to carry out the treatment outlined by the physiotherapist. The purpose of physiotherapy is to prevent loss of muscle tone, to prevent stiffening of joints, and to attempt to overcome these if already present. The cooperation of the patient, particularly in the matter of exercises, is essential, and in most instances the degree of return of function following injuries and orthopedic operations depends to a large extent upon the willingness of the patient to help himself. In each case the treatments and exercises are selected to fit the individual need. Progress is often slow, and it is necessary to keep the patient encouraged.

Rehabilitation

Many orthopedic patients face not only a long period of hospitalization but also a future with a physical handicap.[1] Aid in making adjustment to these should be given to such patients as early as possible, and his fear and anxiety must be allayed. The reason for restrictions upon his activity should be explained and every effort made to increase his confidence in himself and in his future by encouraging him to do actively for himself everything that is permitted. Occupational therapy is a great aid in rehabilitation. It is unfortunate that all too often insufficient consideration is given to the problem, and poor judgment used in the selection of the type of occupational training. It is a sad mistake to provide knitting, basket-making, or needlepoint for a patient who may look on these things as "sissy"; much more will be accomplished if the patient is taught to produce something of which he might have been proud even had he made it before he became handicapped.

Children requiring long-term hospitalization may miss many months or even years of school; in addition, they usually have a physical handicap which is a source of embarrassment. To meet the needs of these children, institutions called "hospital schools" have been established.

SUMMARY

Sprains, dislocations and fractures are wounds of the muscles, joints and bones. The treatment of these makes use of the same principles as are involved in healing of all wounds, notably approximation, immobilization, hemostasis, débridement, control of infection, and good circulation of the blood. The necessary use of devices such as traction and splints, and the long periods involved in achieving the healing of bone bring special problems which need expert nursing care. Rehabilitation must be included in the plan for all patients with serious injuries to the musculoskeletal system.

VOCABULARY REVIEW

crepitus	medullary nail	internal fixation
traction	ischemic palsy	Bradford frame
Kirschner wire	Balkan frame	reduction
	nonunion	

[1] See Brown, pages 766–791.

SUGGESTED READING

1. Chesley, A. J. et al: Home Accident Prevention—A Symposium. Am. J. Pub. Health, *40*:513–524 (May) 1950.
2. Colonna, Paul C.: Regional Orthopedic Surgery. Philadelphia, W. B. Saunders Co., 1950, pp. 1–21.
3. Funsten, Robert V., and Calderwood, Carmelita: Orthopedic Nursing. 2nd Ed. St. Louis, C. V. Mosby Co.. 1949.
4. Hacker, Garnet I.: Medullary Nail. Am. J Nursing, *50*:104–106 (Feb.) 1950
5. Miller, Bernice: Well Leg and Hip Splints. Am. J. Nursing, *48*:572–576 (Sept.) 1948.
6. Moore, Moore, Jr.: Ambulation Following Fractures of the Lower Extremity. Am. J. Nursing, *53*:174–175 (Feb.) 1953.
7. Newton, Kathleen: Basic Needs of the Aged. Am. J. Nursing, *50*:32–35 (Jan.) 1950.
8. Silverstein, Martin A., and Gips, Claudia D.: Skin Care of the Incontinent Patients. Am. J. Nursing, *52*:63–64 (Jan.) 1952.
9. Skinner, Geraldine: Head Traction and the Stryker Frame. Am. J. Nursing, *52*:694–696 (June) 1952.
10. Wilde, Delphine: The Patient in a Spica, Abed and Afoot. Am. J. Nursing, *51*:429–432 (July) 1951.

CHAPTER 45

Inflammatory, Infectious, and Neoplastic Diseases of the Musculoskeletal System

A deplorable amount of human suffering and economic loss results from the ravages of the various disease entities included under the heading of musculoskeletal inflammations and infections. Open wounds acquired by accident may serve as portals of entry for invading bacteria; or microbes, having entered the blood vessels from a focus of infection in the tonsils, teeth, or elsewhere, may be carried to muscles, joints, or bones by the circulating blood. There are some affections which, being obviously inflammatory in character, have been considered to be infectious in origin although the actual infective agent has not been demonstrated. Another group of inflammatory lesions has been thought to be the result of wear and tear during excessive or long use. In all of these, however, the final result, whether due to actual destruction of tissue or to the formation of scars and adhesions, is likely to be the loss of function.

TENOSYNOVITIS

Infection of the tendons and their sheaths usually occurs by the direct extension of an adjacent infectious process, which is often a felon or a furuncle. The acute suppurative tenosynovitis which develops is characterized by great pain on motion of the tendon. Tendons have a relatively poor blood supply, and therefore the local resistance to bacteria is not good. Unless the infection is treated early, tendons are quickly destroyed by the common invaders, the staphylococcus and the streptococcus.

Diagnosis is based upon the systemic signs of infection together with local pain, tenderness over the tendon, and unwillingness of the patient to move the affected part. There is usually some local inflammation, but often this is minimal.

Treatment. The infection must be treated by general systemic measures, antibiotics, and local heat and rest. The tendon sheath should be incised early to permit drainage. As soon as the acute inflammation has subsided, physiotherapy, which includes exercise, massage, and passive motion, must be started in order to bring about restoration of function. When loss of substance occurs as the result of neglect or from a very severe infection, plastic procedures are necessary. It must be remembered that the loss of tendons may mean the loss of the patient's ability to earn a living.

Gonorrheal Tenosynovitis

A common nonsuppurative variety of acute tenosynovitis is due to the gonococcus and often complicates gonorrhea in both male and female. This type may be diagnosed by the suddenness of onset, without evidence of local portal of entry, and by the presence of gonococcal infection of the genital tract. The extensor tendons of the wrist are the ones most often affected. Rest, splinting, diathermy, and antibiotic therapy result in cure.

Tenosynovitis Sicca

Tenosynovitis sicca is a low grade inflammation of tendon and sheath of frequent occurrence; it is probably due to excessive use since there is no evidence of bacterial infection. Motion is possible but is painful, and a characteristic crackling or crepitus is felt over the tendon during motion. As a rule there is little redness or swelling. Simple rest by splinting results in prompt disappearance of the inflammation with relief of symptoms.

DUPUYTREN'S CONTRACTURE

A curious deformity of the hands results from a nodular thickening and shortening of the palmar fascia. This affection, known as Dupuytren's contracture, is not a true inflammation, and no known infectious agent is concerned. It occurs usually in cobblers, mechanics, or others who constantly traumatize the palm of the hand, and, peculiarly enough, the tendency appears to be hereditary. The disabling contracture can be relieved by surgical removal of the diseased palmar fascia.

BURSITIS

Bursas are occasionally the seat of acute suppuration, usually the result of the direct introduction of bacteria into the bursa. Far more common, however, is a chronic low grade bursitis of nonbacterial origin, probably due to excessive wear and tear. An example of this is prepatellar bursitis, known as housemaid's knee. This is a painful affliction, and is cured only by prolonged rest or by excision of the bursa.

The bursas of the elbow (*olecranon*) and shoulder (*subdeltoid*) are also often attacked by this chronic inflammatory process, and the condition proves troublesome to athletes and others who use their arms strenuously.

MYOSITIS

Inflammation of muscle (*myositis*) is relatively uncommon, largely, perhaps, because of the excellent blood supply of this tissue. Bacterial invaders do not thrive unless the muscle is devitalized. Chronic abuse or overuse of muscle is occasionally followed by low grade inflammation and fibrosis. This chronic form of myositis is sometimes seen in the thigh muscles of cavalrymen, or in the arm muscles of professional baseball players.

ARTHRITIS

Inflammation of a joint is both painful and disabling. The common symptom is pain, exacerbated by movement, and on inspection the acutely inflamed joint is seen to be swollen, with obliteration of the normal anatomic prominences. The diseased synovium produces an excess of fluid, distending the joint capsule and causing the extremity to be held in that characteristic semiflexed position which permits the least tension within the joint. Local heat and redness are also observed.

Acute suppurative arthritis is the result of bacterial invasion of the joint and, as in bursitis, may follow a penetrating wound, or may be a blood-borne infection. High fever, leukocytosis, and other systemic responses are usual. Diagnosis is confirmed by aspiration and study of the joint fluid.

An acute but nonsuppurative form of arthritis is caused by the gonococcus; it is important to differentiate this from the suppurative form as the treatment is different. Another variety likely to lead to confusion is seen in acute rheumatic fever, the cause of which is as yet not known. Since nearly any acute febrile illness may be accompanied by painful joints, proper diagnosis is extremely important.

Treatment. The correct treatment of acute suppurative arthritis includes rest, surgical drainage, local heat, immobilization, and antibiotic therapy. In gonococcal arthritis drainage is unnecessary. Early motion of the joint is desirable in order to prevent fixation (*ankylosis*), and therefore active motion is begun as soon as the acute inflammation subsides. Active motion is better than passive motion, for the patient is less likely to harm himself than is the physician or nurse who suffers no personal pain during manipulation of the patient's joint.

The treatment of an acute rheumatic joint or of other joint inflammations of a medical nature such as chronic arthritis, rheumatism, gout, and degenerative arthritis, is nonsurgical in general, but occasionally, as a result of degenerative changes or injury, pieces of cartilage or bone become loose in a joint cavity. Loose bodies are particularly common in the knee, and cause "locking" of the joint. The treatment is surgical removal of the free particles of bone or cartilage.

OSTEOMYELITIS

Acute Form. The acute form of this disease of bone (acute hematogenous osteomyelitis) is a blood-borne bacterial infection, and the commonest pathogen is Staphylococcus aureus. Children are the usual victims. The disease is characterized by the sudden onset of local pain and a severe systemic reaction, including headache, anorexia, nausea, malaise, chills, high fever, and leukocytosis. The local signs are minimal. In the early stages swelling and redness are absent, but the careful examiner discovers one

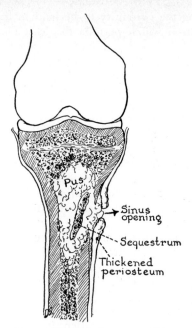

FIGURE 141. Chronic osteomyelitis.

point where pressure over a bone causes exquisite pain, indicating the site of the infection.

It is generally believed that a clump of staphylococci acts as an embolus, plugging one of the tiny end-arteries in a long bone. Deprived of circulation, the local bony tissue is put at a grave disadvantage, and the bacteria multiply rapidly. Cellulitis develops, and since the bone cannot expand, the pressure of the exudation causes much pain. Suppuration occurs within twelve to thirty-six hours. Unless adequate surgical drainage is promptly carried out, the pus ruptures into the marrow cavity and thus spreads throughout the length of the bone; or it breaks through the cortex, elevating and stripping the periosteum from the shaft. In a neglected case both of these sequelae may occur. Diagnosis is based on the symptoms and signs; in the early stages x-ray films show no bony changes.

Treatment. In addition to immediate surgical drainage, treatment includes general measures, antibiotic therapy, and transfusions. Early in the care of the patient the nurse should understand the danger of deformity. The patient usually holds his limb in a flexed position in which there is the least possible strain on the bone and muscles. Foot drop is also apparent early in the disease. The surgeon usually applies a splint of some kind as soon as drainage has been established. This is to hold the limb in an optimal position in order to prevent contracture of the muscles and to add support to the part.

Chronic Form. Chronic osteomyelitis was formerly a terrible affliction, and often persisted, with remissions, during the entire life of many patients who contracted the disease in childhood. Antibiotic therapy has completely changed the outlook for patients with this infection.

The diagnosis of chronic osteomyelitis is easily made by the history of previous infection of the bone, the presence of a persistent, discharging sinus, and the characteristic appearance in the x-ray film of the diseased bone. Frequent acute flare-ups, in which the patient has pain, local inflammation, and fever, are common. Usually due to temporary interruption of drainage of the chronic infection, these exacerbations subside quickly upon the reestablishment of proper openings for the discharge of pus. The nurse should be aware of the great virulence of the organism that is contained in the pus whenever the dressings are changed. The soiled dressings should be placed in a paper bag and burned. She must protect herself and the other patients by thoroughly washing her hands each time she cares for such a patient.

Treatment. Antibiotic therapy, using the agent which is most effective against the bacteria responsible for the infection, surgical drainage of abscess cavities and the removal of pieces of dead bone (*sequestra*) constitute the proper treatment.

TUBERCULOSIS

Modern sanitation and public health measures have done much to reduce the incidence of tuberculosis of the musculoskeletal system, but it is still too common. Tubercle bacilli enter the bones, joints, and tendon sheaths by way of the blood stream from a primary focus of infection, which is usually in the lungs. Tubercles develop, and are followed by the typical cheesy (caseating) destruction of bone or joints. As is characteristic of tuberculous infections, the process is a low grade inflammation, with no redness or local heat, giving rise to the term cold abscess.

Joints and tendon sheaths, when infected, become swollen and painful, and unless healing is brought about, function is lost.

When bone is infected the caseation produces a crumbling disintegration, so that pathologic fracture may occur, or deformity of the bone is produced under weight bearing. Humpback (*gibbus*), now seen less frequently than formerly, is an exaggerated dorsal curvature (*kyphosis*) resulting from the collapse of one or more tuberculous vertebrae. Cold abscesses in the soft tissues adjacent to tuberculous bone occur frequently, and may burrow along tissue planes for considerable distances, ultimately reaching the surface to produce persistent draining sinuses.

Treatment. Tuberculous bones and joints will heal if the patient can develop the proper resistance to the infection. As in all forms of tuberculosis, the most important therapeutic measures are rest, both general and local, and adequate nutrition. Immobilization of the affected parts is essential. This is accomplished by proper splinting and by fusion operations. The treatment is continued over months or years, until adequate healing takes place.

It is common practice to treat patients with tuberculosis of the spine (*Pott's disease*) by immobilization upon a stiff supporting frame (*Bradford frame*). Reduction of the humpback is accomplished by gradual hyperextension. The patient is placed on the frame so that the "hump" is directly over the bend in the frame. If the patient is a child or a restless adult, it may be necessary to use restraint in order that proper position may be maintained. This may be accomplished by the use of a jacket that fits over the chest and shoulders and is tied to the frame; in addition, extension may be applied to the feet. If necessary, the frame may be further bent to increase the degree of hyperextension. The essential point for the nurse to remember is the absolute avoidance of any motion of the back; turning is done in such a way that the patient moves "all in one piece." In the beginning the patient will need help in eating and drinking.

NEOPLASTIC DISEASE

The cells of the various components of the musculoskeletal system are all of connective tissue origin, and the neoplasms arising from them are characteristic in appearance and behavior. The commonest tumor is the fibroma, a benign growth composed of simple connective tissue cells with much extracellular fibrous tissue. Indeed the fibroma is perhaps the tumor that occurs more frequently than any other single type. It is found in any part of the body that has connective tissue, and in the musculoskeletal system it commonly arises from fascia, from a tendon, or from the sheath of a nerve. The symptoms and signs of a fibroma are due solely to the mechanical effect of its size and position. The treatment is simple removal, and cure is certain unless tumor cells are left behind.

Neoplasms arising from muscles or joint structures are rare, despite the large amount of muscular and joint tissue in the body and the constant degree of use to which they are subjected.

Benign tumors of cartilaginous (*chondroma*) or bony (*osteoma*) origin are not uncommon. Although benign, these neoplasms are difficult to cure because it is often impossible to remove them completely without performing a mutilating operation. The chondroma is frequently a multiple tumor, arising simultaneously in several different locations. It is, furthermore, a matter of record that the chondroma, which originally appears to be benign, will, if permitted to grow for several years, often degenerate into a malignant neoplasm.

Sarcoma

Malignant tumors of the connective tissue cells, although not occurring as frequently as malignant epithelial tumors, are nevertheless responsible for many deaths annually. It is a fact that the results of treatment are less successful for the various kinds of sarcoma than for cancer. The tumors are difficult to discover in the early stages, and connective tissue cells are resistant to radium and roentgen irradiation. Sarcoma arises from fascia, tendon, nerve sheath, periosteum, and cartilage. The neoplasm is usually cellular, and the microscopic appearance is sufficiently characteristic to indicate the origin of the growth. Invisible and painless at first, some sarcomas cause symptoms by pressure on nerves, some by reason of the size attained, others because of metastases. Roentgenograms are invaluable in diagnosing these as well as other tumors of the bones.

The type observed most frequently is the spindle-cell *fibrosarcoma,* arising from either fascia, nerve sheath, or periosteum. Less common is the bone sarcoma (*osteosarcoma*) which arises from the osteogenic or osteolytic cells of the periosteum or endosteum. Another form of malignant tumor of bone is the highly malignant small cell *endothelioma* (Ewing's sarcoma). The origin of this neoplasm is obscure, and it differs from the others in being sensitive to radiation therapy.

The bones are frequently the sites of tumor metastases. Car-

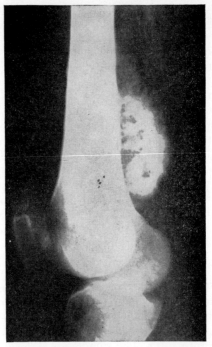

FIGURE 142. X-ray film of osteogenic sarcoma, lower end of femur.

cinomata of such organs as the breast, thyroid, kidney, and prostate often give rise to bony metastases which may be mistaken for primary bone tumors. Differential diagnosis is based upon x-ray appearance, multiplicity of lesions, discovery of a primary tumor elsewhere, or biopsy. Another type of neoplasm, the *myeloma,* may be confused with bone sarcoma because it attacks the bones. This growth arises from the cells of the bone marrow, and may cause widespread destruction of bone.

Bone Cysts

Cystic disease of bone has long been of interest to surgeons, but only recently has some light been thrown on the subject. With the discovery of the part played by the parathyroid hormone in regulating calcium metabolism, it soon became evident that some bone cysts are due to rarefaction of the bone as a result of the loss of calcium from the body caused by hyperparathyroidism. This condition, formerly known as osteitis fibrosa

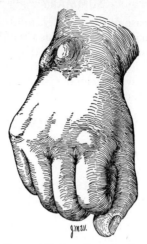

FIGURE 143. Ganglion of wrist.

cystica, is now successfully treated by the removal of parathyroid tumors. Following cessation of the abnormal loss of calcium the cysts disappear. Further discussion of this subject is found in Chapter 34.

GANGLION

It is difficult to classify this common lesion properly. A tumor in the sense that it is a swelling, a ganglion is in no way a neoplasm. Ganglions occur about joints, usually the wrist or ankle, and occasionally the knee. The ganglion is a cyst containing synovial fluid, and under the microscope the wall of the cyst resembles a joint capsule. As a rule, the lesion is painless but when large it may interfere mechanically with joint function. The most reasonable theory of the nature of origin of the ganglion is that it constitutes a herniation or diverticulum of a joint capsule.

The classical method for treating a ganglion was to strike it hard with the family Bible. The blow ruptured the cyst wall and dispersed the fluid. Unfortunately, however, the ganglion thus treated soon returned; permanent cure is effected only by the surgical removal of the cyst wall. Since the ganglion nearly always communicates with the underlying joint cavity, it is essential to find and close the communication in order to prevent recurrence.

SUMMARY

Inflammatory disease of the muscles, joints, and bones, whether infectious or not, may lead to serious disability. It is in the patients suffering from these affections that conservation of function and rehabilitation are most useful. Malignant neoplasms arising from the musculoskeletal system are fortunately not of very frequent occurrence.

VOCABULARY REVIEW

tenosynovitis	*arthritis*	*sequestrum*
bursitis	*osteomyelitis*	*ganglion*

SUGGESTED READING

1. Anderson, Helen C.: Nursing the Patient with Bone and Joint Tuberculosis. Am. J. Nursing, *48*:215–220 (April) 1948.
2. Funsten, Robert V., and Calderwood, Carmelita: Orthopedic Nursing. 2nd Ed. St. Louis, C. V. Mosby Co., 1949.
3. Kilham, Blanche Ann: Nursing Patients with Osteomyelitis. Am. J. Nursing, *50*:19–21 (Jan.) 1950.
4. Krause, Marie V.: Nutrition and Diet Therapy. Philadelphia, W. B. Saunders Co., 1950, pp. 359–368.
5. Leavitt, Harry L.: Bone and Joint Tuberculosis. Am. J. Nursing, *48*:213–214 (April) 1948.
6. Lewin, Philip: Orthopedic Surgery for Nurses, Philadelphia, W. B. Saunders Co., 1947, pp. 187–223.
7. O'Brien, Robert M.: Osteomyelitis. Am. J. Nursing, *50*:17–19 (Jan.) 1950.
8. Young, H. Herman: Surgical Treatment of Arthritis. Am. J. Nursing, *48*:27–28 (Jan.) 1948.

CHAPTER 46

Abdominal Hernia

An external abdominal hernia is the protrusion of abdominal contents through a defect in the abdominal wall. When an opening is present, it is not surprising that omentum, intestine, or other movable viscera should be forced through it, because great pressure develops within the abdomen during such acts as lifting a heavy weight, coughing, sneezing, and the crying of infancy. The local weakness of the abdominal wall is due either to a congenital defect, to a weakness in the arrangement of the anatomic structures, or to the imperfect healing of an operative wound. The two common sites of congenital defect are at the inguinal rings and at the umbilicus. Structural weakness, too, occurs in the abdominal wall at the inguinal rings, and also at the femoral rings, in the lumbar regions, and at the openings in the diaphragm which permit passage of the great vessels and the esophagus. Internal abdominal hernia, on the other hand, is the protrusion of viscera through an abnormal opening in some portion of the mesentery of the alimentary tract; such openings may be due to developmental defect, or may be acquired as the result of injury or operation.

Hernias are classified according to etiology, anatomic location, and degree. If the hernia or the hernial opening in the abdominal wall is present at birth, the hernia is considered to be congenital in origin; all other hernias are considered to be acquired. The common anatomic sites in the order of frequency of their occurrence are inguinal, umbilical, incisional (postoperative), femoral, internal, diaphragmatic, and lumbar. There are other rare types. A hernia is said to be reducible if it is possible, by gentle manipulation and pressure, to replace the protruding abdominal contents within the abdominal cavity; if it is not, the hernia is considered irreducible or incarcerated. When the contents of the hernia are not only irreducible but are so tightly constricted by the hernial opening that the circulation of the contents is impaired, it is a strangulated hernia.

Certain other terms are used in connection with hernias. The hernial ring is composed of the edges of the structures of the abdominal wall between which the hernia has protruded. The hernial sac is the pouch of peritoneum which has been pushed out through the opening by the protruding viscera. The coverings of the hernial sac vary in the different locations according to the anatomy of the region. Some hernias are so large that the abdominal cavity is no longer able to accommodate the protruded viscera; this type is considered to be a hernia which has forfeited the right of domicile.

All operations performed for the repair of hernia (*herniorrhaphy*) are the same in principle. The hernia is reduced, the sac is removed, and an attempt is made to close the defect in the abdominal wall. Success depends upon many things: the type of hernia, the age of the patient, the nature of his tissues, but, above all, upon the perfection of wound healing. Thus in herniorrhaphy there is a special premium upon asepsis, avoidance of tension, and gentle handling of the tissues.

INGUINAL HERNIA

In order to understand the frequency of occurrence of inguinal hernia and the methods of its repair it is necessary to consider briefly both the anatomy and the embryology of the region. During the fetal life of the male the testis migrates from its original site near the kidney, moves down behind the peritoneum, and descends from the abdominal cavity into the scrotum. To do this it must pass through the inguinal canal, a slit-like opening bounded above by the lower margin of the short, lateral abdominal muscles, laterally by the inguinal ligament (*Poupart's ligament*), medially by the lateral border of the rectus muscle, and below by the ramus of the pubic bone. As the testis descends it carries with it a small outpouching of the peritoneum, the spermatic artery and veins, and the duct (*vas deferens*) through which the spermatozoa pass to reach the seminal vesicle. Under normal conditions, by the time birth occurs the connection of this small peritoneal outpouching with the general peritoneal cavity has disappeared, but in a considerable number of infants the connection persists, and thus constitutes a preformed hernial sac. In some of these infants hernias are apparent at birth, but in others protrusion of the abdominal contents (either the omentum or intestine) into the sac does not take place until some strain later in life initiates the process. Thus symptoms and signs of a true congenital inguinal hernia may not appear until the first or second decade of life. Acquired inguinal hernia, on the other hand, usually does not appear until later, and is associated with the thinning and relaxation of the muscles and fascia of the abdominal wall incident to obesity and advanced age. Often the differentiation between the two types is difficult before operation, but during the operation a correct diagnosis can be established because of the different relations of the hernial sac to the spermatic cord. Both congenital and acquired inguinal hernias are often bilateral.

Inguinal hernia is not uncommon in the female, although much less frequent than in the male. The congenital type of hernia does occur because the round ligament of the uterus, the structure embryologically analagous to the male spermatic cord, passes through the inguinal canal to attach to the fascia about the pubic bone.

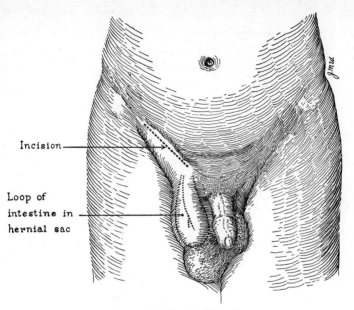

Incision

Loop of
intestine in
hernial sac

FIGURE 144. Inguinal hernia.

The diagnosis of inguinal hernia is usually not difficult. The patient (or his parents or nurse) notices a bulge in the inguinal region which appears on standing or straining, and disappears on lying down. The hernia may descend into the scrotum as far as the testicle; it may be large or small; it may be difficult or impossible to reduce. There is often some discomfort and a dragging feeling, but actual pain is present only, as a rule, when the hernia is strangulated. Palpation of the scrotum, reduction of the hernia, and palpation of the inguinal ring, revealing enlargement and descent of viscera on coughing, confirm the diagnosis.

Treatment

INGUINAL HERNIORRHAPHY

The incision is made just above and parallel to the inguinal (*Poupart's*) ligament. Each layer of tissue is divided and carefully preserved so that it may be used in the repair; the division of these structures permits reduction of the hernia if that has not been possible prior to operation. The peritoneal sac is exposed, dissected free, and excised; the peritoneum is closed flush with the normal boundary of the peritoneal cavity. The various lay-

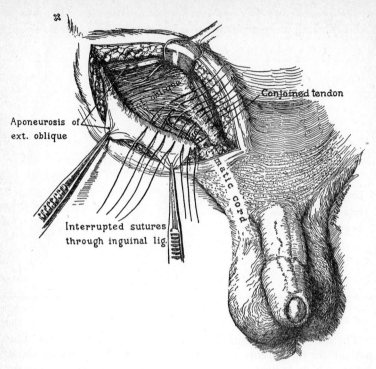

Aponeurosis of
ext. oblique

Conjoined tendon

Interrupted sutures
through inguinal lig.

FIGURE 145. Inguinal herniorrhaphy. The hernial sac has been removed. The
internal oblique muscle and conjoined tendon are being sutured to
the inguinal ligament, over the spermatic cord.

ers of muscle and fascia are then sutured together in an over-
lapping manner (*imbrication*). Since the spermatic cord must
still pass through the abdominal wall in order to reach the testis
it is necessary to leave a small opening, but care is taken to reduce
the size of the opening to fit snugly about the cord. The operation is readily carried out under general, spinal, or local anesthesia, depending upon the condition of the patient and the
preference of the surgeon.

Standard operations for inguinal hernia accomplish the cure
of the condition in more than 95 per cent of those patients who
have small hernias and normal abdominal wall tissues. The
results are less satisfactory in treating patients who have very
large hernial openings and those whose tissues have been weak-

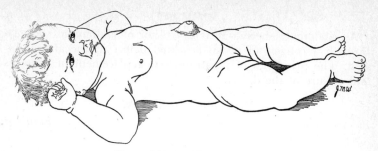

FIGURE 146. Umbilical hernia.

ened by age, obesity, or previous attempts at operative repair. The occurrence of strangulation demands an emergency operation, and, at times, necessitates resection of gangrenous intestine or omentum; infection of the wound is not infrequent in such patients, and the rate of recurrence of the hernia is higher than in uncomplicated cases.

Nursing Care. There is little that is special about the nursing care of patients following inguinal herniorrhaphy. Infants may be dismissed from the hospital as soon as they have recovered from anesthesia, with instructions for the mother to proceed with feedings and care as before operation. Children may remain in the hospital for seventy-two hours, but their activity need not be restricted to bed rest. Adults are requested to ambulate the day after operation; and may leave the hospital in five or six days, by which time the sutures are out, the alimentary tract is functioning normally and there is only a little residual discomfort in the operative area.

Occasionally, a patient will have difficulty in initiating voiding during the first twenty-four hours; catheterization may be necessary.

Children may return to school in ten days or two weeks but should avoid strenuous athletics for about a month. Adults should avoid strenuous exercise or hard labor for about six weeks.

The above plan may be applied to the care of patients after repair of other abdominal hernia except those in which the defect was very large, including those in which stainless steel or tantalum mesh was needed. Such patients may remain in bed for a few days, and should avoid strenuous activity for three months.

SUMMARY

An abdominal hernia is a protrusion of abdominal contents through a congenital or an acquired defect in the abdominal wall. The principles of repair include replacement of contents and closure of the defect.

VOCABULARY REVIEW

incarcerated   *strangulated*   *inguinal*
                              herniorrhaphy

SUGGESTED READING

1. Christopher, Frederick: Textbook of Surgery. 5th Ed. Philadelphia, W. B. Saunders Co., 1949, pp. 1191–1224.
2. Gatch, W. D., and Montgomery, W. F.: The Treatment of External Hernias Containing Gangrenous Bowel. J.A.M.A., *129:*736–739 (Nov. 10) 1945.
3. Watson, L. F.: Hernia. 3rd Ed. St. Louis, C. V. Mosby Co., 1947.
4. Cogswell, H. D., and Czerny, E. W.: Treatment of Hernias in Infants and Small Children. Am. Surgeon, *19:*87–90 (Jan.) 1953.
5. Hagan, William H., and Rhoads, Jonathan E.: Inguinal and Femoral Hernias: A Follow-up Study. Surg., Gynec. & Obst., *96:*226–232 (February) 1953.

Unit XII. NURSING IN SURGERY OF THE REPRODUCTIVE ORGANS

CHAPTER 47

Surgery of the
Male Genital Organs

The organs of reproduction in the male are the penis, the scrotum and its contents (testes and epididymes), the prostate gland, the seminal vesicles, and the connecting tubes (ducts) which provide passage for the spermatozoa in their journey from their point of origin in the testis to emission from the external penile opening (meatus).

The primary function of the penis is copulation; it is richly supplied with nerves and blood vessels, and is composed largely of erectile tissue. The penile urethra, an epithelial-lined tube, serves as the final pathway for both spermatozoa and urine. Emptying into the posterior portion of the urethra are the tiny ducts leading from the prostate and the seminal vesicles. The prostate secretes a glairy fluid which acts as a vehicle for the spermatozoa; the mixture of the two constitutes the semen. The lobes of the prostate gland lie around the urethra just at its junction with the

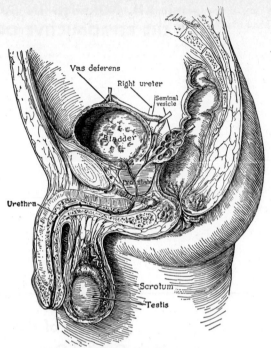

FIGURE 147. Male genital organs.

bladder. The seminal vesicles, one on each side, are located behind and beneath the bladder; these organs act as reservoirs for the spermatozoa, storing them until ejaculation occurs. The vas deferens is the duct which connects the seminal vesicle and testis; it courses laterally and interiorly from the base of the bladder to the inguinal ring, where it becomes incorporated into the spermatic cord, passing through the ring down into the scrotum to the epididymis and testis. The coiled tubules of the epididymis are a second reservoir for mature spermatozoa.

The testis (male gonad) contains the germinal epithelium from which the spermatozoa develop; in addition it contains cells which elaborate the male sex hormones (*androgens*). These hormones begin to appear in quantity at puberty and are responsible for the development of the secondary male sex characteristics, including the deepening of the voice, the growth of hair on the face and chest, the body contours, the awakening of a lively interest in the opposite sex, masculine aggressiveness, and the like. Mature spermatozoa also make their appearance at puberty and the individual becomes capable of reproduction. In the absence of disease or injury to these organs the reproductive power persists for many years; at a later and quite variable age the sex power wanes, and the testes atrophy. One functional testis is sufficient for reproduction, but the loss or maldevelopment of both testes results in the loss of the power; in addition, there is loss of the sex hormone with consequent effects, depending largely upon the age at which the loss occurs.

CONGENITAL AND ACQUIRED DEFORMITIES
Eunuchism

Either maldevelopment or the loss of both testes (*castration*) in infancy results in the development of a eunuch, a sexless man. Such a person has a soft skin, silky hair, no beard, a high-pitched voice, underdeveloped and functionless external genitalia, and lacks the masculine mental attributes. Castration after puberty has somewhat less effect; the reproductive power is lost, of course, but such secondary characteristics as may have already developed tend to remain. There is often, however, a profound psychologic effect upon the individual.

Hermaphrodism

Certain of the lower animals possess the necessary organs for functioning as both male and female, but no human being has ever been proved to be a complete hermaphrodite. At rare intervals, however, a human being has been found who has both a testis and an ovary. Pseudohermaphrodism is less rare; in this condition the person possesses the gonads of one sex but the external genitalia are abnormally developed and may present the appearance of the opposite sex. In such cases it is a not uncommon error to base the diagnosis of sex upon the appearance of the genitalia, an error which has often resulted in the rearing of the child as a member of the wrong sex; later the development of secondary sex characteristics may lead to correction of this error. The genitalia are usually underdeveloped, and operative search for a supposed undescended testis in an individual with a rudimentary penis may lead to the discovery of ovaries. The observation of serious abnormality of the external genitalia in a child should lead to surgical exploration so that the true sex may be determined; following this, plastic corrective procedures can be undertaken upon the genitalia which, although unlikely to restore full reproductive power, will aid greatly in the rehabilitation of the child and in the prevention of serious personality disorders.

Cryptorchidism

In the embryo the development of the testis is closely related to that of the kidney; later in fetal life the testis migrates from its position near the kidney, passing behind the peritoneal cavity to the inguinal ring, and finally descending into the scrotum where it is normally found at birth. In about 4 per cent of male infants, however, the descent of the testis is incomplete on one or both sides; the hidden testis may lie within the abdomen or in the inguinal canal. It was formerly thought that undescended testes would be functionless because of failure to descend, and various surgical procedures were undertaken to bring the testes down into the scrotum. The results of surgery were not invariably satisfactory. Indeed, if untreated, many undescended testes gradually come down just before or at puberty, and a large proportion can be made to descend by administering to the patient a course of injections of the proper hormone (either pituitary or placental gonadotropic hormones. It seems likely that the lack of testicular function in cryptorchidism is due to a deficiency of the proper hormonal stimulation, which is also responsible for the failure to descend, so that a mechanical descent brought about surgically does not of itself bring about testicular function.

Phimosis

In phimosis the foreskin (prepuce) is abnormally tight, so that proper retraction is difficult or impossible. It is a common deformity. Irritation from the resulting uncleanliness leads to infection of the glans (*balanitis*). Phimosis is cured by partial excision of the foreskin (*circumcision*), an operation frequently performed upon infants for prophylaxis or because of religious or tribal custom.

Hypospadias

Hypospadias is a rare deformity in which there is improper closure of the penile urethra, so that there is an opening in the urethra along the under surface of the penis. Delicate plastic surgery is necessary to close the urethra, or to construct a tube to bridge whatever gap may be present. As in any wound of the urethra, precautions are taken to keep the wound clean and dry; a small indwelling catheter is connected to a suction apparatus so that urine is drawn constantly from the bladder and given no opportunity to get into the wound. Sedatives are administered regularly during the first few days after operation in order to prevent the occurrence of erection of the penis, which would put severe tension on the fresh wound.

Chordee

As a result of congenital defect, injury, or disease, fibrous bands or scars may be present in the shaft of the penis, and these, being inelastic, cause a bending of the organ during erection. This deformity, called chordee, may be so severe as to make sexual union impossible. In many instances sufficient relaxation of the band or scar can be obtained by plastic procedures similar to those used elsewhere in the body for relaxation of scars.

Hydrocele

In its descent from the abdominal cavity the testis acquires a sheath of peritoneum. Abnormalities of this developmental process often pave the way for the occurrence of an inguinal hernia, and in other instances a small sac of peritoneum remains in the spermatic cord (the artery and veins of the testis and the vas deferens). Fluid accumulates in this anomalous peritoneal sac, and this is called hydrocele. The fluid-filled cavity varies in size from an almond up to an orange or larger. It is treated properly by surgical excision.

Varicocele

Because of the dependent position of the scrotum and its contents, there is a tendency of the veins of the spermatic cord to dilate and become varicose; this condition is called varicocele. The enlarged veins feel like a bag of worms, and cause a sensation of weight or aching pain. In less severe cases the symptoms are relieved by the wearing of an elastic supporter for the scrotum (suspensory), but sometimes partial excision of the varicose veins is necessary. This operation must be performed very carefully, for injudicious interference with the circulation of the testis results in atrophy. After this operation, as after the operation for hydrocele, an important feature of the care is the wearing of a suspensory until healing is complete, in order to prevent undue swelling and discomfort.

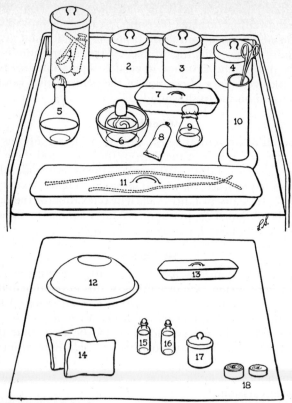

Figure 148. Catheterization set-up for the male patient; equipment is arranged on the upper and lower shelves of table on wheels.

1. Medicine glass, syringe, screw clamp
2. Sterile cotton balls
3. Sterile cotton balls in aqueous Zephiran 1:1000
4. Sterile urine culture tubes
5. Sterile water
6. Alcohol lamp
7. Instruments (sterile)
8. Sterile lubricant
9. Sterile mineral oil
10. Sponge stick in disinfectant solution
11. Sterile urethral catheters
12. Dressing basin
13. Spare instruments
14. Paper bags
15. Tincture of benzoin
16. Ether
17. Unsterile toothpick swabs
18. Adhesive tape, ½ and 1 inch

Nursing Care in Plastic Repair

In many instances the patient is a child who is anxious about his condition. He asks questions and needs a sympathetic and competent nurse to give him explanations in simple terms which

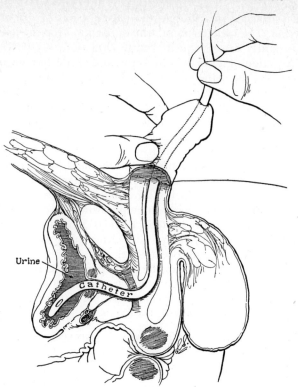

Urine

Catheter

FIGURE 149. Catheterization.

he can easily comprehend. When his questions are answered in a quiet, reassuring manner he will understand that there is no need to be ashamed or to fear ridicule.

Before operation for extensive plastic repair the area that is shaved includes the perineum and genitalia, from the suprapubic region half way down the inner side of the thighs and around the buttocks. The preoperative preparation is like that for general anesthesia.

The delicate plastic surgery used to repair the deformities requires great care. After operation the patient is gently moved from the stretcher to the bed to prevent injury to the wound and disarrangement of the dressings. Placing a bed cradle over the pelvis prevents discomfort from the pressure of the bedclothing. The indwelling catheter that is used to divert the urine from the wound is attached to a straight drainage apparatus with or without suction. The catheter must remain open to keep the operative area constantly dry. Frequent gentle irrigations of the catheter by the injection of a sterile solution with a sterile syringe are useful in keeping the catheter open. Each day the drainage tubing is replaced with clean sterile tubing. Aseptic technic is used because there is at times during the replacement a back-flow of urine which will be contaminated if the tubing is not sterile. Fluids are forced to keep the specific gravity of the urine low. A regular diet is usually well tolerated.

Young adult patients are troubled sometimes by erections after operation. The surgeon usually leaves an order for the nurse to apply an ice cap to the penis for twenty minutes, as required. He instructs the patient, without emphasizing the danger of erection, to call the nurse if he feels there is a beginning erection. In addition, the surgeon may order drugs such as bromides or stilbesterol to reduce the occurrence.

Conscientious adherence to the principles of cleanliness of the wound helps to prevent infection. Dressings are changed when necessary until the wound is healed, and the patient is instructed not to touch the dressings with his hands.

INJURIES OF THE MALE GENITALIA

Wounds of the external genitalia are not uncommon. Unless extensive loss of structure has taken place, genital wounds heal favorably because of the excellent blood supply. Contusion of the testis is a very painful injury, and there is usually gross swelling of the damaged organ. Excellent results follow conservative therapy, which includes rest in bed, the wearing of a suspensory, and the application of cold.

Extensive lacerations of the scrotum occur, usually as the result of catching the trouser and leg of the patient in the moving parts of a machine; the testes are commonly spared. If enough scrotal skin remains to cover the testes the wound can be closed; otherwise the testes must be implanted beneath the skin of the abdominal wall.

Traumatic castration is occasionally seen, especially among battle casualties; for such patients, treatment consists in hemostasis and, later, hormonal-replacement therapy.

Injuries to the internal structures, the vasa, the seminal vesicles, and the prostate, are rare except when incident to operation.

Perhaps the most difficult to treat of injuries to the genitalia is traumatic rupture of the urethra, a rather common complication of severe fractures of the pelvis. Rupture of the urethra may be followed immediately by the extravasation of urine and blood into the subcutaneous tissues of the abdomen and perineum; there may be, also, an external urinary fistula.

INFECTIONS OF THE MALE GENITALIA
Venereal Infections

The treatment of venereal disease in the male, especially gonorrhea, was once the province of the specialist in surgery of the genitourinary tract; this is no longer the case, for the spectacular results obtained by treating patients who have syphilis and gonorrhea with penicillin have made it possible for all physicians to cope with these diseases. It is only the occasional patient with neglected gonorrhea who may need the services of the specialist.

Infections of the Penis

Ulceration of the glans (*balanitis*) occurs when the tightness of the foreskin prevents retraction and cleanliness. The inflammatory process subsides and heals rapidly following division of the tight foreskin, or circumcision, and such local measures as moist heat and cleanliness. Specific lesions of the penis include the chancre of syphilis, the chancroidal ulcer caused by the bacillus of Ducrey, and gonorrheal urethritis. The treatment of these lesions depends upon their proper diagnosis, and is not surgical in any event.

Orchitis, Epididymitis

Inflammation of the testis and epididymis may be acute or chronic. Acute orchitis is caused by the gonococcus, and by the virus of mumps. If the disease is bilateral, sterility often results. Gonococcal orchitis is a complication of gonorrheal urethritis, and is treated with penicillin, rest in bed, and the wearing of a suspensory. There is no specific therapy for the orchitis of mumps. Chronic orchitis is usually a complication of syphilis, and is treated accordingly. Chronic epididymitis, on the other hand, is usually a feature of tuberculosis of the genital tract, which is treated by surgical removal of the affected portions of of the tract if a general survey of the patient does not show evidence of active tuberculosis elsewhere in his body.

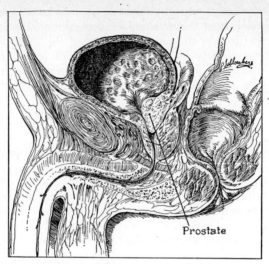

Prostate

FIGURE 150. Benign prostatic hypertrophy.

Vesiculitis, Prostatitis

The seminal vesicles and the prostate may be acutely inflamed as a complication of gonorrhea. After the acute phase has subsided there may remain a chronic infection, difficult to cure. The symptoms of chronic prostatitis are slight, the commonest being a persistent urethral discharge, small in amount. Examination of the prostatic fluid shows white blood cells and occasional bacteria. Chemotherapy and a course of prostatic massage (accomplished by pressure upon the prostate from a finger in the rectum) usually clear up this infection. The seminal vesicles also are occasionally involved in tuberculosis of the genital tract, and in some patients cure follows radical excision of the entire tract (epididymis, vas, and seminal vesicle).

NEOPLASTIC DISEASE OF THE MALE GENITALIA
Benign Prostatic Hypertrophy

This extremely common condition, which occurs in over one third of all men beyond the age of 50, owes its gravity to the location of the prostate gland. The exact cause of the hyperplastic enlargement which the prostate undergoes is not known, but it is probable that it is due to an endocrine disorder, perhaps a male counterpart of the female menopause. In any event, since the prostate is situated at the neck of the urinary bladder surrounding the upper urethra at its junction with the bladder, it is obvious that any significant enlargement of this gland causes obstruction to the outflow of urine. The symptoms of prostatic hypertrophy are frequency of urination, difficult in starting urination, nocturia, and, finally, complete retention of urine. Concomitant with this gradually progressive obstruction is a failure to empty the bladder completely so that there is an increasing amount of residual urine. The other usual complications of urinary obstruction also occur, including hydro-ureter and hydronephrosis, renal damage, urinary infection, and uremia. Diagnosis is established by palpation of the enlarged prostate upon digital rectal examination, and by visualization of the projecting lobes of the prostate as seen through the cystoscope.

PROSTATECTOMY

Surgical removal of the prostate (*prostatectomy*) results in the restoration of the ability to urinate normally. There are three methods of removing the prostate: suprapubic transvesical prostatectomy, perineal prostatectomy and transurethral resection by means of the electrocautery knife through a cytoscope (*resectoscope*). Each of these methods has its advantages and limitations.

Preoperative Care. This is of great importance, for these men as a group are poor surgical risks. Furthermore, it is unsafe to relieve the urinary obstruction suddenly, as renal hemorrhages and failure to secrete urine (*renal shutdown*) may result, with fatal consequence. Release of the urinary back pressure (*decompression*) is carried out gradually, either by means of an indwelling urethral catheter, or by a catheter introduced into the bladder through a suprapubic incision (*suprapubic cystotomy*), attached to a drainage apparatus which can be adjusted to various levels of pressure (Fig. 151). The duration of this period of decompressive drainage depends upon the particular condition and response of the patient, as judged by repeated estimations of his renal function (phenolsulphonephthalein excretion tests). The patient is judged ready for operation when renal function has made maximum improvement and the level of the blood urea has come down to normal. During this period fluids are forced, and antibiotic and chemotherapeutic agents are used to combat the infection of the urinary tract which nearly always complicates obstruction.

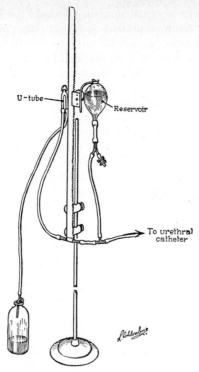

U-tube

Reservoir

To urethral
catheter

FIGURE 151. Decompression apparatus. The bladder is gradually emptied and
the intravesical pressure lowered as the reservoir and U tube are
lowered to the level of the bladder.

Before operation the shaving includes the abdominal, suprapubic and perineal regions. The immediate preoperative preparation is like that for any general or spinal anesthesia, depending
on which type the surgeon has chosen.

Suprapubic Prostatectomy. This operation is preferred by
many urologic surgeons for patients in whom the prostatic enlargement is considerable and projects mainly into the bladder.
General or spinal anesthesia is used. Through a low midline
abdominal incision the bladder is exposed without entering the
peritoneal cavity. The dome of the bladder is incised, bringing
into view the base of the bladder; the projecting lobes of the enlarged prostate are easily seen surrounding the vesical orifice
(outlet of the bladder). Another incision is made, this time
through the lining of the bladder into the capsule of the prostate,

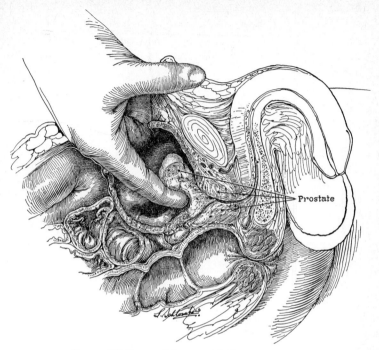

FIGURE 152. Suprapubic transvesical prostatectomy.

and the lobes are enucleated by the surgeon's finger, care being taken not to tear the urethra or the region of the vesical orifice. It is customary during enucleation for the operator to elevate and steady the prostate from below by a finger in the rectum. The prostatic cavity is packed with gauze to control bleeding, an indwelling (mushroom) catheter is placed in the bladder through the wound, and the bladder and abdominal wall are closed in layers by sutures.

On return of the patient to the ward the bladder catheter is immediately connected to an apparatus which exerts very mild suction (Connell apparatus) so that the urine is constantly removed, thus preventing distention of the bladder or extravasation of urine into the wound. The gauze packing is removed forty-eight hours after operation. On about the sixth day after operation an indwelling catheter is inserted and the suprapubic catheter removed, permitting the abdominal wound to heal; when the wound is healed the urethral catheter is removed.

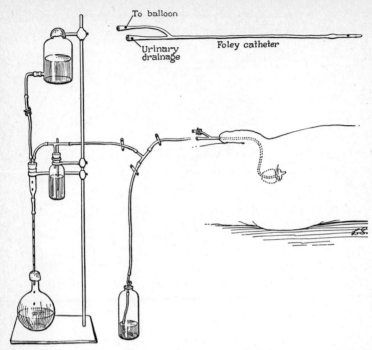

FIGURE 153. Connell suction apparatus. Inflation of the balloon of the Foley catheter prevents the catheter from slipping out of the bladder. The T tube must be secured in the position shown so that urine drops into the drainage bottle and is not drawn into the suction apparatus. The degree of suction is regulated by the rate of drip of of the oil; each drop traps and withdraws a small amount of air.

Perineal Prostatectomy. Division of the vas deferens (*vasectomy*) in the scrotum is often performed as a preliminary step to prostatectomy, for if the vas is not divided, bacteria may enter it as a result of the trauma incident to removal of the prostate; preliminary vasectomy thus prevents the occurrence of acute epididymitis, a painful and troublesome complication. This procedure is easily carried out under local anesthesia the day before prostatectomy.

For perineal prostectomy spinal anesthesia is satisfactory. The patient is placed in the lithotomy position, and an inverted U incision is made around the rectum. Dissection separates the rectum and urethra, and finally exposes the prostate, which is then removed. The perineal wound is sutured, a tube for drain-

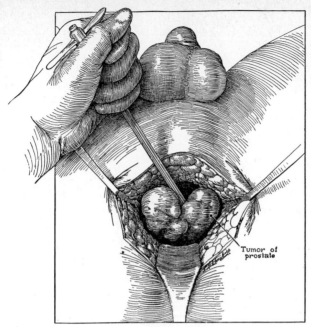

FIGURE 154. Perineal prostatectomy.

age being left in place; an indwelling urethral catheter is inserted for the purpose of keeping the bladder empty and the perineal wound dry.

On the patient's return to the ward the catheter is connected to the suction apparatus. The perineal tube is removed after two days; when the perineal wound is healed the urethral catheter is removed.

Transurethral Resection of the Prostate. For patients who have certain types of prostatic enlargement, notably moderate enlargement of the median lobe with intrusion into the urethra, resection by means of electrical cutting instruments through a modified cystoscope (*resectoscope*) furnishes a highly satisfactory method of treatment. This procedure is particularly useful in elderly, poor-risk patients; the abdominal or perineal wound is avoided, and the period of confinement to bed and hospital is shortened. The preliminary preparation for this operation is the same as for the other types of prostatectomy, with the exception of vasectomy which experience has shown to be unnecessary.

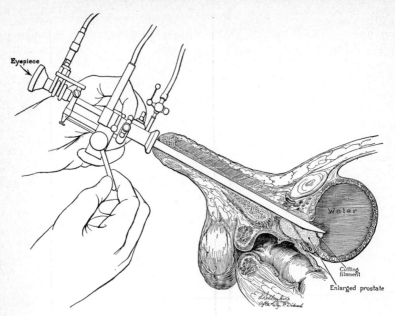

Eyepiece

Water

Cutting filament

Enlarged prostate

FIGURE 155. Transurethral prostatectomy.

Following resection the control of hemorrhage is the most urgent problem. Despite electrocoagulation during the procedure there is often troublesome and persistent bleeding. A Foley catheter, which has at its tip an inflatable rubber bag, is used for the dual purpose of draining the bladder and maintaining hemostatic pressure upon the prostatic wound. Irrigation with physiologic saline is often necessary to remove clots of blood which may obstruct drainage. The catheter is kept in the bladder until the urine is no longer bloodstained, usually three to five days.

A patient who has had a prostatectomy is subject to all the usual postoperative complications, in addition to the special hazards of hemorrhage into the bladder, urinary tract infection, and renal failure. Careful observation and measurement of the urinary output are essential, and frequent examination of the level of urea in the blood and tests of renal function must be made.

Postoperative Nursing Care. These elderly patients have usually been in the hospital for some time in preparation for the operation so that they are familiar with the routine of the ward.

After operation, however, they are apt to become quite confused, whether or not they were ever disoriented before. It is common for them to have the urge to get out of bed. If sideboards are put on the bed, serious injury may be averted.

Intravenous and subcutaneous fluids are given after operation, and when the patient is in a state of shock or has had a spinal anesthesia, the foot of the bed is usually elevated on shock blocks. Fluids are forced as soon as possible on the day of operation; a diet as tolerated is begun the second postoperative day. The catheter is connected either to straight drainage or to a suction apparatus. The drainage tubing must be sterile and is therefore replaced daily. Irrigations of the catheter are done occasionally by the surgeon but are done by the nurse only when the patient has had a transurethral resection. The surgeon changes the first dressing of the perineal wound; thereafter it is the responsibility of the nurse to change the dressings as often as is necessary to keep the patient dry. The dressings are held in place with a modified T binder.

In all perineal operations the incision passes very close to the rectum; if enema tubes or thermometers are passed into the rectum there is danger of puncturing the thin wall.

After operation the patient is sometimes depressed. He may be frightened and bewildered by the numerous procedures that are necessary. An explanation of procedures given before they are started helps him to overcome his feeling of insecurity. He should be encouraged to talk and to ask questions and must receive intelligent answers. When there are questions which the nurse feels she cannot answer the surgeon's help should be sought.

A gathering place, such as a sun porch, where ambulatory patients meet to talk and smoke, is valuable in raising morale. The patient will have more self-confidence when he sees that others in the same or later stages of treatment are able to accept their own situations with ease.

Carcinoma of the Prostate

Cancer of the prostate is of common occurrence among elderly men. If the neoplasm becomes large enough to obstruct the outflow of urine, the symptoms are the same as those of benign prostatic hypertrophy, and about 20 per cent of patients who have obstruction due to prostatic enlargement are found to have carcinoma of the prostate. Many prostatic cancers are extremely invasive, however, and often the presenting symptoms are the result of distant metastases of the prostatic tumor, to bone, brain, or elsewhere. The usual systemic manifestations of malignancy occur, including weight loss, weakness, loss of appetite, and anemia. On examination the prostate is found to be irregularly enlarged and stony hard in consistency. If the tumor has spread beyond the capsule of the gland the examiner can feel that it is fixed to the nearby structures, such as the rectum and base of the bladder. Diagnosis is confirmed by perineal exposure and biopsy of the tumor.

For patients in whom the cancer is thought to be confined within the capsule of the prostate a radical perineal prostatectomy is the proper treatment. When the cancer has spread beyond the capsule, the treatment consists in removal of enough of the tumor by resectoscope to ensure adequate relief of urinary obstruction; this is followed by the implantation of radium or radon tubes for a carefully measured period, in an effort to eradicate the remaining tumor.

It has been found that relief from the pain caused by the invasion of bone by prostatic cancer is obtained in many instances by castration, and that this procedure sometimes produces regression of the malignant process. This discovery, in addition to offering hope of relief to many suffering patients, sheds new light upon the important problem of the causes of neoplastic disease.

Tumors of the Testis

Testicular neoplasms are not common, but the majority of them are malignant and usually occur in young men. Since the tumors arise from the germinal epithelium, many of them are teratomas—neoplasms which contain various tissues and resemble an abortive attempt at the production of a new individual.

Painless enlargement of the testicle should lead to the immediate suspicion of neoplastic disease. Metastases occur early, and often the initial symptoms are due to distant extensions of the tumor. A positive diagnosis is made by biopsy and microscopic examination of the tissue; it is interesting, however, that in many patients having testicular tumors there is a large increase in the excretion of the gonadotropic hormone of the pituitary. This hormone is detected by the Aschheim-Zondek test, the same test used in determination of pregnancy.

Treatment consists in removal of the tumor and testis, the spermatic cord, and the associated lymph glands in the inguinal and retroperitoneal regions of the same side. If these glands have been invaded by the tumor the prognosis is poor. Radiation is to be used following operation.

SUMMARY

Except for injuries, most surgery of the male genital organs is concerned with congenital deformities in the young and neoplastic disease in the older patients. Both categories of patients need much reassurance and encouragement. Constant nursing attention to the management of urinary excretion is required, in addition to the therapy of the nearly always concomitant urinary tract infection.

VOCABULARY REVIEW

castration	*cryptorchidism*	*varicocele*
gonad	*phimosis*	*epididymitis*
androgen	*hypospadias*	*prostatectomy*
hermaphrodite	*hydrocele*	*transurethral*

SUGGESTED READING

1. Brendler, Herbert: Evaluation of Current Treatment of Prostatic Cancer. J. Urol., *68:*734–743 (Oct.) 1952.
2. Buckley, George, and Kearns, John W.: Analysis of Results of Prostate Surgery in 866 Cases. J. Urol., *68:*724–728 (Oct.) 1952.
3. Gross, Robert E., and Cresson, Samuel L.: Treatment of Epispadias: A Report of 18 Cases. J. Urol., *68:*477–488 (Aug.) 1952.
4. Hayes, Basil A.: Retropubic Prostatectomy, Surgical Treatment. Am. J. Nursing, *50:*435–437 (July) 1950.
5. Huggins, Charles: Endocrine Factors in Cancer. J. Urol., *68:*875–884 (Dec.) 1952.
6. Millsap, Juanita G.: Retropubic Prostatectomy, Nursing Care. Am. J. Nursing, *50:*437–438 (July) 1950.
7. Van Schoick, Mildred R., and Huggins, Charles: Carcinoma of the Prostate. Am. J. Nursing, *48:*427–429 (July) 1948.
8. Wright, Lucille, and Prince, Charles L.: Hypospadias, Nursing Care in the Surgical Repair. Am. J. Nursing, *46:*688–689 (Oct.) 1946.
9. Young, H. H.: Cure of Cancer of the Prostate by Radical Perineal Prostatectomy: History Literature and Statistics of Young's Operation. J. Urol., *53:*188–252 (Jan.) 1945.

CHAPTER 48

Gynecology: Introduction

ANATOMY AND PHYSIOLOGY OF THE FEMALE GENITAL TRACT
External Genitalia

The organs comprising the female external genitalia are known collectively as the vulva. These consist of the labia majora, labia minora, clitoris, hymen, vestibule, and Bartholin's glands. The external openings of the urethra and Skene's ducts, although strictly speaking not a part of the external genitalia, are closely related to them and are described with them.

Labia. The two labia majora make up the largest part of the external genitalia. Each is a rounded fold of fatty tissue covered on the outer surface with skin which in turn is covered with hair. The inner surfaces are smooth and composed of mucous membrane. In women who have not had children (nulliparae), the labia majora are in contact; after childbirth they remain separated. The two labia majora are connected posteriorly by a fold of skin, and anteriorly they merge with the larger skin-covered pad of fat lying over the pubic bones and known as the mons veneris.

The labia minora are two smaller folds of mucous membrane which lie within the labia majora. The anterior ends of these folds unite to form the prepuce of the clitoris. The posterior ends blend with the labia majora but are connected with each other by a fold of skin known as the fourchette.

Clitoris. The clitoris is a rudimentary organ corresponding to the penis in the male, situated at the anterior extremity of the labia minora. It is composed of erectile tissue containing numerous blood vessels. The body of the clitoris measures 2 to 3 centimeters in length.

Meatus. The urethral orifice, or meatus, is situated approximately 2 centimeters behind the clitoris. It is a circular opening measuring 4 to 5 millimeters in diameter and is lined with mucous membrane. It is important for the nurse to learn to recognize this opening since it is into the urethra that the catheter must be introduced when a patient is catheterized.

Hymen. The hymen is a circular fold surrounding the entrance to the vagina. In virgins the opening is usually circular and admits a fingertip although it may assume a variety of sizes and shapes. The hymen is generally ruptured at the first sexual intercourse; after childbirth all that remains is a few tags of mucous membrane called carunculae myrtiformes.

Bartholin's Glands. The vulvovaginal or Bartholin's glands are two in number and lie posteriorly on either side of the vagina, close to the outlet. These glands are important since they are frequently involved in gonorrheal infections which may lead to the formation of abscesses or cysts.

Urethra. The urethra is an elastic tube the function of which is to empty the bladder of urine. The average length is 3 to 4 centimeters and the normal caliber is approximately 4 millimeters. At the neck of the bladder the urethra is surrounded by the internal sphincter muscle which controls urination. Throughout its entire course it lies close to the anterior vaginal wall.

Perineum. The perineum is the region between the vagina and the rectum which forms the floor of the genital canal. The principal supporting structures in the perineum which may be injured during childbirth and which may need to be repaired subsequently are the levator ani muscles.

Internal Genitalia

Vagina. The vagina is a musculomembranous tube extending from the vulva to the uterus and connecting the internal and external genitalia. Normally, the vagina points upward and backward, making a right angle with the cervix. The vaginal mucous membrane is thrown up into a number of folds called rugae. Ordinarily the vagina is collapsed, with the anterior and posterior walls in contact except where separated by the cervix. The upper part of the vagina which surrounds the cervix is known as the vaginal vault. The vagina possesses great capacity for distention as is shown by its dilatation to permit the passage of the head of the fetus during childbirth. The urethra lies close in front of the anterior third of the vaginal wall and the bladder lies beneath its upper two-thirds. The posterior part of the vaginal vault (posterior fornix) lies in close proximity to a peritoneal pocket known as the cul-de-sac of Douglas. This relation is important since pelvic abscesses are often drained by opening this cul-de-sac. Lower down, the rectum lies just behind the posterior vaginal

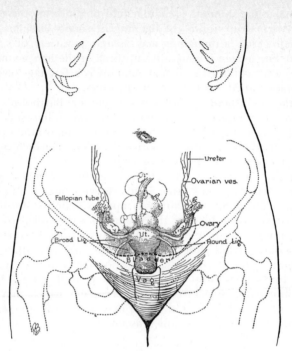

FIGURE 156. Female pelvic organs.

wall, while the lowest part of the vagina lies within the perineum and is closely related to the perineal muscles.

Uterus. The uterus is a hollow, thick-walled, pear-shaped organ composed of smooth muscle. The lower narrower portion is called the cervix and the upper broader portion is called the body or fundus. In a virgin the uterus averages 7½ cm. in length, 5 cm. in width and 2½ cm. in thickness, but after childbirth it is somewhat larger. Normally, the uterus leans anteriorly in the body with the fundus bent forward on the cervix. Its position varies in different individuals, and in the same individual with changes in position and with distention of the bladder. The lower part of the cervix extends into the vagina with the cervical canal opening at its center at the external os. The os is small and circular in nulliparae, whereas in women who have borne children it is usually slitlike. The cervical canal is continuous with the cavity of the body of the uterus; the junction of these two canals is known as the internal os. The length of the entire cavity from the external os to the top of the fundus ranges from 7 to 9 cm. The upper part of the upper uterine cavity is Y-shaped; the two arms of the Y pierce the uterine wall and communicate with the fallopian tubes.

The uterine wall consists of three layers: mucous membrane, which lines the cavity; smooth muscle, which makes up most of the wall; and peritoneum which covers most of the outer surface. Beneath the mucosa of the cervical canal are many branching glands which empty into the canal through small ducts and which secrete clear mucus. The mucous membrane which lines the uterine cavity and produces the menstrual flow is known as the endometrium. It is thicker than the cervical mucosa, measuring 2 to 5 mm. or more in thickness, and contains numerous glands which are simpler in structure than the cervical glands. The glands undergo a definite change during the menstrual cycle which is described more fully in the section on menstruation (p. 584).

Fallopian Tubes. The fallopian tubes are two muscular canals 10 to 12½ cm. long which are attached at their medial ends to the body of the uterus and are approximately the caliber of the average lead pencil in size. Their function is to conduct the egg or ovum from the ovaries to the uterus. The tubes are covered by peritoneum which extends upward from the broad ligaments to surround them and which, between the broad ligaments and the tubes, is known as the mesosalpinx.

Ovaries. The ovaries are two oval bodies about the size of almonds which lie on either side of the uterus on the posterior surface of the broad ligaments. Each ovary is attached along its anterior surface to the broad ligament by a fold of peritoneum and to the uterus by the utero-ovarian ligament. The outer poles of the ovaries are attached to the pelvic wall by two folds known as the infundibulopelvic ligaments, through which the ovarian blood vessels reach the ovaries. The ovary has a tough, white, wrinkled surface. Each consists of two parts, an inner medulla which contains numerous blood vessels, and an outer cortex. Although the function of the medulla is unknown, the cortex contains the secreting structures of the ovary, the graafian follicles.

In its earliest form each of these follicles is a very small, cystlike structure called the primordial follicle which contains an ovum. As the primordial follicle develops, it becomes larger, has a bigger cavity, and a thicker wall composed of granulosa cells. The ovum is situated in the wall of the graafian follicle, the cavity of which is filled with a fluid known as liquor folliculi, containing the estrogenic hormone. This hormone is secreted by the granulosa cells. During active reproductive life several follicles "ripen" each month but usually only one ruptures, permitting the ovum to escape; the remainder of the ripe follicles then degenerate and may become cystic. Such cysts, which never become very large, are known as atretic follicles. After ovulation the follicle which has ruptured becomes filled with a blood clot and is known as a corpus hemorrhagicum. The granulosa cells lining the graafian follicle now change their character and become larger and yellow in color giving a yellow color to the whole structure, which is known as a corpus luteum. Like the graafian follicle this is an organ of internal secretion which secretes, in addition to the estrogenic hormone, another hormone known as progesterone. If pregnancy occurs, the corpus luteum persists and is known as the corpus luteum of pregnancy. If the ovum does not become implanted, the corpus luteum degenerates rapidly, finally becoming a white scar known as a corpus ablicans.

The Menstrual Cycle. Menstruation is the cyclic bleeding from the endometrium or lining of the uterus. It begins at puberty and its function is to prepare the endometrium to receive and nourish the fertilized ovum or egg. In American girls menstruation usually begins between the ages of 11 and 16 years, although it is not unusual for it to begin at an earlier or later age. The average age in the United States is 13 years, whereas in the tropics it is considerably earlier, and in Europe a year or so later.

The menses ordinarily occur at intervals of three to five weeks and the usual duration of the flow is from two to five days. Although the interval between menses is popularly regarded as twenty-eight days, actually the cycle is generally somewhat irregular, and cycles of twenty-one or thirty-five days are not uncommon.

Menstruation does not usually continue during pregnancy, although it sometimes continues during the first few months. It generally ceases between the ages of 40 and 50 years, the cessation being known as the menopause, climacteric, or change of life, and coinciding with the cessation of ovulation.

In addition to the initiation and cessation of the menses, other very extensive changes occur in the body during puberty and the climacteric through the influence of the glands of internal secretion. Examples of these changes which occur at puberty are en-

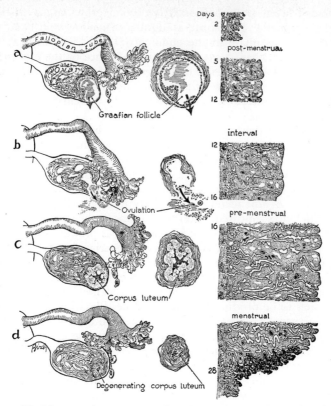

FIGURE 157. Diagram of menstrual cycle. The ovum matures (*a*), and is extruded from the follicle (*b*) (ovulation). The corpus luteum forms (*c*) and the endometrium (at right) is ready for the implantation of a fertilized ovum. In the absence of fertilization, however, the ovum does not become implanted, the corpus luteum degenerates (*d*) and menstruation occurs.

largement of the breasts and uterus and changes in the shape of the body and in the distribution of the hair.

To aid in understanding the menstrual cycle it is necessary to consider the glands of internal secretion which regulate the menses. During the menstrual cycle definite periodic changes take place in the endometrium. When menstruation occurs the superficial endometrial layer, including glands and stroma, sloughs off and is carried out of the uterus with the menstrual flow, leaving only the basal layer. At the end of menstruation the basal layer of the endometrium soon grows much thicker. At this stage the glands are straight and narrow and show no secretion. This phase in the endometrial cycle is known as the postmenstrual stage. Next, under the influence of the estrogenic hormone, which is secreted by the graafian follicles of the ovary, the glands become more dilated and tortuous, although as yet they show no secretion. This is known as the early interval or proliferative stage.

On or about the fourteenth day after the beginning of the last menstruation, one, and sometimes more than one, of the graafian follicles in one or both ovaries ruptures and the ovum or ova are expelled. Within a few hours after the rupture of the follicle, secretion appears in the linings of the endometrial glands. The appearance of this secretion is usually interpreted as a sign that the follicle has ruptured, and is important in the study of sterility since it is an index of ovarian activity. It is produced by the action on the endometrium of a second ovarian hormone, called progesterone, which is secreted by the corpus luteum. In addition to the production of secretion in the glands of the endometrium, progesterone, with the help of the estrogenic hormone, which continues to be produced, causes extreme dilatation and tortuosity in the endometrial glands. Progesterone does not act unless the endometrium has first been prepared by the estrogenic hormone. In the endometrial cycle this stage, from ovulation to the beginning of menstruation, is known as the secretory stage, and its latter portion, for about one week before menstruation, is called the premenstrual stage.

While these changes in the endometrium are occurring, the ovum descends through the fallopian tube. If the fertilized ovum does not become implanted in the endometrium, menstruation occurs. The onset of menstruation coincides with a fall in the level of the estrogenic hormone in the blood, and is thought to be initiated by suppression of the activity of the anterior lobe of the pituitary gland (*hypophysis*), although the exact mechanism is not understood.

The changes in the ovary which are responsible for the production of the estrogenic hormone and progesterone are in turn controlled by the secretions of the anterior lobe of the hypophysis. The first of these secretions, called follicle stimulating hormone (FSH), is responsible for the growth and maturation of the follicle. Under the influence of the second of these hypophyseal hormones, known as the luteinizing hormone (LH), the graafian follicle ruptures, ovulation occurs, and the corpus luteum is formed. A third hypophyseal hormone, LTH, stimulates the corpus luteum to secrete progesterone. It will thus be seen that not only the cyclic changes in the ovary but also the menstrual cycle are indirectly controlled by the hypophysis.

These five hormones (FSH, LH, LTH, estrogen and progesterone) occur in varying quantities in the female blood and urine depending on the age of the woman, the stage in the menstrual cycle when the specimens are obtained, and whether or not the woman is pregnant. One other hormone should be mentioned at this time. This is the chorionic gonadotropic hormone, also known as the anterior pituitary-like hormone (APL). Together with the estrogenic hormone this hormone occurs in large amounts in the urine of pregnant women. It is available commercially in concentrated form and has been used in the treatment of functional uterine bleeding. The Aschheim-Zondek, Friedman, and toad tests for pregnancy are based on the presence in the urine of the APL hormone.

Commercial preparations of most of these hormones are available under a confusing variety of trade names, and are in widespread use in treating symptoms caused or thought to be caused by endocrine imbalance in the female. Some of the preparations are effective when given by mouth but others must be injected into the tissues. In the treatment of menopausal symptoms such as nervousness and hot flushes by far the greatest success has been attained with the estrogenic hormone. This hormone has also been effective in curing gonorrheal vaginitis in children and senile vaginitis in women past the menopause. In both instances it acts by making the lining of the vagina thicker and more resistant to infection. Progesterone has been used successfully in threatened abortion, where it is supposed to relax the uterine muscle, and in certain types of prolonged vaginal bleeding due to a deficiency of this hormone. Other types of functional bleeding have been treated by combined therapy with estrogen and progesterone, with good results in some instances. In addition, sex hormone therapy has been recommended for a multitude of other conditions, often on dubious grounds and with extremely variable results.

PELVIC EXAMINATION

This is, at best, an unpleasant experience for the patient. Much can be done by the nurse to make the examination easier for both

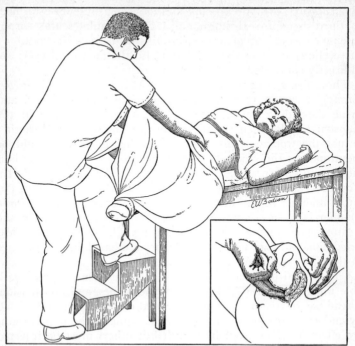

FIGURE 158. Bimanual pelvic examination. Insert shows palpation of uterus.

the patient and the doctor. A sympathetic and reassuring attitude on the nurse's part helps the patient greatly. In addition, proper physical preparation of the patient for examination is very important to the doctor and may mean the difference between a satisfactory and an unsatisfactory examination.

A nurse should always be present during a pelvic examination. In addition to proper preparation of the patient, the nurse should try to have everything ready before the arrival of the gynecologist so the examination will not have to be interrupted. She should further assist by handing the doctor instruments as needed, and by focusing the spotlight while the cervix is being examined.

Equipment. For a pelvic examination the nurse should prepare a tray or small table with the following equipment: good spotlight (if none is available, a flashlight may be used); liquid green soap or lubricating jelly; small gauze sponges; one long Kelly clamp; bivalve vaginal specula, medium and small sizes; cotton

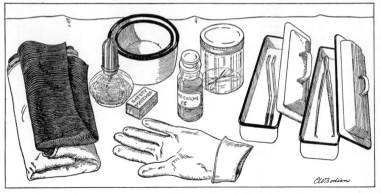

FIGURE 159. Catheterization tray for the female patient.

applicators; two rubber gloves. If a cervical culture is to be taken there should be added: sterile applicators; culture tube; two microscopic slides and cover plates; unsterile normal saline with eyedropper. Since more cervical biopsies are being taken today than ever before, a sterile biopsy forceps should always be included with the equipment.

Preparation of the Patient. The patient's bladder must be empty; therefore, if she is not to be catheterized, she should void before being draped for examination. Pelvic examinations are usually done with the patient in the lithotomy position (on the back, with thighs flexed and legs separated). Examination is most satisfactory if the patient can be placed on a regular examination table; however, if none is available or if she is a bed patient, she is prepared for examination in bed. If the patient is unable to help herself the nurse assists her to undress. All clothing is removed except shoes and stockings. Next, the patient is placed on the examining table with her hips at the edge of the table and her feet put into the stirrups. She is then draped with a sheet folded diagonally across the body with the opposite corners wrapped around her feet. If she is to be examined in bed, she is draped with the sheet in the same manner but the feet rest on the bed instead of in the stirrups; the knees are acutely flexed. The chest is covered with a towel. Occasionally, pelvic examinations are done with the patient in the knee-chest position. The Sims' or lateral position is seldom used at the present time.

Catheterization. In the female it is difficult to obtain a voided specimen of urine which does not contain a few pus cells, even

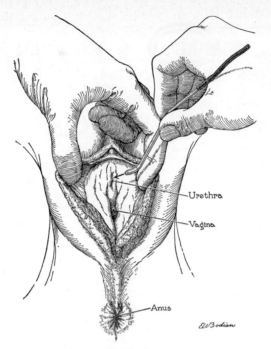

Urethra

Vagina

Anus

FIGURE 160. Catheterization.

though the genitalia were previously cleaned; therefore, many surgeons prefer a catheterized specimen of urine. Another reason for catheterization is inability of the patient to void; this condition is most frequently encountered following operation.

Technic. The equipment necessary to carry out catheterization is shown in Figure 159. After the patient has been draped as for a pelvic examination with dressing towel and rubber under the hips, the dressing towel used to cover the tray is spread out at the foot of the bed and the tray is placed upon it. The catheter and forceps basins and the two enamel bowls are arranged near the patient. The cover of the sterile forceps basin is taken off, and with the sterile forceps three toothpick swabs are removed from the sterile jar. These are placed upright in the sterile basin. The lid of the catheter basin and the top of the Zephiran bottle are removed. After the glove has been put on the left hand, the perineum is exposed and the labia are separated. When the meatus is located the urethral orifice is cleaned by wiping it with a dry toothpick swab in circular motion outward to remove excess mucus. The second toothpick swab is dipped into the Zephiran and inserted slightly into the urethral orifice and rotated carefully. The circular outward motion is continued in cleaning the area for at least 2 cm. in diameter. This procedure is repeated with the third toothpick swab as it was carried out with the second. While the left hand holds the labia steady to guard against contamination, the sterile catheter is picked up, with the right hand, at the junction of the rubber tubing and glass, and is inserted by following the curve of the urethra, first downward and then upward. The urine is drained into the bowl. The catheter should not be moved in any way after it has been inserted. When the bladder is empty the rubber tubing is pinched and the catheter is gently withdrawn. The nurse should examine the catheter carefully before it is sterilized and again before it is inserted. A rubber catheter should be used for children and for pregnant and unconscious patients.

SUMMARY

A knowledge of the anatomy and physiology of the female generative tract is the basis for understanding its disorders. The menstrual cycle and pregnancy are controlled by ovarian activity which, in turn, is directed by hormones secreted by the hypophysis. Routine gynecologic examination includes catheterization and bimanual pelvic examination.

VOCABULARY REVIEW

Bartholin's glands	*menopause*	*uterus*
fallopian tubes	*estrogen*	*cervix*
follicle	*vaginal speculum*	*endometrium*
corpus luteum	*meatus*	*ovary*

CHAPTER 49

Infections of the
Female Genital Tract

GONORRHEA

Gonorrhea is a venereal infection caused by the gonococcus, and is the commonest cause of inflammation of the female genital tract. The causative organism is a biscuit-shaped gram-negative diplococcus which may be identified in pus from patients with the disease by staining or by culture. In the Gram stained smear the gonococci appear as groups of red diplococci inside the pus cells. Since cultures are frequently positive for the gonococcus when smears are negative, cultures as well as smears are taken routinely in many clinics.

The structures in the lower female genital tract which are involved in gonorrheal infections are the urethra, cervix, Bartholin's glands, and Skene's glands. The first two are most commonly infected. The disease is practically always contracted by direct sexual contact although rarely it is acquired innocently. The symptoms appear after an incubation period of three to eight days. The first of these are burning on urination, sometimes associated with frequency, and a purulent yellow discharge from the urethra or cervix or both. If the urethra is infected, the urethral meatus appears reddened, and a drop of pus may sometimes be expressed from it. If the cervix is infected, its surface appears a fiery red upon examination through a speculum, and there is a profuse purulent discharge from the cervical canal.

In suspected cases of gonorrhea, smears and often cultures are made from both the urethra and the cervix. The vaginal mucosa is resistant to the gonococcus during reproductive life; gonorrheal inflammation of the vagina, or vaginitis, occurs only in children or in women past the menopause. The infection in the urethra in adults is usually short-lived and subsides spontaneously in a few days. However, if Skene's glands are involved, the infection there may persist for a long time and may require surgical intervention. Gonorrheal cervicitis is usually very persistent because the gonococci lodge in the depths of the cervical glands, and if untreated the cervical discharge usually continues for many months. After the infection has gone on for three or more weeks it becomes extremely difficult to demonstrate the gonococci even though the infection is still present. If one of Bartholin's glands is infected, it becomes swollen and painful and an abscess may develop. The infection in the gland sometimes becomes chronic, resulting in either a retention cyst or a chronically enlarged gland. Since Bartholin's glands are ordinarily not palpable, a palpable gland is presumptive proof of gonorrheal infection.

Sometimes, when chronic infection of the lower genital tract persists for a long time, warty growths appear on the vulva, in the vagina, or on the cervix. These are known as condylomata acuminata or venereal warts, although they are not always of venereal origin.

Complications

If the gonorrheal infection spreads upward to involve the fallopian tubes, inflammation of the tubes, or salpingitis, a serious complication, occurs. The gonococcus reaches the fallopian tube by way of the endometrium, which becomes temporarily inflamed, but the infection here does not last long. When a fallopian tube becomes infected, it becomes swollen and red, and the lumen is filled with pus. Such a tube may be transformed into a retort-shaped sac of pus of considerable size (*pyosalpinx*), or an abscess made up of both tube and ovary may form (*tubo-ovarian abscess*). Usually in acute salpingitis the pelvic peritoneum becomes inflamed (*pelvic peritonitis*), and in a few cases the peritonitis spreads to involve the entire peritoneum (*generalized peritonitis*). Sometimes an abscess forms in the pelvis outside the fallopian tubes (*pelvic abscess*). Such an abscess usually sinks into the cul-de-sac of Douglas and, if not drained surgically, may rupture into the bladder or rectum.

Patients with acute salpingitis usually appear moderately ill, and complain primarily of lower abdominal pain. If acute salpingitis is treated promptly and vigorously, it sometimes subsides completely, but more often the patient continues to complain of pain. The fallopian tubes usually have been so severely damaged that the lumina are obstructed and sterility results. Many patients continue to have a low grade infection of the fallopian tubes (chronic salpingitis), with persistent or recurrent lower abdominal pain. Eventually, this condition may require surgical removal of one or both fallopian tubes.

Treatment

Acute gonorrhea of the lower genital tract is always treated conservatively with the exception of abscess of Bartholin's glands, which must be drained. The therapy in use at present is a combination of chemotherapy and local therapy. Chemotherapy consists in treatment with one of the sulfa drugs or with penicillin given either intramuscularly or by mouth. In addition, hot douches (110–115° F.) of potassium permanganate 1 to 8000 or P.M.C. powder two or three times a day are usually given at very low pressures since there is danger of spreading the infection upward if high pressures are used. It is not necessary that such patients remain in bed, but violent exercise is to be avoided. Sexual intercourse and alcohol are forbidden. After cessation of treatment, patients with gonorrhea are followed closely by the doctor. At least three negative cervical and urethral smears or cultures must be obtained before the patient can be pronounced cured. Before discharging the.patient as cured, some gynecologists cauterize the cervix to destroy any gonococci which may be lurking in the cervical glands.

Patients with acute gonorrheal salpingitis or gonorrheal peritonitis are acutely ill and are kept in bed at home or preferably in the hospital. They are given the same chemotherapy and douches as patients with lower tract disease, and are kept in low Fowler's position, which tends to keep the infection localized in the pelvis. Care is taken to ensure an adequate fluid intake (2000 to 3000 cc. daily). Sedatives, such as 64 mg. codeine together with 0.6 gm. aspirin or 64 mg. Luminal every four hours are usually prescribed. An ice bag applied intermittently to the lower abdomen frequently gives relief from pain.

Partial isolation of acute gonorrheal cases is necessary, and the bedpan, urinal, towels and bed linen should be carefully isolated. Rubber gloves are worn by the nurse when giving a douche or similar treatments. All concerned must be very careful not to get any pus into the eyes, as the gonococcus causes severe ophthalmia. The best precaution is prompt and thorough hand-scrubbing after each contact with the patient.

Cauterization of the Cervix. This procedure is performed to eradicate chronic infection of the mucous glands of the cervix uteri. Since the cervix can be burned without pain, this operation

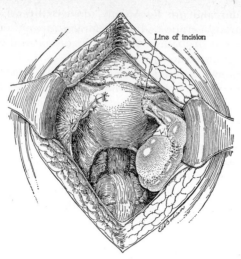

FIGURE 161. Bilateral salpingectomy for hydrosalpinx. The left ovary and tube have already been removed. Dotted line indicates incision for removing diseased right tube. The right ovary will not be removed.

may be done under either local or general anesthesia. If a general anesthetic is necessary, usually gas or sodium pentothal is used. A speculum is inserted and the vaginal mucosa protected from burns with damp sponges. The cervix is seized with a tenaculum and pulled down. The canal and the vaginal surface of the cervix are cauterized with the actual electric cautery, usually eight light, radial strokes like the spokes of a wheel being made.

A variation of this operation, conization of the cervix, has been introduced. In this operation a conical piece of cervical tissue is removed with the electrosurgical unit, a special electrode being used. Following cauterization, or conization, the patients need only such nursing care as is required following anesthesia.

Posterior Colpotomy with Drainage. A pelvic abscess frequently points behind the cervix in the cul-de-sac of Douglas. When this occurs, it is a simple process to drain the abscess through the vagina by making an opening into the cul-de-sac. Two cigarette drains or a long gauze pack is left in the abscess cavity with the ends protruding from the vagina.

Postoperatively these patients are kept in high Fowler's position to expedite drainage from the abscess cavity. Beginning on the third or fourth day after operation the drains are shortened a little each day and are completely removed by the seventh or eighth day after operation. After the drains are out, the patient is given douches or sitz baths. Sulfonamides or one of the antibiotics is generally given postoperatively.

Salpingectomy: Salpingo-oophorectomy. In cases of chronic salpingitis in which lower abdominal pain persists after a fair trial of conservative therapy, at least for several months, the diseased fallopian tube or tubes must sometimes be removed. Occasionally it is found at operation that there is such extensive involvement of the ovary that it, too, must be removed. In young women who have bilateral salpingitis every effort is made to save at least one ovary, because removal of both ovaries produces a surgical menopause. If both fallopian tubes must be removed, a hysterectomy is usually carried out at the same time. If the patient is near the menopausal age it is not so important that the ovaries be preserved. Such operations are usually done under general anesthesia. The nursing care is the same as for other laparotomies.

GONORRHEAL VULVOVAGINITIS

In girls below the age of puberty, gonorrhea runs a completely different course from that in the adult. In childhood the disease is usually acquired by sleeping with infected adults or other infected children, or from infected towels or washcloths. The type of gonorrhea which occurs in children is called gonorrheal vulvovaginitis, because the disease is usually limited to the vulva and vagina. Gonorrheal vulvovaginitis is highly contagious and often spreads through pediatric wards and orphanages. For this reason, strict isolation of infected children is imperative to prevent the spread of the disease.

The symptoms appear three to eight days after exposure. There is a purulent vaginal discharge, and on examination the vulva and vaginal orifice are seen to be reddened and covered with pus. Inspection of the vagina through a Kelly cystoscope shows a similar inflammation of the entire vaginal mucosa and of the surface of the cervix. The vaginal smear and culture are positive for gonococcus.

Treatment. As in adults, penicillin therapy is most successful, and has replaced other forms of therapy.

CERVICITIS

Chronic inflammation of the cervix commonly follows childbirth injury or gonorrheal cervicitis. Among the common manifestations of cervicitis are cervical erosions which appear as red, granular areas surrounding the external os. Actually most so-called lesions are not erosions or ulcers at all, but areas of inflammation, or eversions (turning out of the lining of the cervical canal on the surface of the cervix). Eversions of the cervix give rise to no symptoms unless inflammation is present. The symptom common to all types of inflammation of the cervix is a white vaginal discharge, leukorrhea, which varies considerably in quantity and appearance.

The treatment of erosions and eversions consists of douches, local applications of antiseptics, and cauterization or conization of the cervix. Many patients respond to douches of powder menthol compound or boric acid and alum powders, or some similar preparation, given twice a day. Cauterization of the cervix with silver nitrate or some similar drug is sometimes done. In cases which do not respond to douches, the leukorrhea usually clears up following cauterization with the actual cautery, or conization with the electrosurgical unit.

Lacerations of the cervix are usually the result of childbirth. They may be either unilateral or bilateral, or stellate (star-shaped). Lacerations not immediately repaired after childbirth, in healing leave one or more clefts in the cervix. Usually they are complicated by chronic infection and give rise to leukorrhea. The original treatment of severe chronic cervicitis following childbirth was amputation or operative repair of the cervix. Since the introduction of cauterization by Hunner it has been found that in most cases this procedure clears up the cervicitis and the leukorrhea, making amputation unnecessary. Amputation should not be done during active sexual life since abortion or difficult labor often follows.

PUERPERAL AND POSTABORTAL INFECTIONS

The majority of these infections are due to the streptococcus, although they are sometimes caused by other organisms. All of them have one thing in common, that is, they generally produce cellulitis, an inflammatory reaction characterized by brawny thickening of the soft tissues of the pelvis. Such infections sometimes follow instrumentation such as curettage of the uterus in nonpregnant women; they are rather common following radiation for pelvic cancer. Acute puerperal infections are seldom seen by the gynecologist, but in their later states they come within the realm of gynecology.

Postabortal infections are among the most serious the gynecologist must treat. Most of them follow attempted criminal abortions, in the course of which virulent bacteria are introduced into the uterine cavity. Sometimes such infections follow spontaneous, and occasionally therapeutic, abortions. They may involve the endometrium only, or may extend into and through the uterine wall and into the broad ligaments, in which case the infection is much more serious. The infection spreads, not along the uterine and tubal mucosa as in the case of gonorrhea, but through the veins and lymphatics of the uterine wall and broad ligaments where a thrombophlebitis and lymphangitis are produced. The thrombophlebitis may spread into the femoral vein, causing *phlegmasia alba dolens* (milk leg). If the fallopian tubes are infected, the infection attacks them from without by way of the broad ligaments. The tubal mucosa is affected last, if at all, and for this reason, if the patient recovers, she is less likely to be sterile than if she had had gonococcal salpingitis. Abscesses of the broad ligaments and pelvic or generalized peritonitis may complicate the picture, particularly if instrumental perforation of the uterus has occurred. Infection of the blood stream is common.

Patients with postabortal infections usually appear quite ill, with high fever and, if there is a blood stream infection, chills. There is generally vaginal bleeding or foul-smelling vaginal discharge. If there has been much loss of blood, the patient is probably very anemic. On examination there is usually tenderness and sometimes there are signs of peritonitis over the lower or even the entire abdomen.

Treatment. These patients should be hospitalized and require careful, constant nursing. They are kept in high Fowler's position to prevent the infection from spreading and to improve the drainage from the uterus. An ice bag applied intermittently to the lower abdomen helps to make the patient comfortable. Sedatives such as codeine and aspirin or codeine and Luminal are required. The sulfonamides and antibiotics are given separately or together. It is important that the patient have sufficient fluids, and an intake of 2000 to 3000 cc. a day should be assured; a record of the intake and output is kept. If the patient is vomiting or is unable to take fluids by mouth, intravenous fluids are given. If the patient is anemic, transfusions are necessary until the hemoglobin has reached a satisfactory level. Enemas and strong cathartics sometimes stir up the pelvic infection and should not be given unless absolutely necessary; mild laxatives such as mineral oil or cascara are preferable. If femoral thrombophlebitis is present, the leg is elevated and heparin or Dicumarol therapy is usually started. Under no circumstances is such a leg massaged. Hot gallon douches are usually started ten days or more after abortion or delivery.

Acute puerperal and postabortal infections are, with an occasional exception, always treated conservatively, but subacute or chronic infections may require operation. This is true of abscess of the broad ligaments which persists after several weeks of therapy. Such an abscess is drained by making a low McBurney incision and placing cigarette drains close to the abscess without opening the peritoneum.

In patients who have salpingitis complicating postabortal or puerperal infections and who continue to complain of lower abdominal or pelvic pain after long courses of conservative treatment, removal of the inflamed fallopian tubes may be necessary. The technic and nursing care for this operation are the same as for gonorrheal salpingitis (p. 594).

TUBERCULOSIS OF THE GENITALIA

This is nearly always a local manifestation of a generalized tuberculous infection, with the primary infection located elsewhere in the body. Pelvic tuberculosis may affect the cervix, the endometrium, the fallopian tubes, or the ovaries. Usually the primary lesion lies in the lung or the intestinal tract, with the tubercle bacillus reaching the pelvis by way of the blood stream. Endometritis occurs in about three fourths of the cases of pelvic tuberculosis and salpingitis in almost every case. Tuberculosis is the cause of 5 per cent of all cases of salpingitis. In one third of the cases of pelvic tuberculosis the ovaries as well as the tubes are involved. Tuberculosis of the cervix is rare.

The fallopian tubes may be infected as the result of a generalized tuberculous peritonitis, but more often the tubercle bacilli are carried to the fallopian tubes through the blood stream from a distant focus. Tuberculous peritonitis may be secondary to, as well as the cause of, the salpingitis. Peritonitis is of two forms, the dry form in which the intestines are matted together by dense adhesions, and the wet form in which the abdomen is distended with clear yellow fluid. Genital tuberculosis is notoriously hard to diagnose unless the patient has obvious tuberculosis elsewhere.

Treatment. When tuberculosis of the cervix, the endometrium or the fallopian tubes is proved by pathologic examination, the uterus, tubes, and ovaries are removed if possible. Streptomycin and para-aminosalicylic acid are given after operation.

Nursing Care. In general the nursing care is the same as for patients after other laparotomies. In addition the general supportive care ordered for tuberculous patients, including high caloric diet and rest in bed for a period of several months, is given. It is usually advisable to transfer the patients when convalescent to a tuberculosis sanatorium for further care.

GRANULOMA INGUINALE

This venereal disease is caused by a nonmotile, gram-negative, encapsulated bacillus. The disease is more common in Negroes and is fairly widespread in the southern United States.

The disease is essentially a superficial progressive ulceration of the vulvo-inguinal region which may also involve the lower abdomen and buttocks. The ulcerated areas are covered with red granulation tissue and there is usually considerable purulent discharge. The disease may cause extreme enlargement or elephantiasis of the vulva. The lesions heal with the formation of scar tissue. The disease usually runs a chronic course of many months' or years' duration.

Treatment. Except when elephantiasis is present, the treatment of this disease is medical and consists in intravenous injections of tartar emetic (antimony and potassium tartrate). In advanced cases of elephantiasis, excision of the vulva (*vulvectomy*) must sometimes be done. This condition is not highly infectious and the patient need not be isolated.

LYMPHOGRANULOMA VENEREUM

This venereal disease is most common in the Negro, occurring only occasionally in the white race. It is caused by a filtrable virus and is primarily a chronic infection of the lymphatics, characteristically causing inguinal adenitis in men and rectal stricture in women. Indolent ulcers of the vulva and vagina frequently occur, and there is usually scar tissue at the borders of the ulcers. The ulceration may destroy the urethra in part or entirely, resulting in urethral stricture in the former case and urinary incontinence in the latter. If the lymphatics of the vulva become involved, a chronic lymphedema, producing great enlargement or elephantiasis of the vulva, may result. Inguinal adenitis occurs in women as well as in men, and the inguinal glands may suppurate; such suppurating glands are known as buboes. The disease usually runs a chronic course and tends to burn itself out after a number of years.

The diagnosis is made by the appearance of the lesions and by means of an intradermal test, the Frei test.

Treatment. Treatment in the early stages has been more satisfactory since aureomycin therapy has been introduced. Should the glands suppurate, the buboes are either incised and drained, or the pus is aspirated repeatedly with a syringe and needle, until the adenitis subsides. The surgical treatment of rectal stricture is discussed in Chapter 28, page 324. If elephantiasis of the vulva is extensive, a vulvectomy may be required. Urinary incontinence is treated by transplanting a loop of fascia from the sheath of the rectus abdominis muscle around the urethra.

SPECIAL NURSING PROCEDURES IN PELVIC INFLAMMATORY DISEASE
Douches

Solutions. Those commonly used include: potassium permanganate 1:8000; P.M.C. (powder menthol compound); salt and soda; and boric acid and alum. For cleaning purposes and as routine treatment the solution is 105° F. When a hot gallon douche is ordered (usually for pelvic inflammation) the temperature is from 110 to 115° F.

Equipment. This consists of: irrigation stand or tree; irrigator (rubber bag, enamel can or glass reservoir) with rubber tubing (approximately 36 inches long) with clamp attached; douche nozzle, sterile (sometimes after plastic vaginal operations the surgeon will order the douche given with a rubber catheter); douche pan or bedpan; small rubber sheet and towel; leggings or sheet; two finger cots or a rubber glove.

For convenience the equipment is collected on a tray and inspected for secure fastenings and intact nozzle. Sometimes the surgeon orders a sterile douche; otherwise, it is sufficient to have the equipment clean and only the nozzle sterile. The equipment is brought to the bedside and the irrigation pole put into position at the foot of the bed.

Preparation of the Patient. The patient's cooperation will be increased if she understands the treatment. The sheet is used to cover the patient; the bedcovers are fan-folded to the foot of the bed. For an effective douche the patient should be flat on her back with only one pillow under her head, knees bent, and the soles of her feet planted firmly on the mattress. She is draped as

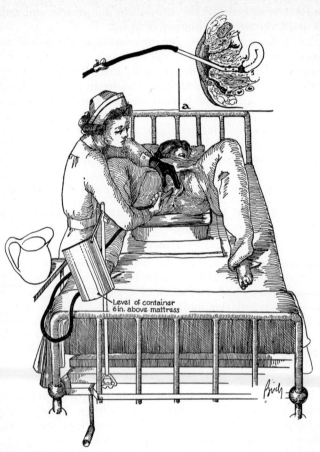

Level of container
6in. above mattress

FIGURE 162. Technic for administering a douche (vaginal irrigation).

for a pelvic examination, with the sheet laid diagonally across her and the corners wrapped around her feet. The small rubber sheet, covered with a towel, is placed under the buttocks to protect the bed. The patient will be more comfortable if a folded treatment towel is placed on the rear edge of the douche pan before it is put under her.

Technic. After another inspection for cracks and rough edges, the nozzle is attached to the tubing without contaminating it. The finger cots are used on the thumb and forefinger of the left hand and these fingers used to separate the labia. Air is expelled from the tubing by allowing some of the solution to run through it. Then the tubing is clamped off and the nozzle gently inserted into the vagina for about 2 inches; an upward and backward motion is used. The clamp is released and the solution allowed to flow slowly. The irrigator should be not higher than 18 inches above the bed. At the conclusion of the douche the nozzle is removed, disconnected, and placed in a basin. The patient is left on the pan for a few minutes to allow all of the fluid to drain out of the vagina.

After-Care. If the patient has had a perineal operation the perineum is carefully dried with sterile cotton pledgets and a sterile perineal pad is applied. After the patient has been made comfortable the equipment is removed, washed and boiled. Charting of the treatment includes time, solution, solution strength, amount, character of return flow, and the patient's reaction should she have one.

SUMMARY

Venereal disease, tuberculosis and criminal abortions cause most of the infections of the female genital tract. As in other infections, treatment is directed at supplementing nature's own defenses. Antibiotic and chemotherapeutic agents are extremely valuable. Surgical procedures are reserved for complications.

VOCABULARY REVIEW

gonorrhea	*vulvovaginitis*	*lymphogranuloma*
colpotomy	*cervicitis*	*cauterization*
salpingectomy	*douche*	

SUGGESTED READING

1. Bundesen, H. N., Plotke, F., and Eisenberg, H.: Psychosomatic Approach to Venereal Disease Control; Chronic Gonorrhea Repeaters. Am. J. Pub. Health, *39:*1535–1540 (Dec.) 1949.
2. Buxton, C. L.: Treatment of Leukoplakia and Kraurosis Vulvae. Geriatrics, *5:*142–146 (May-June) 1950.
3. Hirst, Donald V.: Dangers of Improper Vaginal Douching. Am. J. Obst. & Gynec., *64:*179–183 (July) 1952.
4. Smiley, William L., and Bozeman, Wilfred: Uterine Bleeding in Pelvic Inflammatory Disease. Am. J. Obst. & Gynec., *64:*197–199 (July) 1952.
5. Stokes, John Hinchman, and Taylor, Jane Barbara: Dermatology and Venereology for Nurses. Philadelphia, W. B. Saunders Co., 1948.
6. TeLinde, Richard W.: Operative Gynecology. 2nd Ed. Philadelphia, J. B. Lippincott Co., 1953.
7. Wharton, Lawrence R.: Gynecology Including Female Urology. Philadelphia, W. B. Saunders Co., 1943.

CHAPTER 50

Congenital Deformities;
Sterility; Disorders Due to Pregnancy

CONGENITAL DEFORMITIES

In embryonic life the fallopian tubes, uterus, cervix uteri and upper vagina are formed from the müllerian ducts, two tubular structures which normally join to form a single canal, the uterovaginal canal. This becomes the uterus and upper vagina. The lower part of the vagina is formed by an infolding of the surface of the body of the embryo, which dips in to meet the uterovaginal canal.

Deformities of the Vagina and Hymen

Absence. Congenital absence of the vagina is usually associated with absence or rudimentary development of the uterus and fallopian tubes. Women having this anomaly never menstruate, of course, but the condition is otherwise asymptomatic.

If such a patient wishes to lead a normal sex life, an artificial vagina must be made. This is done by making an opening in the skin at the site of the normal vaginal outlet and lining it with mucous membrane. One method of providing mucous membrane is to bring down a loop of isolated small intestine so that the intestinal mucosa lines the vagina. Another method is to line the artificial vagina with flaps of mucous membrane from the labia. In this case a sterile mold, the size of the desired vagina, is left in place until healing occurs. A modification of this method is to make an artificial cavity, insert the mold, and let the epithelium grow in from the surface to form a lining. In the method most recently described the patient herself makes pressure with a special glass rod against the perineum daily until a vagina of the proper size is formed.

The care of a patient who has had an artificial vagina made is the same as for other vaginal cases. A retention catheter is usually left in the bladder and care must be taken to see that it is draining properly. Care must also be taken lest the mold slip out of place. It is removed approximately two weeks after operation, when the patient is instructed to wear it until the vagina heals completely.

Imperforate Hymen. This is a rare congenital anomaly which results from the failure of the upper and lower parts of the vagina to become connected in fetal life. Usually this abnormality is not noticed until puberty, when external vaginal bleeding fails to occur. The menstrual flow is dammed back and accumulates in the vagina; this is called *hematocolpos*. When the accumulation occurs in the uterine cavity the condition is termed *hematometra* and when in the fallopian tubes, *hematosalpinx*. In hematocolpos the retained blood causes the hymen to bulge outward. The treatment is incision of the hymen and drainage of the accumulated blood.

Double Vagina. A double vagina results from failure of the septum between the vaginal portion of the müllerian ducts to disappear. It is often associated with double cervix and uterus and usually does not require surgical treatment.

Deformities of the Uterus

These anomalies are the result of various degrees of failure of the upper müllerian ducts to fuse. There are several such anomalies including *didelphic uterus* (double uterus and double cervix), *bicornuate uterus* (upper uterus divided into two lateral horns), and *septate uterus* (uterine cavity divided by a longitudinal septum).

These anomalies generally do not require surgical treatment unless they are complicated by pregnancy or produce repeated abortion. If pregnancy occurs in one horn of a bicornuate uterus, normal delivery is impossible and the patient has symptoms like those of a tubal pregnancy. The treatment consists of excision of the pregnant horn. The nursing care is the same as for other patients with pelvic laparotomies.

STERILITY

Failure to conceive may be due to either male or female disability. In the female, obstruction of the fallopian tubes, most often caused by inflammation of the tubes, is the commonest cause of sterility. Obstruction of the cervical canal, either congenital or acquired, retroposition of the uterus, and tumors of the body of the uterus are also causes.

Ovulation occurs about fourteen days after the beginning of the previous menstrual period; the fertile period extends approximately from the twelfth to the sixteenth day of the cycle. It is important that patients understand the span of this fertile period since the other days of the cycle are relatively sterile. It has been shown by Hartman that a few patients sometimes menstruate without ovulating; such patients, of course, are sterile while this condition exists. Other endocrine disturbances, such as hypothyroidism and functional amenorrhea, may also cause sterility.

Examinations. The couple with sterility must be carefully studied according to plan. First the wife is examined to rule out obvious pelvic disease. Next the husband's semen is examined either directly or by the Huhner test. This consists in examination of material from the wife's vagina or cervical canal shortly after intercourse. It should show many motile spermatozoa. If the examination of the husband is satisfactory, a Rubin's test is done on the wife to determine whether the fallopian tubes are patent. This may be done in the doctor's office, but should be carried out with the patient under anesthesia in the hospital if it is thought wise to dilate the cervix at the same time. It is desirable to do a Rubin's test in the second half of the menstrual cycle, so that a biopsy of the endometrium may be performed at the same time, to rule out anovulatory menstruation; absence of secretion in endometrial glands is evidence of this condition. If the patient has retroposition of the uterus, a Smith-Hodge pessary may be inserted to hold the uterus in position. A basal metabolic rate determination to rule out hypothyroidism should be carried out on all patients who complain of sterility. In patients with sterility who need abdominal surgery for some other condition a retrograde Rubin test may be done. Salpingography (x-ray examination of the fallopian tubes after injection of Lipiodol or other opaque medium) is a useful procedure.

Rubin's Test. This test can be carried out in the office without anesthesia, or in the hospital with the patient under anesthesia. After routine clean-up, with the patient in the lithotomy position, the insufflation apparatus is first tested for leaks. The cervix is then seized with a tenaculum and the cannula of the insufflation apparatus inserted into the cervical canal with the rubber nipple against the cervix. The vagina is filled with sterile water to detect improper escape of air back around the cannula and the gas is allowed to run slowly into the tubing. The rate of flow of the gas is estimated by the number of bubbles which pass through the cylinder. The pressure of the gas is noted on the

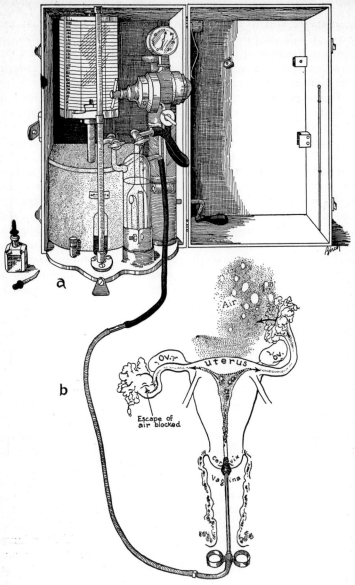

a

b

Air.

ov.

uterus

ov.

Escape of
air blocked

cervix

Vagina

FIGURE 163. Rubin's test (tubal insufflation). The apparatus measures and records the pressure of the air which is pumped into the uterus. If one or both tubes are patent the air pressure does not continue to rise, as the air escapes into the peritoneal cavity.

manometer and is allowed to increase up to 200 mm. of mercury. A fall in pressure indicates patent fallopian tubes. An assistant listens over the abdomen with a stethoscope, and a bubbling or whistling sound confirms the fact that gas is entering the peritoneal cavity.

Treatment. A number of procedures are helpful in treating sterility. If a Rubin's test is unsatisfactory on first attempt it is worth while to repeat it several times, as sometimes a later test is successful. If the basal metabolic rate is low, thyroid extract is given. Rest, and vitamins C and E are sometimes helpful in treating both the sterile husband and wife. If there is cervical stenosis, the cervix should be dilated. If the patient has an anovulatory cycle, pregnant mare's serum (gonadotropin) may be given intravenously when ovulation is due and may cause ovulation in some cases. Plastic operations on the fallopian tubes by the abdominal route in women in whom the fallopian tubes are obstructed lead to pregnancy in a small number of cases (approximately 5 per cent). The results are so poor that these operations are seldom done except in patients who need abdominal operation for some other condition.

RELAXATION AND MALPOSITION OF THE FEMALE GENITALIA

Relaxed Vaginal Outlet

Many women who have had one or more children have relaxation of the vaginal outlet. If the bladder protrudes into the vagina, the condition is known as *cystocele*. If the floor of the urethra also protrudes into the vagina, the condition is known as *urethrocele*. Patients with cystocele and urethrocele may have no symptoms, but many complain of a severe bearing-down sensation in the vagina and a feeling "as if everything were about to drop out." Because of stretching of the floor of the urethra many of these women have partial urinary incontinence when they laugh, cough, or sneeze. When the fascia of the posterior vaginal wall is broken down by childbirth, a herniation of the rectum into the vagina results. This is known as *rectocele*. Some patients with rectocele are asymptomatic; others complain of a bearing-down sensation and many of them are constipated.

Treatment. Patients with relaxation of the vaginal outlet with or without cystocele and rectocele need no treatment if they are

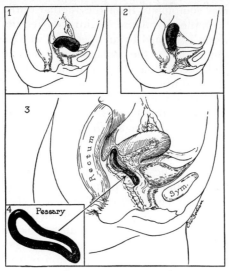

FIGURE 164. *1,* Anteflexion; *2,* retroposition; *3,* uterus held in normal position by pessary; *4,* Smith-Hodge pessary.

asymptomatic; however, the symptoms are often so severe that they are incapacitated and something must be done to correct the condition. If a cystocele exists, it is repaired by means of an operation known as an anterior colporrhaphy. In this operation the bladder is pushed back into place from below and the fascia of the anterior vaginal wall is reconstructed, so that the bladder cannot again prolapse into the vagina. If the patient has relaxation of the vaginal outlet with a rectocele, it is repaired by replacing the rectum and reconstructing the fascia of the posterior vaginal wall. In the course of this operation the separated levator ani muscles are sewed together again so as to reconstruct the perineum.

Uterine Displacements

Prolapse. In association with the relaxed outlet, many women have displacement of the uterus downward into the vagina. This is the result of stretching of the ligaments of the uterus during pregnancy and childbirth, and the condition is known as descensus or prolapse of the uterus. It is spoken of as partial or complete, depending on how far down the uterus comes. If the uterus protrudes completely from the vaginal outlet, the condition is called complete prolapse or third degree descensus. Prolapse of the uterus is treated by an operation which is performed through the vagina, but if the prolapsed uterus is abnormal it is removed through the vagina (vaginal hysterectomy).

Anteflexion. In addition to descensus of the uterus, there are a number of other abnormal positions which the uterus may assume. Sometimes the fundus of the uterus is bent forward on the cervix at a very acute angle; this condition is a congenital abnormality. Patients having acute anteflexion may be asymptomatic but many of them suffer from severe dysmenorrhea, which is treated by dilating the cervical canal under anesthesia. This procedure usually relieves the patient's symptoms temporarily. Anteflexion is usually cured by childbirth.

Retroposition. In about 20 per cent of women the uterus is displaced backward. Retroposition of the uterus may be congenital or may be the result of stretching of the uterine ligaments during pregnancy. Many patients with retroposition of the uterus have no symptoms; in such cases no treatment is necessary. Some, however, complain of severe backache which is worse when they are on their feet. Many also complain of severe dysmenorrhea. In addition, in some instances, retroposition of the uterus is thought to be responsible for sterility.

Treatment. Patients who have severe symptoms are treated, when possible, by manipulation and replacement of the uterus during pelvic examination. The uterus is then held in place by inserting a Smith-Hodge pessary into the vagina. The patient who wears a pessary must take a daily douche and the pessary must be changed at intervals of two months, to prevent irritation of the vaginal wall. The Smith-Hodge pessary is used chiefly as a therapeutic test to determine whether the patient's symptoms will be relieved by replacement of the uterus. Such a test should always be made before a suspension operation is done.

There are several different operations designed to suspend a uterus which is in retroposition and most of them are based on some procedure which shortens the round ligaments. The most commonly performed operation is the modified Gilliam suspension in which the round ligaments are sutured to the fascia of the rectus abdominis muscles, a procedure which is generally successful in correcting retroposition. The nursing care following this operation is the same as for other gynecologic laparotomies.

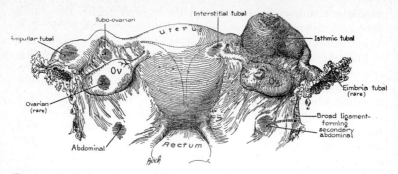

FIGURE 165. Various sites in which extra-uterine pregnancies have occurred. A tubal pregnancy which has just ruptured is shown on the right side.

Fistulas

Vesicovaginal Fistula; Rectovaginal Fistula. Sometimes during childbirth, in the course of a pelvic operation, or following radiation therapy for pelvic disease, the bladder or rectum is injured so that a communication between one of these organs and the vagina results. Such an opening is known as a vesicovaginal or a rectovaginal fistula, and is accompanied by leakage of urine or feces into the vagina.

Treatment. Cure of these fistulas is accomplished by procedures designed to close the opening into the bladder or rectum and cover it with normal vaginal wall. After operation an indwelling catheter is placed in the bladder in order to keep the bladder empty and the wound dry. The nursing care is the same as after vaginal operations. The catheter must be kept open and draining at all times since blocking of the catheter may result in recurrence of the fistula.

EXTRA-UTERINE PREGNANCY

Occasionally a fertilized ovum becomes implanted in the ovary or fallopian tube instead of in the uterus as normally occurs. Such an abnormal pregnancy is known as an ectopic or extrauterine pregnancy, and is caused by an obstruction to the passage of the fertilized ovum through the fallopian tube. As the fertilized ovum grows and enlarges in the fallopian tube, the thin tubal wall becomes tightly stretched. One of two things happens: the wall of the fallopian tube ruptures into the abdominal cavity, or the embryo is extruded into the lumen of the tube and out through the fimbriated end. This latter is known as a tubal abortion, and either rupture or tubal abortion is accompanied by a severe hemorrhage into the peritoneal cavity.

The typical history of a woman with extra-uterine pregnancy is as follows: she misses a menstrual period and perhaps thinks she is pregnant. Several days or weeks later she notices vaginal bleeding which is usually not very profuse. This is followed by a sudden severe pain in the lower abdomen, after which the patient frequently faints. The severe pain and fainting are caused by the sudden hemorrhage into the peritoneal cavity as the tubal pregnancy ruptures or aborts.

Tubal pregnancy is difficult to diagnose before rupture occurs. The diagnosis of tubal pregnancy is always considered when a patient who has missed a period complains of pain in the abdomen. The discovery of a soft mass on one side of the uterus makes the diagnosis more certain. In doubtful cases the diagnosis can often be made by means of culdoscopy. The culdoscope is an instrument resembling a cystoscope; it is introduced through the vagina, behind the cervix, into the peritoneal cavity. The pelvic organs can usually be clearly visualized. Ectopic pregnancy is easy to diagnose after rupture, when the patient presents the typical picture of posthemorrhagic shock. In addition, the abdomen is extremely tender because of the blood in the peritoneal cavity and the umbilicus may be blue in color from the same cause.

Treatment. Ectopic pregnancy is a surgical emergency since the patient may die from hemorrhage if she is not treated promptly. A woman with an ectopic pregnancy which has not ruptured should be operated on before rupture occurs. When a patient with a ruptured ectopic pregnancy reaches the hospital, she is treated first for shock. As soon as she has been given a transfusion and her condition has improved enough to risk surgery, a laparotomy is done and the involved fallopian tube removed. Sometimes the ovary on the same side is damaged and must also be taken out. The nursing care following operation is the same as for other laparotomies.

SUMMARY

The repair of congenital deformities of the female generative tract and the repair of injuries to it resulting from childbirth constitute a large part of gynecology. The rupture of an extra-uterine pregnancy is serious and requires emergency operation.

VOCABULARY REVIEW

hematocolpos   cystocele   ectopic pregnancy
sterility   rectocele   pessary
tubal insufflation colporrhaphy   prolapse
                    vesicovaginal fistula

SUGGESTED READING

1. Brady, Leo, Kurtz, Ethna L., and McLaughlin, Eileen: Essentials of Gynecology. 2nd Ed. New York, The Macmillan Co., 1950.
2. Pisani, Bernard J.: Management of Ectopic Pregnancy with Massive Intraperitoneal Hemorrhage and Shock. Surg., Gynec. & Obst., *95*:149–154 (Aug.) 1952.
3. Longley, Jay R., and Greene, Laurence F.: Urologic Procedures Employed in the Diagnosis of Urinary-Vaginal Fistulas. Surg., Gynec. & Obst., *94*:709–711 (June) 1952.
4. Miller, Norman, and Hyde, Betty: Gynecology and Gynecological Nursing. 2nd Ed. Philadelphia, W. B. Saunders Co., 1949.
5. Wharton, L. R.: Treatment of Certain Congenital Malformations of the Female Genito-Urinary Organs; Resume of Recent Progress. Obst. & Gynec. Surv., *2*:365–374 (June) 1947.

CHAPTER 51

Neoplastic Disease of the Female Genital Tract

BENIGN TUMORS OF THE VULVA

The commonest benign tumors of the vulva are fibromas (connective tissue tumors) and lipomas (fatty tumors). They are treated by excision, which is a simple procedure.

Leukoplakia; Kraurosis Vulvae. Leukoplakia is a disease of the vulva in which the skin becomes thickened and white. Kraurosis vulvae is a shrinking of the subcutaneous tissues which frequently accompanies leukoplakia. Leukoplakia is usually seen in women past the menopause, but sometimes occurs in younger women and is important because it frequently progresses into cancer of the vulva. In leukoplakia the whole vulva may appear shrunken and distorted; the skin is white and shiny and may show cracks. The symptoms are intense itching and burning of the vulva, which are a heavy tax on the nervous system.

Treatment. Mild cases are treated conservatively with soothing ointments, thyroid, estrogenic hormone, vitamin A, x-ray therapy, or subcutaneous injection of the vulva with alcohol. Severe cases are treated surgically by excision of the vulva.

CARCINOMA OF THE VULVA

Cancer of the vulva is a relatively common disease which, in most cases, arises from the squamous epithelium with which the vulva is covered. It is primarily a disease of older women; in about 50 per cent of patients it is preceded by leukoplakia of the vulva. The disease appears first as an ulcer on the vulva which increases in size and assumes a cauliflower-like appearance. It metastasizes early to the inguinal lymph glands. The symptoms are itching and burning of the vulva, although the disease may be asymptomatic in the early stages.

Treatment. If the disease is not too extensive, the treatment is excision of the vulva combined with excision of the inguinal and femoral lymph glands on both sides. This is often followed by deep x-ray therapy. If the disease is too extensive for operation, it is treated with deep x-ray therapy, which may sometimes be combined with radium therapy.

Vulvectomy

General anesthesia is used. Vulvectomy is best done with the electrosurgical cautery since the vulva is highly vascular and bleeds profusely. A circular incision is made at the vaginal orifice and another at the lateral borders of the vulva and the whole vulva is excised. The excision of the inguinal lymph glands is sometimes done at the time of the vulvectomy, and sometimes two weeks later. In this operation an incision is made over the inguinal ligament on each side and the superficial inguinal lymph glands are excised. Then the inguinal ligaments are divided and the deep lymph glands resected.

Nursing Care. The patient usually returns from the operating room with sterile dressings over the vulva as well as over the inguinal regions, and with a retention catheter in the bladder. The catheter should be immediately connected to the straight drainage tubing, and the urinary output charted at regular intervals. The patient is kept flat in bed to prevent pressure on the suture line. When the dressings become soiled, usually on the second or third day, they are removed and a cradle is placed over the patient. If a light cradle is used, the temperature is kept low to prevent burns. Warm perineal irrigations, usually of 1 to 8000 potassium permanganate, are started when the dressings are removed and are given three times daily and as required. About the tenth postoperative day the retention catheter is removed. Some separation of the posterior part of the incision usually takes place but is followed by healing. On the tenth postoperative day the patient is usually gotten out of bed; sitz baths are begun at this time.

BENIGN TUMORS OF THE CERVIX

The only common benign tumor of the cervix is the cervical polyp. This tumor appears as a bright red, round, oval or elongated body which presents at or protrudes from the external os. It usually arises from the lining of the cervical canal rather than the vaginal surface of the cervix. Most cervical polyps are benign, although cancer arises in a polyp occasionally, and early cancer may have a polypoid appearance. The symptoms of cervical polyp are intermenstrual bleeding, which is usually not profuse but is recurrent, and leukorrhea. The latter is due to infection in the cervix or in the polyp.

All cervical polyps should be removed and examined under the microscope to rule out evidence of cancer. Unless the polyp has a broad pedicle or the patient is very nervous, the polyp may be removed in the dispensary or office by clamping it and twisting it off.

MYOMATA UTERI

These tumors, which arise almost exclusively in the body of the uterus, are fibromyomata, that is to say, composed of both smooth muscle and connective tissue. They are usually spoken of as fibroids, and are by far the commonest tumor of the uterus. Their cause is unknown, although there is evidence to indicate that the estrogenic hormone may be a factor in their formation.

Although most myomas are relatively small when encountered, they may attain enormous size. In Cullen's famous case the tumor itself weighed 86 pounds and the patient weighed only 84 pounds after the operation. Myomas are usually spheroid or oval in shape and tend to be multiple. Some are pedunculated and are connected to the uterine wall by a thin pedicle which contains their blood supply. Pedunculated tumors may become attached to an

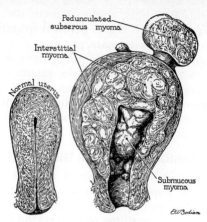

FIGURE 166. Myoma of the uterus.

adjacent organ such as the omentum or intestine from which they receive part of their blood supply. Such myomas are said to be parasitic. Because of insufficient blood supply myomas sometimes become necrotic or cystic. Calcification may occur. Malignant degeneration is discussed in the section on sarcoma of the uterus (p. 623). A closely allied tumor, the adenomyoma, is discussed in the section on endometriosis.

Myomas are frequently asymptomatic, particularly if small. The most important symptom is vaginal bleeding which usually takes the form of prolonged, profuse menstrual flow. The bleeding may be so profuse as to produce a serious anemia. It is unusual for bleeding from myomas to occur after the menopause, when these tumors usually regress. Another group of symptoms such as a bearing-down sensation in the pelvis and frequency of urination are the result of the pressure of the tumor on the surrounding organs. Pressure on the rectum may cause constipation. Fibroid tumors are frequently the cause of sterility and often cause abortion. If large tumors are located in the lower part of the uterus, they may interfere with the birth of the child if pregnancy does occur. Diagnosis is usually not difficult. An enlarged, hard, multinodular uterus is pathognomonic of myomata uteri. Occasionally fibroids cause a soft, symmetrical enlargement of the uterus that is difficult to differentiate from pregnancy. In this case a pregnancy test usually settles the diagnosis. Small submucous fibroids frequently bleed profusely but cannot be felt on

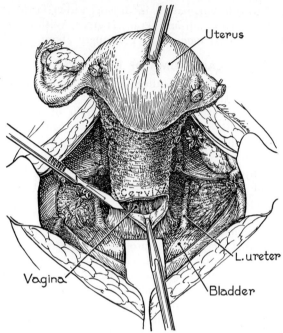

FIGURE 167. Total hysterectomy. The left ovary and tube will not be removed; the stumps of the uterine ligaments and the edges of the peritoneum will be sutured over the suture line which closed the opening in the upper vagina.

pelvic examination. Such tumors can, however, be felt with the curette when the uterine cavity is curetted.

Treatment. The treatment of myomata uteri depends largely upon the age of the patient and the symptoms. Small asymptomatic tumors require no treatment, but the patient should be examined at regular intervals to determine the rate of growth of the tumor. Fibroids usually stop growing and may even decrease in size after the menopause. Tumors which are symptomatic are usually removed together with the uterus (*hysteromyomectomy*). Removal of the myoma alone (*myomectomy*) is sometimes done in patients having only a few tumors who wish to have children. Women near the menopause who have small symptomatic fibroids are sometimes treated with radiation rather than operation, particularly if they are poor operative risks. This treatment is given only after a dilation and curettage has been done to rule out malignant disease. Either deep x-ray therapy or intra-uterine radium therapy is given. With either type of therapy an artificial menopause is brought about.

CARCINOMA OF THE CERVIX

With the exception of cancer of the breast, cancer of the cervix is the commonest malignant tumor in women. Although carcinoma of the cervix is usually thought of as a disease of older women, this is not strictly true. It is not uncommon in women below the age of 35, but the majority of cases occur between the ages of 35 and 50 years. Most gynecologists believe that childbirth injuries to the cervix are a predisposing factor. In 95 per cent of the cases, cancer of the cervix arises from the squamous epithelium covering the cervix. Five per cent are adenocarcinomas which arise from the cervical glands. Carcinoma of the cervix may begin either on the surface or within the cervical canal. Later, either a progressive ulcer or a protruding, fungating tumor appears. In this later stage secondary infection of the tumor with pyogenic bacteria usually occurs and produces a foul-smelling discharge. The disease spreads to the vaginal mucous membrane or to one or both broad ligaments by way of the lymphatics. Later, the tumor may metastasize to the adjacent lymph nodes, or to the vulva, bladder, or rectum. Cases are classified by a standard clinical nomenclature according to the extent of the disease: stage zero, the earliest stage, is that in which the cancer is limited to the cervical epithelium; stage one is that in which the disease is confined to the cervix; stages two, three and four represent progressively more extensive lesions.

Symptoms. The commonest symptom of cancer of the cervix is intermenstrual or postmenopausal bleeding, or leukorrhea, which in the later stages is profuse and foul-smelling. In the early stages bleeding is usually slight, but later extensive hemorrhages may occur. Intermenstrual or postmenopausal bleeding is a danger signal which should always be investigated immediately. In 50 per cent of the cases, postmenopausal bleeding is caused by malignant disease. The diagnosis of cancer of the cervix must always be confirmed by biopsy before treatment is begun. Abnormal bleeding is always an indication for curettage of the uterine cavity and cervical canal, for a hidden cancer may be present even though the cervix appears normal.

Treatment. The standard treatment of cancer of the cervix is irradiation. For suitable, carefully selected patients, however, a radical operation (*panhysterectomy*) achieves good results. Attempts are being made, in addition, to find out if patients with late, widespread disease can be helped by very radical surgical procedures such as pelvic exenteration. In these extensive operations, the entire contents of the pelvis, including the genital organs, bladder, and rectum are removed; the patient is given a permanent colostomy, which is also the route of urinary excretion because the ureters must be transplanted from the bladder into the colon.

Radiation therapy, as used in most clinics, consists of a combination of deep x-ray and radium therapy. The average percentage of the five-year survivals of all patients treated with radiation therapy is 35 per cent. The majority of patients do not seek treatment until the disease is already far advanced (stages three and four); the percentage of cures would be much higher if treatment could be begun in the earlier stages. Therefore, an extensive campaign has been conducted designed to educate the public, so that people with cancer will seek treatment while the disease is still in an early stage.

Radical Panhysterectomy for Carcinoma. General anesthesia is used. This operation is performed through a low midline incision. It differs from the usual conservative panhysterectomy in that as much as possible of the para-uterine tissues, including the pelvic lymph nodes, is removed, together with the entire uterus and both tubes and ovaries. The pelvis is sometimes drained with a vaginal cigarette drain at the end of the operation.

NURSING CARE FOLLOWING RADICAL PANHYSTERECTOMY. Psychologic and emotional factors are important in the care of the patient anticipating hysterectomy. Before admission to the hospital the patient has had an explanation concerning the operation, but many women hesitate to ask the male physician intimate questions. The nurse should try to establish rapport by taking an active interest in the patient to encourage the latter to voice her apprehensions. It is to be expected that a young woman who has not borne children may be very depressed. The mother who already has her family is less concerned about the loss of the uterus and its functions. However, many women have heard tales about the effects of hysterectomy which are likely to cause anxiety unless corrected. Some of the ideas which are common include gaining weight, loss of libido and inability to be a satisfactory mate. Sometimes the patient even has difficulty in accepting the fact that she may never menstruate again. Another reason for emotional distress is the fear of persistent cancer.

The manner of preparing for hysterectomy is the same as that for laparotomy. Postoperatively, the care is also similar to that given to patients with abdominal surgery. Special nursing care is directed toward the prevention of urinary retention. Frequently, there is unavoidable trauma to the bladder which results in loss of muscle tone. Some surgeons instill 1 ounce of 0.5 per cent aqueous mercurochrome into the bladder following the operation. This causes slight irritation to the mucosa, stimulating a desire to void before the bladder becomes distended with urine.

The methods previously described should be used to initiate voiding. It is important that these be started soon after operation for when the bladder is permitted to become distended, the patient becomes increasingly uncomfortable and less able to void. If the patient cannot void, then she must be catheterized. Whenever the patient complains of discomfort, her complaint should be respected and she should be catheterized until she is able to void voluntarily. If the patient voids less than 100 cc. at a time during the first eight hours after operation, she should be catheterized; this should be repeated until she can void larger amounts. Voidings of 100 cc. or more of urine usually signify that the patient has control of bladder function. This is a fairly safe rule but is not always correct. The nurse should examine the patient's abdomen and heed her complaints for, at times, there may be quite a large amount of urine in the bladder. The nurse should make frequent observations when intravenous fluids are given, especially when glucose is given because of its stimulating action upon the kidneys.

Following operation, the preclimacteric patient who has undergone removal of both ovaries will experience "hot flashes." These may occur as early as the fourth or fifth postoperative day. The symptoms of surgical menopause vary but are often more severe than those accompanying normal menopause. "Flashes of heat" are sometimes frequent and hot flushes are troublesome because of sweating which may occur at the time. Other symptoms most commonly manifested are palpitation of the heart, irritability, and frequent attacks of wakefulness. The doctor may order the administration of estrogenic substances which lessens the symptoms. These are not ordered when the patient has cancer because

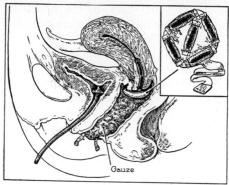

FIGURE 168. Carcinoma of the cervix of the uterus being treated with radium. One radium tube is in the cervical canal, and a pack of tubes, as shown in the insert, is fastened against the surface of the cervix. The bladder is kept empty to prevent a burn, and the gauze packing in the vagina serves to hold back the bladder, vaginal walls, and rectum as much as possible, also to prevent radium burns.

of danger of making the malignancies grow more rapidly. Some doctors prescribe mild sedatives which permit adequate rest and also tend to reduce the symptoms. Some surgeons implant pellets of estrogenic substances into the rectus muscles to control the menopausal syndrome. These may last up to fifteen months, preventing the necessity for intramuscular injection or oral administration of estrogens.

In all cases, the nurse must stress follow-up care. The time for checkup varies with surgeons; the patient should understand when she is to return to her doctor.

Radiation Therapy. In treating carcinoma of the cervix, one or more radium treatments may be given. The radium is usually inserted with the patient under general anesthesia. After dilation of the cervix, a rubber or metal tube containing the radium capsules is inserted into the cervical canal. It is usually fastened in place with a linen or silk suture. If radium is to be applied to the surface of the cervix at the same time, a metal or cloth plaque containing the capsule is placed against the surface of the cervix and is held in place with a gauze vaginal pack. The whole vagina is then packed to prevent the radium from burning the vaginal wall. Lastly, a mushroom catheter is placed in the bladder to keep it collapsed and out of the way of the radium. The patient is then returned to the ward until it is time to remove the radium, when she is taken back to the operating room. The duration of radiation depends on the quantity of radium applied and the total dosage desired.

When the patient returns from the operating room with the radium in place, the retention catheter is connected with the straight drainage tube and the urinary output is measured every three or four hours. Should the catheter fail to drain, the doctor must be notified at once since a full bladder may lead to a radium burn. The patient is kept as quiet as possible in bed to prevent the radium from becoming dislodged. Since radium is expensive, bedpans and bed linen must be carefully examined for radium containers or gauze packs when they are removed. Should a radium applicator be discovered, it should never be touched with the fingers, but always handled with a long instrument. Its discovery must be reported at once. It is advisable for these patients to be kept as far as possible from other patients while the radium is in place. Profuse vaginal bleeding or high fever may occur during treatment and should be reported. Antibiotic therapy is administered routinely while the radium is in place. Sedation is given as needed. Otherwise these patients receive routine care.

CARCINOMA OF THE BODY OF THE UTERUS

In contradistinction to cancer of the cervix, most cases of cancer of the body of the uterus occur after the menopause. A few cases occur at an earlier age, the youngest in the Johns Hopkins series being 28 years old. The ratio of frequency of carcinoma of the body of the uterus to carcinoma of the cervix is one to eight.

Cancer of the body of the uterus is an adenocarcinoma which arises from the endometrial glands. As the tumor grows, it spreads over the endometrium and invades the uterus which, in time, it may perforate. As the tumor increases in size, the body of the uterus enlarges. The tumor sometimes spreads to the fallopian tubes, or to the surfaces of the ovaries, or to the nearby peritoneum. Metastases to the lymph nodes around the bifurcation of the aorta occur late. Metastases to distant organs are found at autopsy in one third of the cases.

Symptoms and Diagnosis. The cardinal symptom of carcinoma of the body of the uterus is abnormal vaginal bleeding. Since most cases occur after the menopause, every case of postmenopausal bleeding must be presumed to be due to carcinoma until proved otherwise. On examination the uterus may feel perfectly normal in early cancer, whereas in more advanced cases the uterus may be enlarged or irregular. In any case, diagnosis must be confirmed by microscopic examination of the uterine curettings.

Treatment. Experience has shown that the best treatment for cancer of the body of the uterus is a combination of radiation and panhysterectomy with removal of both fallopian tubes and ovaries. In treating such a patient, it is customary first to give either intrauterine radium therapy or a course of deep x-ray therapy, and to operate four to six weeks after completion of the radiation. The technic of applying radium to the uterine cavity is somewhat similar to that for treating the cervix. A different applicator is used and the radium is applied to the whole length of the uterine cavity. The nursing care is the same. Postoperative care following panhysterectomy is the same as after other laparotomies. The vaginal cigarette drain if used is removed on the third or fourth postoperative day.

SARCOMA OF THE UTERUS

This is a rare malignant tumor arising in the uterine muscle. Most sarcomas arise in benign myomas and the remainder directly from the uterine muscle. A hard, nodular uterine tumor which bleeds or grows rapidly after the menopause is always suggestive of sarcoma, and should be immediately removed by panhysterectomy. If the pathologic studies of a supposed benign tumor reveal sarcoma, deep x-ray therapy is usually given after operation. The nursing care is the same as for any laparotomy.

OVARIAN CYSTS

Graafian Follicle Cysts. There are many different types of ovarian cysts. The simplest is the graafian follicle cyst, which arises from a follicle which has failed to rupture but, instead, has degenerated and become enlarged. The fluid which fills such a cyst is secreted by the granulosa cells lining it, and is rich in the estrogenic hormone. Sometimes there are many such cysts, causing the ovary to be somewhat enlarged. Such cystic ovaries are often associated with endometrial hyperplasia and with functional uterine bleeding.

Corpus Luteum Cysts, and Hematomas. Another type of cyst which is associated with the graafian follicle is the corpus luteum cyst. The corpus luteum is always cystic, but sometimes the cavity at the center is abnormally large, so that the ovary is increased in size. Such a structure is known as a corpus luteum cyst if it is filled with clear fluid. If it is filled with blood, as sometimes occurs, it is spoken of as a corpus luteum hematoma. These are often associated with pain or with menstrual irregularities, and such cases may be difficult to differentiate from appendicitis or ectopic pregnancy.

Serous Cysts. A type of larger ovarian cyst has a single cavity and is filled with clear fluid; this is the simple serous cyst.

Cystadenomas. These are a group of more complicated tumors which at times attain large size. These may have one or more separate cavities; tumors with several cavities are spoken of as multilocular. Cystadenomas may have a smooth lining but sometimes the lining is covered with many small projecting nodules; such tumors are spoken of as papillary. If they contain a thin watery fluid, they are described as serous; if the fluid is gelatinous, they are called pseudomucinous cystadenomas. In the serous type in particular the papillary structures at times spread to the neighboring abdominal organs, and the abdomen may become filled with fluid; these complications sometimes subside when the ovarian tumor is removed by the surgeon.

Dermoid Cysts. These tumors contain many different tissues having separate origins, which eventuate in such varied structures as hair, glands, teeth, and bone. Dermoids are really separate individuals growing inside the ovary, and are thought to arise early in embryonic life. Dermoid cysts seldom become larger than grapefruit, and are usually benign. Teratomas are related tumors which also contain many different tissues; however, these are always solid tumors, and are nearly always malignant.

OVARIAN CARCINOMA

Cancer of the ovary originates directly from the normal epithelial tissues of the ovary, or from a previously existing benign ovarian tumor. It may also be a metastasis from a cancer of the gastrointestinal tract, in which case it is spoken of as a Krukenberg tumor. Secondary carcinoma of the ovary may also originate in the uterus or fallopian tube. Fifteen per cent of all ovarian tumors are malignant. Grossly they are either solid or cystic; the cystic tumors usually contain much papillary material. These tumors spread most commonly to the neighboring organs by way of the peritoneum, and large quantities of fluid may accumulate in the peritoneal cavity. In cases where the carcinoma is inoperable, the fluid may need to be drained off (*paracentesis*) at frequent intervals. More than five barrels of fluid were removed from one such patient over a period of several years.

Fibromas. A word may be said about ovarian tumors which arise from connective tissue. These are called fibromas. They are solid tumors which sometimes become fairly large, and are commonly associated with ascites, and sometimes with hydrothorax. Malignant tumors of connective tissue origin are rare.

Granulosa Cell Tumor; Arrhenoblastoma. The granulosa cell tumor is a feminizing, and arrhenoblastoma a masculinizing tumor. Both arise from primitive cells having in the first instance feminine, and in the second, masculine characteristics. The granulosa cell tumor secretes the estrogenic hormone, the arrhenoblastoma secretes the male sex hormone. If a granulosa cell tumor appears before puberty, early or precocious puberty results. If it occurs after the menopause, regular menstruation sometimes reappears after many years of amenorrhea. Appearance of an arrhenoblastoma in a normal woman produces such changes as atrophy of the breasts, increase in body hair, change in the voice, cessation of the menses, and enlargement of the clitoris. In both types of tumors the symptoms disappear when the tumor is successfully removed.

Treatment of Ovarian Tumors

The treatment of ovarian tumors depends on the type of tumor. Graafian follicle and corpus luteum cysts usually require no treatment. The other neoplastic tumors of the ovary, if they have attained any size, must be removed surgically when the diagnosis is made. It is usually necessary to remove the fallopian tube together with the ovary on the affected side. In cases of carcinoma of the ovary, both ovaries, and the uterus also if possible, are removed, regardless of whether metastases are present or not. Such patients should always be operated on, no matter how hopeless the situation may appear to be, since surgery presents the only hope of cure. Deep x-ray therapy is usually given after operation, and is sometimes beneficial.

ENDOMETRIOSIS

One interesting cyst with which all nurses should be familiar is the endometrial cyst. Such cysts are filled with chocolate-colored fluid, and are often described as "chocolate cysts." The fluid is really old blood, which owes its presence to the fact that the cyst walls contain endometrial tissue like that lining the uterine cavity. Whenever the patient menstruates, bleeding takes place into the cyst, where the blood gradually accumulates. This condition is also known as endometriosis of the ovary. The ovary, however, is not the only place where endometriosis occurs: it is also found in the uterine wall, which may be riddled with patches of endometriosis. In some cases, these form discrete tumor masses, appearing grossly much like simple myomas but showing typical endometrial tissue on microscopic examination. Other locations in which endometriosis is often found are the outer surface of the uterus, the fallopian tubes, rectovaginal septum, uterosacral ligaments, sigmoid colon, vagina, bladder, and umbilicus.

There has been much speculation as to the origin of endometriosis, and a number of theories have been advanced in an attempt to explain this disease. The theory of Sampson is ingenious, and probably accounts for some cases at least. Sampson believed that endometriosis is caused by menstruation backward through the fallopian tubes into the pelvis, and that bits of endometrium are carried along with the flow, finally becoming implanted on the pelvic organs. This theory is supported by the fact that retrograde menstruation has been observed in people with retrodisplacement of the uterus, and that endometriosis is commoner in such individuals. A second theory supposes that endometrium can be formed from another pelvic tissue called germinal epithelium by a process known as metaplasia.

Bleeding into the pelvis occurs from all the areas of endometriosis as long as menstruation continues. The blood is irritating to the peritoneal surfaces, and causes severe pain at the time of menstruation. It also causes dense adhesions to form between the pelvic organs. When endometriosis occurs in the umbilicus or bladder or in operative scars, as it sometimes does, the patient has external bleeding from these locations. The commonest symptom complex is progressively more severe dysmenorrhea associated with *menorrhagia* (prolonged profuse menstrual periods). After a time the pain usually becomes so severe that the patient demands relief. The symptoms generally subside after an artificial or surgical menopause has been brought about.

Treatment. In young women with endometriosis the attempt is usually made first to control the patient's symptoms with sedatives. Should operation become necessary, as it often does, the operator tries to save sufficient ovarian tissue so that the patient may have children. Such a patient is advised to have her family as soon as possible, since sterility often results as the disease progresses. In addition to removal of as many of the endometrial implants as possible, both ovaries are removed from women near the menopause, for castration stops the progress of the disease and often causes any remaining implants to atrophy. Patients who are poor operative risks are sometimes treated with radiation therapy, once the diagnosis has been established. This type of therapy has the same result as castration.

SUMMARY

Cancer of the female generative tract is the most common form of cancer in women; happily, it can be detected early and cured completely if women will have regular and adequate gynecologic examination.

VOCABULARY REVIEW

leukoplakia	*panhysterectomy*	*exenteration*
vulvectomy	*cystadenoma*	*curettage*
myoma	*endometriosis*	

SUGGESTED READING

1. Cancer Nursing, A Manual for Public Health Nurses. Federal Security Agency and New York State Department of Health, 1950.
2. A Cancer Source Book for Nurses. American Cancer Society, Inc., New York, 1950.
3. Delaplaine, Robert W. et al.: Effective Control of the Surgical Menopause by Estradiol Pellet Implantation at the Time of Surgery. Surg., Gynec. & Obst., *94:*323–333 (March) 1952.
4. Duker, Teresa: Nursing Care in X-ray Therapy of Cancer and Allied Diseases. Pub. Health Nursing, *44:*680–683 (December) 1952.
5. McLaughlin, Eileen: Nursing Care in Hysterectomy. Am. J. Nursing, *50:* 295–298 (May) 1950.
6. Nolan, James F., and DuSault, Lucille: The Elimination of Untoward Radiation Sequelae in the Treatment of Carcinoma of the Uterine Cervix. Surg., Gynec. & Obst., *94:*539–542 (May) 1952.
7. Ranney, Brooks: Endometriosis. Am. J. Nursing, *52:*1465–1466 (December) 1952.
8. TeLinde, Richard W.: Hysterectomy. Am. J. Nursing, *50:*293–295 (May) 1950.
9. Tyronne, Curtis, and Weed, John C.: Hysterectomy. A Personal Experience with Two Thousand Consecutive Cases in Private Practice. Ann. Surg., *133:* 819–829 (June) 1951.
10. Walker, Elizabeth: Cytologic Test for Cancer. Am. J. Nursing, *49:*43–45 (January) 1949.

CHAPTER 52

Communicable Diseases in Surgery

Only a small portion of the large subject of communicable disease is of surgical importance. Although any surgical patient may contract such communicable diseases as measles, mumps, and the like, the treatment of these diseases is medical. The fact that the initial phase of some of them may give rise to abdominal or other symptoms and signs which simulate surgical conditions, especially in children, has been mentioned (p. 247). In the course of certain of the communicable diseases, however, complications sometimes arise that require surgical treatment. Among these are intestinal perforation due to typhoid, contractures of extremities resulting from poliomyelitis, empyema caused by pneumonia, and pelvic abscess secondary to gonorrhea in the female. There are many more, and considerable discussion of them has already appeared in this text.

Strictly speaking, the ordinary surgical infections, such as those caused by the introduction of the common pyogenic bacteria into the tissues, are not communicable diseases in the sense that measles and chickenpox are; they may be and often are, however, spread from one patient to another, and this was the rule rather than the exception prior to the introduction and adoption of the principles of antisepsis and asepsis. It is always necessary to exercise extreme care when treating patients who have septic wounds in order to prevent the transfer of virulent bacteria to an uninfected patient. Many of the medical communicable diseases are transmitted by the bites of insects or larger animals, and some are spread by mechanical contact with excreta. This is also true of the surgical infections about to be discussed.

RABIES (HYDROPHOBIA)

This virus disease is fatal to man and animals. The virus is present in the saliva of the infected animal, and is thus transmitted by its bite. Rabies most commonly infects the dog, but it is also found, though rarely, in the cat, horse, cow, fox, wolf, and some others. The name hydrophobia is a misnomer; the rabid animal does not fear water but is unable to swallow because of spasm of the pharyngeal muscles. The disease has a varying incubation period, usually forty to sixty days.

Treatment. When treatment by the Pasteur method is given before the disease develops, rabies is averted; after the onset no form of treatment is successful. The Pasteur treatment consists in the inoculation of the patient with several increasing doses of material prepared from the spinal cord of infected animals. If a person is bitten by a dog, or any other animal, an immediate effort must be made to secure the animal. If it appears ill, examination of the brain must be made; if the animal remains perfectly healthy during an observation period of several weeks, there is no danger of rabies. If the animal cannot be located, however, or if it is found to be rabid, the Pasteur treatment must be given to the patient at once.

TETANUS

This disease, commonly known as lockjaw, is characterized by spasm (tetanic contraction) of the muscles of the body. Depending upon the degree of intoxication, some or all of the muscles are affected, thus interfering with opening the mouth, swallowing, moving the extremities, or even breathing. In severe cases the patient dies as a result of respiratory paralysis, or of exhaustion from the prolonged muscular contraction. The tetanus bacillus produces this disease by manufacturing a powerful poison (tetanus toxin) that affects the nervous system. This microorganism is a strict anaerobe, and also has the ability to form spores; these are difficult to kill and under the proper conditions develop into the toxin-producing bacilli. Commonly found in the feces of animals, and occasionally in those of man, these spores are widely distributed, and are generally present in streets and fertilized fields. The usual manner of human infection is through a puncture wound, made perhaps by stepping on a nail or running a contaminated splinter through the skin. The bacilli do not stir up much inflammatory reaction in the tissues, and do not spread, remaining where inoculated; the toxin produced is then absorbed and carried throughout the body in the lymphatics and in the blood stream, and thus reaches the nervous system. As a minute amount of this toxin may cause death, the successful treatment of tetanus depends upon the neutralization of the toxin before a lethal amount reaches the central nervous system.

Prevention. Since the disease has a high mortality rate, prevention is of the utmost importance. The accidental introduction of spores or bacilli is difficult to prevent, but fortunately two adequate methods exist for neutralization of tetanus toxin. The first of these is the administration of tetanus antitoxin, a serum prepared from animals (horse, cow, rabbit, pig) to which repeated small sublethal doses of tetanus toxin have been given. These animals develop immunity, and by transfer of their serum to the patient, temporary immunity is considered. It is important to note that although antitoxin neutralizes toxin it does not destroy the bacilli; these, if permitted to do so, will continue to manufacture toxin, so that the antitoxin will afford only temporary safety. Following the use of antitoxin minor degrees of serum sickness are common, including fever, urticara (hives), and painful joints. More serious reactions are associated with edema and respiratory obstruction; these require prompt medical attention.

A second and better method of preventing tetanus is by active immunization, which produces permanent immunity to the toxin. This immunization is accomplished by a course of toxoid inoculations, similar to the method employed in diphtheria immunization. Active immunization is employed in the armed forces and has been spectacularly successful in preventing tetanus among the wounded. Eventually, when all children receive tetanus toxoid, there will be little need for antitoxin, and tetanus will become rare. At present, however, in the case of every civilian having a wound in which the spores may be present tetanus antitoxin must be administered, unless he has previously been immunized, and in sufficient amount. The antitoxin, of course, is animal serum; patients must therefore be tested carefully for sensitivity to avoid severe serum reactions.

Treatment. Active treatment is necessary when tetanus has already developed. The patients should receive large doses of antitoxin by several routes: locally about the wound, intravenously, and also by injection into the spinal cord, so as to neutralize quickly as much as possible of the already existing toxin. The wound should be excised *en bloc* in order to remove the tetanus bacilli, thus preventing the manufacture of additional toxin.

Nursing Care. As even slight stimulation excites a convulsion, absolute silence is advisable. Sedatives are needed to relax the muscle spasm; at times general anesthesia is necessary. Convulsions can be controlled to some degree by the use of barbiturates and Avertin. Narcotics, especially morphine, tend to depress the respirations so that they are rarely used. Patients in respiratory distress are given oxygen; all patients need special attention to nutrition and fluids. When the jaws are not completely locked, fluids may be given by mouth. A rubber tip should be placed at the end of the drinking tube or Asepto syringe so that biting of the glass is prevented if the patient has a muscle spasm during the feeding. When the jaws are locked or when the patient is reluctant to take fluids by mouth it is advisable to feed the patient through a tube introduced into the stomach through the nose. High caloric feedings should be given frequently in small amounts (200 cc. or less). The advantages of this are that there is only slight disturbance of the patient and there is no danger of aspiration.

The urinary output should be watched carefully. The patient is usually incontinent of urine so that frequent bathing with soap and water is essential to prevent bedsores. Recovery, when it occurs, is slow and gradual; by degrees the spasticity of the muscles disappears.

In patients who are very seriously ill, with spasms interfering with adequate respiration, it has been found possible to tide them over the critical period by achieving paralysis of the contracted muscles by the use of curare. A tracheotomy is performed so that a clear airway can be maintained, and the patient is placed in a respirator to accomplish aeration of the lungs.[1]

GAS BACILLUS INFECTION

There is a group of spore-bearing pathogenic anaerobes which produce gas as well as toxins. Of these, the organism most commonly encountered is the Welch bacillus. Such putrefactive anaerobes thrive especially well in wounds where there is much crushed muscle or deficient circulation; here the bacteria grow fast and the infectious process spreads rapidly. The spores of this group are found in the feces of man and animals, and are widely distributed in nature. Infections are apt to occur in severe wounds as, for example, compound fractures of the leg which are contaminated by soil or by dirty underclothing. The clinical picture is marked by sudden acceleration of pulse and rise in temperature, and by the appearance of bubbles of gas in the tissues. These bubbles may be seen in x-ray films, or are discovered by the characteristic *crepitus,* a sign in which palpation of the tissues gives rise to a crackling sensation similar to that observed in feeling excelsior through tissue paper. Unless measures are taken to stop the spread of the infection, death will probably occur in a few hours.

Treatment. Once the infection has become clinically recognizable, only amputation or the wide excision of the infected tissues saves life. Here, too, the most important measure is proper prophylaxis. The value of careful débridement in order to prevent such infections was established in World War I. Crushed or devascularized tissue must be removed. Huge doses of antibiotic agents, especially penicillin, are administered immediately upon beginning the treatment of the type of wound in which a gas infection might develop, especially a compound fracture. Antitoxic sera are also available and should be used, but their value is questionable.

Nursing Care. Patients having infections due to spore-bearing bacilli must be strictly isolated. Spores are difficult to kill and may survive in dust for long periods of time, ready to become active as soon as introduced into favorable surroundings. In the ward every precaution must be taken to prevent the transfer of bacilli or spores to uninfected patients; if possible the infected patient should be in a private room. Gowns and rubber gloves should be worn by all in attendance; if practicable, these at-

[1] For nursing care of the patient in a respirator see Brown, pages 150–155.

tendants should be relieved from duties with other patients. Linen, dishes, and utensils must be sterilized, and dressings burned. The bag containing the soiled linen in the room should be placed in a clean bag before it is taken to the laundry to prevent the linen from acting as a source of contamination while it is being transported. The nurse assisting with the dressing should place the soiled dressings in a paper bag. This bag should be placed in a clean bag provided by a clean nurse outside of the door, and taken at once to the incinerator. When there is no autoclave available in the ward for the sterilization of gloves, it is convenient to use a pressure cooker such as is ordinarily used in the canning of foods. The patient should not be released from isolation until repeated cultures from his wounds are sterile; he should then be transferred to a new bed, and his old bed and room disinfected. It is only by the conscientious observance of such strict measures that the disastrous transfer of spores to other patients can be prevented. Aside from the isolation precautions, the nursing care is that of an acutely ill, toxic patient.

SKIN DIPHTHERIA

The occurrence of virulent Klebs-Loeffler bacillus, the causative agent of diphtheria, has been commonly observed in the past by pediatricians in ulcers of the extremities of patients known to have had recent diphtheria or exposure to it. In World War II widespread outbreaks of this same lesion occurred in adults. It is likely that the organism is a secondary invader of an already existing break in the skin; in any event, large necrotic ulcers occur, usually on the lower leg, and from these the diphtheria bacillus may be cultured. These bacteria are toxin-producers, and paralyses of various nerves or cardiac damage sometimes results from absorption of their toxin. Another serious complication is that the patient with such a lesion may be the source of an epidemic of pharyngeal diphtheria.

Treatment. Treatment consists in rigid isolation of the patient, the local and systemic injection of diphtheria antitoxin, and such surgery as may be needed to heal the ulcer.

OTHER INFECTIONS

Infections due to some of the higher bacteria, the fungi, yeasts, and molds, are of surgical significance, though fortunately of rare occurrence. This group includes Actinomyces, Sporothrix, Blastomyces, and Coccidioides. These infectious agents produce granulomatous or ulcerative lesions which, if untreated, usually progress gradually to a fatal ending. It is fortunate that antibiotic and chemotherapeutic agents are now available which can favorably influence some of these infections. Surgical intervention is indicated when abscesses form, or when necrotic tissue needs removal.

SUMMARY

Certain of the communicable diseases are of surgical significance. The surgeon who treats a dog bite must advise the Pasteur treatment to prevent rabies if the animal was or might be rabid. Every wound in which anaerobes might grow could result in tetanus; it is to be hoped that the entire population will be protected against this eventuality.

VOCABULARY REVIEW

rabies	*antitoxin*	*blastomycosis*
tetanus	*tularemia*	*toxoid*
spore	*actinomycosis*	

SUGGESTED READING

1. Christopher, Frederick: A Textbook of Surgery. 5th Ed. Philadelphia, W. B. Saunders Co., 1949, p. 86.
2. Firor, Warfield M.: The Treatment and Prevention of Tetanus. Am. J. Surg., *46:*450–453 (Dec.) 1939.
3. Shaughnessy, H. J., and Zichis, J.: Prevention of Experimental Rabies. J.A.M.A., *123:*528–533 (Oct. 30) 1943.
4. Top, Franklin H.: Newer Drugs in the Treatment of Communicable Disease. Am. J. Nursing, *49:*700–704 (Nov.) 1949.